Horizons in Medicine

number **10**

Edited by

Gareth Williams MA MD MRCP

Professor of Medicine, University of Liverpool

Honorary Consultant Physician, University Hospital Aintree

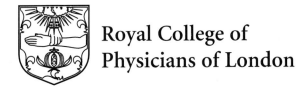

Publisher's Acknowledgements

The Royal College of Physicians is pleased to acknowledge generous support towards the cost of production of this book from:

Novartis Pharmaceuticals

Knoll Pharmceuticals

SmithKline Beecham

Hoescht Marion Roussell Ltd

The Editor, Professor Gareth Williams was responsible for compiling the programme for the conference upon which this book is based. The College is indebted to him for his rigorous editing and to all the contributors to this volume for allowing their papers to be included and for taking the time to prepare them for publication.

Royal College of Physicians of London
11 St Andrews Place, London NW1 4LE

Registered Charity No. 210508

ISBN 1 86016 0824

Typeset by Dan-Set Graphics, Telford, Shropshire
Printed in Great Britain by The Lavenham Press Ltd, Sudbury, Suffolk

British Library Cataloguing in Publication Data
A catalogue record of this book is available from the British Library

Editor's dedication

To Caroline, Timothy, Joanna, Sally and Pippa

Preface

Not many people look at the preface to a medical book – so, if you've started, please read on. The main purpose of a preface is, of course, to tempt the unwary to dip into the book and possibly even buy a copy (ideally, several copies). So how can the tenth volume of *Horizons in Medicine* justify its fight for your attention?

There are four main reasons. Firstly, it will bring you right up to date on key topics that span a broad spectrum of medicine and clinical science. Secondly, and crucially, you will probably enjoy the experience, unlike many other exercises in Continuing Medical Education. Thirdly, it is an extremely attractive book which will beautify any bookshelf and will look particularly impressive if left open on a desk or coffee table. Finally, in hard financial terms, it is outstandingly good value for money.

Each volume of *Horizons in Medicine* is distilled from the lectures presented at the corresponding Advanced Medicine Conference, held each spring at the Royal College of Physicians. The 1998 Conference observed the noble traditions of wide coverage (in this case, from the most superficial layers of the skin to the darkest recesses of the brain) and of selecting contributors who are not only experts in their field but are also gifted at communicating the importance, clinical relevance and excitement of what they do. We believe that we have succeeded in maintaining the excellence in scope, content and literacy for which this series has become famous.

At the same time, we have also broken new ground: for the first time, volume 10 is in full colour throughout. We hope that this change will bring *Horizons* to an even wider readership, and will help to shape the future for the series.

You may be prepared to concede that it looks good, but are you persuaded that this book will be useful to you? We think so. The topics covered are important and of general interest to doctors of all disciplines and at all stages of their career. All the chapters are carefully designed and written to be accessible to non-specialists. The book should therefore appeal to everyone in medicine, from students and MRCP candidates who want clear reviews and gems to stun their examiners, right through to those same examiners, trying to keep up to date and satisfy their curiosity about what is going on outside their speciality.

Editors who survive a book like this are generally prematurely aged, virtually friendless and indebted to an embarrassingly long list of people, without whom the enterprise would have sunk without trace. I am eternally grateful to the following, some of whom still speak to me.

Above all, the contributors, for the excellence of their contributions and their prompt and generous responses to the unreasonable demands of the editor. Christine Greenwood, for her secretarial expertise, efficiency and good humour, all of which far exceed any bounds of duty. The entire production team of the College's Publications Unit, who have made this such an attractive book. Our sponsors –

Novartis, Knoll, SmithKline Beecham and Hoescht Marion Roussell Ltd – for the generosity of their financial support which helped us to cover the additional costs of rapid publication in full colour. And finally, my wife and family, for letting me do this in the first place.

GARETH WILLIAMS
Liverpool
December 1998

Contributors

DAVID BACK *Professor of Pharmacy, Department of Pharmacology & Therapeutics, University of Liverpool, Ashton Street, Liverpool L69 3BX*

MICHAEL BARRY *Consultant Physician, National Medicines Information Centre, Pharmacoeconomic Centre, St James's Hospital, James's Street, Dublin 8*

PETER H BAYLIS *Dean of Medicine, The Medical School, University of Newcastle upon Tyne, Framlington Place, Newcastle upon Tyne NE2 4HH*

ALASDAIR BRECKENRIDGE *Professor of Pharmacy, Department of Pharmacology & Therapeutics, University of Liverpool, Ashton Street, Liverpool L69 3BX*

KEITH AV CARTWRIGHT *Professor of Clinical Microbiology, Group Director, Public Health Laboratory Service, Directorate Office, Gloucestershire Royal Hospital, Great Western Road, Gloucester GL1 3NN*

DAVID CHADWICK *Professor of Neurology, University of Liverpool, Walton Centre for Neurology and Neurosurgery, Lower Lane, Liverpool L9 7LJ*

RICHARD N CLAYTON *Professor, Head of Department of Medicine, Keele University and North Staffordshire Hospital, Thornburrow Drive, Hartshill, Stoke on Trent, Staffordshire ST4 7QB*

LAURIE CRAY *Patient, Wirral Hospital NHS Trust*

MICHAEL DOHERTY *Professor of Rheumatology, Rheumatology Unit, City Hospital, Hucknall Road, Nottingham NG5 1PB*

SIR COLIN DOLLERY *Consultant, SmithKline Beecham Pharmaceuticals, New Frontiers Science Park (South), Third Avenue, Harlow, Essex CM19 5AW*

RICHARD HT EDWARDS *Professor of Research and Development in Health and Social Care, University of Wales College of Medicine, Cardiff CF4 4XN*

CELIA EMERY *Research Fellow, University Section of Respiratory Medicine, University of Sheffield, Medical School, Beech Hill Road, Sheffield S10 2RX*

PAUL EMERY *ARC Professor of Rheumatology, Rheumatology & Rehabilitation Research Unit, University of Leeds, 36 Clarendon Road, Leeds LS2 9JT*

MICHAEL JG FARTHING *Professor of Gastroenterology, Director, Digestives Diseases Research Centre, St Bartholomew's & The Royal London School of Medicine and Dentistry, Turner Street, London E1 2AD*

JAMES FERGUSON *Consultant Dermatologist, Photodermatology Unit, University of Dundee, Ninewells Hospital, Dundee DD1 9SY*

JOHN V FORRESTER *Professor of Ophthalmology, Honorary Consultant, Head of Department of Ophthalmology, University of Aberdeen, Medical School, Foresterhill, Aberdeen AB25 2ZD*

RICHARD SJ FRACKOWIAK *Dean, Institute of Neurology, The National Hospital for Neurology and Neurosurgery, Queen Square, London WC1N 3BG*

PETER FRIEDMANN *Professor of Dermatology, Dermatology Unit, University Medicine, Level F, Centre Block, Southampton General Hospital, Tremona Road, Southampton SO16 6YD*

MARK GARDINER *Professor of Paediatrics, Head of Department of Paediatrics, The Rayne Institute, University Street, London WC1E 6JJ*

DUNCAN GEDDES *Professor of Respiratory Medicine/Consultant Physician, Royal Brompton Hospital, Sydney Street, London SW3 6NP*

ANTHONY H GERSHLICK *Consultant Cardiologist, Honorary Senior Lecturer, Department of Academic Cardiology, University of Leicester, Clinical Sciences Wing, Glenfield General Hospital, Leicester LE3 9QP*

TIM HIGENBOTTAM *Professor of Respiratory Medicine, University Section of Respiratory Medicine, University of Sheffield, Medical School, Beech Hill Road, Sheffield S10 2RX*

DAVID HOSKING *Consultant and Professor of Mineral Metabolism, Division of Mineral Metabolism, Nottingham City Hospital NHS Trust, Hucknall Road, Nottingham NG5 1PB*

COLIN D JOHNSON *Reader in Surgery, University Surgical Unit, Southampton General Hospital, Tremona Road, Southampton SO16 6YD*

JOHN A KANIS *Professor and Director, Centre for Metabolic Bone Diseases, WHO Collaborating Centre, University of Sheffield Medical School, Beech Hill Road, Sheffield S10 2RX*

TOM KENNEDY *Consultant Physician and Rheumatologist, Wirral Hospital NHS Trust, Arrowe Park Road, Upton , Wirral L49 5PE*

RACHEL M KNOTT *Senior Research Fellow, Department of Ophthalmology, Medical School, Foresterhill, Aberdeen AB25 2ZD*

FOO LEONG LI-SAW-HEE *University Department of Medicine, City Hospital NHS Trust, Dudley Road, Birmingham B18 7QH*

GREGORY YH LIP *Consultant Cardiologist and Senior Lecturer, University Department of Medicine, City Hospital NHS Trust, Dudley Road, Birmingham B18 7QH*

EUGENE V McCLOSKEY *Senior Clinical Research Fellow, Centre for Metabolic Bone Diseases, WHO Collaborating Centre, University of Sheffield Medical School, Beech Hill Road, Sheffield S10 2RX*

KENNETH EL McCOLL *Professor of Gastroenterology, Department of Medicine and Therapeutics, University of Glasgow, Gardiner Institute, Western Infirmary, Glasgow G11 6NT*

STEVEN J McNULTY *Clinical Research Fellow, Diabetes & Endocrinology, Clinical Research Group, University Clinical Departments, University Hospital Aintree, Longmoor Lane, Liverpool L9 7AL*

CELIA MOSS *Consultant Dermatologist, Birmingham Children's Hospital NHS Trust, Steelhouse Lane, Birmingham B4 6NL*

MARK B PEPYS *Professor of Immunological Medicine, Department of Medicine, Imperial College School of Medicine, Hammersmith Hospital, Du Cane Road, London W12 0NN*

JONATHAN L REES *Professor of Dermatology, Department of Dermatology, Medical School, Framlington Place, Newcastle upon Tyne NE2 4HH*

JONATHAN M RHODES *Professor of Medicine, Gastroenterology Research Group, University Clinical Departments of Medicine, University of Liverpool, Duncan Building, Daulby Street, Liverpool L69 3GA*

PETER SANDERCOCK *Department of Clinical Neurosciences, Western General Hospital, Edinburgh EH4 2XU*

ELAINE SHOWALTER *Professor of English, Department of English, Princeton University, Princeton, New Jersey 08544 1016, USA*

CHARLES RJ SINGER *Consultant Haematologist, Directorate of Pathology, Royal United Hospital Bath NHS Trust, Royal United Hospital, Combe Park, Bath BA1 3NG*

GLENN C TELLING *Group Leader, Prion Disease Group, MRC Unit, Department of Neurogenetics, Imperial College of Science, Technology and Medicine, St Mary's, Norfolk Place, London W12 1PG*

JITEN P VORA *Consultant Physician/Endocrinologist, Diabetes Unit, Royal Liverpool University Hospitals, Prescot Street, Liverpool L7 8XP*

SIR DAVID J WEATHERALL *Regius Professor of Medicine, Institute of Molecular Medicine, John Radcliffe Hospital, Headington, Oxford OX3 9DS*

SIMON WESSELY *Professor of Epidemiological and Liaison Psychiatry, Academic Department of Psychological Medicine, King's College School of Medicine & Dentistry, Institute of Psychiatry, 103 Denmark Hill, London SE5 8AF*

JOHN WILDING *Senior Lecturer in Medicine, Honorary Consultant Physician, Diabetes and Endocrinology Clinical Research Unit, University Clinical Departments, University Hospital Aintree, Longmoor Lane, Liverpool L9 7AL*

GARETH WILLIAMS *Professor of Medicine, University of Liverpool and Honorary Consultant Physician, University Hospital Aintree, Longmoor Lane, Liverpool L9 7AL*

NICHOLAS A WRIGHT *Deputy Prinicipal and Vice-Principal for Research, Imperial College School of Medicine, The Hammersmith Hospital, Du Cane Road, London W12 0NN*

Contents

Preface v

List of contributors vii

RHEUMATOLOGY AND BONE DISEASE

Treatment of rheumatoid arthritis: new drugs, new hopes 1
Paul Emery

Osteoarthritis: new thoughts about an old disease 15
Michael Doherty

Osteoporosis 29
John A Kanis & Eugene V McCloskey

Paget's disease 41
David Hosking

A case of bleeding gums 55
Tom Kennedy & Laurie Cray

GASTROENTEROLOGY AND NUTRITION

Acute pancreatitis: a conceptual framework for better management . . . 67
Colin D Johnson

***Helicobacter pylori* infection and its role in human disease** 81
Kenneth EL McColl

Diet and colon cancer 93
Jonathan M Rhodes

New prospects for the management of obesity: from molecular targets to novel drugs 109
Gareth Williams & Steven J McNulty

The Croonian Lecture
Bugs and guts: it's good to talk? 129
Michael J G Farthing

DERMATOLOGY

Sun, skin and cancer: from oncogenes to red-hair genes 141
Jonathan L Rees

Atopic Eczema 155
Peter Friedmann

Management of psoriasis: recent developments in phototherapy 169
James Ferguson

Genetic skin disorders 177
Celia Moss

ENDOCRINOLOGY AND METABOLISM

Acromegaly: a fresh look at its outcome and management 189
Richard N Clayton

Hyponatraemia 207
Peter H Baylis

Diabetic retinopathy: what goes wrong in the retina? 223
John V Forrester & Rachel M Knott

New drugs for the treatment of diabetes and its complications 237
John Wilding

Diabetic nephropathy: natural history and treatment 253
Jiten P Vora

NEUROLOGY

Epilepsy: new understanding from new genes 275
Mark Gardiner

Use of new anti-epileptic drugs 287
David Chadwick

Imaging the brain at work 297
Richard S J Frackowiak

Management of acute stroke 315
Peter Sandercock

CARDIORESPIRATORY DISEASE

Emerging concepts in the management of acute myocardial infarction . . 329
Anthony H Gershlick

Atrial fibrillation and its management 343
Gregory Y H Lip & Foo Leong Li-Saw-Hee

Primary pulmonary hypertension 361
Tim Higenbottam & Celia Emery

Cystic fibrosis 381
Duncan Geddes

The Lumleian Lecture
C-reactive protein and amyloidosis: from proteins to drugs? 397
Mark B Pepys

INFECTIOUS DISEASES AND HAEMATOLOGY

Prion diseases of man and other species 415
Glenn C Telling

Investigation and early management of meningococcal disease 429
Keith AV Cartwright

Is HIV now treatable? 443
Michael Barry, David Back & Alasdair Breckenridge

The Watson-Smith Lecture
Intestinal stem-cell repertoire: from normal gut development to the origins of colonic cancer 457
Nicholas A Wright

Myeloma and other plasma cell dyscrasias: new ideas about pathogenesis and treatment 475
Charles RJ Singer

A MISCELLANY

Modern drug design: from combinatorial chemistry to high-throughput screening 491
Colin Dollery

Chronic fatigue syndrome: a true illness or a social and political issue? . 503
Simon Wessely & Elaine Showalter *(Introduction by Richard HT Edwards)*

Gene therapy: the beginning of the end or the end of the beginning? . . . 517
David J Weatherall

Publisher's note

Professor Alastair Compston submitted a paper for this volume but it was not included at the editor's discretion, and will now form part of his chapter on demyelinating disease in the 11th edition of *Brain's Diseases of the Nervous System* to be published by Oxford University Press.

Treatment of rheumatoid arthritis: new drugs, new hopes

Paul Emery

□ INTRODUCTION

Rheumatoid arthritis is a ubiquitous disease affecting around 1% of adults. It is characterised initially by synovitis of the hands, particularly the metacarpophalangeal joints, with inflammation spreading to involve other synovial joints and eventually causing destruction of cartilage and bone (see Figs 1–3). It has become clear that rheumatoid arthritis, as well as damaging joints, has an important metabolic impact elsewhere in the body. If left untreated, the active inflammatory process can produce major systemic catabolic effects, including loss of bone mineral in the spine and other sites remote from affected joints (secondary osteoporosis) and weight loss in some cases, together with an intense acute-phase response [1,2] (see Fig. 4). The overall level of joint inflammation correlates both with the severity of systemic damage (as measured by secondary osteoporosis and the magnitude of the acute-phase response) and with articular manifestations such as the number of radiological erosions and the rate of functional deterioration [1]. As the severity of inflammation produces a proportional and measurable amount of damage, it is now possible to quantitate the progression of the disease, and also to estimate the costs of not treating the disease actively.

Better understanding of the mechanisms of both local and systemic effects of rheumatoid arthritis – which are related to different inflammatory mediators – has stimulated the search for rational new drug therapy, and this will be the focus for this chapter.

□ PATHOGENESIS OF RHEUMATOID ARTHRITIS

Rheumatoid arthritis is thought to be an autoimmune disease in which T-lymphocytes play a central role (Fig. 3). The autoantigen that provokes the immune attack on the joint tissues is not known; one possible candidate is collagen (possibly type II collagen). The synovium and related tissues in acute rheumatoid arthritis are the site of intense immune activity. The release of cytokines such as tumour necrosis factor-α (TNF-α) and interleukins-1 and -6 (IL-1, IL-6) from activated lymphocytes and macrophages is crucial in initiating and sustaining synovitis (see Figs 3–5).

These pro-inflammatory cytokines, especially TNF-α and IL-1β, are important in causing both local inflammation and damage (synovitis, loss of cartilage and bone), some of which is probably inflicted by the cytokine-stimulated release of protease enzymes from activated leukocytes. Cytokines, notably TNF-α, IL-1β and IL-6, entering the circulation also mediate the systemic effects of rheumatoid arthritis.

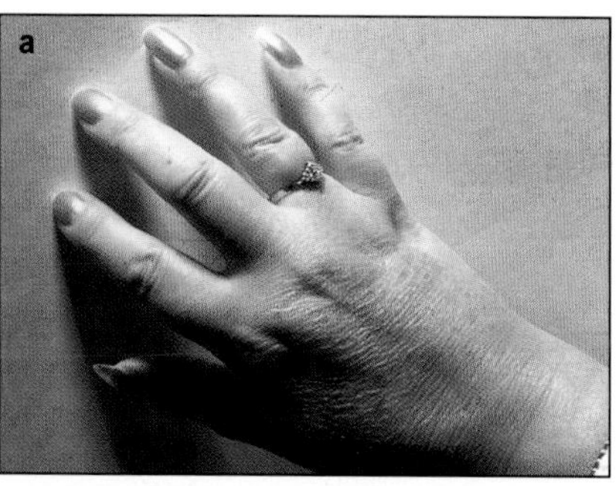

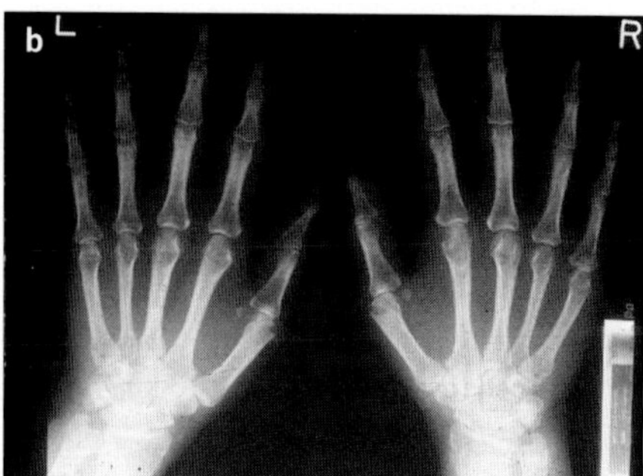

Fig. 1 Early rheumatoid arthritis, showing **(a)** clinical appearance illustrating the minimal soft tissue swelling of metacarpo-phalangeal joints, and **(b)** radiology showing soft tissue changes only.

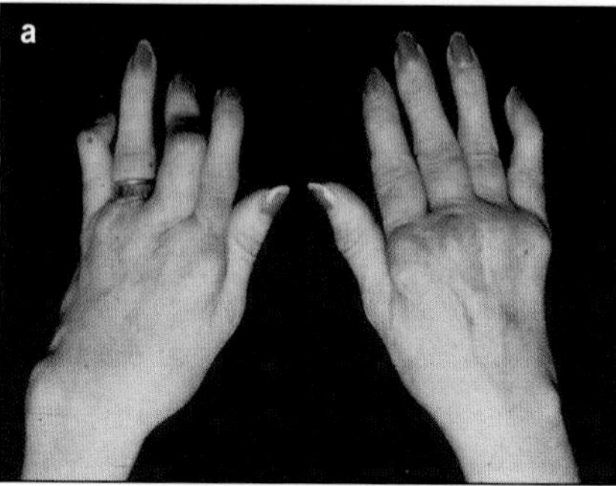

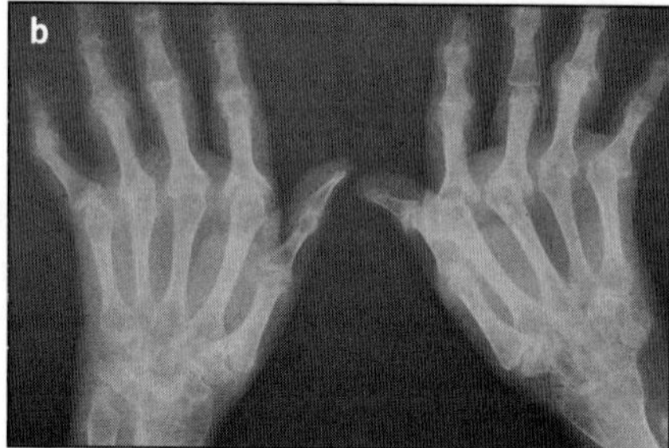

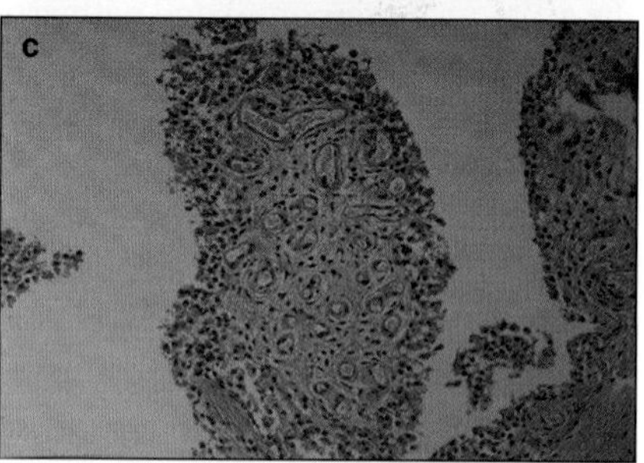

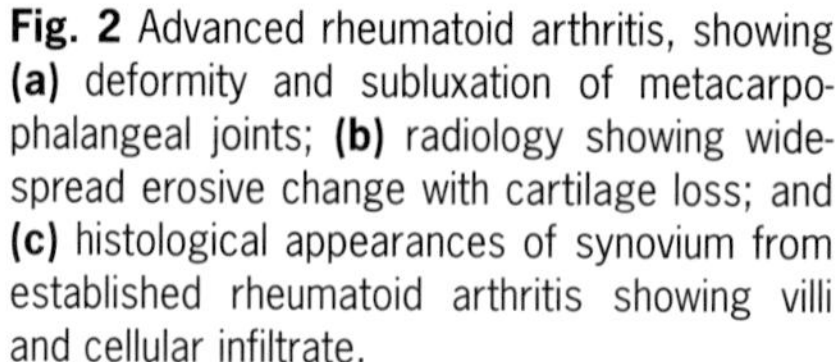

Fig. 2 Advanced rheumatoid arthritis, showing **(a)** deformity and subluxation of metacarpo-phalangeal joints; **(b)** radiology showing widespread erosive change with cartilage loss; and **(c)** histological appearances of synovium from established rheumatoid arthritis showing villi and cellular infiltrate.

Local inflammation and pain are also perpetuated by various prostaglandins, notably PGE2. However, prostaglandins have little influence on the systemic response. Prostaglandin production is inhibited by the non-steroidal anti-inflammatory drugs (NSAIDs), which block COX-2, the inducible form of cyclo-oxygenase (see below). NSAIDs can therefore decrease inflammation in affected joints, alleviating symptoms such as pain and swelling, but have no effect on the acute-phase response or extra-articular complications such as osteoporosis of the spine, which are largely cytokine-mediated; neither do NSAIDs slow the progression of the disease itself, or the development of peri-articular erosions (see Fig. 4). By contrast, drugs that block the release or actions of cytokines might be expected to suppress the signs of inflammation and also to modify some of the processes that underlie active joint disease and the systemic complications of rheumatoid arthritis. Consistent with this are the observations that all the disease-modifying anti-rheumatic drugs (DMARDs) share the common property

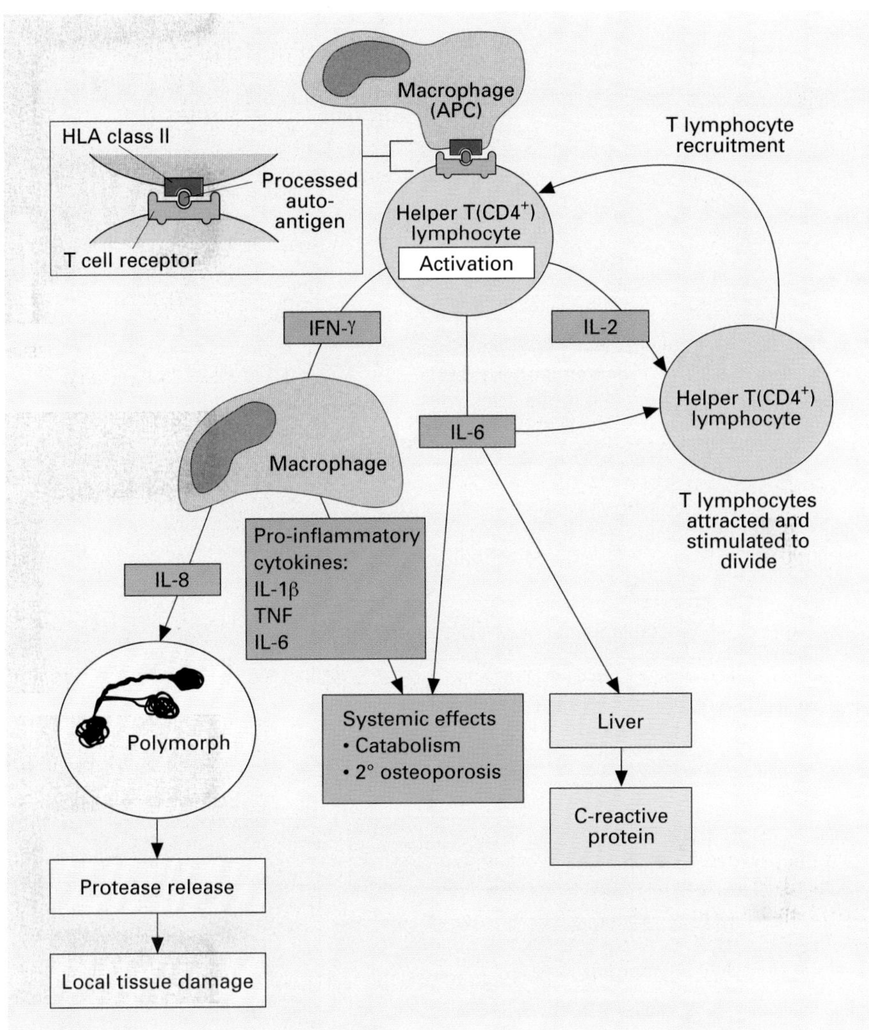

Fig. 3 Immune cells and cytokines in rheumatoid arthritis. T helper lymphocytes are activated by macrophages presenting autoantigen in assocation with HLA class II antigen. Cytokines including interferon-γ (IFN-γ) and interleukins (IL)-1β, -2 and -6 mediate both local and systemic inflammatory effects.

of blocking cytokine release, and that all agents that have been shown to inhibit cytokine release, or that interfere with the receptors for the pro-inflammatory cytokines, also have positive effects in preventing joint damage.

☐ RATIONAL DRUG THERAPY OF RHEUMATOID ARTHRITIS

These observations suggest the functional classification of anti-rheumatic drugs, which is shown in Table 1. For comparison, a list of established drugs used to treat the disease, and some of the newer agents in clinical development, is shown in Table 2.

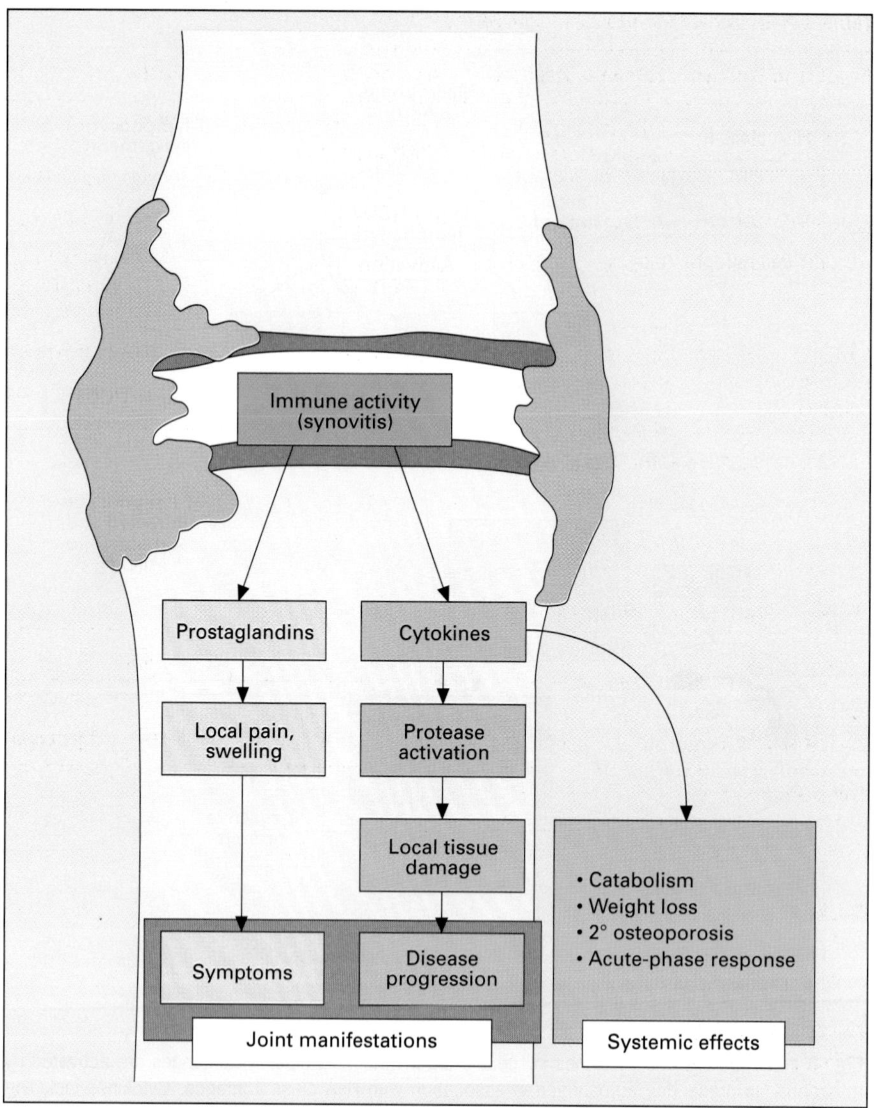

Fig. 4 Local joint and systemic inflammation in rheumatoid arthritis.

This account will focus on some of the novel agents, namely specific inhibitors of the cyclo-oxygenase isoform COX-2, and certain 'biological' therapeutic agents that modulate the production or activity of the cytokines produced in inflamed joints.

COX-2 selective inhibitors

Cyclo-oxgenase is the rate-limiting enzyme in the synthesis of prostaglandins from their precursor, arachidonic acid. There are two isoforms of the enzyme. COX-1 is

Table 1 A functional classification of anti-rheumatic drugs.

Aspects of disease	Outcome measure	Mediators	Drugs
Symptoms (pain)	Self-reported (e.g. visual analogue scale)	Prostaglandins Other molecules	NSAIDs COX-2 inhibitors Analgesics
Joint inflammation	Swollen joint score	Cytokines	Cytokine inhibitors
Joint destruction	Imaging (X-rays, MRI)	Cytokines Proteases	Cytokine inhibitors Protease inhibitors DMARDs
Systemic inflammatory response	Acute-phase proteins (eg C-reactive protein)	Cytokines	Cytokine inhibitors

NSAIDs, non-steroidal anti-inflammatory drugs; DMARDs, disease-modifying anti-rheumatic drugs.

Table 2 Drugs used to treat RA: established and in clinical development.

		Effects on:		
Class and name	**Mode of action**	**Joint symptoms**	**Joint disease**	**Systemic**
Anti-inflammatory				
• NSAIDs	Inhibit COX-2 (and -1)	+	–	–
• COX-2 inhibitors	Inhibit COX-2 only	+	–	–
Glucocorticoids				
• Oral		+	+	+
• Intra-articular		+	+	–
Disease-modifying				
• Immunosuppressives		+	+	+
Methotrexate		+	+	+
Cyclosporin				
• Other				
Hydroxychloroquine				
Sulphasalazine				
• 'Biological' agents				
Anti-T-cell (CD4) Mab		+	+	+
IL-1 receptor antagonist		+	+	+
TNF-α Mab (CA2)		+	+	+
TNF-α receptor antagonists		+	+	+
Anti-inflammatory cytokines (rh IL-10, -11 -4)				
Oral collagen	Induce tolerance	+	+	+

COX, cyclo-oxygenase; IL, interleukin; Mab, monoclonal antibodies; TNF, tumour necrosis factor; rh, recombinant human.

constitutively expressed in the stomach and other sites, where prostaglandins act to maintain the integrity of the mucosa and protect against peptic ulceration; drugs that inhibit COX-1 are therefore ulcerogenic. COX-2 is upregulated in inflamed tissues (virtually all cells express COX-2) and is therefore the logical target for drugs to alleviate the local inflammatory manifestations of rheumatoid arthritis. The explosion in knowledge about COX-2 has revealed that it is also constitutively expressed in certain sites (kidney, brain), and it is thought to play major roles in promoting gastrointestinal neoplasia, in ovulation and ovum implantation, and in various functions in the brain and the renal medulla.

Conventional NSAIDs inhibit both COX-1 and COX-2 and therefore have adverse effects, particular in the stomach (ulceration) and kidney (sodium and water retention, reduced glomerular filtration), and inhibit platelet aggregation. Specific inhibitors of COX-2 are currently under development. Those available at present show preference for inhibition of the COX-2 isoform, while two highly specific drugs (with at least 100-fold greater affinity for COX-2 than COX-1), namely celecoxib and MK966, are in phase III of clinical development [3].

'Biological' therapies

Recent advances in molecular technology have made it possible to identify distinct immune cell subsets, cell markers and products that contribute to the pathogenic process that leads to rheumatoid arthritis (see Figs 3 and 5). These cells and markers have been the subject of targeted therapy, particularly using monoclonal antibody technology. The aim of many of these approaches has been to induce 'immune tolerance' against the presumed autoantigens, and thus to abort the immune cascade and its production of damaging cytokines.

Cellular targets

The recognition of the central role of T-cells in the pathogenesis of rheumatoid arthritis (see Fig. 5) identified them as one of the first targets for immunotherapy. In theory, inactivating the T-helper (CD4-positive) lymphocytes should induce immune tolerance. A variety of anti-T-lymphocyte monoclonal antibodies has been studied in humans. Several open studies have demonstrated efficacy, but fewer have shown convincing responses when the antibodies were administered double-blind (reviewed in [4]). A major factor limiting efficacy has been toxicity, notably first-dose reactions and vasculitis, particularly with high dosages; because of this, no study has yet been able to give the optimal duration of therapy that is likely to achieve the aim of tolerance.

Cytokine targets

Because of the central role of the pro-inflammatory cytokines, IL-1β and TNF-α in the pathogenesis of the local and generalised effects of rheumatoid arthritis, many studies have aimed to inhibit or block their production.

There is some evidence that TNF-α is at the top of the hierarchy of mediators of

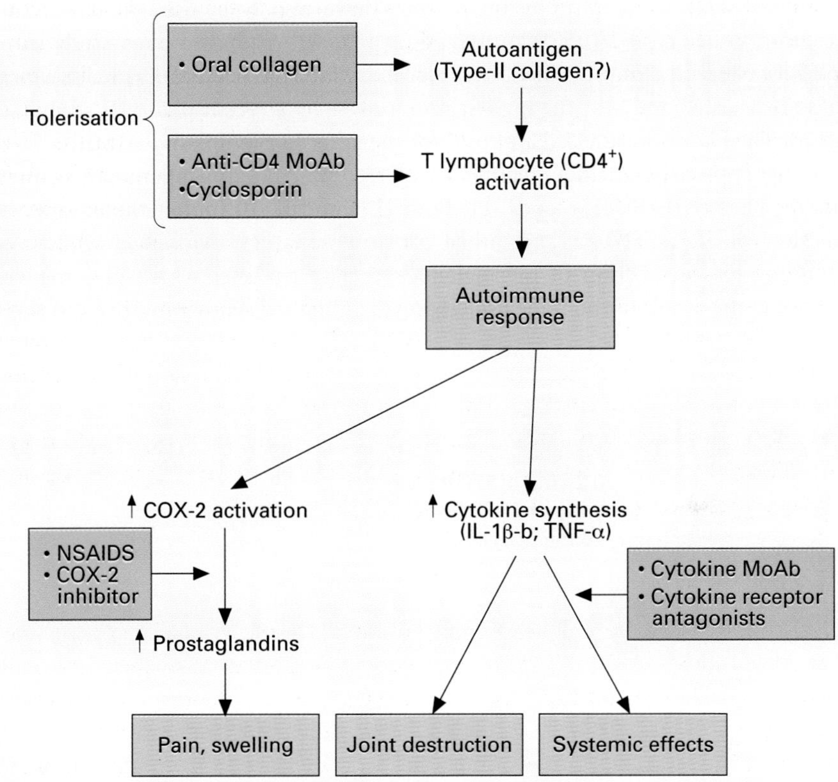

Fig. 5 Some potential points of intervention in the pathogenesis of rheumatoid arthritis.

systemic inflammation, while IL-1β may be more important in causing tissue destruction. These hypothesese remain to be confirmed in clinical practice, though there is some support from the studies described below.

A peptide that acts as an antagonist at the IL-1 receptor (recombinant human IL1 Ra) has been given by subcutaneous injection. A phase II study showed a favourable dose-response relationship, with effective reductions in the acute-phase protein levels and in the radiological score of joint damage. It is now being tested in combination with methotrexate.

The chimeric human monoclonal antibody, cA2, is directed against TNF-α. An initial study showed dramatic efficacy [5], particularly in reducing fatigue; however, tachyphylaxis tended to occur, with diminishing responses to successive infusions of the monoclonal antibody. Furthermore, the drug-induced antibody formation, particularly antinuclear antibody and anticardiolipin antibodies. Fortunately, a recent 12-week phase II study of cA2 given together with various doses of methotrexate has demonstrated a synergistic effect, and has shown that high-dose methotrexate and cA2 inhibit the production of treatment-induced antibodies. A 12-month phase III study is now in progress. In the US, cA2 has recently received approval for use as a single agent in Crohn's disease.

Soluble TNF-α receptor fusion proteins have also been used to block TNF receptors, either type 1 (p55/60) or type 2 (p75/80). A phase I open study using TNFR:Fc p80 found improvement over placebo, which has been confirmed in a large phase II trial [6] and – at the highest dose only – by a recent phase III study (see Fig. 6). The FDA have advised approval for the latter in rheumatoid arthritis.

Other approaches include treatment with recombinant anti-inflammatory interleukins, namely IL-10, IL-4 or IL-11. Both IL-4 and IL-10 inhibit the release and function of IL-1, TNF-α and other pro-inflammatory cytokines, while also inhibiting the production of the metalloproteinase enzymes which may mediate damage to the cartilage and bone underlying the inflamed synovium. IL-4 and IL-10

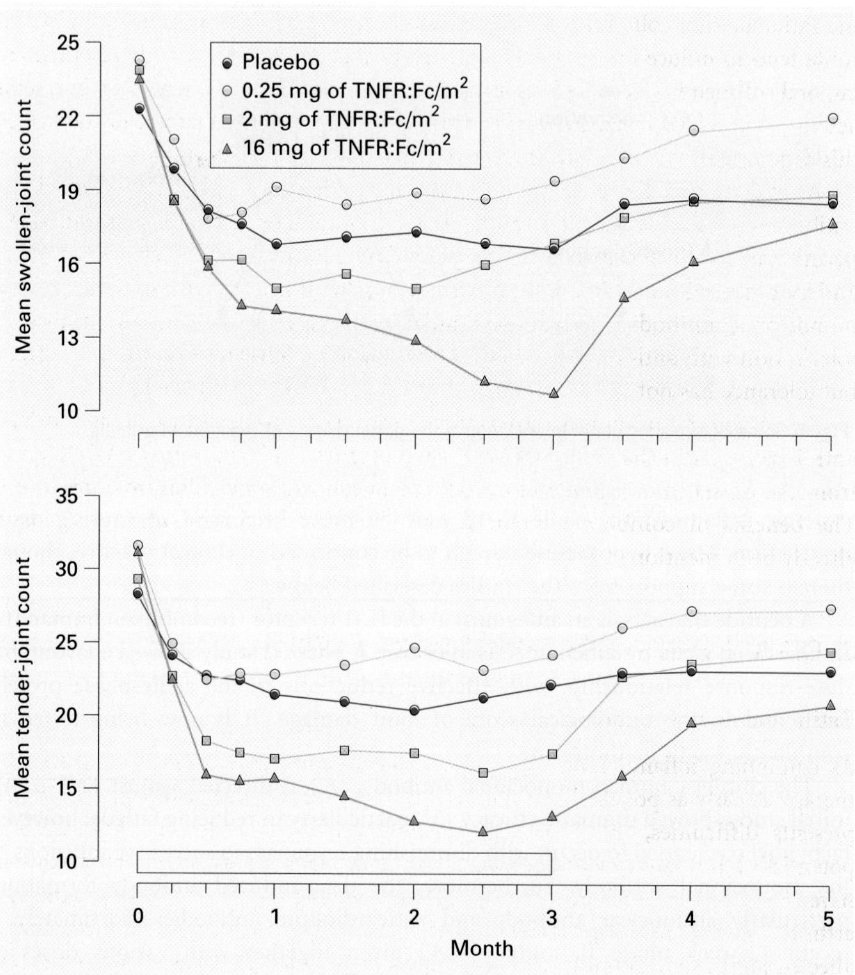

Fig. 6 Effects of recombinant human TNF-α receptor fusion protein (TNFR:Fc) in patients with rheumatoid arthritis, showing dose-related improvements in joint swelling (*upper panel*) and tenderness (*lower panel*). (Redrawn from Moreland *et al* [6], with kind permission of the Editor of *New England Journal of Medicine.*)

can be viewed as natural buffers or modulators of the potentially destructive pro-inflammatory cytokines. IL-11 is an anti-inflammatory cytokine that reduces the production of TNF-α in response to IL-1, IL-12, IL-6 and nitric oxide. Clinical trials of all these molecules are currently in progress.

Other approaches to immune tolerance

The fact that long-term remission does not occur with the 'biological' therapies, even when these are effective in the short term, has stimulated the search for other tolerising treatments which could reset the immune system, thus fundamentally and permanently altering the disease process.

One approach has involved the use of collagen administered orally, and is based on the rationale that collagen is a putative autoantigen and that antigens given by this route tend to induce immune tolerance rather than an active antibody response. So far, oral collagen has been tested for its ability to suppress the rebound flare in disease activity that occurs in rheumatoid arthritis patients treated with methotrexate when this drug is withdrawn; unfortunately, results to date have been disappointing.

As already noted above, prolonged therapy with anti-T-cell (CD4) monoclonal antibodies has been attempted, but treatment has not been given for long enough to permit any definitive conclusion. One potentially promising approach is to combine anti-cytokine with anti-T-cell treatment. In a pilot study, we have tested anti-TNF monoclonal antibodies to suppress inflammation, with the aim of promoting tolerisation with anti-T-cell antibodies; this study has shown some additive effects, but tolerance has not yet been achieved. (Morgan, *et al*: unpublished.)

A regimen of conventional drugs that effectively combines anti-cytokine with an anti-T-cell agent is the combination of methotrexate with cyclosporin. When given from the outset, this regimen has produced promising results, but no cures as yet. The benefits of combining methotrexate with anti-TNF antibodies (cA2) have already been mentioned above.

□ GENERAL PRINCIPLES OF MANAGEMENT: A NEW LOOK

Rationale for early treatment

As continuing inflammation leads to cumulative damage, it seems logical to start therapy as early as possible, and this view is now generally accepted. However, it also presents difficulties, in that early aggressive therapy may be inappropriate and potentially hazardous for patients whose long-term prognosis is relatively good. Criteria have recently been developed that can predict the long-term outcome of rheumatoid arthritis, for both radiological measures of joint damage (erosions) and the function of affected joints. One example of this approach is the staging classification for patients with persistent inflammatory symmetrical arthritis (PISA), which has been developed from two longitudinal studies [7–10]. This scheme provides a practical basis for classifying patients early in the natural history of their disease, and is increasingly being used to target therapy at those who are likely to have a poor prognosis (see Table 3).

Table 3 PISA (Persistent Inflammatory Symmetrical Arthritis) staging classification.

Feature	Score
• Raised HAQ*: 6–11	1
12–24	2
• Elevated ESR (>x mm/1hr)	1
• Rheumatoid factor positive	1
• Presence of shared epitope	1
• Female gender	1

TOTAL SCORE

Total Score	Prognosis
0	Good
1–3	Intermediate
>3	Poor

HAQ = health assessment questionnaire (measure of function); shared epitope = conserved sequence of amino acids on gene encoding HLA DR molecule, associated with RA.

Overall, the development of clinically useful prognostic markers and outcome measures, and the advent of therapies with proven efficacy, have allowed adequate cost-benefit analyses of various therapies to be undertaken. There is already a general move to using intensive treatments earlier in selected patients with rheumatoid arthritis, and it is likely that this strategy will continue to be refined.

New developments in joint imaging

It has until recently been difficult to evaluate accurately the extent of damage to joints in rheumatoid arthritis. Conventional radiographs are relatively insensitive for early changes, and not sufficiently specific later in the disease.

One reason for the poor outcome noted in many studies is that, even at an early stage of the disease, there may already be substantial and possibly irreversible damage. Indeed, magnetic resonance imaging (MRI) has shown significant bony changes in most patients with rheumatoid arthritis, after a mean duration of only a few weeks (see Fig. 7). Interestingly, these studies confirmed the pathogenic primacy of synovitis, as the bony changes were not seen in its absence.

The availability of specialised imaging techniques – using coordinated studies of MRI, dual-emission X-ray absorptiometry (DEXA), ultrasound and arthroscopy – should accelerate our understanding of the natural history of rheumatoid arthritis, and perhaps of the mode of action of drugs designed to treat it. For example, the combined use of arthroscopy and MRI has shown a strong correlation between

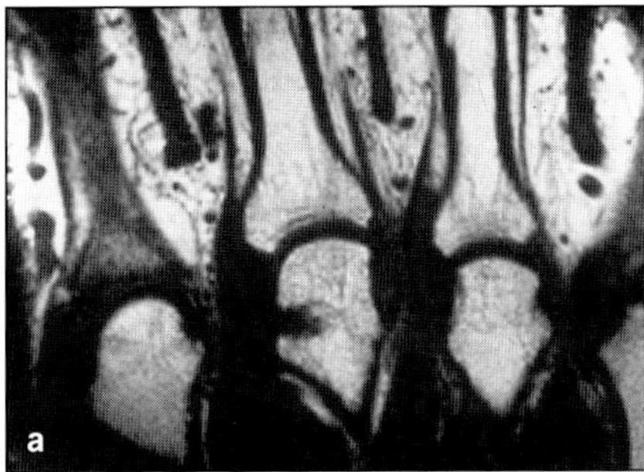

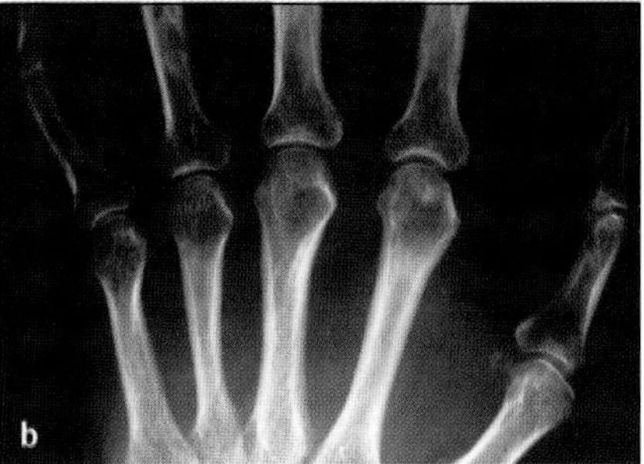

Fig. 7 Comparison of **(a)** magnetic resonance imaging (MRI) and **(b)** plain radiology in early rheumatoid arthritis, showing bony damage (oedema) and synovitis detectable by MRI that is not apparent with conventional radiographic methods.

histological and structural features of disease, during a study of intra-articular anti- CD4 monoclonal antibodies.

Combination therapy with available agents

Many disease-modifying anti-rheumatic drugs have been used to treat rheumatoid arthritis, with variable success. At present, it is not possible to predict which patients will respond to a single DMARD. It has been suggested that a combination of agents may be more effective, with a more rapid induction of response and additive or synergistic effects achieved with lower doses and hence fewer side effects.

Initial studies of combination therapy used unselected patients and combinations of drugs which have now fallen out of favour; a meta-analysis showed no benefit from combination therapy in these circumstances [11]. Refinements have been suggested, with the targeting of treatment in one of two ways: patients are either identified as having a poor prognosis from the outset of disease (see above and Table 3) or by virtue of having failed or only partially responded to monotherapy.

The strategies for combination therapy are now termed 'step-up' and 'step-down'. Step-up is the addition of a second agent when there is no response to an initial drug. The step-down approach, which is applied particularly to patients with a poor prognosis, uses multiple drugs which are progressively withdrawn as the disease comes under control. Examples of the step-up strategy include the addition of methotrexate in partial responders to sulphasalazine [12], which showed that the continuation of sulphasalazine was helpful for these patients (see Fig. 8). Another study of triple therapy, which examined increasing doses of methotrexate in combination with sulphasalazine and hydroxychloroquine, found increased efficacy – and, interestingly, less toxicity – in the triple-therapy group compared with the other treatment arms that included fewer drugs [13].

Two studies have selected patients with particularly poor prognosis, namely the COBRA study [14] and the Leeds study [15]. Both have shown that additional therapy produces further benefit, and that the toxicity of the disease was greater than the combined toxicity of the chosen drugs. The COBRA study followed the

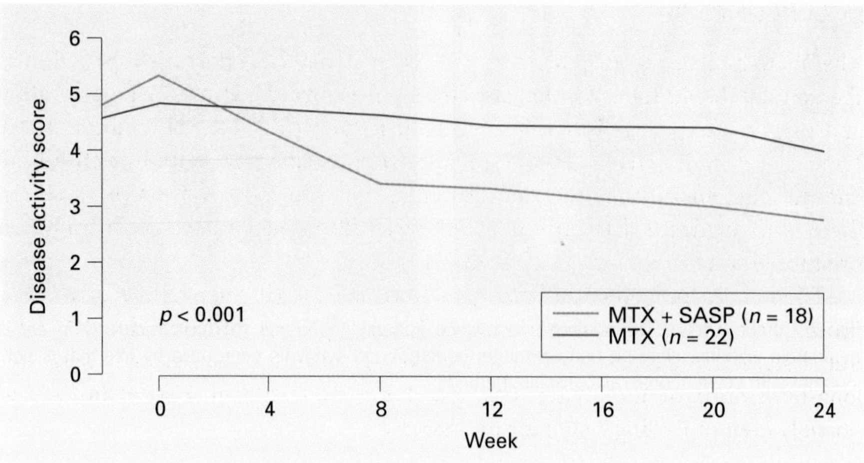

Fig. 8 'Step-up' approach in the treatment of rheumatoid arthritis. The addition of sulphasalazine to partial methotrexate responders. (Data from Haagsma *et al* [12], with permission of the Editor of *British Journal of Rheumatology.*)

step-down approach, with the administration of high-dose corticosteroid plus methotrexate and sulphasalazine from the outset, with the first two drugs being withdrawn after 6 months. This regimen was compared with sulphasalazine alone; the patients treated with triple therapy showed a significant improvement in erosion score after 1 year, a benefit that persisted up to 2 years; however, measures of clinical disease activity of arthritis returned to comparator levels after 12 months.

The Leeds study focused on subjects with very poor prognosis, treated from the outset with a combination of intra-articular steroids, methotrexate and cyclosporin, the latter chosen because of its potentially synergistic action; the comparator was sulphasalazine [15]. The central findings were that the response rate to triple therapy was higher, with the greatest benefit after 1 year, and that the dropout rate was low because of better efficacy.

Glucocorticoids: new strategies for old drugs

Glucocorticoids have been studied for many years in rheumatoid arthritis, and are undoubtedly effective in treating the disease; unfortunately, their benefits are short-term, while their potentially harmful side effects (including loss of bone mineral) are long-term. Recently, one study examined the effects of adding glucocorticoids to standard DMARD, and showed a small but significant improvement in radiographic indices of damage, but no improvement on function or disease activity [16].

Glucocorticoids were included in the COBRA studies [14], which showed a beneficial reduction in radiological erosions; there was a reduction in bone mass in the steroid-treated group, but this did not reach significance. The Leeds study, using intra-articular steroid injections, showed no additional loss of bone density in patients receiving this treatment.

☐ CONCLUSIONS

Rheumatoid arthritis is potentially a treatable disease, and existing and new therapies are being applied systematically with the aims of suppressing inflammation and preventing damage in the joint, and of reducing the systemic complications. From recent studies, it is clear that inflammation and damage are intimately linked, and that therapies that control inflammation can reduce damage. As yet, however, there is no evidence that early interventions with available intensive therapy can produce long-term remissions or a cure [17].

The search for biological agents, targeted at specific links in the pathogenic process that leads to joint destruction, has already provided encouraging data from initial studies in patients, and should make us optimistic that we can realise our long-term aims of modifying the natural history of rheumatoid arthritis, and possibly even of finding a cure for the disease.

Drug classification

	Modifies	Outcome measures	Mediators	Drugs
I	Symptoms	Visual analogue scale	Prostaglandins + other molecules	COX-2 inhibitors Analgesics
II	Inflammation		Prostaglandins	COX-2 inhibitors
	• Local	Swollen joint count		
	• Systemic	Acute-phase response	Cytokines	Cytokine inhibitors (including conventional DMARDs)
III	Structure	Radiology + (MRI)	Cytokines Proteinases	DMARDs Metalloproteinase inhibitors

Feaures of COX-2 preferential and specific drugs

PREFERENTIAL (or Selective)	SPECIFIC
In vitro	*In vitro*
Better profile of COX-2 inhibition than COX-2	No inhibition of COX-1 throughout therapeutic range of COX-2 inhibition*
In vivo	
Reduced dose-dependent effect on platelets, renal blood flow and gastrointestinal toxicity compared with non-preferential drugs	No effect on platelets, no effect on COX-2 mediated renal function (GFR) Little if any gastrointestinal toxicity

*This equates to a greater than 2 log difference in IC_{50} for COX-1/2 in whole blood assay.

REFERENCES

1 Devlin J, Gough A, Huisoon A, *et al.* The acute phase and function in early rheumatoid arthritis: C-reactive protein levels correlate with functional outcome. *J Rheumatology* 1997: **24**; 9–13.

2 Gough AK, Lilley J, Eyre S, *et al.* Generalised bone loss in patients with early rheumatoid arthritis occurs early and relates to disease activity. *Lancet* 1994: **344**; 23–7.

3 Lipsky P. Cycloxygenase research: advances with clinical implications. In: Pemery XX, ed. *Fast Facts: Rheumatology Highlights 1997*. Oxford: Health Press, 1998.

4 Moreland LW, Bucy RP, Pratt PW, *et al.* Use of chimeric monoclonal anti-CD4 in patients with refractory rheumatoid arthritis. *Arthritis Rheum* 1993; **36**: 307–18.

5 Elliott MJ, Maini RN, Feldmann M, *et al.* A randomised double-blind comparison of chimeric monoclonal antibody to tumour necrosis factor alpha (cA2) versus placebo in rheumatoid arthritis. *Lancet* 1994: **344**; 1105–10.

6 Moreland LW, Baumgartner SW, Schiff MH, *et al.* Treatment of rheumatoid arthritis with a recombinant human tumour necrosis factor receptor (p75)-Fc fusion protein. *N Engl J Med* 1997: **337**; 141–7.

7 van Leeuwen MA, van Rijswijk MH, van der Heijude DMFM, *et al.* The acute-phase response in relation to radiographic progression in early rheumatoid arthritis: a prospective study during the first three years of the disease. *Br J Rheumatol* 1993; **32**(suppl 3): 3–8.

8 Emery P. The optimal management of early rheumatoid arthritis: the key to preventing disability (review). *Br J Rheumatol* 1994; **33**: 765–8.

9 Emery P, Salmon M, Bradley H, *et al.* Genetically determined factors as predictors of radiological change in patients with early symmetrical arthritis. *British Medical Journal.* 1992; **305**: 1387–9.

10 Gough AK, Faint JM, Salmon M, *et al.* Genetic typing of patients with inflammatory arthritis at presentation is predicative of outcome. *Arthritis and Rheumatis*m. 1994; **37**: 1166–70.

11 Felson DT, Anderson JJ, Meenan RF. The efficacy and toxicity of combination therapy in rheumatoid arthritis: a meta-analysis. *Arthritis Rheum* 1994: **37**; 1487–91.

12 Haagsma CJ, van Rlel PL, de Rooij DJRAM, *et al.* Combination of methotrexate and sulphasalazine vs methotrexate alone: a randomised open clinical trial in rheumatoid arthritis patients resistant to sulphasalazine therapy. *Br J Rheumatol* 1994; **33**: 1049–55.

13 O'Dell JR, Haire CE, Eriksson N, *et al.* Treatment of rheumatoid arthritis with methotrexate alone, sulphasalazine and hydroxychloroquine or a combination of all three medications. *N Engl J Med* 1996; 334: 1287–91.

14 Boers M, Verhoeven AC, Markusse HM, *et al.* Randomised comparison of combined step-down prednisolone, methotrexate and sulphasalazine, with sulphasalazine alone in early rheumatoid arthritis. *Lancet* 1997: **350**; 309–18.

15 Proudman SM, Richardson C, Green MJ, *et al.* Treatment of poor prognosis early rheumatoid arthritis: conventional therapy with sulphasalazine vs aggressive therapy with methotrexate, cyclosporin A and intra-articular corticosteroids. *Arthritis Rheum* 1997; Abb suppl (968); S192.

16 Kirwan JR, The Arthritis and Rheumatism Council Low Dose Glucocorticoid Study Group. The effect of glucocorticoids and drug destruction in rheumatoid arthritis. *N Engl J Med* 1996: **35**; 2–4.

17 Emery P. Rheumatoid arthritis: not yet curable with early intensive therapy (review). *Lancet* 1997: **350**; 304–5.

Osteoarthritis: new thoughts about an old disease

Michael Doherty

□ INTRODUCTION

Osteoarthritis (OA) is by far the commonest condition to affect human synovial joints. It is a major cause of locomotor pain, the single most important cause of disability and handicap from arthritis, and an important health care challenge with major resource implications. Its strong association with ageing, combined with the increasing right shift in age distribution of the Western community, will make OA an even greater health issue in the next millennium. Important research advances over the past decade have led to a change in our perspective of OA. Previously considered a 'wear and tear' or 'degenerative' disease that has to be accepted as an inevitable consequence of trauma and ageing, OA is increasingly viewed as a dynamic, essentially reparative process with exciting potential for strategies to intervene in the pathogenic sequence of events.

□ NATURE OF OSTEOARTHRITIS

In advancing the hypothesis that OA represents active repair rather than passive degeneration, three observations are particularly worthy of emphasis.

First, OA has been present throughout our evolutionary history and a similar condition occurs in other animals with synovial joints that fuse their epiphyses in maturity.

Second, OA is a dynamic, metabolically active process at the tissue level (Fig. 1). Although focal loss of hyaline cartilage is a hallmark of OA, chondrocytes, especially early in OA, increase their metabolic rate, produce more cartilage matrix components, and increase in number to form chondrocyte 'clones'. There is florid production of new bone through the ossification of newly formed fibrocartilage (enchondral ossification), particularly at the joint periphery (marginal osteophyte). The synovium hypertrophies, and its outer layer, the capsule, slowly thickens and tightens. Osteochondral bodies often form in the synovium, appearing on radiographs as calcified 'loose bodies'; these originate either from chondroid metaplasia of synoviocytes, or by secondary growth of detached cartilage fragments engulfed by synovium. It therefore appears that all the joint components are trying to produce new tissue. Although the net balance results in hyaline cartilage loss, this is focal rather than widespread, and the slow remodelling of bone ends and the capsular thickening help to redistribute the load across the joint and so maintain joint stability. Periarticular changes include bursitis, enthesopathy (ie abnormality of entheses, the sites of attachment of fibrous structures – ligament, tendon, capsule – into the periosteum and bone) and atrophy of type II muscle fibres.

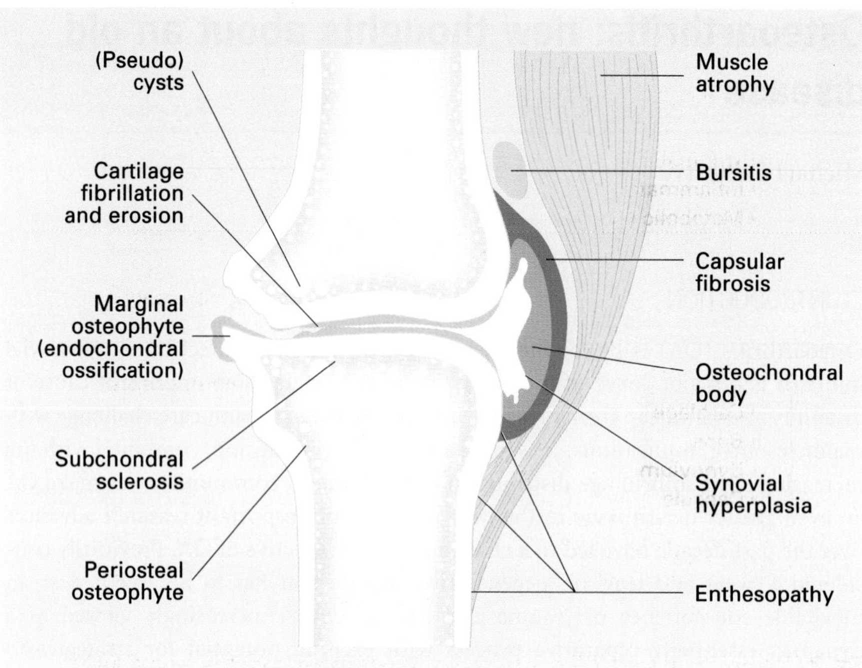

Fig. 1 Changes occurring in the joint affected by OA. (From *Colour Atlas and Text of Osteoarthritis*; see Further Reading section.)

Third, in the community clinical and radiographic features of OA are very common in adults aged over 50 years, showing increased prevalence with each decade. However, in most instances OA occurs without any symptoms or disability. In those with problematic OA, symptoms are commonly phasic, often originate from periarticular sites (bursitis, enthesopathy – especially around the knee and hip), and are usually associated with a good prognosis, especially in small joints such as in the hand.

All these features – phylogenetic preservation, increased biosynthetic activity of joint tissues, discordance between symptoms and presence of OA, and its generally good outcome – suggest that OA reflects the inherent repair process of synovial joints (Fig. 2). A wide variety of insults may trigger the need for repair. Some are obvious, such as major joint trauma; ligament rupture and instability; inflammatory joint disease (rheumatoid and juvenile chronic arthritis); or rare metabolic diseases (eg ochronosis and osteopetrosis) that compromise cartilage or bone. More often, however, specific insults cannot be recognised.

Once the repair process is triggered, all joint tissues (cartilage, bone, synovium, capsule) take part in the response. The outcome will depend on the balance between the severity and chronicity of the insults, and the efficiency of the repair process. In most instances, the slow repair process wins and leads to a 'compensated' situation, with altered joint structure but no symptoms or disability. In some cases, however,

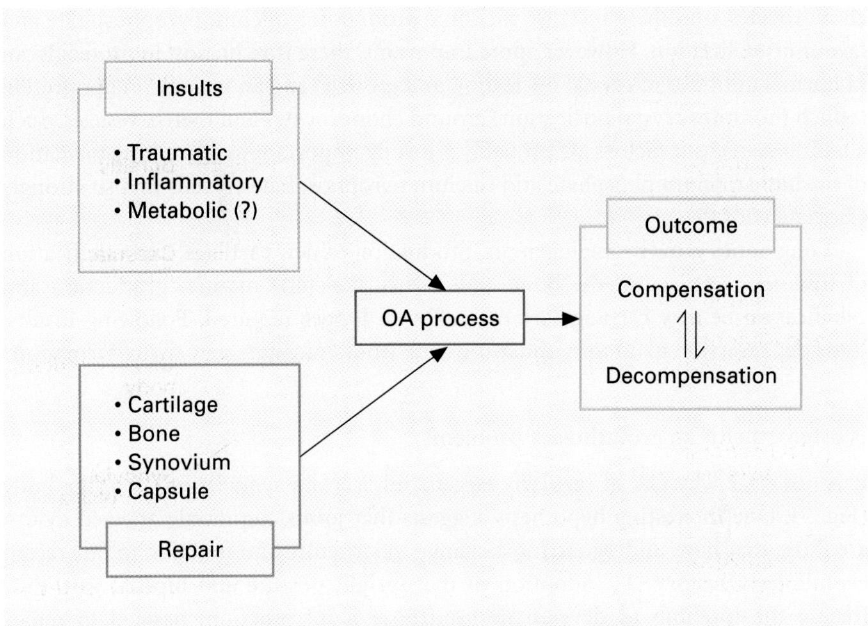

Fig. 2 Diagrammatic representation of OA as the inherent repair process of synovial joints.

perhaps due to an overwhelming insult and/or poor repair, the process cannot compensate, resulting in progressive tissue loss, pain and disability. Such an interpretation in part explains the marked heterogeneity of OA, with differences in environmental (extrinsic) and constitutional (intrinsic) triggering factors, and varying efficiency of the repair process, all of which would encourage diversity of clinical patterns and outcomes.

The perspective of OA as a repair process with varying success, comprising 'subsets' with differing aetiopathogenesis, fits well with other histological and biochemical observations. For example, certain chondroitin sulphate epitopes (eg CS 3-B-3) expressed on aggrecan in immature cartilage are absent from normal mature adult cartilage, but are re-expressed as 'neo-epitopes' in OA cartilage. Aggrecan is the very high molecular weight unit comprising hyaluronan to which are attached core protein chains with keratan sulphate and chondroitin sulphate joined to them; aggrecan is the principal macromolecule of the cartilage matrix. Similarly, angiogenesis, an important component of immature (growing) but not adult locomotor tissues, again becomes prominent in OA joints, as does the deposition in cartilage of calcium crystals, mostly partially carbonate-substituted hydroxyapatite. Calcium crystals deposit in articular (hyaline) and fibrocartilage of synovial joints. Crystals can then be shed from cartilage to be secondarily taken up by synovium and capsule. It is therefore possible that the cartilage and bone in OA revert to a more immature state that is better geared towards production of new tissue. The factors that regulate cartilage calcification (chondrocalcinosis) remain unclear. OA cartilage contains raised pyrophosphate levels, reflecting increased metabolic activity of chondrocytes, and these increase the ionic product for calcium pyrophosphate and favour crystallisation. However, more important, there is reduction in proteoglycan (a normal inhibitor of crystal nucleation and growth) and an increase in lipoprotein (which promotes crystal nucleation) around chondrocytes and matrix vesicles. Such alterations in tissue factors are probably critically important in promoting formation of the basic calcium phosphate and calcium pyrophosphate crystals that so strongly associate with OA.

Long bones grow by angiogenesis, production of new cartilage, and calcification of this new cartilage at the bone ends. Once skeletally mature, production and calcification of new cartilage are normally no longer required. Following insults, however, reversion to a more immature state would facilitate new tissue formation.

Is osteoarthritis an evolutionary problem?

It is not clear why OA so regularly targets only certain synovial joints in the body (Fig. 3). One interesting hypothesis suggests that joints commonly affected by OA are those that have undergone most change in structure and function in our recent evolutionary history [1]. Adoption of the upright posture and bipedal gait, thus freeing the forelimb to develop multipurpose hand function, has led to major changes in thumb bases, finger joints, knees, hips, apophyseal joints of the lower cervical and lumbar spine, and the first metatarsophalangeal joints particularly. These sites, therefore, may not yet be fully adapted to their new functions and have little mechanical reserve in the face of insult. This intriguing hypothesis is so far supported by the varying distribution of OA in other species.

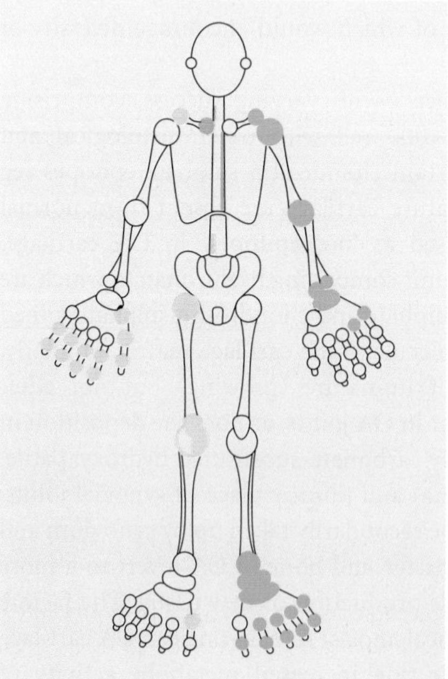

Fig. 3 Distribution of OA; common target sites are shown on the left, relatively protected sites on the right.

Risk factors for development of osteoarthritis

A number of risk factors have now been identified. These may be broadly grouped into constitutional (systemic) changes and local, predominantly mechanical factors (Fig. 4). It is clear that risk factors vary according to joint site, and that factors relating to initiation of OA may differ from those relating to its progression.

Ageing is a general risk factor for OA at all sites, though this is unexplained; age-related changes in cartilage (eg reduced water content) differ from those of OA (eg increased water content). A somewhat defeatist explanation is that we simply encounter more insults (extrinsic and intrinsic) to our joints the longer we live, and that ageing results in declining efficiency of our repair process. An alternative, more optimistic hypothesis is that gradual, age-related declines in muscle strength and joint proprioception may tip previously 'compensated' OA into 'decompensated', symptomatic OA [2]. Since muscle strength and proprioception are both amenable to intervention through exercise, this hypothesis, if correct, clearly has important implications for primary prevention.

The diversity of systemic and local risk factors that may operate at different joints is clearly illustrated by the examples of nodal generalised osteoarthritis (NGOA), and OA that affects the knee and hip.

Nodal generalised osteoarthritis is the best defined of the clinical subsets of OA that have been identified. NGOA is characterised by:

- OA affecting many interphalangeal joints of the fingers
- Heberden's and Bouchard's nodes (Fig. 5)
- a strong female preponderance

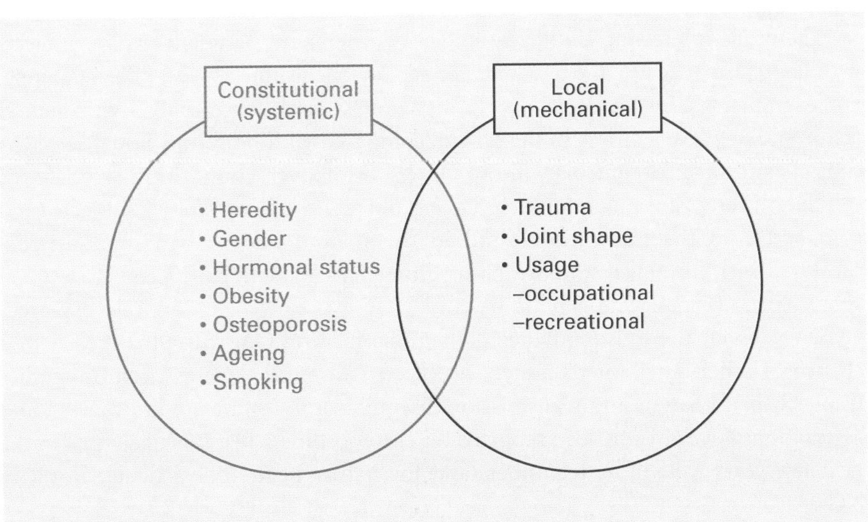

Fig. 4 General and local risk factors for OA (see also Tables 1 and 2); 'hormonal status' refers to the balance or changing levels of sex hormones around the menopause, a time commonly associated with the onset of NGOA.

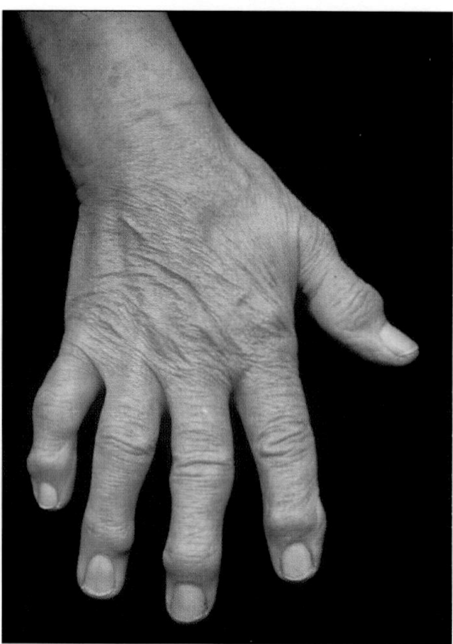

Fig. 5 Nodal OA showing Heberden's nodes posterolaterally over distal, and Bouchard's nodes over proximal, interphalangeal joints. Note the characteristic lateral deviation at some joints (reflecting focal rather than diffuse cartilage loss); because of capsular thickening and bone remodelling, such joints usually remain stable.

- □ marked familial predisposition
- □ peak onset of nodes and hand OA around middle age
- □ good eventual functional outcome for OA affecting the hands
- □ increased predisposition to bilateral knee OA in later life.

There are interesting pathophysiological differences between NGOA subjects with hand and knee OA and age- and gender-matched subjects with knee OA alone. For example, NGOA subjects have a high (50%) prevalence of IgG rheumatoid factor and low levels of IgA in the serum, compared with both non-nodal knee OA subjects and normal controls without OA [3]. Moreover, chondroitin sulphate 6:4 sulphation ratios are much lower in knee synovial fluid from NGOA subjects (and comparable to the low ratios found in rheumatoid knees) than in non-nodal subjects. Such findings support basic differences in aetiopathogenesis between subsets of knee OA. The genetic basis of NGOA is now being actively explored. NGOA is by far the most convincingly familial form of OA, with an almost 1 in 2 chance of inheritance for daughters of affected women. Gene association studies using sib-pair analysis and transmission disequilibrium testing are in progress, and associations have already been reported on chromosome 2 [4]. It is likely that in the next few years we will better understand the nature of the polyarticular insult in NGOA.

The knee is the commonest large joint to be affected by OA, with up to 25% of women aged over 70 years showing radiographic changes. Involvement is usually bilateral, particularly in women and in the elderly. Although OA may affect the knee as a mono- or pauci-articular problem, this site shows strong association with hand OA (Fig. 5). Risk factors for knee OA are summarised in Table 1. Obesity is a major risk factor at this site for symptoms as well as for development and progression of radiographic change, obese women having up to a fourfold increased risk of knee

Table 1 Risk factors for knee osteoarthritis

	Increase risk	Decrease risk
Development	Female	Smoking
	Ageing	
	Obesity	
	Nodal hand OA	
	Knee trauma, instability	
	Occupation (eg football ie, repetitive knee-bending)	
Progression	Knee chondrocalcinosis	
	Knee effusion	
	? NSAIDs	
	? Low levels of dietary antioxidants	

OA [5]. Curiously, smoking has a significant negative association, even after adjusting for factors such as the lower body weight in smokers, alcohol intake, exercise and other lifestyle variables. Recent data from the Framingham study suggest that diets low in vitamins C, A and E (antioxidants) are associated with a greater risk of progression of radiographic change [6]. It seems, therefore, that avoidance of obesity and maintenance of good nutrition could have a major impact on knee OA in the community. A further important lifestyle factor that is gaining increased attention is exercise. Locomotor tissues are built to move; if there is insufficient motion and usage, all the tissues of the joint (cartilage, bone, muscles) undergo atrophy, and the capsule tightens. At the other extreme, however, excessive usage may traumatise any or all of the joint tissues and lead to damage. Current data suggest that traumatic overuse of joints in professional athletes, soccer players and certain occupations (eg mining and farming) increases the risk of OA at certain sites, notably the knee. There is also increasing evidence that less severe but regular excessive load-bearing on flexed knees may predispose to knee OA.

Risk factors for the hip are shown in Table 2. Comparison between factors at these two lower-limb large joints show important differences. For example, men and women are equally affected by hip OA; although obesity is not a risk factor for its development, it is a risk factor for its progression.

Viewing OA as a repair process, it is not surprising that there is frequently discordance between symptoms, disability and structural change (Fig. 6). Such discordance varies according to joint site. Concordance is best at the hip and then at the knee; concordance is poor at the hand and worst at spinal apophyseal joints. At the knee, it is apparent that there are different associations for pain/disability and for

Table 2 Risk factors for hip osteoarthritis

	Increase risk	Decrease risk
Development	Caucasian Ageing Structural alteration (eg Perthes' acetabular dysplasia) Occupation (eg farming)	Osteoporosis Smoking
Progression	Superior pole OA Obesity Knee chondrocalcinosis ? NSAIDs	

structural change. For example, high scores of anxiety and depression and poor quadriceps strength both show good correlations with pain and/or disability, but not with structural change.

□ MANAGEMENT OF OSTEOARTHRITIS

The key objectives in the management of OA are:

- patient education
- pain relief
- optimisation of function
- modification of the disease process

Locomotor pain, including that relating to OA, is a complex problem requiring a holistic, 'total patient' approach. Symptoms and functional impairment relating to OA change with time and in response to interventions, and it follows that patients must be reviewed reasonably frequently to assess progress and to revise the management plan if necessary.

Non-pharmacological management

A number of non-pharmacological strategies may significantly reduce pain and improve function (Table 3). Education of the patient is safe and cost-effective and can have important and prolonged benefits on pain and disability – comparable, for example, to those of oral non-steroidal anti-inflammatory drugs (NSAIDs). Education can be given as part of a package such as the arthritis self-management course [7] of six weekly two-hour sessions in small groups of 15–20 patients, covering a wide range of topics to help in understanding and coping with the disease (see Table 3). Such programmes have been shown to reduce pain scores by up to 20% and reduce disability, and to have persisting benefit without reinforcement for time periods of up to 4 years.

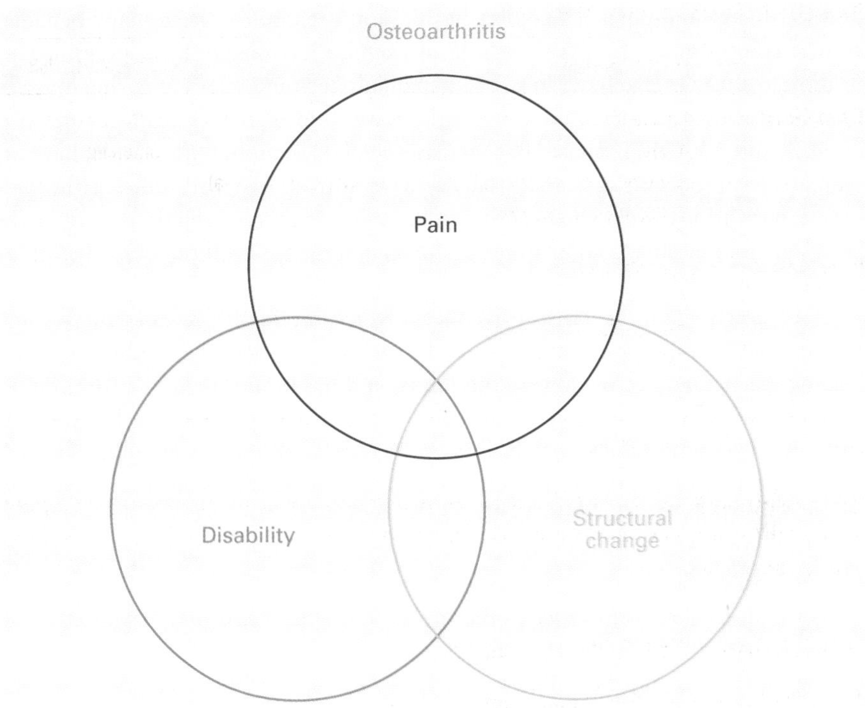

Fig. 6 Concordance between symptoms (pain), disability and structural change in osteoarthritis is not always good, especially for small joints.

Effective education can also be delivered without personal contact, for example by an interactive computer programme, which can be suitable even for older subjects. Telephone contact from a non-medical professional (eg a secretary, research nurse etc), once a month for 12 months, has also been shown to reduce pain and improve function in patients with lower limb OA, and to be cost-neutral [8].

Table 3 Non-pharmacological management of osteoarthritis

	Arthritis self-management course
Education; improved self efficacy	Pathophysiology of OA
Regular telephone contact	Principles of exercise and relaxation
Exercise; strengthening, aerobic fitness	Joint protection
Reduced adverse mechanical factors (eg weight loss, shoes, insoles)	Work simplification
Local physical measures:	Pacing daily activities
non-invasive (eg heat, cold)	Details of treatments
invasive (tidal lavage)	Good nutrition
	Problem solving
	Communication skills with doctors and allied health professionals
	Pain management

Movement is important for joint health, and exercise can have many benefits, even if compromised by OA. The role of exercise has mainly been examined in relation to knee OA. Exercises to strengthen quadriceps and relax hamstring muscles have been shown to increase local muscle power and to reduce pain, for up to 6 months. Interestingly, exercise that increases general aeorobic fitness may have an even greater impact on pain and disability, at least in short-term studies. How long such interventions work is currently under study. Even very elderly patients have been shown to be able to adopt appropriate regular exercise without exacerbation of symptoms or risk.

It is clearly common sense to reduce adverse mechanical factors on a compromised OA joint. For example, weight loss in obese patients can reduce pressure loading, particularly across lower limb joints, and has been shown in a community setting to reduce pain and to reduce the risk of structural progression. The problem, of course, is how to achieve weight loss in the obese, but there is growing evidence that a combination of appropriate dietary advice with exercise is more effective than either used alone. Appropriate footwear (ie thick but soft soles, no elevated heel, broad forefoot, soft uppers) can also help symptoms of knee and hip OA, as can wedged insoles to correct varus strain.

Local physical measures such as the application of heat and cold may be effective analgesics. More invasive local measures, such as tidal lavage of the knee (running through a litre or more of saline), which can be done without arthroscopy or a general anaesthetic, has also been shown to be beneficial, although the mechanism remains obscure.

Drug therapy

A current classification of drugs used in OA is shown in Table 4 [9]. Traditionally, drug therapy has concentrated on pain relief, but novel agents that aim to modify the disease process itself are now under investigation.

Table 4 Classification of drugs used to treat osteoarthritis

Symptom-modifying drugs	Disease-modifying drugs
Rapid onset	**Currently under investigation**
Simple analgesics (paracetamol)	Oral tetracycline
NSAIDs	Intra-articular hyaluronan
Intra-articular steroid injections	Oral or local intra-articular injection of metalloproteinase inhibitors
Prolonged onset	
Intra-articular hyaluronan	
Oral chondroitin sulphate	
Oral diacerrhein	

Symptom-modifying drugs

For reducing pain, a good case can be made for trying full-dose paracetamol in the first instance (1 g three or four times daily). Several studies show that paracetamol is as effective as an oral NSAID for many patients, and is clearly considerably safer. The use of combined analgesics (usually paracetamol plus a codeine derivative) may give more pain relief than paracetamol, but the higher incidence of side-effects often limits their use.

Topical NSAIDs are very popular with patients, and there is evidence that they significantly reduce knee pain, compared with carrier cream alone. Since most patients with OA have symptoms at only one or a few joints at any time, such local treatment is rational. Some NSAID is absorbed systemically, but blood levels (the dominant determinant of major toxicity) are much lower than those derived from oral NSAIDs, which argues in favour of this route of delivery. Topical capsaicin (which specifically depletes substance P, the neurotransmitter in the C fibres that transmit pain) also reduces pain from knee and hand OA, and again is very safe.

Several randomised controlled trials have shown intra-articular steroid to be effective for knee OA, but pain relief is temporary and lasts only 2–6 weeks. There are no apparent clinical predictors of response to intra-articular steroid; although one study reports the presence of an effusion to confer greater benefit, this may relate more to better accuracy of injection into a knee with an effusion rather than to greater efficacy *per se* [10]. Intra-articular injection of hyaluronan, of several molecular weights, has recently been licensed in the UK for symptom relief in knee OA. Hyaluronan occurs in many tissues throughout the body. In the synovial joint, it is secreted by synoviocytes into synovial fluid (giving it its characteristic high viscosity), and it is also synthesised by chondrocytes, forming the axial component of the large aggrecan molecules. Hyaluronan has many interesting physicochemical properties that include modulation of cellular (synoviocyte and chondrocyte) function, altered viscoelastic properties of synovial fluid, adhesion to nociceptors possibly to reduce pain perception, mopping up of reactive oxygen species etc. How it works to reduce pain in OA remains unclear but its pain relief is delayed in onset (occurring after several weeks of weekly injections compared with the much quicker response from an intra-articular steroid injection). Hyaluronan preparations probably can give a degree of pain relief similar to that of intra-articular steroid, though the effect takes 3–5 weeks to occur and may last longer (several months); unfortunately hyaluronan needs to be given in courses of 3–5 weekly injections, which poses logistic problems. Diacerrhein is given orally and has a delayed onset of symptom benefit (≥4 weeks). It is able to stimulate prostaglandin E2 synthesis in chondrocytes and inhibits the effects of interleukin-1 on chondrocytes. It is currently available in mainland Europe, but not in the UK.

A number of guidelines [11] support the following order for using symptom-modifying drugs in OA:

- First-line: full-dose paracetamol
- Second: topical creams

- Third: compound analgesics or an oral NSAID (try low-dose ibuprofen first)
- Fourth: intra-articular steroid to be used as an adjunct to treatment, eg to tide a patient over an important short-term life event or to encourage initiation of other therapy such as exercise.

Disease-modifying drugs

A number of trials of potential disease modifiers are in progress and their results are awaited with interest. Examples include oral tetracyclines (which have many biological effects, including inhibition of matrix metalloproteinases; there is animal work to support a beneficial disease-modifying effect in experimental OA), intra-articular hyaluronan, or metalloproteinase inhibitors (some of which are available in oral form though others need to be given by local intra-articular injection). At present, however, the only evidence that drugs can modify the natural history is for oral NSAIDs, and this is an observation suggesting that oral indomethacin or diclofenac may hasten rather than retard cartilage loss at the knee [12]. Several predominantly retrospective studies support the old concept of 'analgesic hip', and various oral NSAIDs can reduce heterotopic new bone formation following hip replacement if given at regular daily doses for 6–8 weeks following surgery (Fig. 7). This dramatic effect on new bone formation in response to surgical insult has raised serious concerns over the impact that such NSAIDs might have on the slower bone remodelling that occurs in OA.

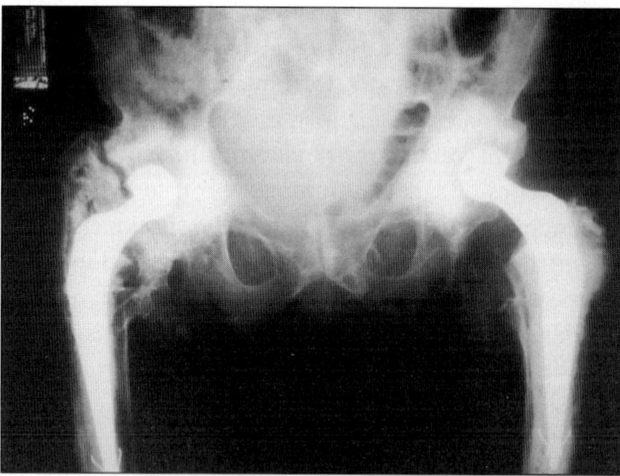

Fig. 7 Hip radiograph of a patient who developed florid heterotopic new bone formation following initial right hip replacement. Regular oral NSAID (diclofenac) taken for 6 weeks following left total hip replacement prevented heterotopic new bone formation on that side.

IS PRIMARY PREVENTION OF OSTEOARTHRITIS FEASIBLE?

Clearly, primary prevention of OA is desirable. A good case can be made for several strategies, including:

- Reduction in obesity, which could have a major impact on the prevalence of knee OA in an ageing community

- □ Encouragement of aerobic exercise throughout life, which would also facilitate a reduction in obesity
- □ Avoidance of overt trauma to joints, through appropriate precautions in high-risk occupations and recreation.

Apart from a healthy, well-balanced diet that maintains a reasonable body weight, the intriguing evidence for the importance of normal levels of micronutrients (eg vitamins A, E and C) has already been mentioned [6]. Appropriate nutrition, weight control and exercise obviously links in with the health of other major body systems, particularly metabolic and cardiorespiratory. The problem of how to implement such a public health programme, however, continues to tax health departments in all Western countries.

REFERENCES

1 Hutton C. Generalised osteoarthritis: an evolutionary problem? *Lancet* 1987; **i**: 1463–5.

2 Slemenda C, Brandt KD, Heilman DK, *et al.* Quadriceps weakness and osteoarthritis of the knee. *Ann Intern Med* 1997; **127**: 97–104.

3 Hopkinson ND, Powell RJ, Doherty M. Autoantibodies, immunoglobulins and Gm allotypes in nodal generalised osteoarthritis. *Br J Rheumatol* 1992; **31**: 605–8.

4 Wright GD, Hughes AE, Regan M, Doherty M. Association of two loci on chromosome 2q with nodal osteoarthritis. *Ann Rheum Dis* 1996; **55**: 317–9.

5 Anderson J, Felson DT. Factors associated with osteoarthritis of the knee in the first National Health and Nutrition Examination Survey (NHANES 1). *Am J Epidemiol* 1988; **128**: 179–89.

6 McAlindon TE, Jacques P, Zhang Y, *et al.* Do antioxidant micro nutrients protect against the development and progression of knee osteoarthritis? *Arthritis Rheum* 1996; **39**: 648–56.

7 Lorig KR, Mazonson PD, Holman HR. Evidence suggesting that health education for self-management in patients with chronic arthritis has sustained health benefits while reducing health care costs. *Arthritis Rheum* 1993; **36**: 439–46.

8 Weinberger M, Tierney WM, Cowper PA, *et al.* Cost-effectiveness of increased telephone contact for patients with osteoarthritis. *Arthritis Rheum* 1993; **36**: 243–6.

9 Group for the Respect of Ethics and Excellence in Science (GREES). Recommendations for the registration of drugs used in the treatment of osteoarthritis. *Ann Rheum Dis* 1996; **55**: 552–7.

10 Jones A, Doherty M. Intra-articular corticosteroids are effective in osteoarthritis but there are no clinical predictors of response. *Ann Rheum Dis* 1996; **55**: 829–32.

11 Hochberg MC, Altman RD, Brandt KD, *et al.* Guidelines for the medical management of osteoarthritis. II. Osteoarthritis of the knee. *Arthritis Rheum* 1995; **38**: 1541–6.

12 Huskisson EC, Berry H, Gishen P, *et al.* Effects of anti-inflammatory drugs on the progression of osteoarthritis of the knee. *J Rheumatol* 1995; **22**: 1941–6.

FURTHER READING

Brandt KD, Doherty M, Lohmander LS (Eds). *Osteoarthritis.* London: Oxford University Press, 1998.

Doherty M (Ed). *Colour Atlas and Text of Osteoarthritis.* London: Mosby Wolfe, 1994.

☐ MULTIPLE CHOICE QUESTIONS

1 Characteristic features of the osteoarthritis process:
 (a) Global loss of hyaline cartilage
 (b) Marginal new bone formation
 (c) Reduced water content of cartilage
 (d) Increased calcium crystal deposition in cartilage
 (e) Capsular weakness and joint instability

2 Common target sites for osteoarthritis:
 (a) The 1st carpo-metacarpal joint
 (b) The radiocarpal joint
 (c) The glenohumeral joint
 (d) The acromio-clavicular joint
 (e) The great toe interphalangeal joint

3 Nodal generalised osteoarthritis is characterised by:
 (a) Polyarticular finger interphalangeal joint osteoarthritis
 (b) Poor outcome for hand symptoms and disability
 (c) Autosomal dominant inheritance
 (d) Peak onset of hand involvement in post-retirement years
 (e) Supero-lateral nodes and radial/ulnar deviation of finger interphalangeal joints

4 Positive risk factors for development of knee osteoarthritis:
 (a) Female gender and ageing
 (b) Low peak bone mass
 (c) Obesity
 (d) Smoking
 (e) Farming

5 Interventions shown to reduce pain and disability in symptomatic knee osteoarthritis:
 (a) Regular, increased impact loading
 (b) Quadriceps strengthening exercises
 (c) Increased aerobic/fitness training
 (d) Oral capsaicin
 (e) Supplements of vitamins A, E and C

ANSWERS

1a False	2a True	3a True	4a True	5a False
b True	b False	b False	b False	b True
c False	c False	c False	c True	c True
d True	d True	d False	d False	d False
e False	e False	e True	e False	e False

Osteoporosis

John A Kanis and Eugene V McCloskey

□ INTRODUCTION

Osteoporosis is increasingly recognised as a major challenge to public health [1]. A great deal is now known about its aetiology and, in particular, the importance of gonadal deficiency at the menopause in women. In addition, numerous lifestyle factors have been shown to contribute to osteoporosis. Knowledge has now advanced significantly in this therapeutic area, and many agents are now available to treat the condition. Despite these significant advances, there remain many challenges to be overcome, and these will be reviewed in this chapter.

□ DEFINITION OF OSTEOPOROSIS

Osteoporosis can be viewed conceptually as a systemic disease, characterised by low bone mass and microarchitectural deterioration of bone tissue that lead to increased bone fragility and susceptibility to fracture. Microarchitectural deterioration and bone fragility are difficult to measure *in vivo*, and the practical definition of osteoporosis therefore depends on the assessment of bone mineral density. Bone mineral density can now be accurately measured by a variety of absorptiometric techniques. Of these, the most information is provided by dual-energy x-ray absorptiometry (DXA), which is suitable for measuring bone density in the whole skeleton or in specific sites, particularly those susceptible to fracture.

As discussed below, women are much more susceptible than men to the clinical complications of osteoporosis, and most systematic studies of bone mineral density have been undertaken in females. Bone mineral density in the young healthy female population is normally distributed (Fig. 1). Osteoporosis in women is generally defined in terms of this reference range [2], as a bone mineral density that is lower than 2.5 standard deviations below the mean value in healthy young females [3]. The use of standard deviation units rather than absolute units overcomes some of the problems of using different types of equipment. When defined in this way, approximately 15% of Caucasian women have osteoporosis of the forearm, spine or hip, and approximately 30% will have osteoporosis at any of these sites. This is approximately equivalent to the proportion of the female population at risk from fractures. Bone mineral density declines with age, and individual values at specific sites can similarly be related to the age-adjusted reference range (see Fig. 2).

The assessment of bone mineral density gives an index of fracture risk, which approximately doubles for each standard deviation decrease in bone density [4]. This gradient of risk is as strong as that derived from measuring blood pressure to predict stroke, and significantly better than that relating serum cholesterol

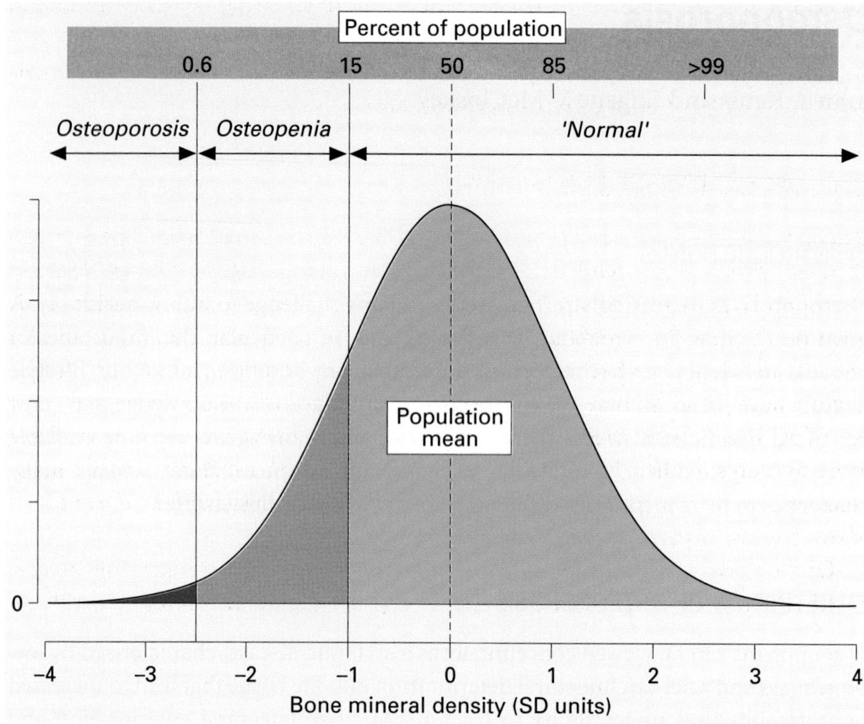

Fig. 1 Distribution of bone mineral density in premenopausal adult women. Osteoporosis is defined as a bone mineral density at least 2.5 standard deviations below the mean of the young female population. Low bone mass (osteopenia) denotes values lying between 1 and 2.5 standard deviations below the mean [2].

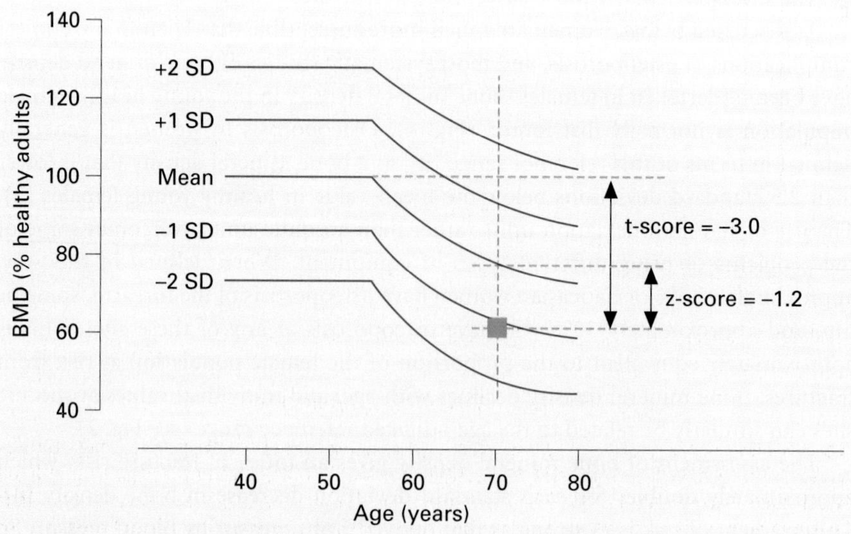

Fig. 2 Age-related reference range for bone mineral density in women.

concentrations to the risk of myocardial infarction in men (Fig. 3). As in the case of blood pressure, however, the test lacks sensitivity [1]: a low bone mineral density is of high predictive value for a future fracture, but fractures also occur in many individuals with a 'normal' bone mineral density.

□ COMPLICATIONS OF OSTEOPOROSIS

Osteoporosis itself is asymptomatic unless fractures occur. Because bone density decreases progressively with age, particularly in women (Fig. 2), the incidence of osteoporosis increases in an exponential manner (Fig. 4). Many osteoporotic fractures also show exponential age-related increases. The most vulnerable sites for fracture are the wrist, vertebral bodies and hip. The lifetime risk of an osteoporotic fracture at any one of these sites is approximately 15% in Western women after the age of 50 years, and approximately one in three Western women will have one or more fractures in their lifetime. This is comparable to the lifetime risk of cardiovascular disease in women – a statistic that highlights the magnitude of the problem of osteoporosis in the community.

Of the various osteoporotic fractures, hip fracture carries the greatest morbidity, mortality and socioeconomic cost. For example, the annual direct hospital costs for

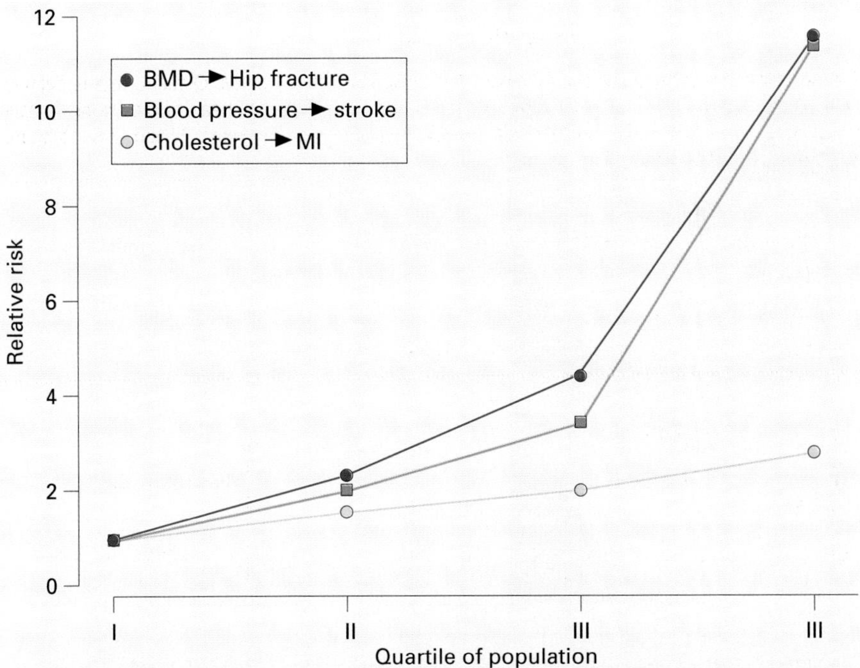

Fig. 3 Relative risk of clinical outcomes according to measurement of risk factors categorised by quartiles. Those in the lowest quartile are assigned a risk of 1.0. The 25% of the population with the lowest bone mineral density (BMD) has a greater than 10-fold increase in hip fracture risk. BMD measurements have as powerful a predictive value for hip fracture as does blood pressure for stroke, and are stronger than serum cholesterol for myocardial infarction (MI) in men [2].

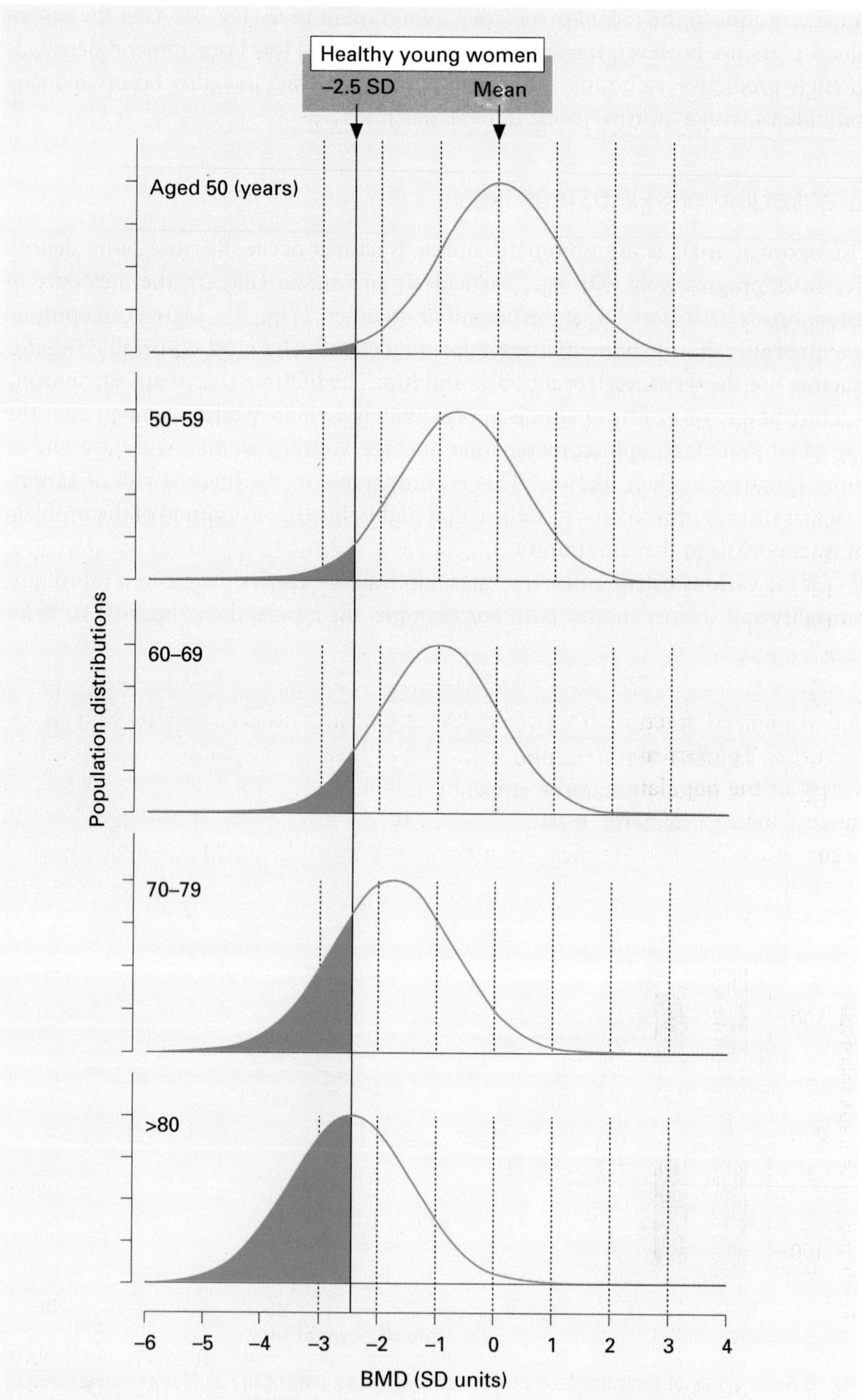

Fig. 4 Bone mineral density (BMD) in women at different ages and the frequency of osteoporosis. As the mean value for BMD decreases with age the prevalence of osteoporosis increases exponentially [2].

fracture in England and Wales currently amount to £220 million, of which nearly 90% is accounted for by hip fractures. Because hip fractures invariably require hospital admission, much more is known about the epidemiology of hip fracture in various communities than is the case for vertebral fracture or Colles fracture.

□ OSTEOPOROSIS IN THE FUTURE

Osteoporosis is a disease of ageing, and life expectancy is increasing all over the world. The increase in life expectancy is particularly marked in Southeast Asia, where robust predictions indicate that the numbers of elderly (over 65 years of age) will increase 2-fold by the year 2025 (Fig. 5). The burden of osteoporosis is likely to increase not only for this reason, but also owing to an independent increase in the age- and sex-specific incidence of osteoporosis. This latter phenomenon is unexplained, but a plausible hypothesis has related it to the decreasing level of everyday physical activity in the community [5]. Variations in the age- and sex-specific incidence of osteoporosis may also explain the wide range in risk of hip fracture in different communities [6,7]; for example, age-standardised data from Europe show that the risk of hip fracture in different European countries varies by more than 10-fold (Fig. 6). This may also be explained by differences in the levels of routine physical activity.

These factors are likely to cause steep increases in the incidence of osteoporosis and its related fractures that will have important implications for health care resources. The increase in the incidence of hip fracture that can be expected due to ageing of the population will more than double during the next 35 years [8]. If a modest increase of <1% in age- and sex-specific incidence of osteoporosis also occurs – as it has done in the past in many regions of the world – then the number

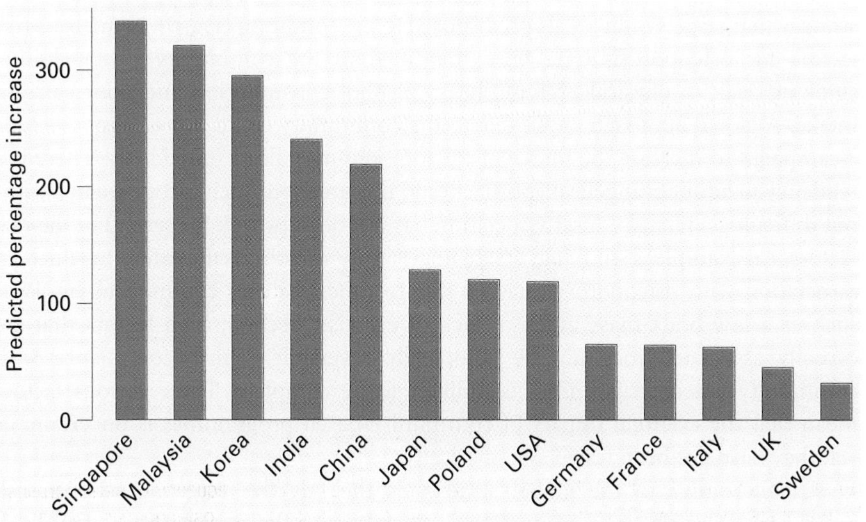

Fig. 5 Projected increase in the elderly community between 1990 and 2025.

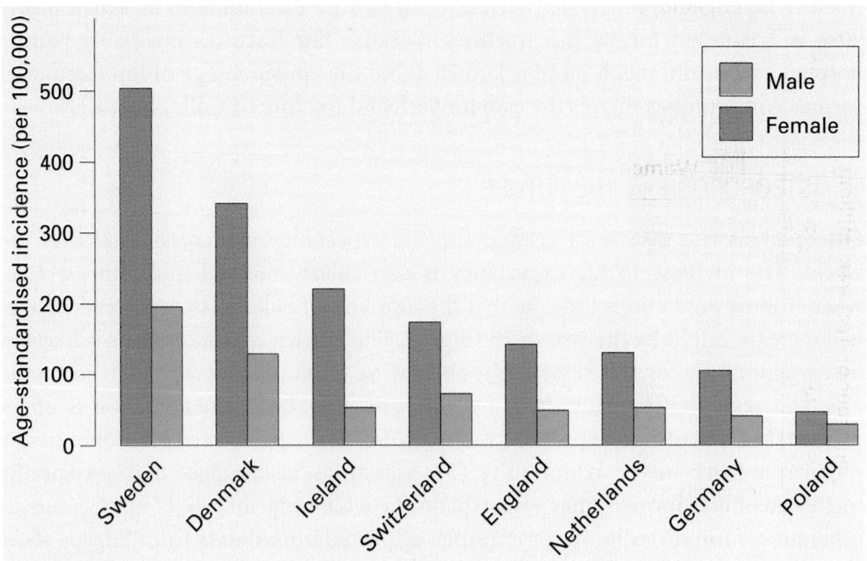

Fig. 6 Age-standardised risk of hip fracture in different European countries [6].

of hip fractures is likely to triple (Fig. 7). In Europe, hip fracture at present accounts for one-fifth of all orthopaedic admissions, so in the very near future hospital resources will be markedly stressed.

□ TREATMENT STRATEGIES FOR OSTEOPOROSIS

Management strategies for osteoporosis have focused on either global approaches that aim to reduce the risks of osteoporosis in the community at large, or a 'high risk' strategy that targets individuals predisposed to the condition (Fig. 8). Numerous risk factors for osteoporosis have been identified in the community [2], including smoking, lack of physical exercise, heavy alcohol consumption and poor calcium intake. A global approach applicable to the community could, for example include a campaign to increase the intake of calcium amongst all its individuals. There is a tendency to adopt evangelical approaches in this area, but such tactics are not without difficulties. First, a causal association has not been proven for several of the risk factors. An example is smoking, where uncertainty surrounds the extent to which an association with osteoporosis may be due to other features common in smokers, such as a low body mass index or lack of exercise. Second, even factors that are causally associated may not be completely reversible. Third, compliance with community-based programmes is unlikely to be complete. These various factors mean that the eventual impact of community-based programmes is uncertain; as yet, they have not been tested systematically.

An alternative to the global strategy is the selective targeting of high-risk individuals. The aim is to identify those members of the community most at risk from osteoporosis or from fractures and to bring effective therapeutic interventions

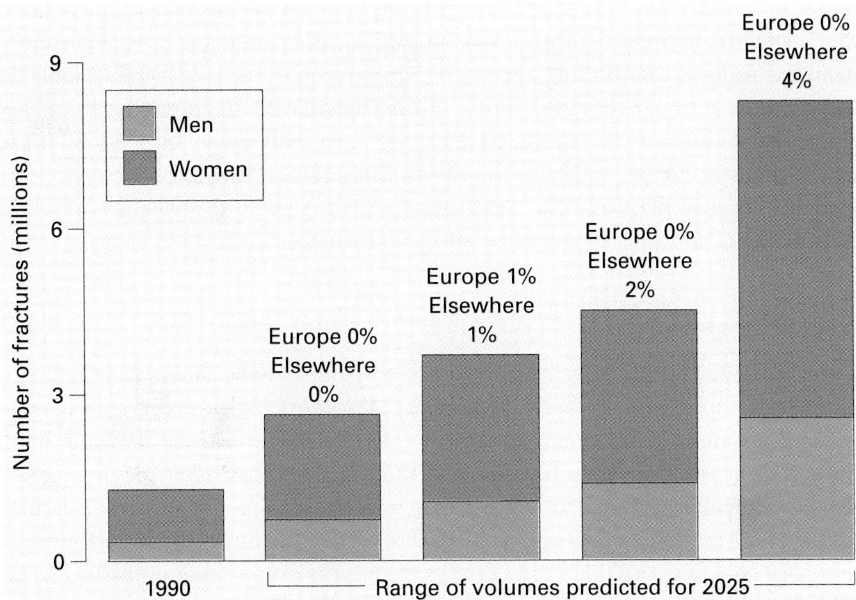

Fig. 7. Number of hip fractures worldwide in 1990 and the number estimated for 2025 according to assumptions concerning possible increases in age-specific incidence of hip fracture, shown for Europe and North America ('Europe') and other countries ('Elsewhere'). Hip fractures will more than double to 2.6 million in 2025, assuming no change in age-specific rates. With various assumptions concerning secular trends, the number of hip fractures in 2050 could range between 4.5 and 21.3 million. (From Gullberg *et al* [8])

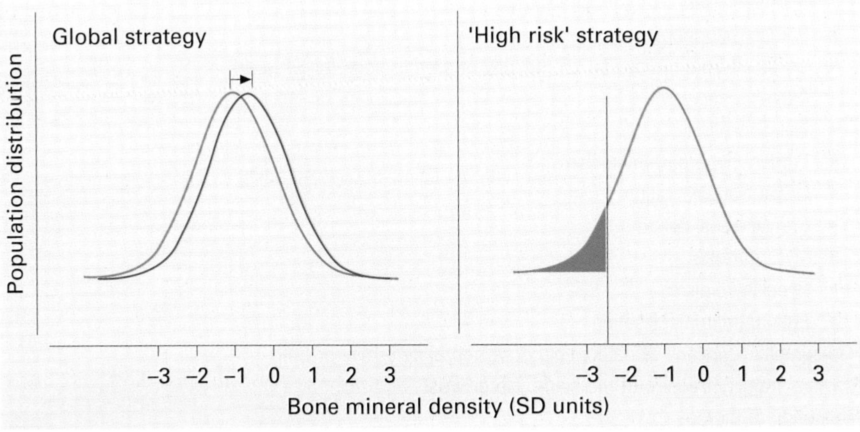

Fig. 8 Treatment strategies for osteoporosis. The global approach aims to shift bone mineral density to the right in the entire population, whereas the high-risk approach identifies individuals at particular risk of osteoporosis.

to bear on them. There is at present no clear rationale for the mass screening of bone mineral density in order to target interventions [1], and patients at risk are currently identified using a case-finding approach. Several important risk factors (Table 1) identify those at high risk from fracture [9]. In centres with diagnostic facilities, it is appropriate to measure bone mineral density in such individuals, since not all those with strong risk factors will have the disease. In addition, the assessment of bone mineral density permits the quantification of risk and provides baseline measurements on which to assess the effects of treatment.

Drugs to treat osteoporosis

A wide variety of agents is available for the treatment of osteoporosis [2]. In women, particularly those with an early menopause, the most logical intervention is to consider hormone replacement treatment (HRT). HRT effectively prevents bone loss and decreases the risk of fracture, and there is also substantial epidemiological and experimental evidence to suggest that it decreases the risk of cardiovascular disease [1]. The main drawback is poor compliance owing to the resumption of menstrual bleeding, and there have also been concerns over a possibly enhanced risk of breast cancer which, even if genuine, is small. The development of combined continuous regimens of HRT has decreased the frequency of unwanted menstrual bleeding, and a variety of oestrogen analogues is being developed which may avoid the risk of adverse effects on breast tissue. A major problem with the widespread use of HRT at the time of the menopause is that long-term treatment, for up to 10 years, is usually recommended. The question arises as to what happens to bone mass when

Table 1 Clinical indications for bone densitometry.

Presence of strong risk factors

- Premature menopause (<45 years)
- Prolonged secondary amenorrhoea
- Primary hypogonadism
- Corticosteroid therapy (>7.5 mg/day of prednisolone for ≥1 year)
- Anorexia nervosa
- Malabsorption
- Primary hyperparathyroidism
- Organ transplantation
- Chronic renal failure
- Myelomatosis
- Hyperthyroidism
- Prolonged immobilisation

Radiographic evidence of osteopenia or vertebral deformity or both

Previous fragility fracture of the spine, hip or wrist

Monitoring of therapy

- Hormone replacement therapy in established osteoporosis
- Newer agents (bisphosphonates, calcitonins, vitamin D and derivatives, sodium fluoride)

treatment is stopped. If 'catch up' bone loss occurs, the ultimate effect on bone density and therefore on hip fracture rates may be trivial (Fig. 9). For this reason, interventions in the elderly may be more worthwhile, at least for hip fracture risk.

Many interventions other than HRT are now available and have been tested in the elderly (Table 2). They are all capable of at least slowing the rate of bone loss and, in some instances, can induce increments in skeletal mass that are sustained for the duration of treatment.

The use of bone mineral density measurements to target intervention specifically on those proven to have substantially reduced values improves the cost-effectiveness of all but the cheapest treatment (ie HRT). Conversely, the lack of diagnostic facilities in many countries [9] presents major problems for the widespread introduction of a rational and effective approach to the management of osteoporosis.

The case-finding strategy has been formalised in Europe [10], and similar guidelines are in preparation for the UK. An advantage of this approach is that treatments are targeted at those at very high risk, although it will miss many individuals who will sustain fragility fractures. There will be a need, therefore, to develop screening strategies which should perhaps be targeted at the elderly, in whom the risk is greatest and the dividends of treatment more cost-effective.

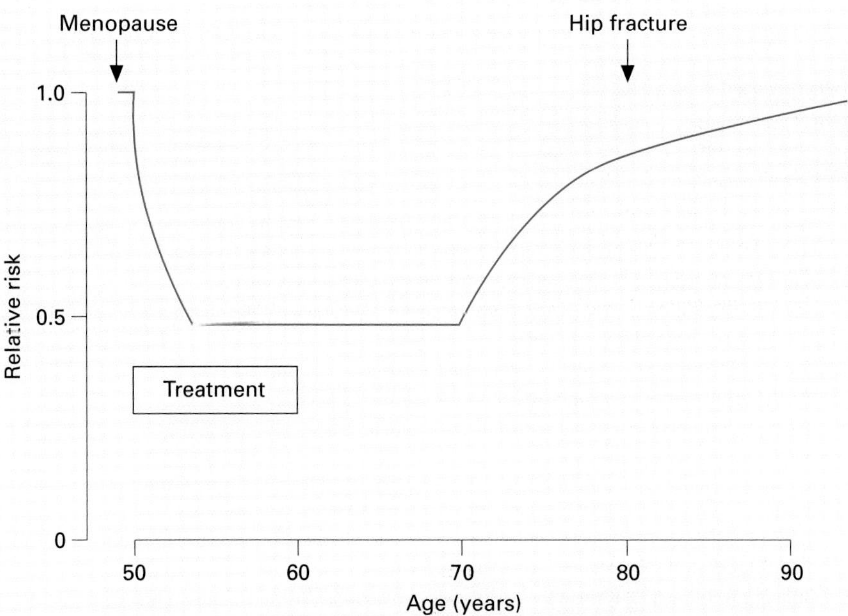

Fig. 9 Effect of a hypothetical treatment on hip fracture risk. Treatment for 10 years at the time of the menopause decreases the risk by 50%. If the protective effect wears off after treatment is stopped, the effect on hip fracture risk is attenuated since hip fractures occur on average at the age of 80 years [2].

Table 2 Agents used in the treatment of osteoporosis.

Inhibitors of bone turnover

- Oestrogens
- Anti-oestrogens (raloxifene, tamoxifen* and others under development)
- Tibolone
- Progestogens
- Calcitonins (salmon, eel, human)
- Bisphosphonates
  - Alendronate
  - Clodronate*
  - Etidronate
  - Pamidronate*
- Vitamin D derivatives
  - Calciferol and cholecalciferol
  - Calcitriol
  - Alfacalcidol
- Ipriflavone*
- Calcium

Stimulators of bone formation

- Fluorides*
  - Sodium fluoride
  - Monofluorophosphate
- Anabolic steroids*
  - Stanozolol
  - Oxandrolone
  - Nandrolone

*Generally used in specialist units.

REFERENCES

1 World Health Organisation. Assessment of fracture risk and its application to screening for postmenopausal osteoporosis. *WHO Technical Report Series*, 843. Geneva: WHO, 1994.

2 Kanis JA. *Textbook of Osteoporosis.* Oxford: Blackwell Science, 1996.

3 Kanis JA, Melton LJ, Christiansen C, Johnston CC, Khaltaev N. The diagnosis of osteoporosis. *J Bone Miner Res* 1994; **9**: 1137–41.

4 Marshall D, Johnell O, Wedel H. Meta-analysis of how well measures of bone mineral density predict occurrence of osteoporotic fractures. *Br Med J* 1996; **312**: 1254–9.

5 Johnell O, Gullberg B, Kanis JA, *et al.* Risk factors for hip fracture in European women. *J Bone Miner Res* 1995; **10**: 1902–5.

6 Johnell O, Gullberg B, Allender A, Kanis JA, and the MEDOS Study Group. The apparent incidence of hip fracture in Europe. *Osteoporos Int* 1992; **2**: 298–302.

7 Elffors L, Allander E, Kanis JA, *et al.* The variable incidence of hip fracture in southern Europe: the MEDOS study. *Osteoporos Int* 1994; **4**: 253–63.

8 Gullberg B, Johnell O, Kanis JA. World-wide projections for hip fracture. *Osteoporos Int* 1997; **7**: 407–13.

9 Compston JE, Cooper C, Kanis JA. Bone densitometry in clinical practice. *Br Med J* 1995; **310**: 1507–10.

10 Kanis JA, Delmas P, Burckhardt P, Cooper C, Torgerson D, on behalf of the EFFO. Guidelines for diagnosis and management of osteoporosis. *Osteoporos Int* 1997; **7**: 390–406.

□ MULTIPLE CHOICE QUESTIONS

1 Osteoporosis:
  (a) Is more common than breast cancer
  (b) Is defined as a fragility fracture
  (c) Is always symptomatic
  (d) Is increasing in prevalence
  (e) Is essentially untreatable

2 Hip fracture:
  (a) Costs less than other osteoporotic fractures
  (b) Gives rise to mortality
  (c) Varies by less than 3-fold between countries
  (d) Occurs most frequently between the menopause and 70 years of age
  (e) Is increasing in frequency

3 Bone mineral density:
  (a) Remains stable with age in adults
  (b) Predicts fracture risk
  (c) Can be used to monitor treatment
  (d) Is not a diagnostic test for osteoporosis
  (e) Should be measured in all women at menopause

4 Treatment of osteoporosis:
  (a) Is feasible using a global strategy
  (b) Should be offered to all women
  (c) Could be managed by screening the population
  (d) Includes the use of fluoride
  (e) Should be considered in patients with premature menopause

ANSWERS

1a True
b False
c False
d True
e False

2a False
b True
c False
d False
e True

3a False
b True
c True
d False
e False

4a False
b False
c False
d True
e True

Paget's disease

David Hosking

□ INTRODUCTION

The characteristic feature of Paget's disease is greatly accelerated bone remodelling, which causes normal lamellar bone to be gradually replaced by mechanically compromised woven bone (Fig. 1). This results in the clinical manifestations of bone pain, deformity and fracture. Over the last decade, there have been major advances in understanding the pathogenesis of Paget's disease. This, together with specific therapies that modulate remodelling, have extended the goals of treatment beyond purely symptomatic relief to the long-term control of the disease process itself.

□ PATHOGENESIS OF PAGET'S DISEASE

Many studies, ranging from epidemiology to molecular biology, suggest that Paget's disease is caused by environmental triggers, possibly infections, acting in genetically predisposed individuals.

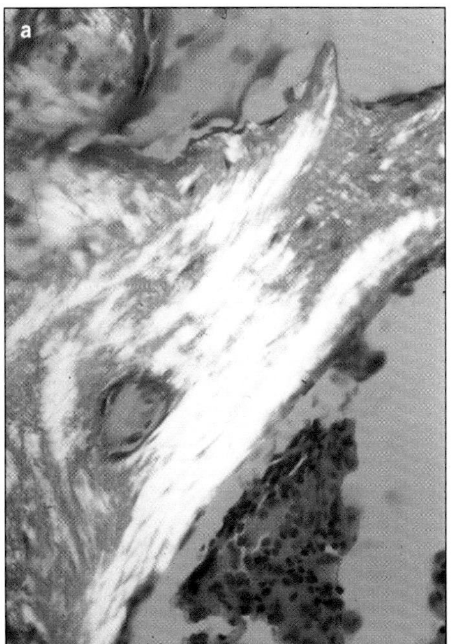

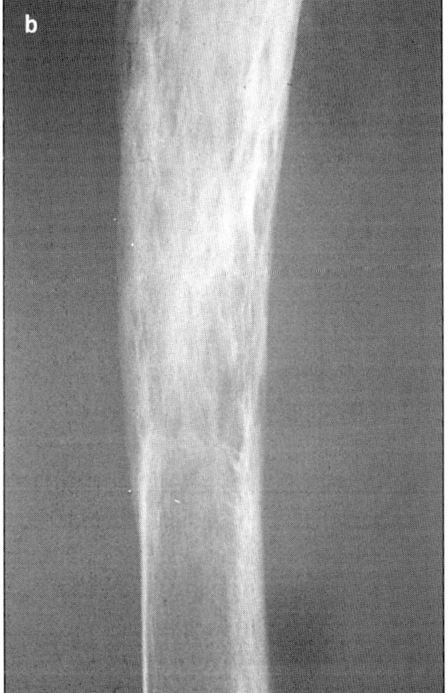

Fig. 1 (a) Bone biopsy sample showing lamellar bone (white) and woven bone (purple). **(b)** Radiograph of shaft of femur, showing transition between woven (top) and lamellar (bottom) bone.

Virus infection

The primary abnormality in Paget's disease resides in the osteoclast which shows a variety of ultrastructural changes and is responsible for excessive resorption of lamellar bone [1]. Bone formation is also increased, but the preservation of normal osteoblast morphology indicates that this is an appropriate response, coupled to the increased resorption (Fig. 2). A high proportion of pagetic osteoclasts contain nuclear inclusions similar to nucleocapsids of DNA viruses of the paramyxovirus class. Although specific viruses have not been definitely identified, immunocytochemical and *in situ* hybridisation studies have suggested that the most likely candidates are measles, respiratory syncytial virus or canine distemper virus [2,3]. However, their true pathogenetic significance is uncertain but mRNA for these viruses is expressed in osteoclasts and also in osteoblasts, osteocytes and mononuclear cells in the pagetic lesion. This may provide an explanation for the enhanced growth induced in early osteoclast precursors ('colony forming unit-granulocyte, macrophage'; CFU-GM) by pagetic stromal cells. On the other hand, intact virus has not been isolated from any of these cell lines, nor has it proved possible to transmit infection to normal cells by coculture. This might suggest that the virus has a replication defect, but would still be able to have a pathogenetic role as it could be transmitted through the osteoclast population by fusion of mature osteoclasts with early precursors. Measles virus transcripts have also been identified in bone marrow

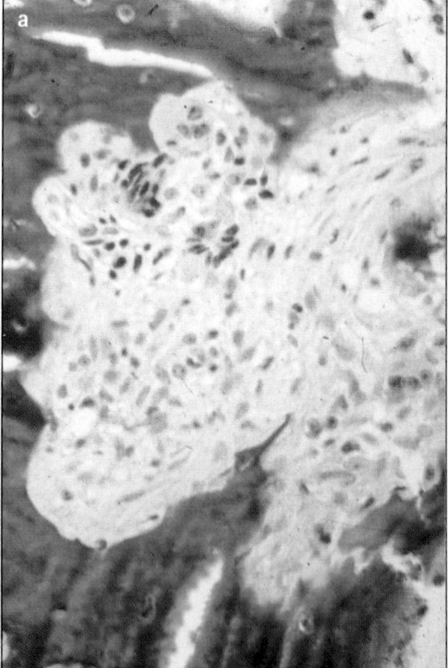

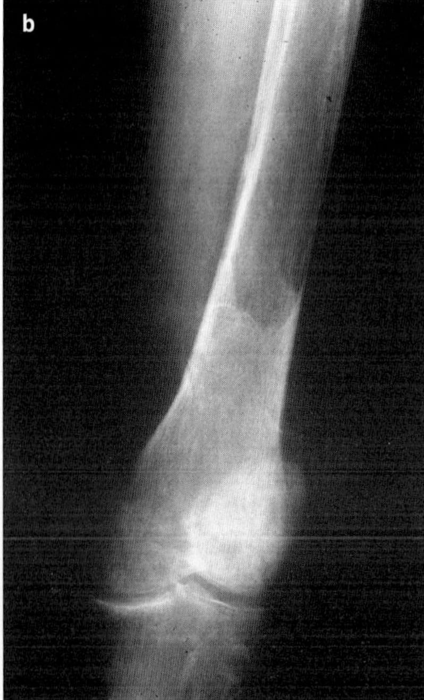

Fig. 2 (a) Bone biopsy showing increased osteoclastic bone resorption and increased osteoblastic surface (bottom right-hand corner). **(b)** Radiograph of shaft of femur showing resorption front extending down diaphysis towards the femoral condyle.

mononuclear cells and osteoclast precursors (CFU-GM) from affected patients; these mRNA sequences can also be demonstrated in peripheral blood samples from pagetic subjects [2,3]. Haematogenous spread of such cells might explain the patchy skeletal distribution of the disease.

Genetic and cellular mechanisms

Epidemiological studies have shown that approximately 15% of patients with Paget's disease have an affected first-degree relative, thus suggesting a genetic susceptibility. Although the cellular mechanisms underpinning the increase in osteoclastic activity in Paget's disease are uncertain, some potential connections between virus infection and genetic predisposition have been identified. An interesting possibility is that a paramyxovirus infection, through the production of reactive oxygen species, might stimulate the expression of proto-oncogenes such as Bcl-2 [4]. This particular proto-oncogene is of particular interest because it is a suppressor of programmed cell death (apoptosis) and known to be upregulated (specifically in the osteoclast) in Paget's disease. Overexpression of Bcl-2 could therefore prolong the lifespan of the osteoclast (Fig. 3). Moreover, the gene for Bcl-2 has been mapped to chromosome 18q, which is also the susceptibility locus for the rare condition of familial expansile osteolysis which bears some similarities to Paget's disease [3]. One link between the viral and genetic aetiologies might therefore be through an inherited defect in the control mechanism which normally suppresses Bcl-2 production. By leading to unopposed Bcl-2 overexpression, virus infection would result in extended osteoclast survival, greater potential for fusion of precursors with affected osteoclasts, and ultimately increased bone resorption (Fig. 4). How these changes might relate to the other known regulators of osteoclast function such as the interleukins (IL)-1, IL-6 and macrophage-colony stimulating factor (M-CSF) is currently unknown [5].

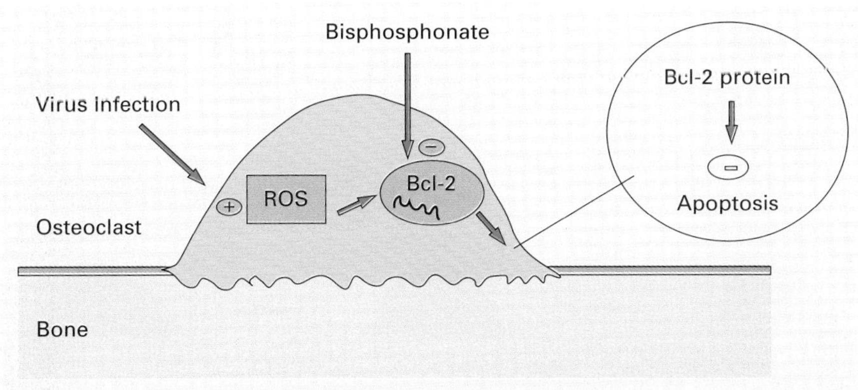

Fig. 3 Possible interactions between viruses and apoptosis in the osteoclast, and their roles in the pathogenesis of Paget's disease. Apoptosis is inhibited by the product of the Bcl-2 proto-oncogene, which is one possible site of action of the bisphosphonates which reduce osteoclast activity and survival (ROS = reactive oxygen species).

These processes may also provide clues about the cellular mode of action of the bisphosphonates, which are now the cornerstone of treatment of Paget's disease. These agents cross cell membranes poorly and probably enter the osteoclast by endocytosis during resorption of exposed bone surfaces on to which bisphosphonates are adsorbed. Bisphosphonates may trigger a variety of intracellular processes leading to accelerated apoptosis of osteoclasts and thus inhibition of resorption – none of these is necessarily mutually exclusive. Certain bisphosphonates (eg clodronate) may be metabolised to non-hydrolysable analogues of ATP which inhibit a variety of metabolic pathways. By contrast, pamidronate and other amino-bisphosphonates inhibit enzymes of the mevalonate pathway, and so disrupt the biosynthesis of sterols required for normal structure and function of cell membranes [6].

Bisphosphonates also cause a loss of both Bcl-2 activity and activation of a family of cystine proteases (caspases) which mediate an irreversible step in the apoptotic process. The ability of these drugs to promote apoptosis may therefore offset the stimulatory effects of virus infection on osteoclasts, with the net result that bone resorption is inhibited.

Epidemiological data and secular trends

Paget's disease shows striking geographical localisation and temporal variation, consistent with an important aetiological role of environmental factors. Studies in the UK conducted over 20 years ago showed a particularly high prevalence (about 5%) in the Lancashire mill towns. A recent survey of some of the same towns has shown a decrease in prevalence to about 3% among men and women aged over 55 years. It seems likely that the severity of the disease – both in terms of its biochemical activity and the extent of skeletal involvement – has also declined over the last two decades.

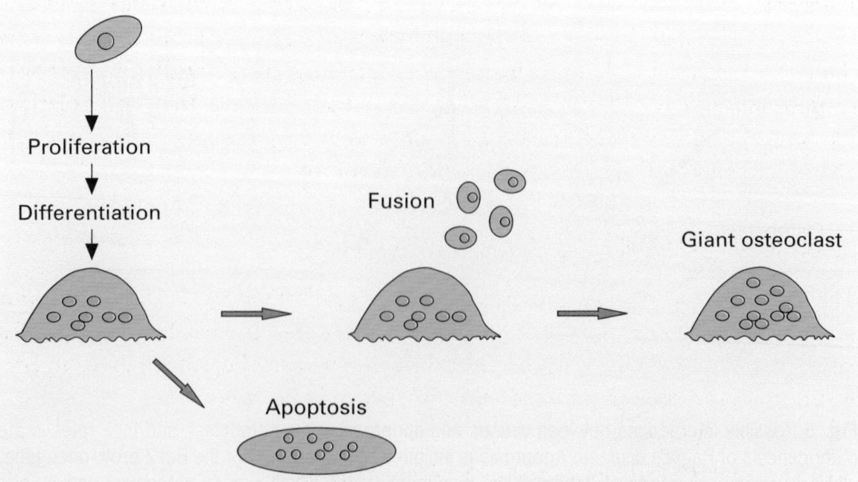

Fig. 4 The osteoclast cycle in Paget's disease.

A recent survey from New Zealand [7] found that, despite an increase in the size of the susceptible population and increased referral rate to a specialist clinic, there has been a fall in the number of new patients with biochemically highly active disease. Moreover, the age of newly referred patients has risen steadily over the years, while the proportion of those with extensive disease (>20% skeletal involvement on bone scintigraphy) has also declined. Similar changes are also apparent in the UK and have an important bearing on the strategy for current disease management.

☐ CLINICAL FEATURES

The main symptoms of Paget's disease are pain and deformity, the latter sometimes giving rise to neurological compression syndromes or predisposing to long-bone fractures (Figs 5–7) [8].

Bone pain is the commonest presenting symptom; it may have a number of components, including increased vascularity and periosteal distortion due to abnormal architecture or deformity. The main clinical problem is to distinguish bone pain from that originating from adjacent joints. Many patients with Paget's disease are elderly and therefore prone to degenerative joint disease, which may itself be initiated or exacerbated by the presence of peri-articular pagetic involvement. While both types of pain are worse on weight bearing, that due to Paget's disease is also present at rest. This distinction has to be clinical, since biochemical and radiographic tests do not reliably differentiate between these sources of pain.

The abnormal pagetic bone architecture also leads to a bowing deformity of long bones (Fig. 6); this increases the mechanical strain on adjacent joints and leads to pain, either directly or indirectly, through the development of degenerative joint disease. As weight-bearing bones such as the femur and tibia become increasingly bowed, they develop stress fractures over the convex border which may become painful or extend to produce the characteristic transverse complete fracture.

Deformity of the spine may lead to a variety of neurological entrapment syndromes either due to direct compression or through a vascular steal syndrome (Fig. 7a). Cranial or facial deformity may be obvious physically, but changes at the skull base can result in internal hydrocephalus or long-tract neurological signs as a consequence of basilar invagination (Fig. 7b). Cranial nerve palsies, particularly of the ocular (III, IV and VI cranial nerves) and auditory nerves, may also occur due to encroachment of the disease into their exit foraminae.

☐ GENERAL TREATMENT OF PAGET'S DISEASE

The management of Paget's disease has been transformed by the introduction of potent osteoclast inhibitors such as the calcitonins and the bisphosphonates. The latter are now pre-eminent in current treatment strategies because of their superior potency, convenience of administration and general tolerability.

Structure and mechanism of action of bisphosphonates

The structures of the bisphosphonates currently licensed for the treatment of Paget's

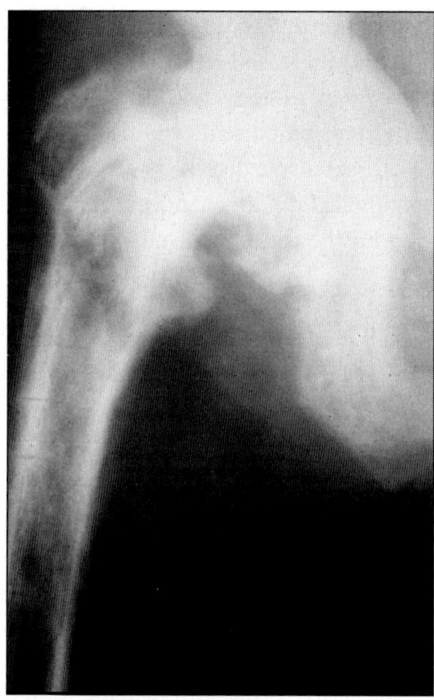

Fig. 5 Radiograph of hip joint and proximal femur showing osteoarthritis of hip and bowing deformity of femoral shaft with stress fractures on the lateral cortical margin.

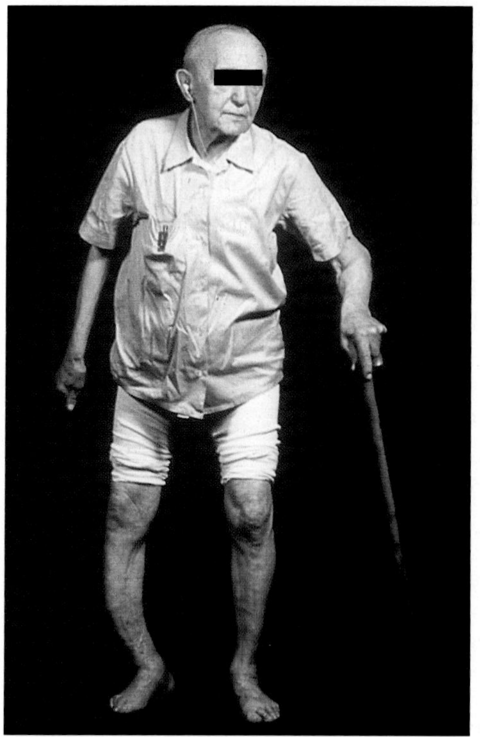

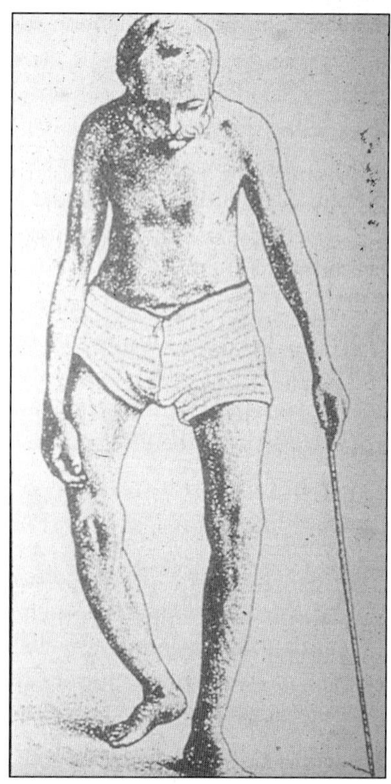

Fig. 6 A patient with Paget's disease showing bowed right tibia.

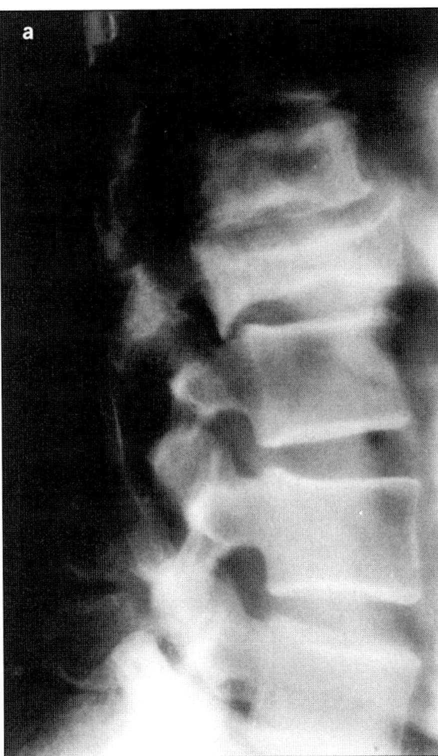

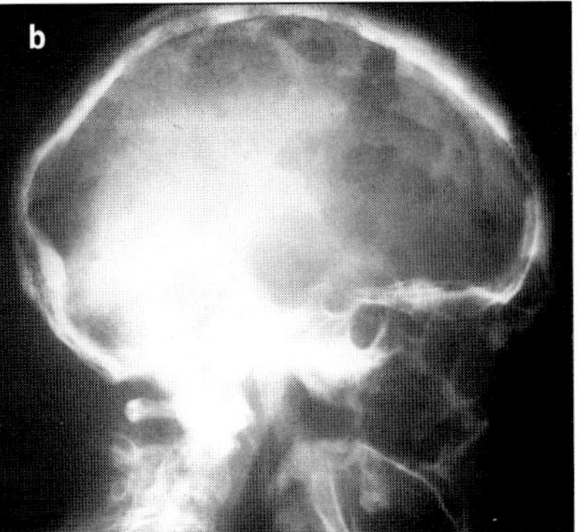

Fig. 7 Radiological changes of Paget's disease **(a)** in the spine; **(b)** in the skull.

disease or undergoing clinical trials are shown in Fig. 8. The major determinant of potency is the structure of the carbon side chain (R); elongation of the chain to 3–4 carbon atoms with terminal coupling of an amino group or ring structure may increase potency 5,000–10,000 fold compared with etidronate. This has led to the use of smaller doses, with consequent broadening of the safety margin between the desired and the unwanted effects of the drugs. In particular, defective mineralisation, which was a problem with the high-dose or prolonged treatments required with etidronate, does not occur with the newer bisphosphonates.

The mechanism by which bisphosphonates inhibit osteoclastic resorption is summarised in Fig. 9. Once the lining cells retract to expose the bone surface, bisphosphonate binds to the hydroxyapatite of the bone mineral. The drug is subsequently released as the osteoclast acidifies the underlying resorption cleft, and is then taken up into the ruffled border region of the osteoclast. As mentioned above, bisphosphonates may inhibit bone resorption through various mechanisms that may differ between individual members of this class. They may:

- exert intracellular effects, including inhibition of protein tyrosine phosphatases and/or proton transport in membrane vesicles;
- reduce resorption through an effect on osteoclast formation, fusion or apoptosis; or

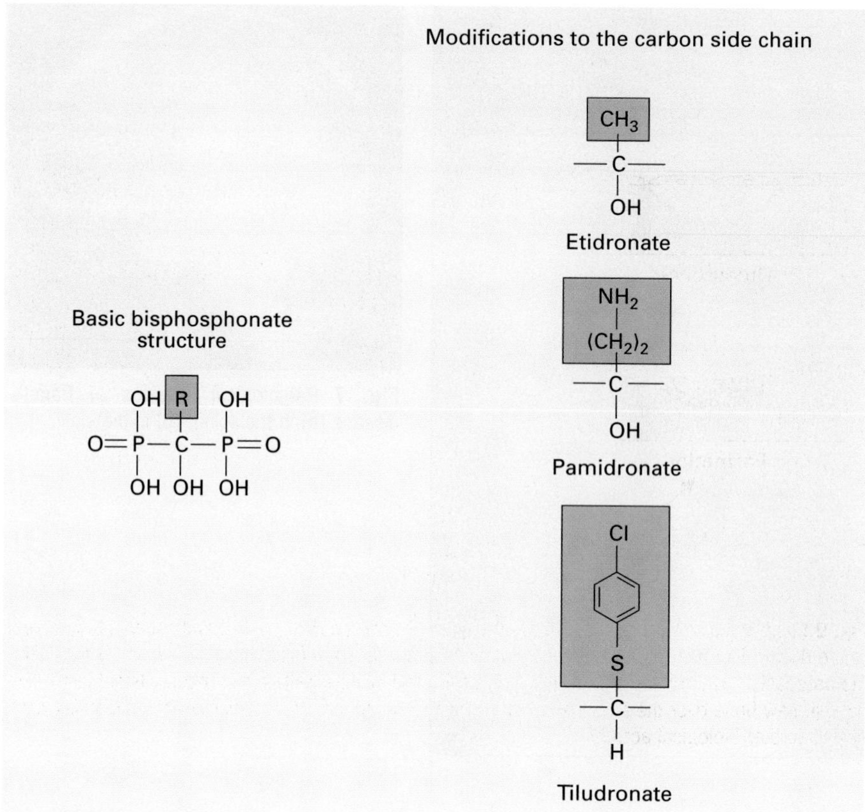

Fig. 8 Structures of three bisphosphonates currently licensed in the UK for the treatment of Paget's disease.

- □ modulate the production of inhibitors of osteoclastic recruitment by osteoblasts [5].

Following the reversal phase that precedes new bone formation (see Fig. 9), osteoblasts deposit osteoid on the bisphosphonate remaining in the resorption cavity. After mineralisation, the buried drug becomes biologically unavailable until this site is re-excavated by a later phase of remodelling. The bone formed during bisphosphonate therapy has a normal lamellar pattern, which replaces the woven bone of the untreated condition [9]. The prolonged remission observed after bisphosphonate treatment [10] suggests that the buried drug may be released relatively soon after deposition because of the focal nature of Paget's disease, and then further inhibit resorption at that site.

Dose-response relationships and practical aspects of treatment

The high rate of bone turnover makes Paget's disease an ideal model for evaluating the dose-response relationship for novel bisphosphonates, and detailed data are

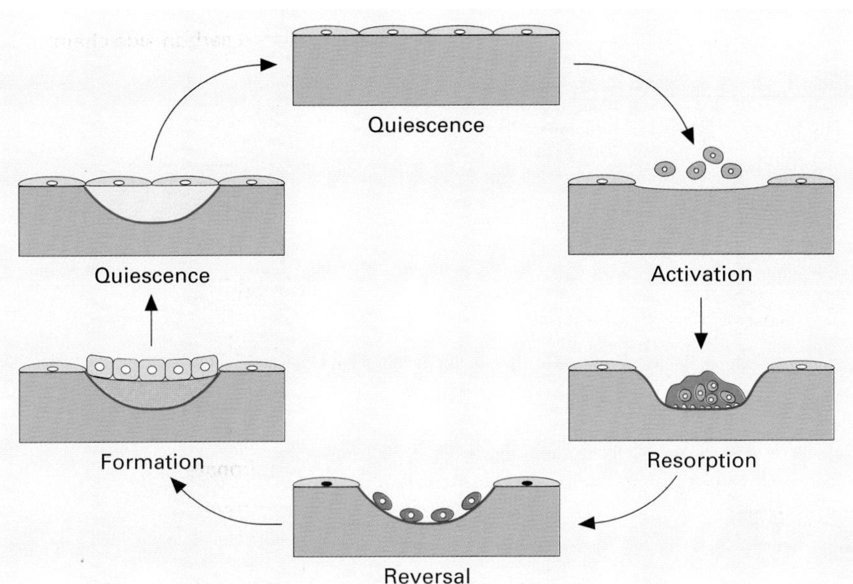

Fig. 9 Mechanism of action of bisphosphonates on the remodelling cycle. Bisphosphonate is bound to the bone mineral surface exposed by osteoclastic resorption (shown in red) and is taken up into the osteoclast, where it inhibits osteoclast activity and inhibits further resorption. Osteoblasts then deposit new bone over the bisphosphonate which since no longer in contact with remodelling cells has no further biological activity.

available for all current agents. The maximum tolerated dose is generally determined by the presence of gastrointestinal effects such as dyspepsia or diarrhoea, although these symptoms are not solely related to dose. Figures 10 and 11 summarise the response to optimal doses of bisphosphonates licensed for the treatment of Paget's disease (or which have undergone randomised trials). Response should be evaluated in terms both of the percentage reduction in excess bone turnover (ie the pretreatment value minus the mean value of the reference range) (Fig. 10) and of the proportion of patients who achieve normal bone turnover (usually measured as serum alkaline phosphatase) (Fig. 11).

The target of normal bone turnover is important, since there is now clear evidence that this will be followed by a more prolonged remission of disease activity [10]. The probability of achieving this with a fixed dose and duration of treatment depends both on the potency of the bisphosphonate and on the pretreatment activity (Fig. 11). Etidronate and tiludronate appear less potent in normalising bone turnover than risedronate and alendronate [11,12], while the intravenous route of administration of pamidronate gives more scope for delivering a higher dose to the bone surface [13,14]. However, when compounds are compared in terms of the percentage reduction of excess alkaline phosphatase, most of the current agents produce an 80–90% reduction within six months.

As the potency of available bisphosphonates has increased and the prevalence of

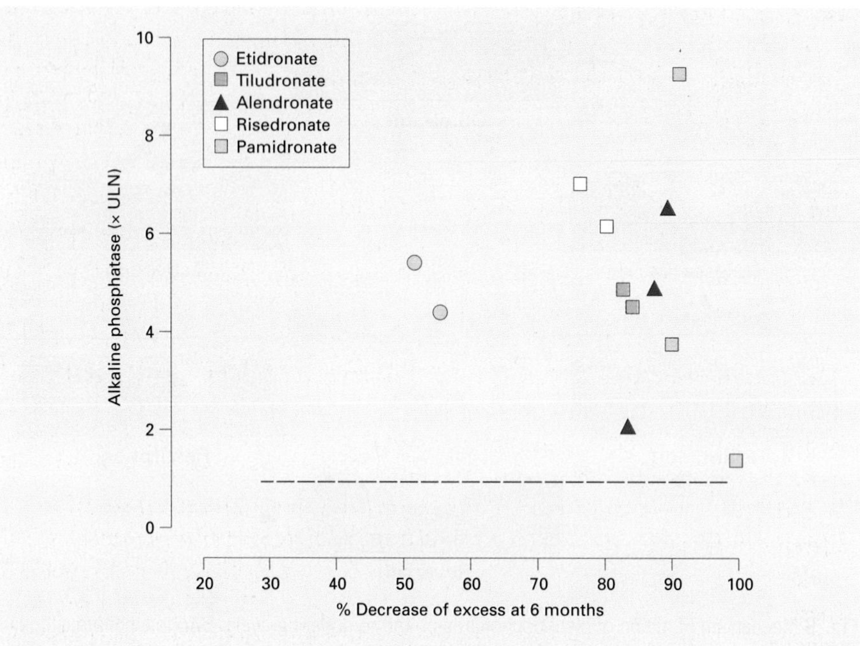

Fig. 10 Response to currently available bisphosphonates. Summary of results from randomised trials of bisphosphonates in Paget's disease (ULN = upper limit of normal).

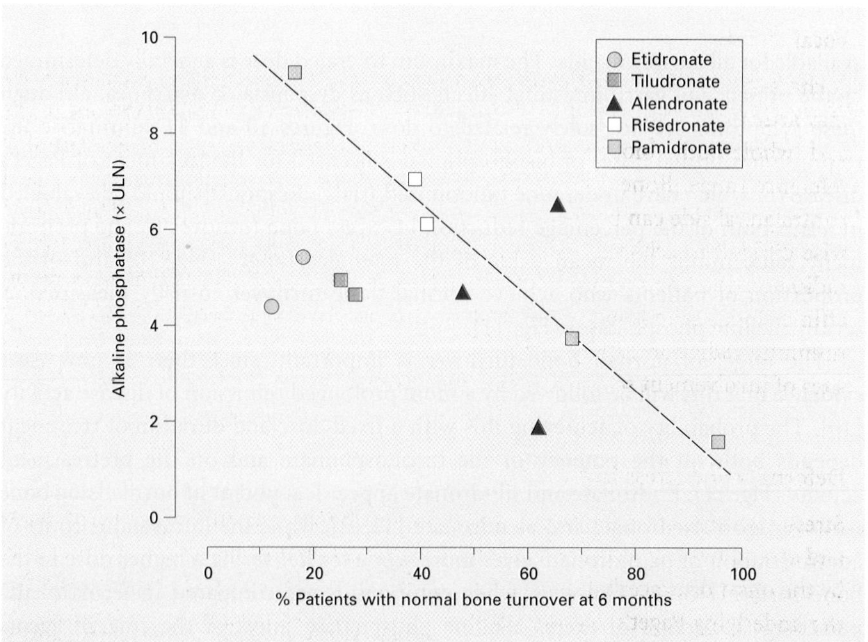

Fig. 11 Proportion of patients who achieve normal bone turnover in relation to pretreatment levels of alkaline phosphatase (ULN = upper limit of normal)

side effects reduced, the tendency has been to aim to reduce measures of bone turnover to well within the normal range [13]. The rationale for this strategy is that the probability of approaching pre-pagetic disease level of bone turnover (which is unknown), and thus achieving a prolonged remission, will increase progressively as bone turnover falls within the reference range.

The realisation of this goal has become more feasible with recent studies of intermittent regimens of bisphosphonate administration. Despite the generalisations above, patients with Paget's disease show considerable individual variations in response. The most cost-effective approach to achieving normal bone turnover is to give a relatively short course of treatment over approximately three months, and then pause to allow bone turnover to establish a new steady state. Alkaline phosphatase, the most readily available marker of disease activity, continues to decline for 6–8 weeks after stopping bisphosphonate, so an interruption of treatment for three months seems a reasonable approach. If bone turnover remains elevated above the target value, the cycle can be repeated.

Monitoring changes in bone turnover when alkaline phosphatase lies within the reference range may be one of the few indications for use of the newer bone turnover markers such as bone-specific alkaline phosphatase or deoxypyridinoline cross-links. These are more specific for bone remodelling than total alkaline phosphatase or urinary hydroxyproline excretion and have a tighter reference range [15], but otherwise have few advantages in routine clinical use that might justify their extra cost.

□ SPECIFIC CLINICAL PROBLEMS IN MANAGEMENT

Focal disease

A characteristic feature of Paget's disease is its focal distribution. Severe symptoms may arise from a limited focus of disease, where the volume of affected bone is small and 'whole-body' biochemical markers of disease activity may remain within the reference range. Bone scintigraphy to compare focal uptake with the non-affected contralateral side can be used to assess local disease activity (Fig. 12). This is otherwise difficult to achieve except by biopsy, which is only rarely appropriate [8]. The radionuclide technetium methylene diphosphonate (TcMDP) is taken up with high affinity by pagetic bone and is widely used for bone scanning in this disease. To minimise radiation exposure, a lower dose of TcMDP should be used and limited sites of involvement scanned for a longer period.

Deformity and stress fractures

Stress fractures are common and usually asymptomatic, but may become painful and extend to form a complete transverse fracture. Such extension is often preceded by the onset or exacerbation of pain, and it may be difficult to distinguish this from the underlying Paget's disease. Localising the region of maximum tenderness with a radio-opaque skin marker can allow congruence between the site of symptoms and radiographic evidence of a stress fracture to be assessed.

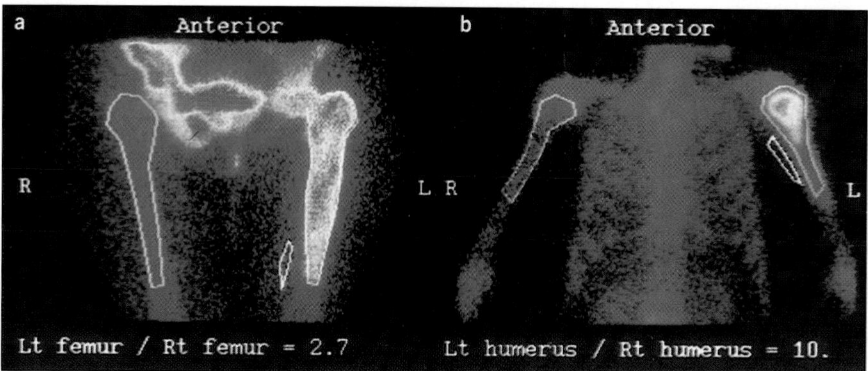

Fig. 12 Bone scans showing **(a)** increased uptake in left femur and right pelvis. The area of interest is highlighted and measures the relative increase in uptake showing 2.7 times as much activity in the left femur as the right; **(b)** similar quantification in the left humerus showing 10 times as much activity as the right humerus.

Histologically, stress fractures are the focus of increased bone remodelling but they may remain in a state of dynamic equilibrium for many years without evidence of extension. They appear 'hot' on a bone scan; this has an important bearing on treatment as the increased bone blood flow at this site may encourage preferential uptake of bisphosphonate. The risk of extension cannot be assessed biochemically, and bone turnover markers may be normal in patients with rapidly worsening fissure fractures.

Reduction in bone remodelling by over-enthusiastic treatment with bisphosphonates may disrupt the previous equilibrium and cause stress fractures to extend. It is, therefore, important to obtain high-quality radiographs of all affected weight-bearing bones before starting treatment. The development of pain localised to the site of a known fissure fracture is an indication for bed-rest and stopping treatment to allow the symptoms to subside. Treatment can then be re-introduced, but at a lower dose – particularly important with the use of intravenous bisphosphonates such as pamidronate. In the presence of known fissure fractures, it is probably wise to begin with a lower dose (15–30 mg pamidronate), and give a longer course of treatment with the aim of reducing measures of bone turnover to the upper part of the reference range. The radiographic appearances of fissure fractures do not improve with medical treatment and will heal only after surgical correction of the deformity.

REFERENCES

1 Rebel A, Malkani K, Basle M, Bregeon C. Osteoclast ultrastructure in Paget's disease. *Calcif Tissue Res* 1976; **20**: 187–99.

2 Reddy SY, Singer FR, Mallette L, Roodman GD. Detection of measles virus nucleocapsid transcripts in circulating blood cells from patients with Paget's disease. *J Bone Min Res* 1996; **11**: 1602–7.

3 Roodman GD. Paget's disease and osteoclast biology. *Bone* 1996; **19**: 209–12.

4 Mee AP, Hillarby C, Selby PL, *et al.* Up-regulation of Bcl-2 mRNA in Paget's disease: the link between viral infection and genetic susceptibility. *Bone* 1997; **20** (Suppl 4) IOS.

5 Suda T, Nakamura I, Jimi E, Takahashi N. Regulation of osteoclast function. *J Bone Min Res* 1997; **12**: 869–79.

6 Luckman SP, Hughes DE, Chilton KM, *et al.* Bisphosphonates act by inhibiting protein prenylation. *J Bone Min Res* 1997; **12** (Suppl 1): S194.

7 Cundy T, McAnulty K, Wattie D, *et al.* Evidence for secular change in Paget's disease. *Bone* 1997; **20**: 69–71.

8 Hosking DJ, Meunier PJ, Ringe JI, *et al.* Paget's disease of bone: diagnosis and management. *Br Med J* 1996; **312**: 491–4.

9 Reid IR, Nicholson GC, Weinstein RS, *et al.* Biochemical and radiological improvement in Paget's disease of bone treated with alendronate: a randomised placebo-controlled trial. *Am J Med* 1996; **171**: 341–8.

10 Patel S, Stone MD, Coupland C, Hosking DJ. Determinants of remission of Paget's disease. *J Bone Min Res* 1995; **8**: 1467–73.

11 Siris E, Weinstein RS, Altman R, *et al.* Comparative study of alendronate versus etidronate for the treatment of Paget's disease of bone. *J Clin Endocrinol Metab* 1996; **81**: 961–7.

12 Roux C, Gennari C, Farrerons J, *et al.* Comparative, prospective, double blind, multicentre study of the efficacy of tiludronate and etidronate in the treatment of Paget's disease of bone. *Arthritis Rheum* 1995; **38**: 851–8.

13 Harinck HIJ, Papoulos SE, Blanksma HI, *et al.* Paget's disease of bone: early and late responses to three different modes of treatment with aminohydroxypropylidene bisphosphonate (APD). *Br Med J* 1987; **295**: 1301–5.

14 Gutteridge DH, Retallack RW, Ward LC, *et al.* Clinical, biochemical, haematological and radiographic responses in Paget's disease following intravenous pamidronate disodium: a 2-year study. *Bone* 1996; **19**: 387–94.

15 Alvarez L, Guanabens N, Peris P, *et al.* Discriminative value of biochemical markers of bone turnover in assessing the activity of Paget's disease. *J Bone Min Res* 1995; **10**: 458–65.

☐ MULTIPLE CHOICE QUESTIONS

1 Paget's disease:

(a) Is most probably due to a single gene defect
(b) Is due to a recent infection with canine distemper virus
(c) Is becoming more common
(d) Tends to present at an older age
(e) Involves more of the skeleton in new cases

2 Bisphosphonate treatment:

(a) Has a direct effect on both osteoblasts and osteoclasts
(b) Should be given continuously to maintain disease control
(c) Reduces alkaline phosphatase and hydroxyproline to the same degree
(d) Should be discontinued when symptoms are controlled
(e) Is more effective than calcitonin in controlling bone turnover

3 Serum alkaline phosphatase and urinary hydroxyproline excretion:

(a) Are always elevated in symptomatic Paget's disease
(b) Are not as good as the newer specific markers such as bone specific alkaline phosphatase and pyridinoline cross links
(c) Are more specific than symptoms in monitoring response

(d) Will predict the probability of relapse when treatment is stopped
(e) In the untreated patient predict the probability of long-term complications

ANSWERS

1a False	2a False	3a False
b False	b False	b False
c False	c True	c True
d True	d False	d True
e False	e True	e False

A case of bleeding gums

Tom Kennedy and Laurie Cray

□ CASE PRESENTATION

A 22 year old teacher was originally seen in the maxillofacial department, referred by her general practitioner with a 3-week history of swollen bleeding gums. She was also noted to be suffering from a blocked sinus for 1 week, with some headache. Clinically, she appeared pale and there was palpable cervical lymphadenopathy. Examination of her mouth demonstrated hyperplastic ulcerated inflamed gums (see Fig. 1). A gum biopsy and full blood count were taken.

Three days after the initial presentation, she was admitted with a tentative diagnosis of leukaemia. It was also recorded that she had lost weight, although the extent was not clear, and that she had right-sided earache with some discharge from the external auditory meatus. She complained of arthralgia in both knees and the right elbow. There was no other past medical or family history of note. She was a non-smoker and drank 8 units of alcohol per week.

On examination she looked unwell and pale, with an oral temperature of 37°C and tender cervical lymphadenopathy. Her pulse was 100/min and regular, and her blood pressure 100/60 mmHg. Her heart sounds were normal. The respiratory, abdominal and neurological examination was normal, and no significant skin or joint abnormalities were noted. There was a mucopurulent discharge from the right ear.

Initial investigations and progress

The results of the initial blood and biochemical investigations are summarised in Tables 1 and 2. Biochemical profile was normal apart from a very mild elevation of liver enzymes, and her renal function was also normal. The admission chest radiograph showed a vague rounded shadow in the left mid-zone, 3 cm in diameter, adjacent to the hilum (see Fig. 2). The preliminary histology report of the gum biopsy showed acute gingivitis with no evidence of malignancy (see Fig. 3).

On the sixth day after admission, a vasculitic-type rash developed over her lower limbs (see Fig. 4). The arthralgias were more marked but no synovitis was present. Examination of her ears and nose showed erythema and granulation tissue in the right ear and both nasal cavities; swabs and biopsies were taken. Further investigations included a computed tomography (CT) scan of her chest which showed a mass 4 cm in diameter extending from and merging with the left hilum. The posterior margin was sharp, suggesting that it was bounded by the oblique fissure. The left hilar glands were bulky but there was no mediastinal lymphadenopathy (see Fig. 5). CT scans of the head showed normal frontal sinuses, but with mucosal thickening

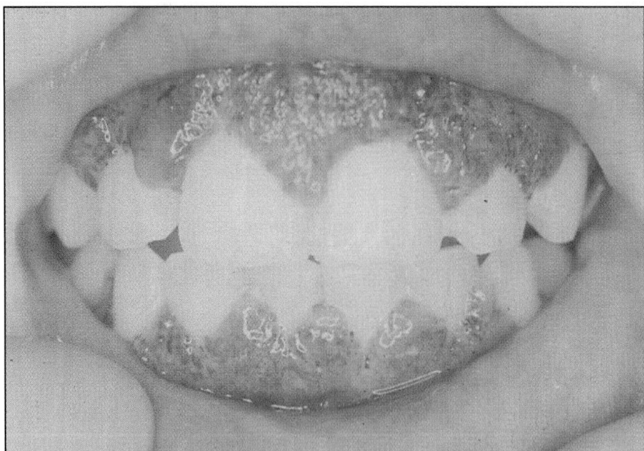

Fig. 1 Inflamed gums at presentation.

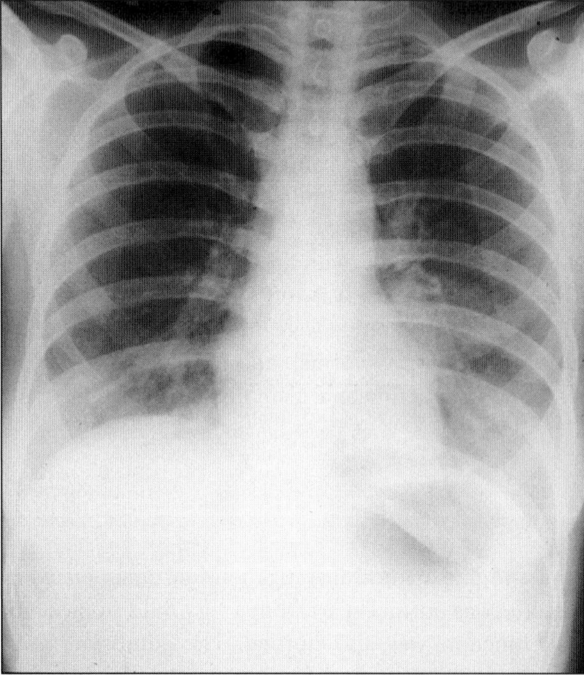

Fig. 2 Chest radiograph at presentation showing left mid-zone shadow 3 cm in diameter.

that was extensive in the right maxillary sinus, (especially at the base) and was also present in the left antrum, ethmoid and sphenoid sinus and to a lesser extent in the nasal cavity (see Fig. 6). Ultrasound examination of the upper abdomen was normal.

The autoimmune profile (see Table 3) initially showed significantly raised c-anti-neutrophil cytoplasmic antibody (ANCA) (PR3) at 76 units (normal range 0–10), rising to 87 units 3 days later. The p-ANCA was negative. The nasal and ear swabs did not grow any pathological bacteria.

The histology of the biopsy from the left nostril showed necrosis with a dense mixed inflammatory cell infiltrate containing numerous polymorphonuclear

Table 1 Patient L.C.: initial investigations.

Haemoglobin	13.0 g/dl
White cell count	14.1×10^9/l
• neutrophils	12.4
• monocytes	0.4
Platelets	423×10^9/l
International normalised ratio	1.1
Activated partial thromboplastin time	29 s (normal range 25–40 s)
Fibrinogen	8.7 g/l
Plasma viscosity	2.20 mPa/s (normal range 1.5–1.72)

Table 2 Patient L.C.: biochemistry tests.

Renal function	normal
Creatinine clearance	96 ml/min
Liver function tests	
• Alkaline phosphatase	86 iu/l (normal range 30–90)
• Aspartate aminotransferase	32 iu/l (0–31)
• Gamma-glutamyltransferase	24 iu/l (7–32)
• Albumin	37 g/l (36–52)
• Globulin	39 g/l (21–37)
Complement	
C3	1.52 g/l (normal range 0.75–1.65)
C4	0.20 g/l (0.20–0.65)

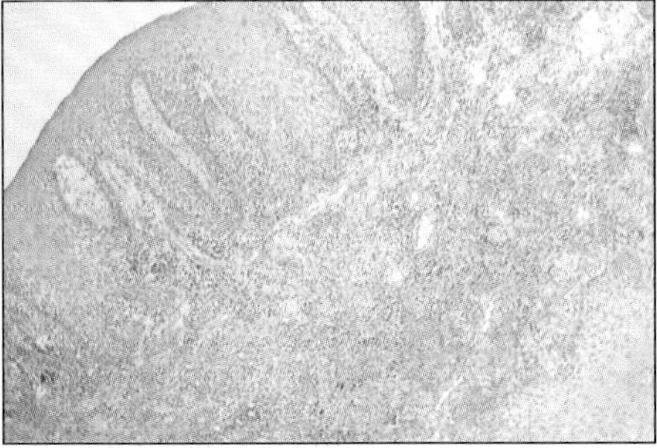

Fig. 3 Histology of gum mucosa, showing elongated rete ridges, acanthosis and a dense inflammatory cell infiltrate (low power magnification).

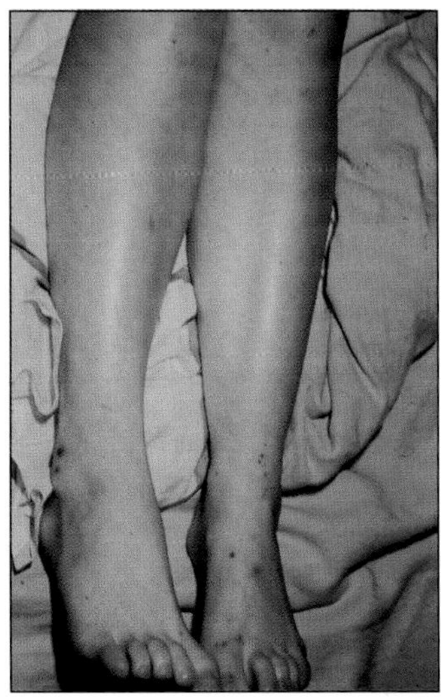

Fig. 4 Vasculitic-type rash on legs, 9 days after presentation.

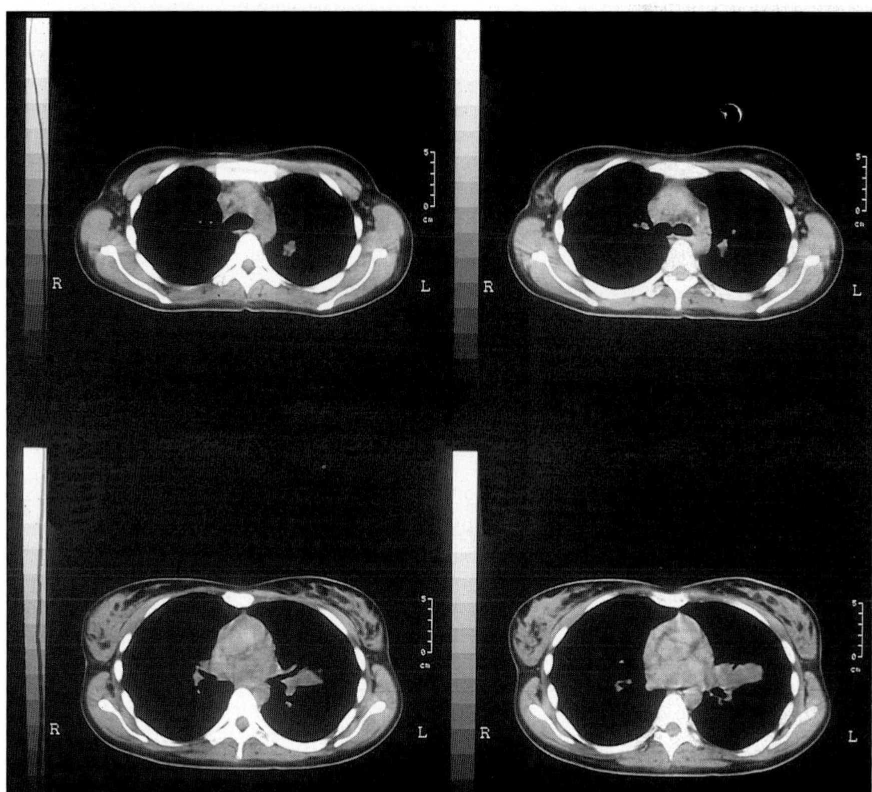

Fig. 5 Chest CT scan, showing 4 cm mass in left mid-zone; the oblique fissure limits the posterior margin of the mass.

Table 3 Patient L.C.: autoimmune test results.

Autoantibody screen	negative (gastric parietal 1,280)
Rheumatoid arthritis latex	negative
Extractable nuclear antigens screen	negative
c-anti-neutrophil cytoplasmic antibody screen	positive
c-ANCA (PR3)	76 units (on admission)
	87 units (3 days after admission)
	negative (24 days after admission)
p-ANCA screen	negative
Anti-glomerular basement membrane	negative

leukocytes, plasma cells and lymphocytes (see Fig. 7). Acute inflammatory cells and histocytes infiltrate many of the vessels. Scanty multinucleated cells are present within both the stroma and the vessel walls. Fibrin is deposited in vessel walls and in the surrounding tissue. Several poorly defined epithelioid cell granulomata are

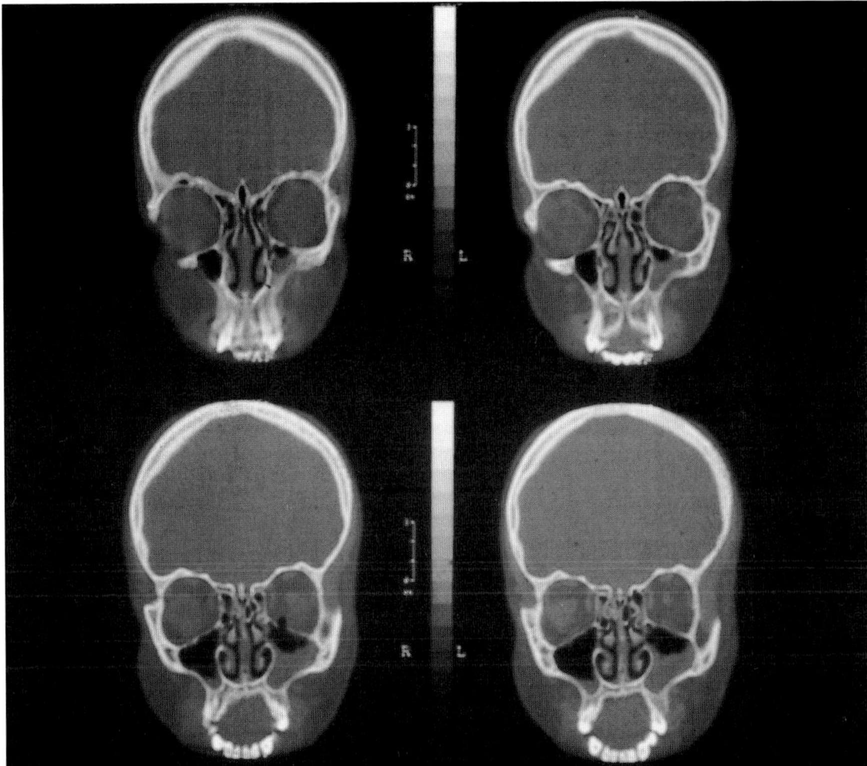

Fig. 6 CT scan, showing extensive mucosal thickening in most of the paranasal sinuses.

scattered within the inflamed submucosa (see Fig. 8). The features are those of a marked granulomatous vasculitis, consistent with Wegener's granulomatosis.

Diagnosis and management

A diagnosis of Wegener's granulomatosis was made (see Table 4). Treatment was started on day 6 of admission with methyl prednisolone, given as three 500 mg intravenous boluses during 5 days. This was followed with oral prednisolone 60 mg daily from day 14, and oral cyclophosphamide 50 mg daily was started the next day. In view of risk of infertility with this treatment, and following discussion with Mr Peter Brinsden, Bourn Hall Clinic, Cambridge, ovarian biopsies were taken at laparoscopy on day 27 after admission. Ovarian tissue has been cryopreserved with the aim of allowing conception at a later date.

Soon after starting the prednisolone, there was rapid improvement. The vasculitic rash settled. A repeat CT scan of her chest 6 weeks after admission showed considerable regression of the left mid-zone mass and no mediastinal lymphadenopathy (see Fig. 8). Her c-ANCA has been negative since 3 months after admission. She was treated with a reducing course of prednisolone, reaching 7.5 mg

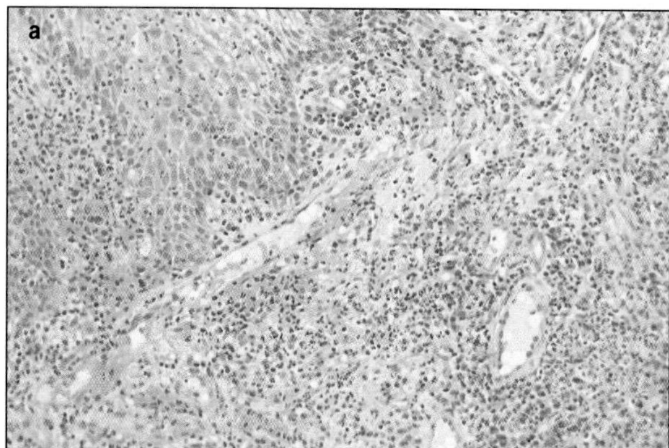

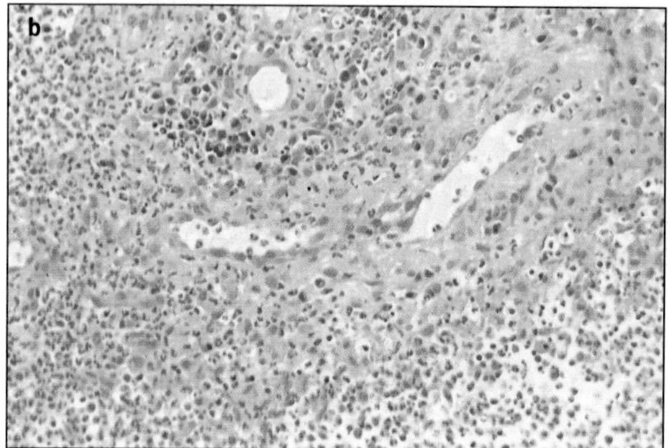

Fig. 7 Nasal biopsies, showing **(a)** epithelioid granuloma, fibrinoid necrosis and inflammatory cell infiltration and **(b)** a higher-power view of a granuloma (high power magnification).

Table 4 Clinical features of Wegener's granulomatosis. (From Hughes GRV. *Connective tissue disease.* Oxford: Blackwell Scientific Publications, 1977.)

	% of cases at presentation
Lung involvement	100
• modular and/or cavitating infiltrates	
• granulomatous vasculitis	
Sinuses	90
• sinusitis	
• necrotising granulomata	
Kidneys	
• focal nephritis	80
Joints	
• fleeting arthralgia	60
Ears	
• crusting	70
• serous otitis media	40
Skin	
• vasculitic rash	16
Weight loss	16

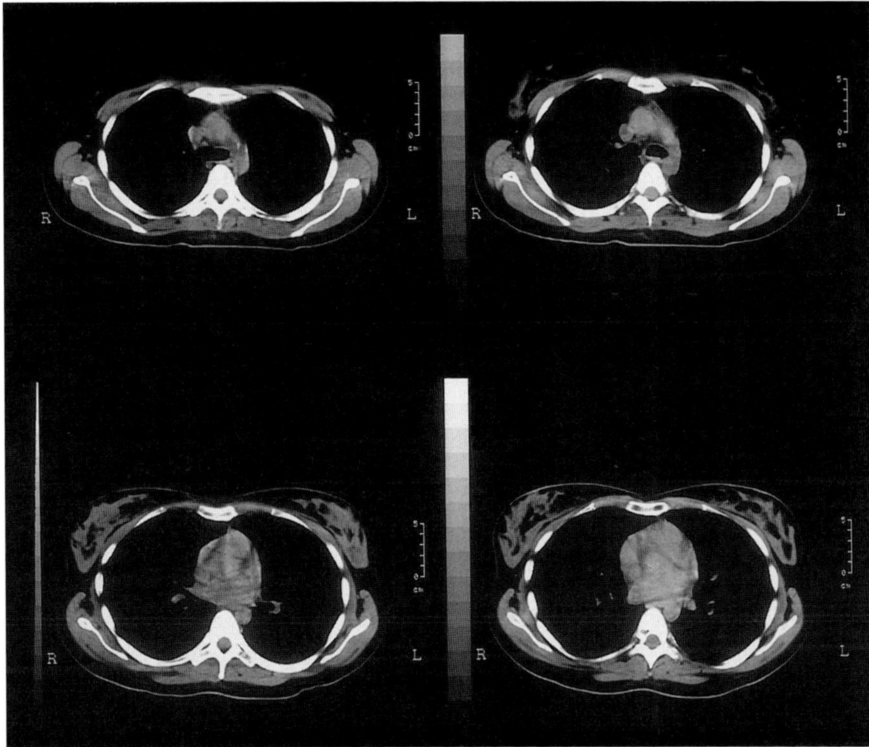

Fig. 8 Chest CT scan, 6 weeks after presentation, showing almost complete resolution of previously demonstrated left mid-zone mass.

daily after 6 months and finally being withdrawn after 17 months. The cyclophosphamide was initially increased to 100 mg daily to allow reduction of the prednisolone dosage which caused her to become cushingoid. Cyclophosphamide was reduced after 17 months to 50 mg daily, and she continues with this dose at the time of writing 25 months after presentation. Apart from some mild nasal crusting and fatigue, she remains symptomatically well and has had no significant intercurrent infections.

□ DISCUSSION

The treatment protocol (see Table 5) developed by Fauci and colleagues [1] has dramatically improved the outlook for patients with Wegener's granulomatosis, from 90% mortality in 2 years and a mean survival of 5 months, to 87% survival during a mean follow-up of 8 years. However, the treatment regimen is toxic, with rates of 46–55% for severe infection (including *Pneumocystis carinii* pneumonia), 33–54% for amenorrhoea and up to 34% for haemorrhagic cystitis. There is a 2.4-fold overall increase in cancer risk, with relative risks of 33 and 11 for bladder cancer and lymphoma respectively [1–4].

Table 5 Fauci's protocol for the treatment of Wegener's granulomatosis [1].

To induce remission

- Oral cyclophosphamide 2 mg/kg daily
- Prednisolone 1 mg/kg daily

Maintenance

- Cyclophosphamide 2 mg/kg maintained until 1 year after clinical and laboratory remission, then tapered by 25 mg decrements every 2–3 months
- Prednisolone continued for 2–4 weeks, then converted to alternate days, then gradually reduced as clinical condition allows

Monitoring

- Ensured leucocyte count never fell below 3–3.5 x 103 (generally performed every 2–4 days); leucocyte count slope monitored to predict lowest counts and adjust dose

Alternative treatment protocols have, therefore, been developed and tested. A recent trial compared pulsed intravenous cyclophosphamide with the Fauci oral regime [2]. There were fewer side effects with the pulsed therapy but remission was achieved in only 48%, compared with 71% with the oral daily regime. Using methotrexate 0.3 mg/kg per week to a maximum of 15 mg weekly, 71% of patients achieved remission but 36% relapsed with a median time to relapse of 29 months [5]. In each of these studies, remission (defined as no clinical or laboratory evidence of disease) has been induced, and treatment then continued for 1 year before gradually reducing the drugs. An alternative approach has been to achieve remission with oral cyclophosphamide and then to use weekly intravenous methotrexate with or without oral prednisolone to maintain it [6]. This regimen, with methotrexate alone, induced remission in 86% of patients and, with the addition of prednisolone, in 91%; use of trimethoprim/sulphoxazole without prednisolone achieved remission in 58% of patients, whereas in the trimethoprim/sulphoxazole plus low-dose prednisolone group all 8 patients had a recurrence of disease acitivity [6]. The ECSYSVASTRIAL group (European Community Study Group of Therapeutic Trials in Vasculitis) is currently undertaking studies using azathioprine [7].

A crucial management step in this particular case has been to store ovarian tissue to facilitate pregnancy at a later date, because of the known detrimental effects of cyclophosphamide on female fertility. Studies in patients with systemic lupus erythematosus have demonstrated that the risk of ovarian failure is 12–83%, depending on whether cyclophosphamide was given orally or intravenously [8,9]. Older age at onset and longer treatment, together with a greater degree of marrow suppression (as judged by the lowest neutrophil count), further increased the risk. Furthermore, the risk of early menopause, before the age of 40, is increased to 41%. The risk of iatrogenic infertility is not confined to cyclophosphamide (see Table 6).

We took the opportunity to collect and store laparoscopic ovarian biopsies. Although the techniques to mature unstimulated ovarian tissue have not yet been perfected in humans, we hope and expect that this will become feasible. In certain situations where chemotherapy is planned in the future, it may be possible to stimulate the ovaries and freeze oocytes for later assisted conception. Patients,

Table 6 Cytotoxic drugs that may or may not cause gamete failure and infertility in men and women.

	Women	Men
Nitrogen mustards, including cyclophosphamide	Yes	Yes
Chlorambucil	Yes	Yes
Busulphan	Yes	Yes
Bleomycin	Yes	Unknown
Vinca alkaloids	Yes	No? (vincristine is safe)
Methotrexate	No	No
5-Fluorouracil	No	No
6-Mercaptopurine	No	No

whether female or male, should never have to look back with anger and resentment because they were not properly advised about their fertility before undergoing chemotherapy.

Wegener's granulomatosis is no longer a fatal disease but there is a high relapse rate and current therapies are toxic. As with all rare diseases, it is difficult to undertake randomised controlled trials but these are mandatory and, with the international collaboration achieved through the ECSYSVASTRIAL group, this may now be possible.

ACKNOWLEDGEMENTS

I would like to thank Miss Laurie Cray, our patient, for allowing her problems to be so openly discussed and for her willingness to participate so fully in the presentation. I am also very grateful to my colleagues at Wirral Hospital Trust, Dr Mano George (Consultant Rheumatologist), Dr Joyce Magennis (Consultant Radiologist), Dr Hani Zakhour (Consultant Histopathologist) and Mr Peter Brinsden (Medical Director, Bourn Hall Clinic, Bourn, Cambridge) for their most helpful advice in the management of this case and the preparation of this report.

REFERENCES

1 Fauci AS, Haynes BF, Katz P, Wolff SM. Wegener's granulomatosis: prospective clinical and therapeutic experience with 85 patients for 21 years. *Ann Intern Med* 1983; **98**: 76–85.

2 Guillevin L, Cordier J-F, Lhote F, *et al.* A prospective multicenter randomised trial comparing steroids and pulse cyclophosphamide versus steroids and oral cyclophosphamide in the treatment of Wegener's granulomatosis. *Arthritis Rheum* 1997; **40**: 2187–98.

3 Hoffman GS, Kerr GS, Leavitt RY, *et al.* Wegener granulomatosis: an analysis of 158 patients. *Ann Intern Med* 1992; **116**: 488–98.

4 Hoffman GS. Treatment of Wegener's granulomatosis: time to change the standard of care? *Arthritis Rheum* 1997; **40**: 2099–104.

5 Sneller MC, Hoffman GS, Talar-Williams C, *et al.* An analysis of forty-two Wegener's granulomatosis patients treated with methotrexate and prednisolone. *Arthritis Rheum* 1995; **38**: 608–13.

6 De Groot K, Reinhold-Keller E, Tatsis E, *et al.* Therapy for the maintenance of remission in sixty-five patients with Wegener's granulomatosis. *Arthritis Rheum* 1996; **39**: 2052–61.

7 Rasmussen N, Jayne DRW, Abramowicz D, *et al.* European therapeutic trials in ANCA-associated systemic vasculitis: disease scoring, consensus regimens and proposed clinical trials. *Clin Exp Immunol* 1995; **101**: 29–34.

8 Wang CL, Wang F, Bosco JJ. Ovarian failure in oral cyclophosphamide treatment for systemic lupus erythematosus. *Lupus* 1995; **4**: 11–4.

9 McDermott EM, Powell RJ. Incidence of ovarian failure in systemic lupus erythematosus after treatment with pulse cyclophosphamide. *Ann Rheum Dis* 1996; **55**: 224–9.

☐ MULTIPLE CHOICE QUESTIONS

1 Presenting symptoms in the majority of patients with Wegener's granulomatosis:
(a) Sinusitis
(b) Ear crusting
(c) Pulmonary infiltrates
(d) Weight loss
(e) Rash

2 c-ANCA may be positive in patients with:
(a) Systemic lupus erythematosus
(b) Wegener's granulomatosis
(c) Diabetes
(d) Multiple sclerosis
(e) Microscopic polyarteritis

3 Treatments that reduce the risk of steroid-related osteoporosis:
(a) Hormone replacement therapy
(b) Fluoride
(c) Cyclical etidronate
(d) Calcium with vitamin D
(e) Calcium alone

4 Drugs linked to gamete failure in premenopausal women:
(a) Busulphan
(b) Cyclophosphamide
(c) Bleomycin
(d) Methotrexate
(e) 5-Fluorouracil

5 Statements about cyclophosphamide:
(a) Haemorrhagic cystitis occurs in 5% of patients
(b) The overall increased risk of cancer is less than 5-fold
(c) Cyclophosphamide does not cause male infertility
(d) In patients with Wegener's granulomatosis, cyclophosphamide and prednisolone therapy may induce remission in 90% of patients but relapse occurs in 40% of patients
(e) *Pneumocystis carinii* is a common cause of serious infection in patients with Wegener's granulomatosis treated with cyclophosphamide

ANSWERS

1	2	3	4	5
1a True (67%)	2a False	3a True	4a True	5a False *(20–34%)*
b True (70%)	b True	b False	b True	b True *(2.4×)*
c False *(a sign; not symptom)*	c False	c True	c True	c False
d False (16%)	d False	d True	d False	d True
e False (13%)	e True	e False	e False	e True

Acute pancreatitis: a conceptual framework for better management

Colin D Johnson

□ INTRODUCTION

Acute pancreatitis is a common and important abdominal emergency. Its incidence in the UK is between 100 and 250 per million and it carries an overall mortality of 10%. Its pathogenesis has been poorly understood, which has meant that its management has been more empirical than rational. One of the main unanswered questions has been how inflammation in a relatively small organ can cause such catastrophic systemic sequelae, including hypotension and shock, pulmonary oedema and septicaemia with gut commensal bacteria. As these problems are major contributors to mortality and morbidity in acute pancreatitis, this area has been an important focus for research into the condition.

Fortunately, some of the underlying pathogenic mechanisms are now being elucidated. This chapter will examine the current understanding of the factors causing the local and systemic complications of acute pancreatitis, and will use this as a framework to describe some new approaches to rational clinical management of the disease.

□ PATHOGENIC MECHANISMS IN ACUTE PANCREATITIS

Many conditions and agents can precipitate acute pancreatitis (Fig. 1), of which the most common in the UK are gallstones and alcohol. It is now apparent that these factors induce acinar-cell damage in various ways, and that oxidative stress and inflammatory mediators lie on the final common pathway that leads to inflammation of the gland and the systemic sequelae.

Events within the pancreas

Acute pancreatitis shows all the features of acute inflammation, with heavy infiltration by polymorphs (which can be seen crossing the capillary wall and entering the substance of the gland) and necrosis in severe cases (see Fig. 2). This is reflected by oedema and swelling of the pancreas, visible macroscopically and on CT or MR imaging (Fig. 3). In severe cases, with pancreatic necrosis, there is failure of enhancement of the pancreas on dynamic CT.

A long-held concept was that acute pancreatitis is due to release of activated proteases and other enzymes within the pancreas, leading to autodigestion. This was the rationale for the now-abandoned practice of treating the disease with protease inhibitors, notably aprotinin (Trasylol). It is now clear that, although enzyme

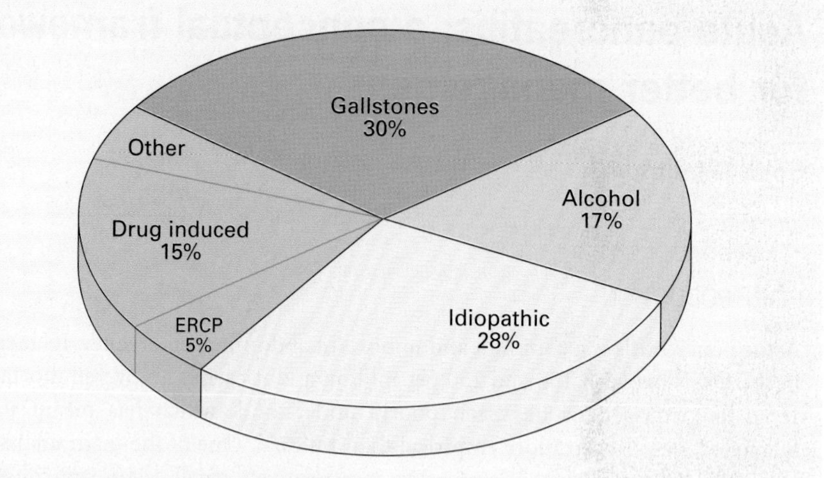

Fig. 1 Pie chart of causes of acute pancreatitis in the UK.

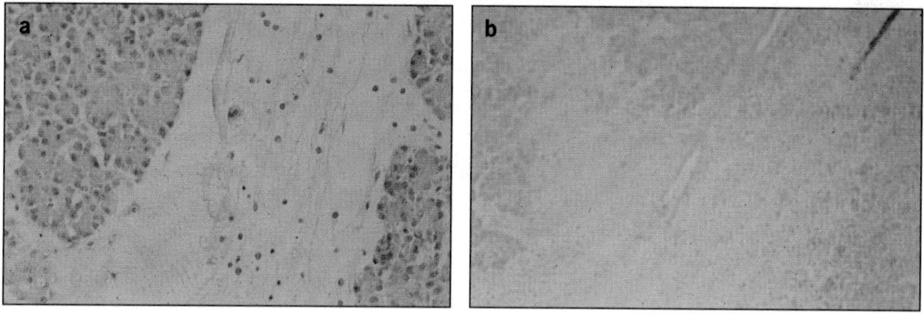

Fig. 2 Histology of acute pancreatitis: **(a)** acute inflammation, showing heavy polymorph neutrophil infiltration; **(b)** extensive pancreatic necrosis.

activation and release may occur as a result of acinar-cell damage, it is more likely to be an epiphenomenon rather than the cause of the damage.

Instead, there is now growing evidence that oxidative stress, mediated by oxygen free-radicals, is responsible.

Patients with acute pancreatitis are depleted in various important antioxidants [1], and several groups have now reported reductions in total antioxidant capacity of the blood during the acute phase (<12 h) of the disease. We have found increased levels of superoxide dismutase, an enzyme that scavenges free radicals and which is up-regulated in response to oxidative stress, in patients with acute pancreatitis [2]. Moreover, plasma levels of malondialdehyde, a product of lipid peroxidation due to free-radical attack, are raised within 12 h of admission to hospital, in proportion to the clinical severity of the disease [3] (Fig. 4).

The suggested sequence of events that leads to inflammation and polymorph neutrophil infiltration in the pancreas is shown in Fig. 5.

Oxidative stress releases oxygen-derived free radicals from injured cells, and these together with other products of cell breakdown are strongly chemotactic for

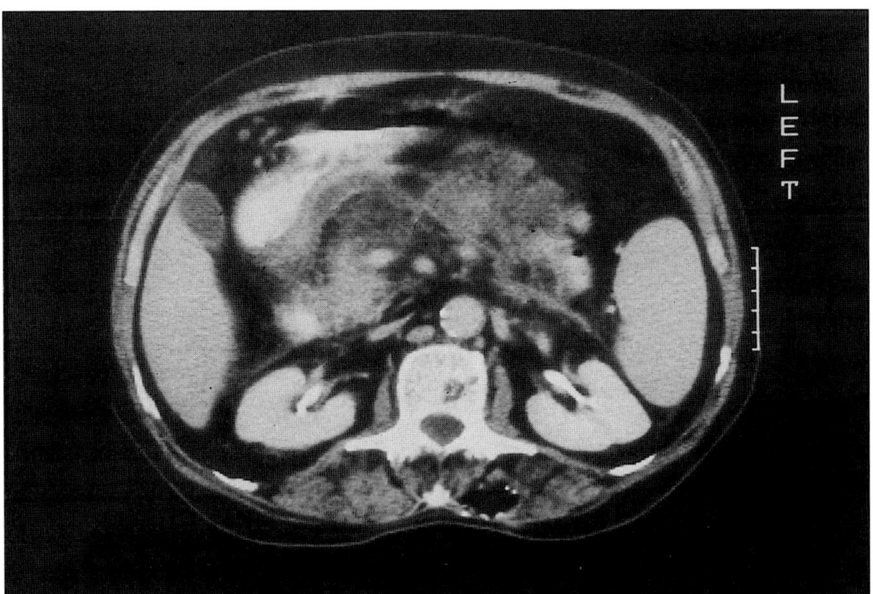

Fig. 3 CT scan of abdomen, showing marked oedema of the pancreas in a patient with mild acute pancreatitis.

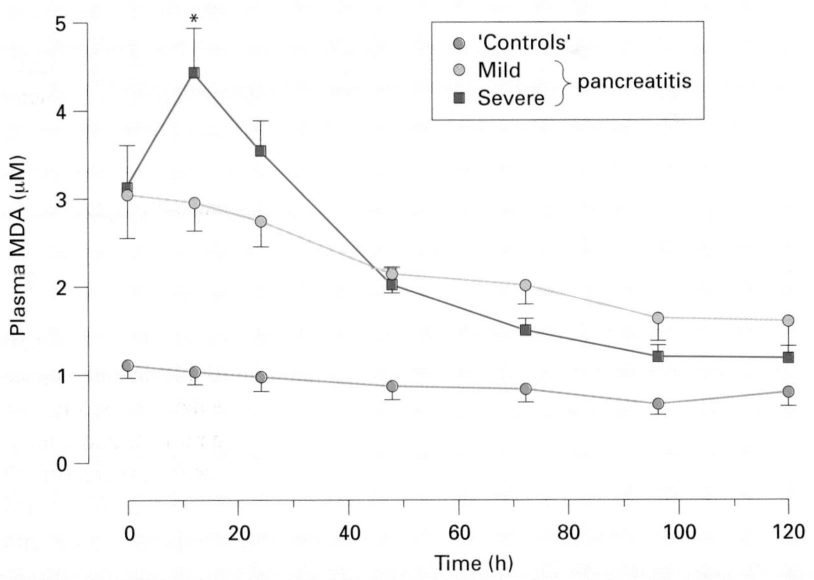

Fig. 4 Plasma malondialdehyde (MDA) concentrations in patients with mild and severe acute pancreatitis, compared with controls with unrelated abdominal inflammatory conditions. Error bars are SEM. Overall levels in both mild and severe pancreatitis are significantly higher than in controls (ANOVA $p<0.05$); $^{*}p<0.05$ for severe vs mild. (From reference 3).

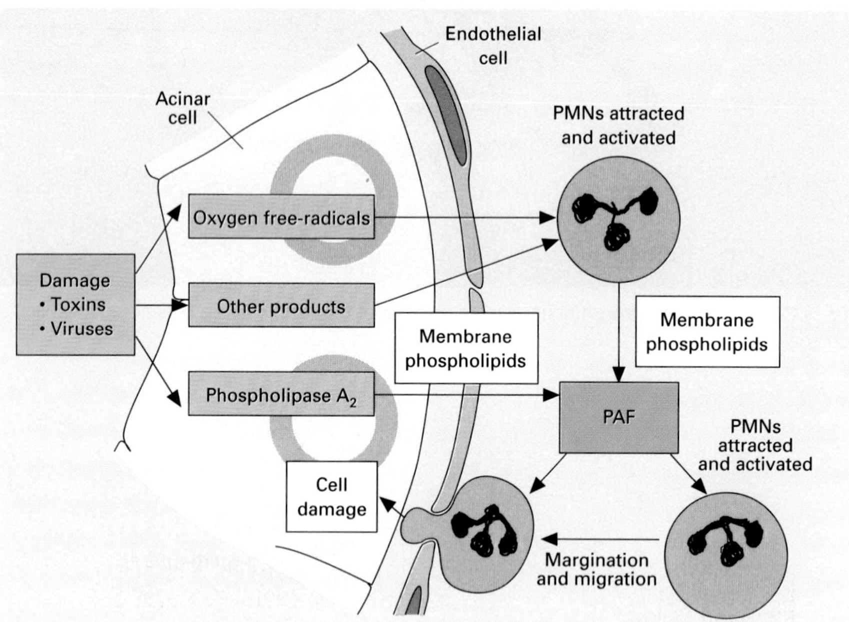

Fig. 5 Mechanisms of damage to the pancreas in acute pancreatitis. Note the central role of platelet-activating factor (PAF), which also mediates some of the systemic complications.

neutrophils. Attracted neutrophils adhere to the endothelium of pancreatic capillaries (margination) and then migrate into the gland. The neutrophils are activated and release platelet-activating factor (PAF), a small lipid based mediator which plays a central role in both local and systemic responses, by cleaving it from phospholipids in cell membranes; phospholipase A_2 produced by damaged acinar cells also generates PAF in this way. PAF, originally named for its ability to aggregate platelets, is a crucial mediator of the local inflammatory response, causing the capillary leakage that leads to oedema of the pancreas and stimulating the immigration and activation of neutrophils in a positive-feedback fashion. Its wider effects on the endothelium are reflected by pulmonary oedema, loss of intravascular volume, and entry of gut bacteria into the circulation (see below). The pathogenic properties of PAF have recently been reviewed in detail [4].

Systemic events

These result from circulating mediators released by local inflammation within the pancreas, and can be attributed to a 'systemic inflammatory response syndrome' and to the entry of gut bacteria to the circulation (Fig. 6).

In the lung, increased endothelial permeability leads to interstitial oedema, with the 'shock lung' appearance of adult respiratory distress syndrome (Fig. 7), and impaired gas transfer; pleural effusions, which indicate a poor prognosis, also arise in this way. Systemic effects include generalised capillary leakage, with peripheral oedema, hypovolaemia and hypotension. These factors together impair gut perfusion, damaging the gut mucosal barrier, which in turn allows increased

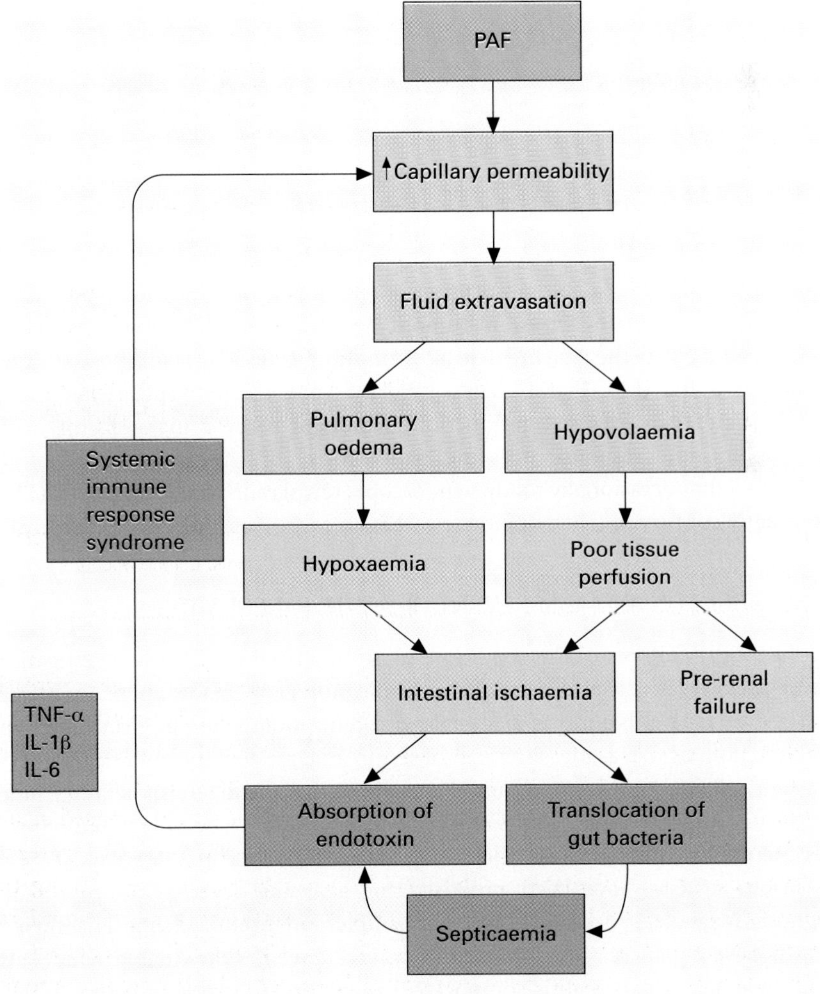

Fig. 6 Pathogenetic pathways leading to the systemic immune response and extra-pancreatic complications of acute pancreatitis.

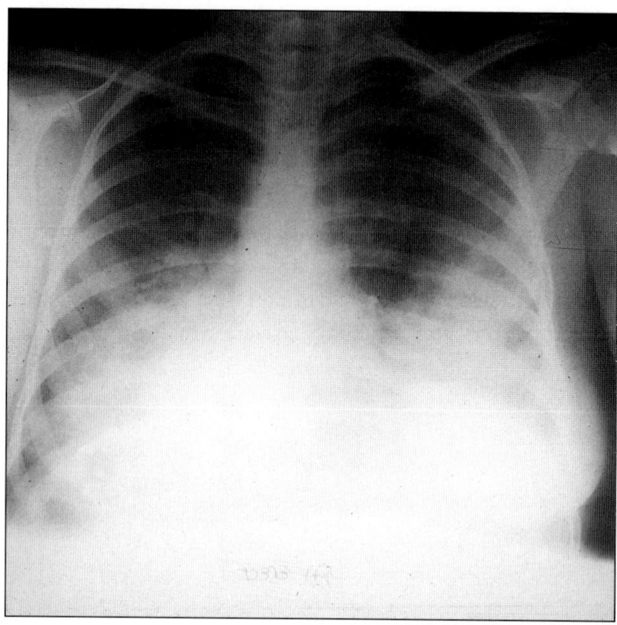

Fig. 7 Chest X-ray showing typical appearance of adult respiratory distress syndrome.

translocation of bacteria, and absorption of endotoxin, into the bloodstream. The endotoxaemia stimulates release of tumour necrosis factor-α (TNF-α) by monocytes, which triggers the systemic release from monocytes and neutrophils of interleukin (IL)-8 and IL-6 (Fig. 8). These cytokines mediate the acute inflammatory response, and their excessive production is thought to be a major factor in the systemic immune response of acute pancreatitis [5]. A careful study of the pancreatitis that occasionally follows endoscopic retrograde pancreatography (ERP) has recently confirmed that cytokine release is an early event [6].

□ INVESTIGATION AND ASSESSMENT OF ACUTE PANCREATITIS

The diagnostic features of the condition are summarised in Table 1. Investigations aim to assess severity as well as confirm the diagnosis and should therefore include chest X-ray, arterial blood gas analysis and careful monitoring of electrolytes and renal function, as well as measurement of serum amylase activity and imaging of the pancreas (see Fig. 3). It is important to remember that the diagnosis is *not* excluded by a normal amylase value. This is especially true if there is a delay between onset of pain and presentation: amylase values may return to normal in 2 or 3 days.

Various criteria have been proposed for assessing severity and to predict prognosis in acute pancreatitis, and one simple and useful scheme is shown in Table 2. 'Severe' pancreatitis is defined in criteria agreed at the Atlanta symposium [7] as an attack of pancreatitis complicated by any organ or system failure, or by a local complication (pancreatic or peripancreatic necrosis, pancreatic abscess or pseudocyst). Patients categorised as at high risk of complications by clinical

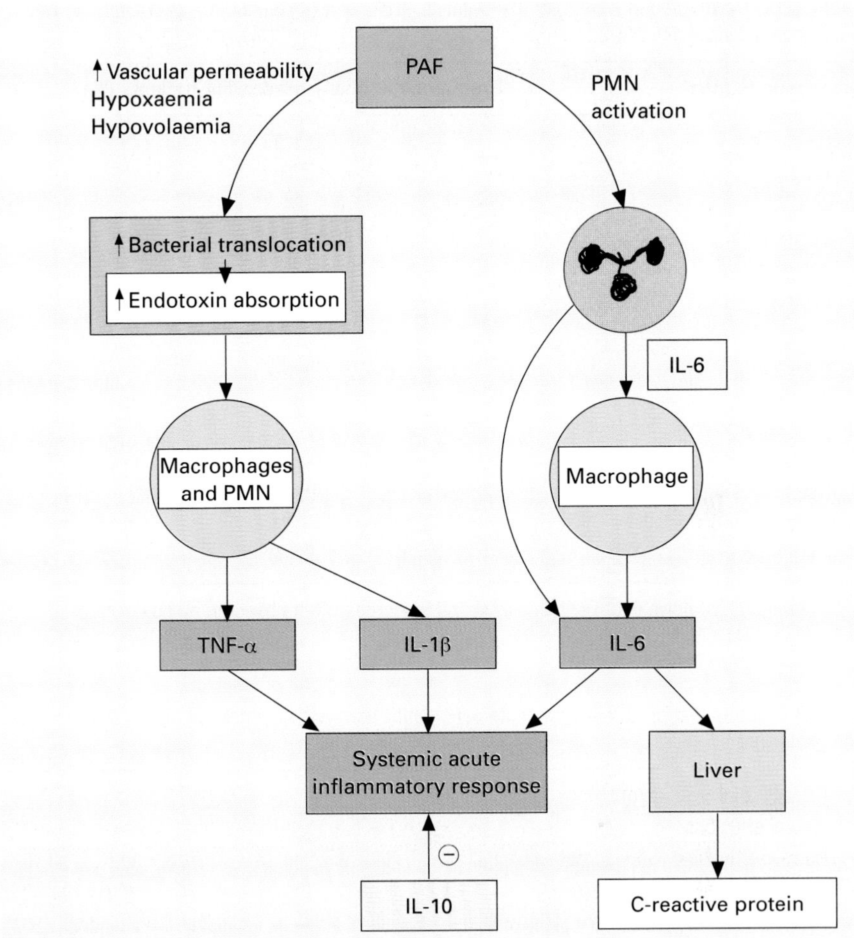

Fig. 8 Roles of PAF and pro-inflammatory mediators (TNF-α, IL-1β, IL-6) in the systemic immune activation of acute pancreatitis. IL-10 may inhibit these responses. C-reactive protein levels predict the severity of pancreatitis (see Table 2).

assessment, prognostic markers such as elevated C-reactive protein (>120 mg/l) or multiple factor scoring systems (Ranson [8], Glasgow [9], APACHE II [10,11]) are termed 'predicted severe pancreatitis'. These patients require aggressive fluid resuscitation, oxygen supplementation, prophylactic antibiotics and other preventive measures outlined below. Clinical signs helpful for prediction of severity include obesity [12–15], pleural effusion [16] and bruising in the flanks (the Grey Turner sign) due to extravasation of blood in the pancreatic bed, which has long been associated with a poor outcome (Fig. 9).

☐ RATIONAL MANAGEMENT OF ACUTE PANCREATITIS

A full discussion of current management standards for severe acute pancreatitis has

Table 1 Diagnostic features of acute pancreatitis. (Data from Hatful D. 4th year Study in Depth, Southampton University, 1992.)

Diagnostic feature	Frequency in newly presenting patients (%)
Epigastric pain	90–95
Vomiting	78
Nausea	90
Abdominal pain	
upper	25
central	5
lower	8
radiating to back	50–60
Ecchymosis	<5
Elevated enzyme levels in plasma	
Amylase >3 × ULN	90–95
Lipase >2 × ULN	95–99
Pancreatic oedema on US or CT scan	100
Pleural effusion	5–10

ULN, upper limit of normal range; US, ultrasound (pancreas often obscured by bowel gas).

Table 2 Features that predict severe acute pancreatitis (carrying high risks of organ failure or local complications).

- Obesity (BMI >30 kg/m^2)
- Pleural effusions
- Body-wall bruising (Grey Turner sign)
- C-reactive protein >120 mg/l
- APACHE II score ≥6 (see text [10])

Criteria agreed at an International Consensus Meeting, Santorini, Greece, September 1997.

recently been published [17], and these are summarised in Table 3. It includes the role of standard interventions such as endoscopic sphincterotomy and surgical debridement, which are beyond the scope of this chapter. Here, we shall focus on interventions that relate to the pathogenic model outlined above. Several events occurring in the pancreas and systemically are suitable targets for therapeutic intervention. Prevention of hypotension and hypovolaemia is paramount. Infected necrosis can be prevented by timely antibiotic prophylaxis, while gut barrier function may be supported by relatively small amounts of enteral nutrition. The deleterious effects of various pro-inflammatory cytokines, notably TNF-α and PAF, could be blocked by antagonists at their receptors; conversely, the anti-inflammatory cytokine IL-10 has been shown by experimental work in animal models to ameliorate the effects of acute pancreatitis.

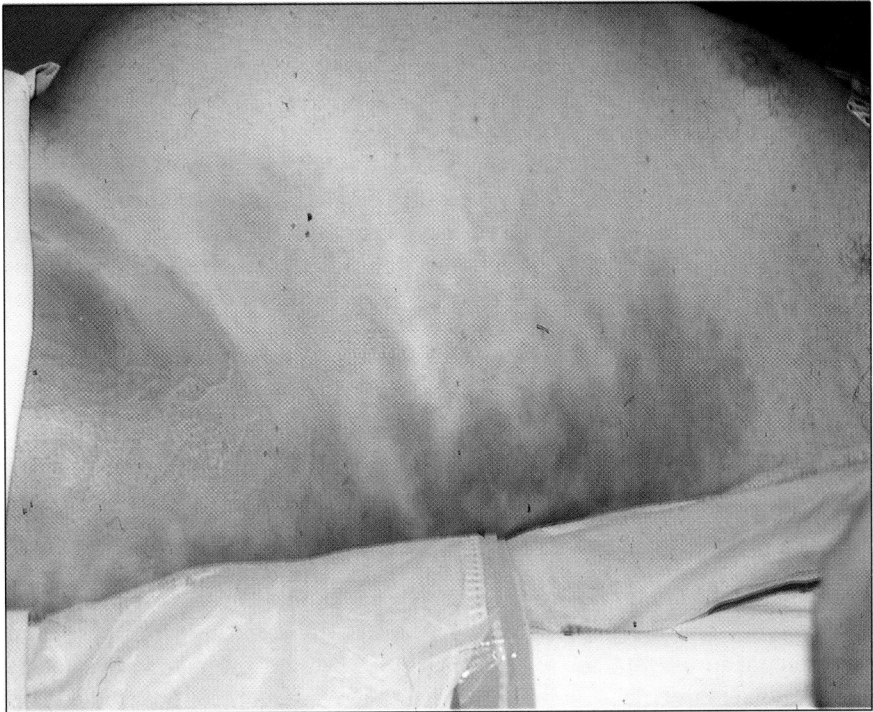

Fig. 9 The Grey Turner sign of bruising in the flanks; this is due to extravasation of blood into the pancreatic bed and denotes severe acute pancreatitis.

Table 3 Principles of the management of acute pancreatitis [17].

General supportive measures – all patients

- Fluid repletion
- Adequate oxygenation
- Analgesia

Preventive measures – all predicted severe cases

- Enteral feeding (nasojejunal or nasogastric tube)
- Prophylactic antibiotics (broad-spectrum, including anaerobe cover)
- Treat gallstones (early ERCP in predicted severe cases with known gallstones, in gall bladder or common bile duct)

Treat complications – all severe cases

- Support systems failure (inotropes, ventilation, dialysis, etc)
- Detect pancreatic necrosis (if no better after 7 days)
- Detect infected necrosis by fine-needle aspiration
- Debride necrosis (if infected; if condition worsens)

General supportive measures: circulatory and respiratory support

The dangers of hypovolaemia, due to fluid extravasation, cannot be overestimated. Hypovolaemia impairs the perfusion of vital organs and so contributes to organ failure and the translocation of gut bacteria into the circulation. Pulmonary oedema impairs gas transfer, which further compounds the effect of hypovolaemia.

All patients with severe acute pancreatitis should therefore be managed with aggressive fluid replacement. Those with hypotension and/or oliguria whose blood pressure and urine output do not improve immediately require a central venous pressure line to monitor rapid fluid replacement. A mixture of synthetic colloid and crystalloid should be given.

Supplemental oxygen should be given to all patients with severe pancreatitis. A face mask or nasal catheter is generally sufficient, but blood gas estimations should be performed frequently in the early stages and ventilatory support considered if respiratory function worsens.

Enteral nutrition

Another time-honoured dogma in this area has now been disproved. It is not necessary to drain the stomach via a nasogastric tube and resort to parenteral nutrition in an attempt to 'rest the pancreas', because the pancreas is totally unresponsive to external stimuli during the acute phase. Indeed, two studies have shown that enteral nutrition (generally given via a nasojejunal tube) is not only safer and cheaper than parenteral nutrition but is itself therapeutic and leads to a reduced incidence of infective complications and of surgical intervention [18,19]. Enteral feeding may help to maintain the barrier function of the gut, preventing bacterial translocation. Standard enteral formulation should be used; full feeding volumes are probably not necessary as it appears that a small nutrient load is sufficient to maintain gut mucosal integrity.

Antibiotic prophylaxis

There has been considerable controversy about the role of prophylactic antibiotics. For many years they were thought to be of no value, on the basis of inadequate studies conducted in the 1970s. The current consensus is that prophylactic antibiotics have an important role to play in the prevention of infective complications [20]. There are four randomised studies in the literature which overall show a convincing reduction in mortality in patients with severe pancreatitis who received antibiotics. This is consistent with an important pathogenic role of bacteria translocating from the gut to the bloodstream.

Patients with predicted severe pancreatitis should therefore be given intravenous antibiotics, which should be broad-spectrum and also cover gut anaerobes. Most regimens include a cephalosporin (this class featured in most of the randomised trials); our unit routinely employs cefuroxime and metronidazole.

Selective gut decontamination using oral paste and enteral and rectal administration of non-absorbed broad-spectrum antibiotics and fungicides has been proposed for the prevention of infection in these patients. However, the only study to test this hypothesis also included intravenous cefotaxime treatment for a mean period of 7 days after recruitment to the study, and it is therefore not possible to attribute the observed benefit with confidence to gut decontamination.

PAF antagonists

The crucial role of PAF in mediating both pancreatic damage and the life-threatening systemic sequelae [4] suggests that blocking the PAF receptor with a specific antagonist would be therapeutically beneficial. There is now sound experimental evidence from animal models to support this approach, and initial clinical experience is also encouraging.

The PAF receptor is a typical membrane-spanning cytokine receptor, and a specific antagonist, lexipafant, has been investigated in Phase II clinical trials of acute pancreatitis. A small initial trial [21] showed that treatment for 5 days with lexipafant significantly reduced the incidence of organ failure, which was confirmed in a larger study (50 patients) of one week's treatment [22]. In the latter study, three of 24 lexipafant-treated patients died, compared with six of 26 in the placebo group, but the numbers were too small to assess any statistical significance of this difference.

A multicentre study of 290 patients with severe pancreatitis, conducted in the UK, has recently suggested that treatment with lexipafant may be effective in reducing mortality when given early [23]. This study failed to show any effect of lexipafant on the incidence of organ failure, perhaps because 40% of patients recruited already had organ failure at entry to the study. There was a significant reduction in the number of patients with 'sepsis', defined as evidence of organ failure associated with any proven bacterial infection (Fig. 10). Although lexipafant treatment did not significantly decrease overall mortality, it was halved in patients treated within 48 hours of onset of pain (Table 4). As would be expected from the supposed mechanism of action, early intervention was more beneficial. There was also a significant correlation between short duration of symptoms and therapeutic benefit. This *post hoc* analysis requires confirmation by a prospective study, which is currently in progress.

□ CONCLUSIONS

An improved understanding of the pathogenesis of acute pancreatitis, and particularly the role of the inflammatory response in systemic complications, is now leading to improved therapy. The origin of infection from the gut has underwritten prophylactic antibiotic therapy, and provides a rationale for enteral nutrition early in the attack. The systemic immune response and its impact on other organs can be diminished by use of the PAF antagonist lexipafant. Other immune antagonists or anti-inflammatory cytokines (eg IL-10) may ultimately be developed, and may work in synergy with this agent. It is not clear at present whether these various strategies which are effective alone may be even more beneficial when used in combination.

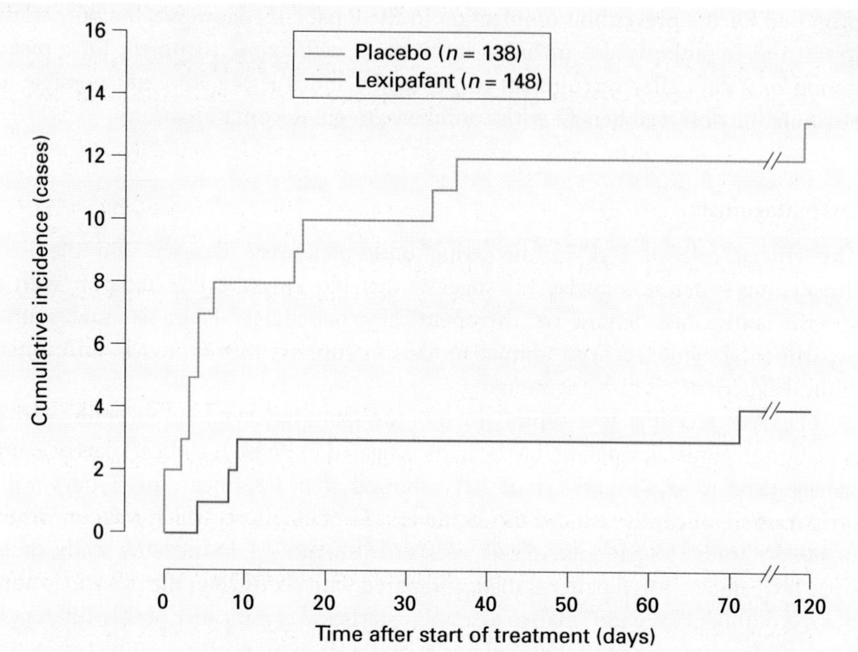

Fig. 10 Cumulative incidence of sepsis (defined as organ failure with positive bacterial cultures) in a clinical trial of 7 days lexipafant treatment vs placebo; p=0.016. (Data from reference 23.)

Table 4 Mortality in a placebo-controlled, randomised trial of lexipafant in 290 patients with severe acute pancreatitis [23]; mortality was significantly decreased when lexipafant was started within 48 h of the onset of pain, but not in the treated group overall.

	All patients		**Early treatment**	
	placebo	**lexipafant**	**placebo**	**lexipafant**
Total number	138	151	98	107
Exclusions*	3	4	3	3
Deaths from pancreatitis:				
• number	21	14	17	8†
• % mortality	17	10	18	8†

*Included deaths from unrelated causes.
† p = 0.03 vs placebo group.

REFERENCES

1 Scott P, Bruce C, Schofield D, Shiel N, Braganza JM, McCloy RM. Vitamin C status in patients with acute pancreatitis. *Br J Surg* 1993; **80**: 750–4.

2 Marchand L. Antioxidants in acute pancreatitis. 4th year Study in Depth. University of Southampton, 1997.

3 Marchand LJC, Gough AC, Johnson CD. Malondialdehyde and prognosis in acute pancreatitis. *Digestion* 1997; **58** (Suppl 2): 35.

4 Johnson CD. Platelet activating factor and PAF antagonists in acute pancreatitis. *Digestive Surg* 1999 (in press).
5 Kingsnorth AN. Role of cytokines and their inhibitors in acute pancreatitis. *Gut* 1997; **40**: 1–4.
6 Messman H, Vogt W, Holstege A, *et al.* Post ERP pancreatitis as a model for cytokine induced acute phase response in acute pancreatitis. *Gut* 1997; **40**: 80–5.
7 Bradley EL. A clinically based classification system for acute pancreatitis. Summary of the Atlanta symposium. *Arch Surg* 1993; **128**: 586–90.
8 Ranson JHC. The timing of biliary surgery in acute pancreatitis. *Ann Surg* 1979; **189**: 654–62.
9 Osbourne DH, Imrie CW, Carter DC. Biliary surgery in the same admission for gallstone associated acute pancreatitis. *Br J Surg* 1981; **68**: 758–61.
10 Knaus WA, Draper EA, Wagner DP, Zimmerman JE. APACHE II: a severity of disease classification. *Crit Care Med* 1985; **13**: 818–29.
11 Larvin M, McMahon MJ. APACHE-II score for assessment and monitoring of acute pancreatitis. *Lancet* 1989; **ii**: 201–5.
12 Lankisch PG, Schirren CA. Increased body weight as a prognostic parameter for complications in the course of acute pancreatitis. *Pancreas* 1990; **5**: 626–9.
13 Porter KA, Banks PA. Obesity as a predictor of severity in acute pancreatitis. *Int J Pancreatol* 1991; **10**: 247–52.
14 Funnell IC, Bornman PC, Weakley SP, Terblanche J, Marks IN. Obesity: an important prognostic factor in acute pancreatitis. *Br J Surg* 1993; **80**: 484–6.
15 Toh SKC, Walters J, Johnson CD. APACHE-0 a new predictor of severity in acute pancreatitis. *Gut* 1996; **38** (Suppl 1): A35.
16 Talamini G, Bassi C, Falconi M, *et al.* Risk of death from acute pancreatitis. *Int J Pancreatol* 1996; **19**: 15–24.
17 Glazer G, Mann DV, and the British Society of Gastroenterology working group. UK guidelines for the management of acute pancreatitis. *Gut* 1998; **42**(Suppl 2).
18 Kalferentzos F, Kehagias J, Mead N, Kokkinis K, Gogos CA. Enteral feeding is superior to parenteral nutrition in severe acute pancreatitis: results of a randomised prospective trial. *Br J Surg* 1997; **84**: 1665–9.
19 Windsor AJC, Kanwar S, Li AJK, *et al.* Compared with parenteral nutrition, enteral feeding attenuates the acute phase response and improves disease severity in acute pancreatitis. *Gut* 1998; **42**: 431–5.
20 Powell JJ, Miles R, Siriwardena A. Antibiotic prophylaxis in the initial management of severe acute pancreatitis. *Br J Surg* 1998; **85**: 582–7.
21 Kingsnorth AN, Galloway SW, Formela LJ. Randomised double-blind phase II trial of lexipafant, a platelet-activating factor antagonist, in human acute pancreatitis. *Br J Surg* 1995; **82**: 1414–20.
22 McKay CJ, Curran F, Sharples C, Baxter JN, Imrie CW. Prospective placebo-controlled randomised trial of lexipafant in predicted severe acute pancreatitis. *Br J Surg* 1997; **84**: 1239–43.
23 Toh SKC, for the British Acute Pancreatitis Study Group. Lexipafant, a platelet activating factor (PAF) antagonist, reduces mortality in a randomised, placebo-controlled study in patients with severe acute pancreatitis. *Gut* 1997; **40** (Suppl 1): A12.

□ MULTIPLE CHOICE QUESTIONS

1 The actions of platelet-activating factor (PAF) include:
(a) Formation of platelet aggregates
(b) Increased capillary permeability
(c) Increased deformability of red blood cells
(d) Activation of neutrophils
(e) Release of phospholipase A_2

2 In severe acute pancreatitis:
(a) Enteral feeding is contraindicated
(b) Parenteral feeding reduces serious complications
(c) Pleural effusions may be present
(d) The serum amylase may be normal
(e) CT scanning is useful to show oedema of the gland

3 In acute pancreatitis, prophylactic antibiotics:
(a) Should be given to all patients
(b) Should include broad-spectrum cover
(c) Antagonise the effects of PAF
(d) Reduce mortality in severe acute pancreatitis
(e) Should be stopped after 48 hours

4 In the treatment of acute pancreatitis:
(a) The protease inhibitor aprotinin decreases mortality
(b) The PAF antagonist lexipafant reduces overall mortality
(c) Lexipafant reduces the severity of organ failure
(d) Colloid solutions are contraindicated
(e) Ventilation may be required

5 Early action in severe acute pancreatitis should include:
(a) Aggressive fluid replacement
(b) Frequent measurement of urine volume
(c) Routine oxygen supplements
(d) Routine placement of central venous pressure and arterial pressure lines
(e) Draining the stomach via a nasogastric tube

ANSWERS

1a True	2a False	3a False	4a False	5a True
b True	b False	b True	b False	b True
c False	c True	c False	c True	c True
d True	d True	d True	d False	d False
e False	e True	e False	e True	e False

Helicobacter pylori infection and its role in human disease

Kenneth E L McColl

□ INTRODUCTION

Helicobacter pylori is a flagellated bacterium that colonises the gastric mucosa of approximately half the world's human population (Fig. 1). Its prevalence in the Western world rises progressively with age, from 10% in children under 10 years of age to more than 60% in subjects aged over 60. Its prevalence is also related to the socioeconomic status of the population and particularly to living conditions during childhood. Current evidence suggests that the infection is acquired early in life and then persists indefinitely. The chances of contracting the infection in childhood are higher in areas of socioeconomic deprivation, while the rising prevalence with age may represent a cohort effect due to the generally poorer childhood environment experienced by the older population.

The bacterium is found within the mucus layer of the gastric mucosa and adhering to the luminal surface of the epithelial cells (Fig. 2). It does not invade the underlying mucosa, but stimulates infiltration of the mucosa by both acute and chronic inflammatory cells, producing the histological features of gastritis, even in the absence of ulceration (Fig. 2). Half the population of the world, therefore, have this organism in the stomach and an accompanying histological gastritis.

The stomach constantly secretes acid, one of whose main functions may be to kill the bacteria that are constantly swallowed within food and so provide one of the body's first lines of defence against enteric infections (see chapter 10). *H. pylori* is unique in being able to survive in this highly acidic environment. It is largely protected by its exceptionally high content of the enzyme urease, which converts urea in the gastric juice into carbon dioxide and ammonia, a strong alkali.

Its high urease activity is exploited in two tests to diagnose *H. pylori* infection. The urea breath test involves giving patients a drink containing urea labelled either with the stable non-radioactive isotope ^{13}C or the radioactive isotope ^{14}C, and then monitoring the excretion of the relevant isotope in carbon dioxide exhaled 20 minutes later. In the urease slide test, a biopsy of gastric mucosa obtained at endoscopy is placed in a small well containing urea and a pH-sensitive dye whose colour changes when the pH is raised by the organism's synthesis of ammonia. Other means of diagnosing the infection include measuring specific antibodies against *H. pylori* in the serum, and histological examination or culture of gastric biopsies.

The genome of *H. pylori* has now been sequenced [1]. Although relatively small (1.7 Mb, less than half the size of the genome of *E. coli*), it contains several likely determinants of pathogenicity and specific features that might enable it to survive in the hostile environment of the stomach; these include high degrees of variability in the genes encoding surface proteins, which could help to protect it against the

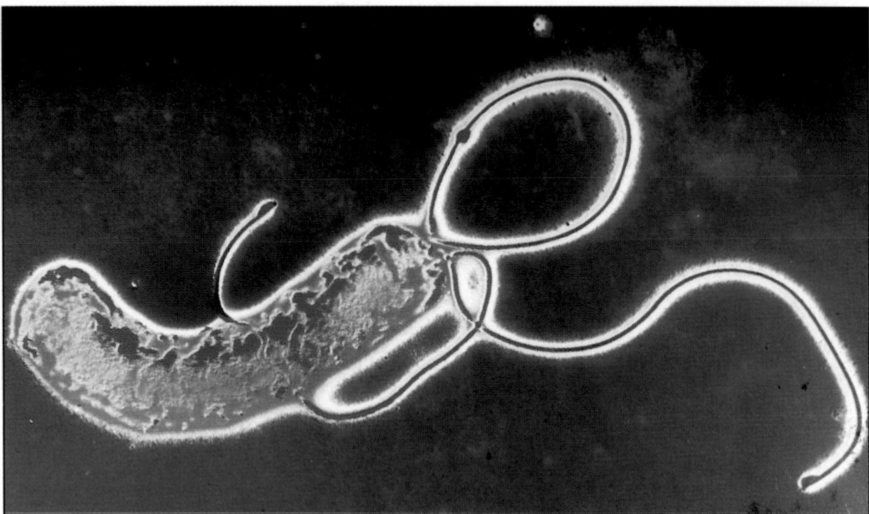

Fig. 1 *Helicobacter pylori* (scanning electron micrograph).

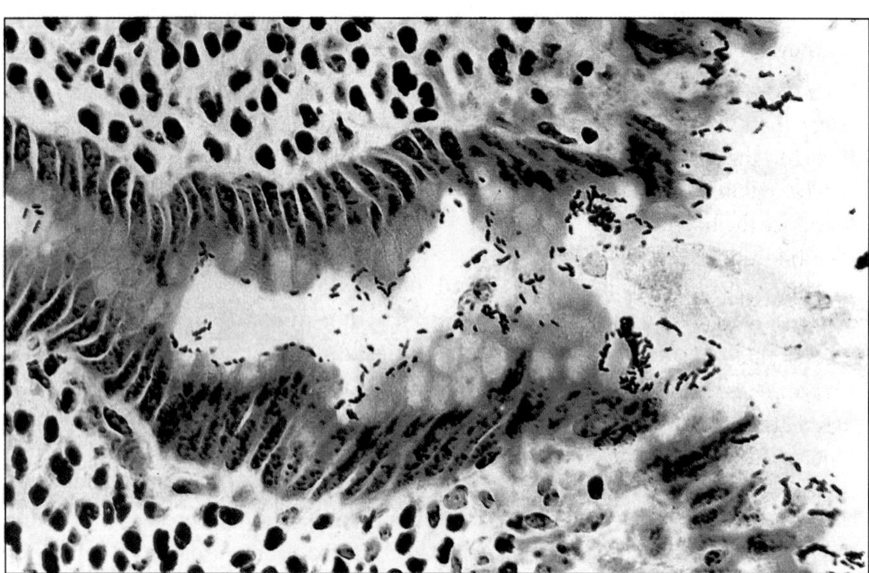

Fig. 2 Histological features of *C. pylori* infection in the stomach. Showing: organisms lying on the gastric mucosa, with underlying inflammation, marked mucosal atrophy, the change associated with the development of gastric cancer and gastric lymphoma (MALToma).

host's immune defences. Genes relevant to human disease include *cag* (cytotoxin-association gene), which encodes a high-molecular-weight protein of unknown function but which is associated more severe histological gastritis and an increased incidence of developing significant clinical diseases such as peptic ulcer or gastric cancer. The genome sequence is available on the Internet, at http://www.tigr.org/tdb/mdb/hpdb/hpdb.html.

□ *H. PYLORI* AND GASTROINTESTINAL DISEASES

Since its recognition in 1986, *H. pylori* infection has been strongly implicated in various upper gastrointestinal disorders. There is now compelling evidence that it is important in the aetiology of peptic ulcer disease, gastric cancer and gastric lymphoma, and it may also be involved in the pathogenesis of non-ulcer dyspepsia. The role of the infection in these disorders will be discussed in turn.

Duodenal ulcer disease

Duodenal ulceration is a common clinical condition that affects 10% of the population at some time in their life. *H. pylori* infection is found in more than 95% of duodenal ulcer patients. Eradication of the infection leads to healing of the ulcer and will prevent its recurrence in over 90% of cases; by contrast, over 90% of duodenal ulcers healed with conventional anti-secretory medication will recur within 12 months of stopping therapy [2,3]. Eradication of *H. pylori* infection is also effective in curing duodenal ulcers that have been complicated by bleeding, and prevents the recurrence of haemorrhage [4].

Pathogenic mechanisms of *H. pylori* infection

The mechanism by which infection causes duodenal ulceration has recently become clear [5]. In ulcer patients, the infection and accompanying inflammation are confined to the distal stomach (antrum), with little if any involvement of the proximal body region (see Figs 3 and 4). Neuroendocrine G cells of the gastric antrum produce the hormone gastrin which stimulates the parietal cells in the mucosa lining the body of the stomach to secrete acid. Acid secretion is decreased by a low pH within the antrum, as this inhibits further gastrin release. This acid inhibitory control of gastrin release is mediated via the release of somatostatin by D cells which are situated close to the G cells. *H. pylori* infection and/or inflammation of the antrum results in depletion of somatostatin and consequently loss of the acid-mediated inhibitory control of gastrin release. The increased gastrin stimulates increased secretion of acid by the healthy body mucosa. The resulting increased duodenal acid load results in progressive duodenal mucosal damage and ultimately ulceration. Strains of *H. pylori* that express *cag* and the S1a variant of vacA are more likely to result in duodenal ulceration.

Eradicating *H. pylori* infection lowers gastrin levels and thus acid secretion, leading to healing of the duodenal ulceration, and this is now the recommended first-line treatment for patients with duodenal ulcer disease. This strategy is highly effective in preventing relapse of the duodenal ulceration, but has less impact on the dyspeptic symptoms which are usually the main (or only) reason for the patient seeking medical treatment. Almost 50% of duodenal ulcer patients continue to experience dyspepsia following successful eradication of the infection and ulcer healing [6]. The reason for this is unclear; dyspepsia may be partly related to coexisting causes such as gastro-oesophageal reflux disease which are not helped by eradicating the infection, or to unknown irreversible changes that might be induced by the infection or other factors related to ulceration or its treatment.

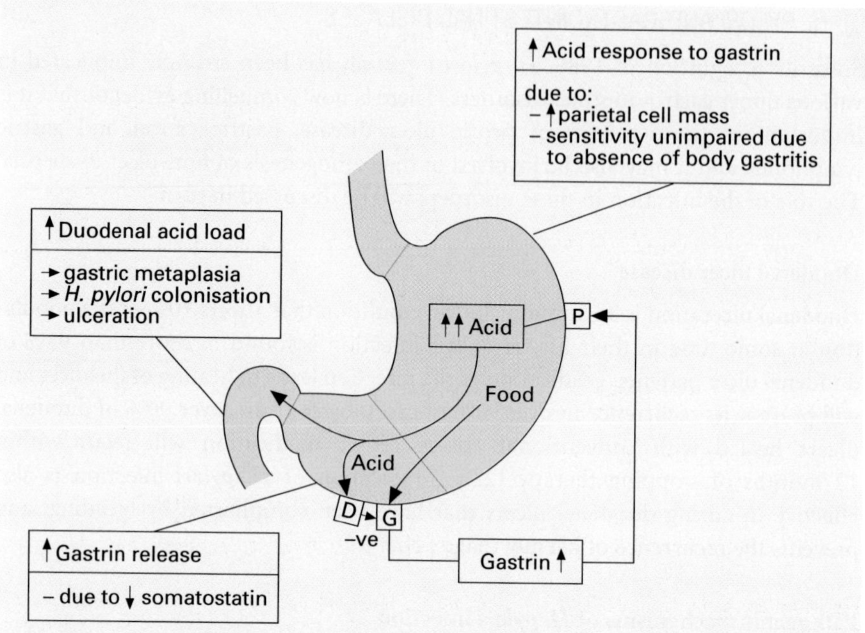

Fig. 3 Role of *H. pylori* infection on pathophysiology of duodenal ulceration. In duodenal ulcer patients the antral infection and or associated inflammation decreases somatostatin production and thus impairs the acid-mediated inhibitory control of gastrin release. The increased gastrin stimulates increased acid secretion by the healthy uninflamed body mucosa. The resulting increased duodenal acid load leads to progressive damage to the duodenal mucosa and ultimately ulceration.

Gastric ulcer disease

Gastric ulcers have long been recognised as having a different aetiology from those in the duodenum. Gastric ulcers are not associated with excess acid secretion; indeed, many gastric ulcer patients are hypochlorhydric. In addition, gastric ulcers are frequently related to the use of non-steroidal anti-inflammatory drugs (NSAIDs).

H. pylori infection is present in most patients with gastric ulcers that are not associated with NSAIDs; in these cases, eradication of the infection prevents relapse of the ulcer disease [7]. By contrast, the role of eradicating *H. pylori* infection in treating or preventing gastric ulcers related to NSAIDs remains unclear [8].

Gastric cancer

There is now very strong evidence that *H. pylori* infection plays a key role in the sequence of events that leads to cancer of the body or antrum of the stomach. Case-control prospective studies have shown an increased risk of developing these cancers in subjects who are seropositive for *H. pylori* infection [9]. Interestingly, *H. pylori* infection is not associated with an increased risk of cancer of the cardia or gastro-oesophageal junction [10].

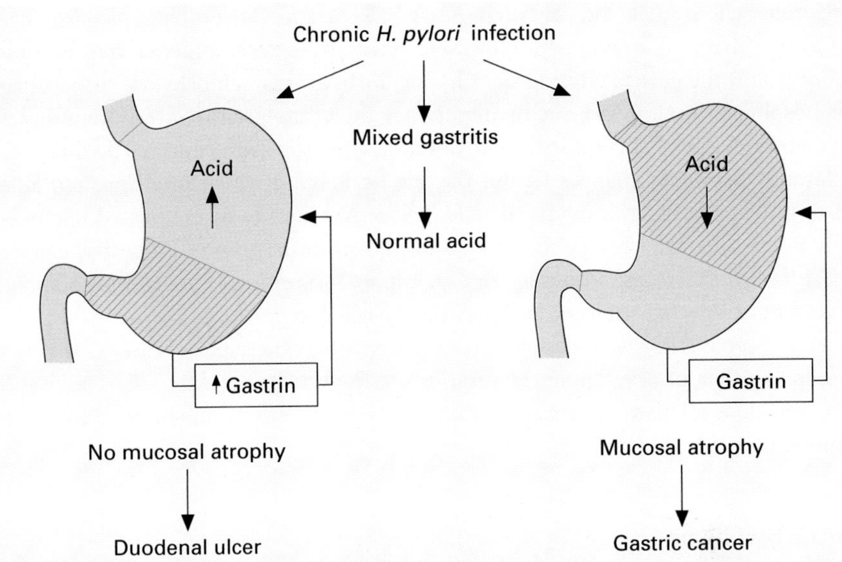

Fig. 4 Different outcomes of *H. pylori* infection. In some subjects, infection predominantly affects the antrum, producing a non-atrophic gastritis that increases gastrin secretion and thus stimulates acid secretion; this predisposes to duodenal ulceration (see Fig. 3). Others develop gastritis of the body region of the stomach accompanied by atrophy and this decreases acid secretion. This form of gastritis carries an increased risk of gastric cancer. Other subjects show inflammation of the antrum and body region and have no overall change in acid secretion.

Possible mechanisms by which the infection contributes to the development of gastric cancer are becoming clearer. In some subjects, *H. pylori* infection and the accompanying inflammation cause structural damage to the gastric epithelium, with atrophy and intestinal metaplasia that extend from the antrum into the acid-secreting body of the stomach. This impairs acid secretion, and these subjects develop hypochlorhydria or even achlorhydria. It has long been recognised that cancer of the body and antrum of the stomach develops against a background of atrophy and hypochlorydria, though the reason is unknown. The inflammatory process that destroys the epithelium may also induce neoplastic changes; alternatively, or additionally, hypochlorhydria may allow colonisation of the gastric lumen by bacteria that synthesise potentially carcinogenic nitrosamines.

It is not clear why some subjects develop an antral-confined gastritis with acid hypersecretion, while others develop gastritis that involves the entire stomach and is associated with acid hyposecretion (Fig. 4). It may be related to dietary factors, such as lack of vitamin C or increased salt intake, which could favour more severe and atrophic gastritis. Genetic factors are also likely to be important: subjects with a family history of gastric cancer are more likely to develop atrophy and hypochlorhydria in response to *H. pylori* infection, particularly if more than one relative has suffered from cancer [11]. The concomitant development of autoimmune responses against the parietal cells could also influence the extent of mucosal damage.

Serological studies indicate that nearly all gastric cancer patients have had *H. pylori* infection previously. However, once the gastric mucosa has become atrophic and the gastric environment hypochlorhydric or achlorhydric, it becomes less hospitable to *H. pylori*; such patients may therefore lose the infection and may have no evidence of current infection when they present with cancer. The infection apparently produces changes within the gastric mucosa which predispose to later development of cancer, implying that *H. pylori* may have to be eradicated relatively early in life – before irreversible changes occur – in order to prevent gastric cancer. This prevention strategy would involve widespread screening of the community and treatment of infected subjects, and may not be feasible.

First-degree relatives of gastric cancer patients may be a special case, as they are at increased risk of developing the tumour themselves. It therefore seems advisable to screen close relatives of cancer patients for *H. pylori* infection, and to eradicate it if present.

Gastric lymphoma

Mucosa-associated lymphoid tissue (MALT) is normally not found within the gastric mucosa, but may develop in patients infected with *H. pylori*. As MALT may undergo neoplastic change, *H. pylori* infection has been implicated in the development of the rare gastric lymphoma, also known as primary non-Hodgkin's lymphoma of the stomach or 'MALToma' (see Fig. 2). MALTomas apparently arise from clonal expansion of B lymphocytes within the lymphoid infiltrate that characterises the chronic gastritis associated with *H. pylori* infection [12]. Much excitement has recently been generated by the observation that eradicating *H. pylori* infection in patients with low-grade MALT lymphoma results in regression and complete disappearance of the tumour in the majority of cases [13]. Eradication therapy is now recommended as first-line treatment for such patients.

Non-ulcer dyspepsia

Dyspepsia is a common condition, affecting 10–30% of the general population. Endoscopic investigation of dyspeptic subjects reveals ulcer disease in approximately 20% and gastro-oesophageal reflux disease in 25%, but over 50% show no macroscopic abnormality; these patients are referred to as suffering from 'non-ulcer dyspepsia'. *H. pylori* infection and associated histological gastritis are present in about 50% of such subjects, a prevalence that is 5–10% higher than in the asymptomatic population. In a large placebo-controlled, randomised trial, we recently demonstrated symptomatic benefits of eradicating *H. pylori* in patients with non-ulcer dyspepsia [14]; one year later, 21% of patients treated with anti-*H. pylori* therapy were asymptomatic, compared with only 7% of those who received placebo. These results indicate that *H. pylori* infection is a cause of symptoms in a subgroup of *H. pylori* infected patients presenting with non-ulcer dyspepsia. Interestingly, the only factor found to predict a beneficial response to eradication treatment was a short duration of dyspepsia: 29% of patients with dyspepsia for less than five years were cured, compared with only 12% in those with a longer history. Some previous studies have also found symptomatic benefit from eradicating *H. pylori* in patients with non-ulcer dyspepsia, but other studies observed no benefit. It appears, therefore, that the symptomatic benefit of eradicating *H. pylori* infection in patients with non-ulcer dyspepsia is confined to a relatively small subgroup of such patients.

Gastro-oesophageal reflux disease

Current evidence indicates that *H. pylori* infection does not play any role in the aetiology of gastro-oesophageal reflux disease, the commonest identifiable cause of dyspepsia. Indeed, one study has suggested that eradication of *H. pylori* in ulcer patients might actually lead to reflux disease [15]. However, this may represent coexistent reflux that becomes more apparent when anti-secretory therapy is withdrawn, which is known to cause marked rebound acid hypersecretion, particularly in the absence of *H. pylori* infection. At present, therefore, there is no evidence that eradicating *H. pylori* infection will improve symptoms in patients with confirmed gastro-oesophageal reflux.

Recent studies have raised concerns about potentially deleterious interactions between *H. pylori* infection and long-term treatment with proton-pump inhibitors, which are frequently used to control gastro-oesophageal reflux disease [16]. Drug-induced inhibition of acid secretion alters the distribution of *H. pylori* associated gastritis in the stomach, causing it to extend from the antrum into the body in the distribution found in patients who develop gastric cancer. One study (which has been criticised because of inappropriate controls) also suggested that proton-pump inhibitor therapy may lead to gastric atrophy in *H. pylori* infected subjects. Accordingly, some groups recommend that patients with gastro-oesophageal reflux disease should be checked for *H. pylori* infection before prescribing long-term proton-pump inhibitor therapy, and any infection eradicated. It is also becoming recognised that proton-pump inhibitors are less effective in controlling intragastric acidity in *H. pylori* negative subjects. In patients with *H. pylori* infection, proton-pump inhibitor therapy maintains intragastric pH at near neutral levels, whereas pH is significantly lower in *H. pylori* negative subjects [17]; this is because the body gastritis which develops in *H. pylori* positive subjects during proton-pump inhibitor therapy further inhibits the ability of the mucosa to secrete acid and thus enhances the action of the drug.

At present, definitive advice cannot be given concerning eradication of *H. pylori* before starting long-term proton-pump inhibitor therapy in reflux disease, although this would seem a reasonable approach, especially in view of the increasing evidence that the infection causes various harmful effects on the upper gastrointestinal tract.

There is no evidence to implicate *H. pylori* infection in the development of carcinoma of the gastro-oesophageal junction, which is a recognised complication of severe reflux.

☐ PRACTICAL ASPECTS OF *H. PYLORI* ERADICATION THERAPY

Selection of patients

At present, there is clear evidence that eradication of *H. pylori* infection benefits patients with duodenal ulcers, gastric ulcers and low-grade gastric lymphoma (Table 1). Some studies have found symptomatic benefit in a subgroup of patients with non-ulcer dyspepsia. Eradicating the infection from first-degree relatives of patients with a strong family history of gastric cancer would also seem wise, but there is not yet direct evidence that this will prevent cancer. More research is required into the interaction between proton-pump inhibitor therapy and *H. pylori* infection in reflux disease.

Treatment and follow-up for *H. pylori* infection

Numerous studies have now shown that the most effective first-line treatment for eradication of *H. pylori* is one week of triple therapy, comprising a proton-pump inhibitor plus two antibiotics. The most commonly used antibiotics are amoxycillin, metronidazole and clarithromycin. These triple therapy regimens eradicate infection in 85–95% of cases.

Eradication of infection is best confirmed by performing a urea breath test at least four weeks after finishing treatment. If the infection persists, a further course of triple therapy using different antibiotics can then be given. Failure of eradication may be due to bacterial resistance, which may develop against both metronidazole and clarithromycin but is rarely seen with amoxycillin. For this reason, second-line treatment should again use amoxycillin but substitute metronidazole for clarithromycin (or vice versa).

Successful eradication of the infection should be confirmed routinely in all patients with previously complicated duodenal ulcer disease, in all patients with persisting symptoms, and in those who have no dyspeptic symptoms to indicate successful therapy (eg relatives of gastric cancer patients). Because of the possibility of underlying cancer, all gastric ulcer patients should have a repeat endoscopy following eradication therapy, to confirm that the infection has cleared and to take further biopsies to exclude neoplasia.

Table 1 Which patients benefit from eradication of *H. pylori* infection?

Duodenal ulcer	Yes
Gastric ulcer	Yes
Gastric MALT lymphoma	Yes
Non-ulcer dyspepsia	Only subgroup
Family history of gastric Ca	Probably
Gastro-oesophageal reflux disease	No

☐ IMPLICATIONS FOR THE INVESTIGATION OF DYSPEPSIA

Awareness of *H. pylori* infection has transformed the treatment of dyspeptic disease, and may also influence the investigation of some patients with dyspepsia. Recent studies indicate that non-invasive tests of *H. pylori* status are valuable in predicting endoscopic finding in patients presenting with dyspepsia [18] (Fig. 5). In those with a positive non-invasive *H. pylori* test (urea breath test or serology), there is a 20–40% chance of underlying ulcer disease. By contrast, those who test negative have only a less than 5% probability of ulcer disease, and the only likely endoscopic abnormality is oesophagitis (in about 20%).

It has been suggested that such non-invasive tests could determine the management of dyspeptic patients. Those with a positive *H. pylori* test could be given eradication therapy empirically to treat underlying ulcer disease or non-ulcer dyspepsia; only those with persisting or troublesome symptoms after successful eradication would be considered for further investigation. In addition, dyspeptic subjects with a negative *H. pylori* test could be reassured that they are very unlikely to have an ulcer and that the probable diagnosis is reflux disease, for which they should be treated empirically. Such an approach could reduce the increasing demand for upper gastrointestinal endoscopy, a costly and uncomfortable invasive procedure.

It should be emphasised, however, that this non-endoscopic strategy for managing dyspepsia should be limited to patients less than 50 years of age and who have no features or risk factors of underlying malignancy. These include weight loss, dysphagia, anaemia, family history of gastric cancer or gastric surgery, bleeding or persisting vomiting. In addition, patients receiving NSAIDs would be unsuitable for

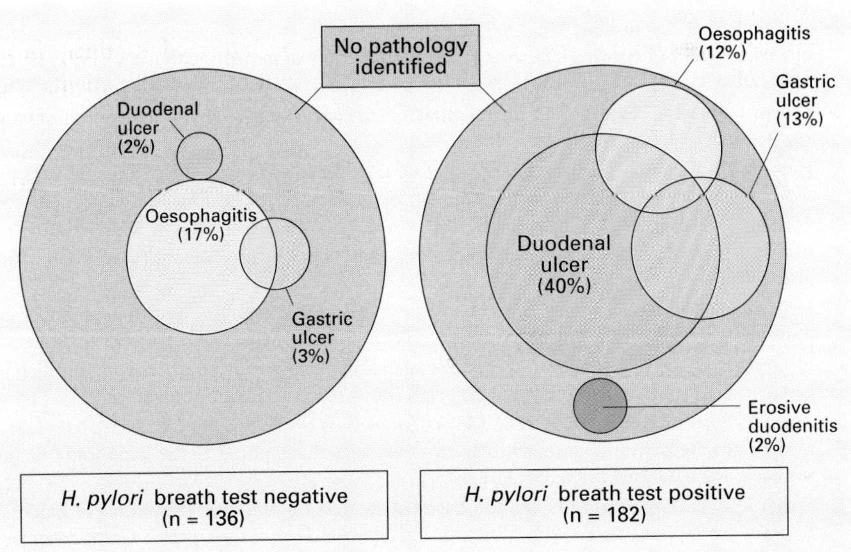

Fig. 5 Endoscopic findings in dyspeptic patients, according to whether the ^{14}C-urea breath test for *H. pylori* infection was negative or positive.

this approach as they may develop severe ulcer disease in the absence of *H. pylori* infection.

Currently, studies are under way to assess the relative merits of endoscopy and non-invasive *H. pylori* testing in young patients presenting with dyspepsia.

□ CONCLUSIONS

Since the discovery of *H. pylori* only 12 years ago, our understanding of the aetiology of several common and important upper gastrointestinal diseases has been transformed. This new knowledge has given us the ability to cure a substantial proportion of these common diseases and may radically change our approach to the investigation of dyspepsia. Interest is now turning to other potential adverse effects of this common infection in subjects without dyspeptic disease, and to whether we should ultimately aim to eradicate *H. pylori* from mankind.

REFERENCES

1 Tomb JF, White D, Kerlavage AR, *et al.* The complete genome sequence of the gastric pathogen *Helicobacter pylori. Nature* 1997; **388:** 539–47.

2 Marshall BJ, Goodwin CS, Warren JR, *et al.* Prospective double-blind trial of duodenal ulcer relapse after eradication of *Campylobacter pylori. Lancet* 1988; **ii:** 1437–41.

3 Hentschel E, Brandstatter G, Dragosics B, *et al.* Effect of ranitidine and amoxycillin plus metronidazole on the eradication of *Helicobacter pylori* and the recurrence of duodenal ulcer. *N Engl J Med* 1993; **328:** 308–12.

4 Graham DY, Hepps KS, Ramirez FC, *et al.* Treatment of *Helicobacter pylori* reduces the rate of rebleeding in peptic ulcer disease. *Scand J Gastroenterol* 1993; **28:** 939–42.

5 McColl KEL, El-Omar E, Gillen D, Banerjee S. The role of *Helicobacter pylori* in the pathophysiology of duodenal ulcer disease and gastric cancer. *Semin Gastroenterol Dis* 1997; **8:** 142–55.

6 McColl KEL, El-Nujumi A, Murray S, *et al.* Assessment of symptomatic response as predictor of *Helicobacter pylori* status following eradication therapy in patients with ulcer. *Gut* 1998; **42:** 618–22.

7 Labenz J, Borsch G. Evidence for the essential role of *Helicobacter pylori* in gastric ulcer disease. *Gut* 1994; **35:** 19–22.

8 Hawkey CJ, Karrasch JA, Szczepanski L, *et al.* Omeprazole compared with misoprostol for ulcers associated with nonsteroidal antiinflammatory drugs. *N Engl J Med* 1998; **338:** 727–34.

9 Forman D, Newell D G, Fullerton F, *et al.* Association between infection with *Helicobacter pylori* and risk of gastric cancer: evidence from a prospective investigation. *Br Med J* June 1991; **302:** 1302–5.

10 Hansen SE, Vollset K, Melby S, *et al.* Gastric mucosal atrophy is a strong predictor of non-cardia gastric cancer but not of cardia cancer (abstract). *Gastroenterology* 1998; **114.**

11 El-Omar E, Orien K, El-Nujumi A, *et al.* Prevalence of atrophy and hypochlorhydria is high in gastric cancer relatives and related to *H. pylori* status (abstract) *Gastroenterology* 1998; **114.**

12 Zucca E, Bertoni F, Roggero E, *et al.* Molecular analysis of the progression from *Helicobacter pylori* associated chronic gastritis to mucosa-associated lymphoid tissue lymphoma of the stomach. *N Engl J Med* 1998; **338:** 804–10.

13 Weber DM, Dimopoulos MA, Anandu DP, *et al.* Regression of gastric lymphoma of mucosa-associated lymphoid tissue with antibiotic therapy for *Helicobacter pylori. Gastroenterology* 1994; **107:** 1835–8.

14 McColl KEL, Murray K, El-Omar E, *et al.* Symptomatic benefit from eradicating *Helicobacter pylori* infection in patients with non-ulcer dyspepsia. *N Engl J Med* 1998; **339:** 1869–74.

15 Labenz J, Blum AL, Bayerdörffer E, *et al.* Curing *Helicobacter pylori* infection in patients with duodenal ulcer may provoke reflux esophagitis. *Gastroenterology* 1997; **112**: 1442–7.

16 Kuipers EJ, Lee A, Klinkenberg-Knol EC, Meuwissen SGM. The development of atrophic gastritis: *Helicobacter pylori* and the effects of acid suppressive therapy (review). *Aliment Pharmacol Ther* 1995; **9**: 331–40.

17 Labenz J, Tillenburg B, Peitz U, *et al. Helicobacter pylori* augments the pH-increasing effect of omeprazole in patients with duodenal ulcer. *Gastroenterology* 1996; **110**: 725–32.

18 McColl KEL, El-Nujumi A, Murray L, *et al.* The *Helicobacter pylori* breath test: a surrogate marker for peptic ulcer disease in dyspeptic patients. *Gut* 1997; **40**: 302–6.

☐ MULTIPLE CHOICE QUESTIONS

1 *Helicobacter pylori* infection is associated with an increased risk of developing:
- (a) Adenocarcinoma of the gastro-oesophageal junction (cardia)
- (b) Adenocarcinoma of the mid or distal stomach
- (c) Gastric MALT lymphoma
- (d) Gastro-oesophageal reflux disease
- (e) Gastric ulcer

2 *Helicobacter pylori* infection can result in:
- (a) Increased gastric acid secretion
- (b) Decreased gastric acid secretion
- (c) Increased serum gastrin
- (d) Gastric atrophy
- (e) Gastric metaplasia of duodenal mucosa

3 Eradication of *Helicobacter pylori* infection:
- (a) Produces resolution of symptoms in most patients with non-ulcer dyspepsia
- (b) Prevents recurrence of ulceration in 90% of duodenal ulcer patients
- (c) May result in regression of gastric MALT lymphoma
- (d) Is recommended in all subjects with a positive *H. pylori* test
- (e) Is best achieved by prescribing a seven-day course of omeprazole plus amoxycillin

ANSWERS

1a False	2a True	3a False
b True	b True	b True
c True	c True	c True
d False	d True	d False
e True	e True	e False

Diet and colon cancer

Jonathan M Rhodes

□ INTRODUCTION

Colon cancer is, after lung cancer, the second commonest cancer-related cause of death. For many years, it has been widely accepted that environmental influences, especially diet, are its major aetiological factors. Unfortunately, the dietary factors that might cause or prevent it have not yet been determined with certainty, making it difficult to give clear advice that might substantially reduce the risk.

□ EVIDENCE FOR ENVIRONMENTAL FACTORS

Doll and Peto, in a classic epidemiological review in 1981, pointed out that the known incidence of colon cancer varied markedly between countries; for example, the incidence in those under 65 years old in Connecticut, USA, was 10 times that in Nigeria [1]. They deduced that about 90% of the colon cancer risk in the USA was environmentally determined, probably by diet. The strong effect of environment has also been demonstrated in studies of migrant populations, including the four-fold increase in cancer of the colon and rectum in Japanese who had migrated to Hawaii [2] (Fig. 1).

□ THE FIBRE STORY: DANGERS OF OVERENTHUSIASTIC EXTRAPOLATION

Dennis Burkitt first drew attention to the large stool bulk of indigenous Africans, who have very low rates of colon cancer. A striking negative correlation between colon cancer risk and stool weight was confirmed by Cummings *et al* [4] in a study of 23 population groups in 12 countries (Fig. 2). This study also demonstrated a correlation between stool weight and dietary non-starch polysaccharide (fibre) content and, together with similar studies, led to the conclusion that a high fibre intake would protect against colon cancer.

With time, however, the fibre story has become less convincing. There is strong epidemiological evidence for a protective effect of vegetable consumption, with 23 of 28 studies reviewed by Potter [5] supporting this view. Similar studies of cereal fibre, however, showed no association in seven studies, a protective effect in only two, and increased risk in three [3]. Studies in animal cancer models are similarly inconclusive, some showing increased cancer rates with cereal fibre and no effect of inert bulking agents. It now seems likely that the apparent protective effect of vegetable consumption is not related simply to fibre content, and that dietary fibre supplementation (eg with bran) will not necessarily protect against colon cancer.

An alternative hypothesis, initially plausible, was that the protective effect of

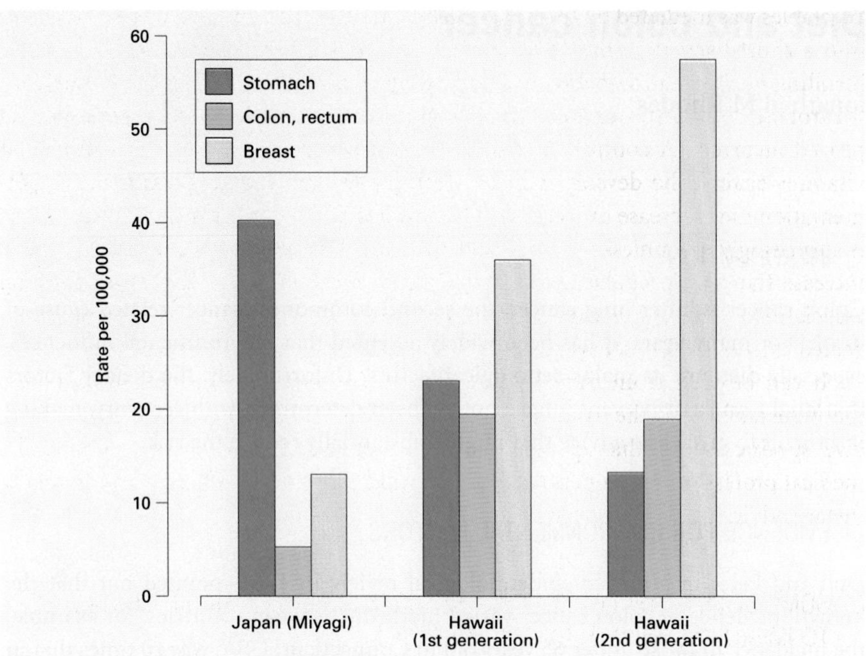

Fig. 1 Cancer incidence for selected cancers in Japanese women by generation in Hawaii and Japan, 1968–77 (from Ref [3]; data age-adjusted to the world standard population from Ref [2]).

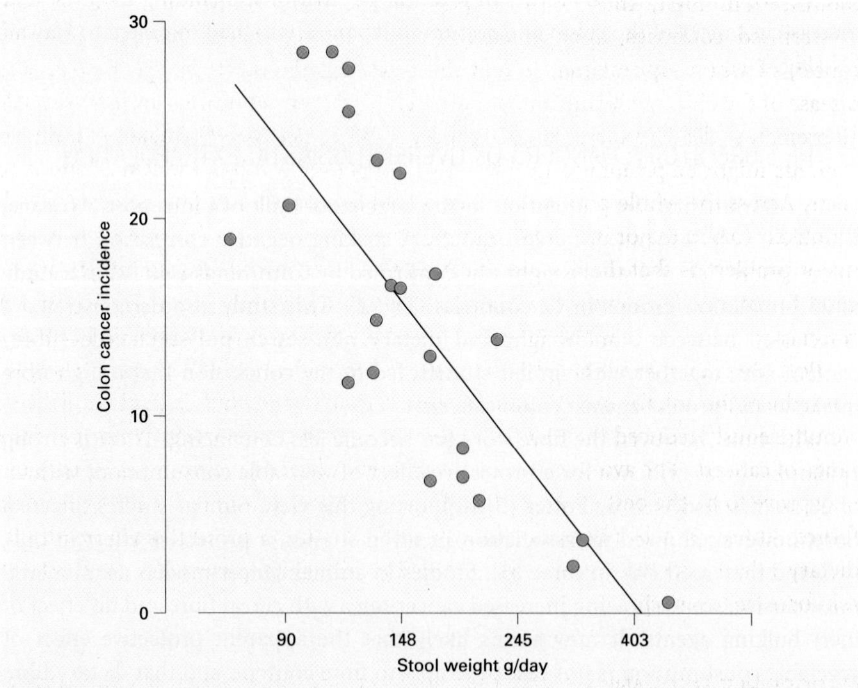

Fig. 2 Colon cancer incidence per 100,000 versus stool weight. Data from 23 population groups in 12 countries (from Ref [4] by permission of *Gastroenterology*).

vegetables was mediated by their antioxidant vitamin content. This was extrapolated into a short-lived experiment to market chocolate-coated carrots, in the hope of instilling healthy eating habits at an early age. Carrots are rich in the antioxidant β-carotene, but unfortunately the assumptions underlying this experiment all proved incorrect. A controlled trial has shown no protective effect of antioxidant vitamins against the development of colon polyps [6]; indeed β-carotene supplementation may increase cancer risk. Also, the availability of β-carotene from carrots is surprisingly low unless they have been cooked. Finally, the chocolate coating will increase the calorie intake and favour obesity, and both these factors have strong associations with colon cancer. Overall, encouraging children to eat chocolate-coated carrots might increase rather than reduce their risk for colon cancer.

It can be seen from this that we must have a detailed understanding of the mechanisms behind the associations between diet and colon cancer before we can give specific rather than general dietary recommendations to the public. The medical profession has not enhanced its reputation by the conflicting and changing dietary advice that it has given in the past.

☐ SOME SIMPLE BUT DEPRESSING STATISTICS: FUNDAMENTAL OBSTACLES TO IMPROVING HEALTH BY ALTERING DIET

Even when the associations between diet and colon cancer are understood, substantial practical problems will make it difficult to improve survival through dietary modification. First, there is a simple but formidable arithmetic obstacle. In Westernised countries, approximately 6% of the population develop colorectal cancer, of whom approximately half die from the disease. It is, on the whole, a disease of the elderly; the median age of affected patients at death is over 60 years. If all premature deaths from colorectal cancer could be prevented by dietary modification, life might be prolonged in this 3% of the population by a median of about 10 years. Across the whole population, this would amount to just four months, which is unlikely to be a major incentive to change the dietary habits of the nation. Another major problem is that dietary modification that prevents one disease might not be good for others; for example, a high meat intake apparently increases the risk for colon cancer, but there is also evidence that it protects against oesophageal cancer.

Both these arguments suggest that a dietary modification will have most impact if it reduces the risk for more than one disease. Indeed, the ideal would be a diet that simultaneously reduced the risk for ischaemic heart disease together with that for a range of cancers. The avoidance of obesity scores well in this respect (see below) and may prove to be the best evidence-based advice that we can offer for the foreseeable future. Although it has been notoriously difficult to prevent or reverse obesity by dietary advice, concentrating on the benefits of cancer prevention may help to reinforce this message.

☐ POSSIBLE MECHANISMS FOR DIETARY EFFECTS ON COLON CANCER RATES

Advances in molecular biology have greatly clarified the mechanisms that underlie the development of colon cancer. Central to this has been the increasing evidence in support of stepwise mutations in the adenoma-carcinoma sequence, as originally proposed by Hill *et al* [7] and expanded by Vogelstein [8] (Fig. 3). The basis of this hypothesis is that five or six mutations must occur in a stem cell before an invasive cancer develops. Since these mutations are most likely to occur during cell division, the risk for colon cancer development is determined at the cellular level by three factors: the mutation rate, the mitosis rate and apoptosis (programmed cell death) which can potentially rescue the situation by removing a mutated stem cell. Dietary factors may modulate colon cancer risk by affecting any of these processes, either directly or by altering the formation or metabolism of other agents that influence them. This makes it very difficult to screen foodstuffs for cancer risk. Simple bacterial screening tests for mutagenesis (eg the Ames test) are negative for some potent carcinogens such as asbestos, and even colon cell-based systems will miss the interactions that occur in the whole animal, for example between food, bile and bacteria.

The situation is further complicated by possible genetically determined variations in host response, such as malfunction in DNA repair genes (as in hereditary non-polyposis colon cancer) or inherited alterations in the metabolism of a pro-carcinogen. For example, it has been suggested that fast acetylators may be at greater risk when they eat meat, because N-acetylation of the heterocyclic amines produced when meat is burnt (barbecued) can produce a highly mutagenic metabolite that readily forms DNA adducts (Fig. 4).

Many substances in food are carcinogenic *in vitro* or in animal models, but their relative importance in human cancers is unknown. These include polycyclic hydrocarbons, present in foods that have been cooked at high temperature and particularly in smoked foods; N-nitroso compounds, found especially in preserved foods to which nitrites have been added; and heterocyclic amines, produced by the

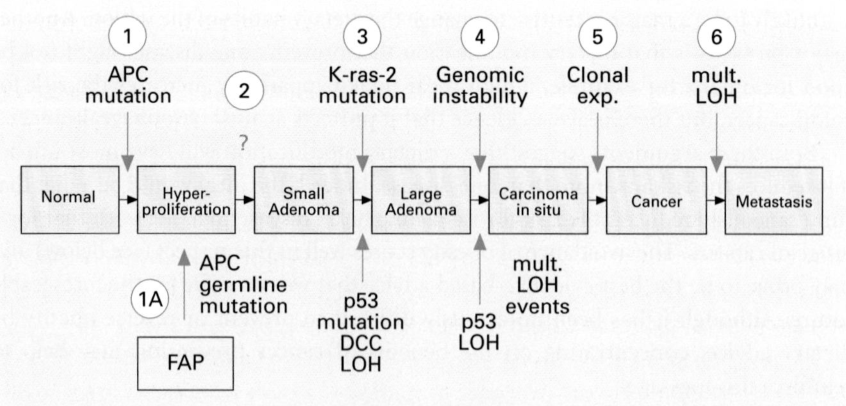

Fig. 3 Vogelstein hypothesis for multi-step aetiology of colon cancer (from Ref [9] by permission of the National Cancer Institute and Oxford University Press). APC = gene for adenomatous polyposis coli; FAP = familial adenomatous polyposis; DCC = gene 'deleted in colonic cancer'; LOH = loss of heterozygosity (ie resulting in loss of the only normally functioning allele).

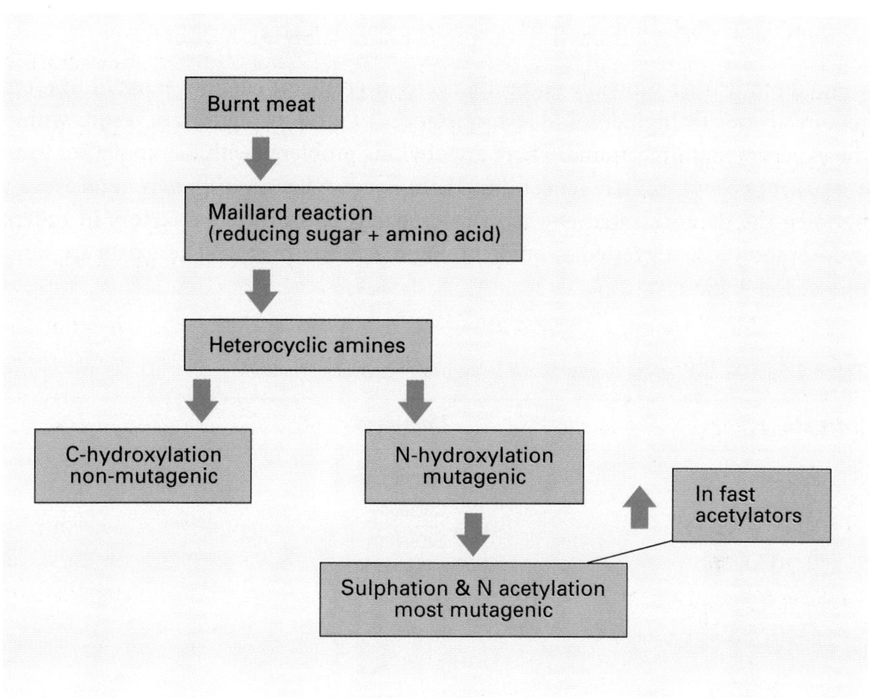

Fig. 4 A potential gene/environmental interaction: acetylator status and burnt meat.

Maillard reaction between reducing sugars and amino acids when meat is burnt. In addition, Hill [10] and others have noted the potential for the intestinal bacterial flora to produce endogenous carcinogens.

High fat intake is one of the most consistent dietary correlates with colon cancer, and this has focused research on the carcinogenic effects of secondary bile acids such as deoxycholate and lithocholate; these are released following bacterial deconjugation of bile and are present in increased amounts in response to a high fat intake. An alternative hypothesis, proposed by Morotomi *et al* [11], is that fat is a source of diacylglycerol, an important component of the signalling cascade which results in proliferation of epithelial cells.

Finally, severe dietary deficiencies of methionine, choline and folate have all been shown to increase the risk of DNA methylation abnormalities under experimental conditions, and epidemiological studies have reported a lower colon cancer rate in association with high intakes of folate and methionine.

The ways in which dietary components might counteract the effects of carcinogens are at least as numerous as the possible mechanisms for the carcinogens themselves. For example, protective factors could inhibit carcinogens by inactivating them (eg isothiocyanates and glucosinolates) or blocking their formation (eg ascorbate), by suppressing DNA synthesis (eg carotenoids) or by inducing apoptosis (eg short-chain fatty acids produced by bacterial fermentation of fibre) [5].

☐ EVIDENCE FROM FEEDING STUDIES IN EXPERIMENTAL MODELS

Animal models are probably better than *in vitro* tests for carcinogenicity but often require artificially high doses of test substances to produce significant results within the experimental time-frame. There are obvious problems with extrapolation from animal models to human cancer, but there is generally an impressive consistency between the demonstrated effects of carcinogens and protective factors in rodent models and those suggested by epidemiological studies in man. These data are summarised in Table 1.

Table 1 Factors that affect experimental large bowel cancer in rodents.

Increase	Decrease
Bile diversion	Wheat bran
Cholestyramine	Cellulose
Colitis	Selenium
Butyrate	Vitamin C
Vitamin A deficiency	Vitamin E
Wheat bran (during initiation)	Beta carotene
Corn bran	Antibiotics
Neomycin	Indomethacin
	Cabbage
	Diallyl sulfide (garlic)

From Ref [12] by permission of J B Lippincott.

☐ EPIDEMIOLOGICAL EVIDENCE FOR DIETARY FACTORS

As the situation *in vivo* is so complex, evidence for links between a food and colon cancer can best be gained initially from epidemiological studies, and then followed by *in vitro* and animal studies to assess the possible mechanisms underlying any significant correlation.

Comparisons between national cancer rates and diet can be based on 'food disappearance' statistics (ie sales of specific items of food which are assumed to approximate to their consumption). These show a strong correlation between meat consumption and colon cancer risk (Fig. 5), though it was pointed out by Armstrong and Doll in 1975 [13] that similar correlations could also be shown between colon cancer risk and gross national product and that these effects may be attributable to affluence and overeating rather than to any specific foodstuff.

More specific information about individual foods can be obtained from case-control or cohort studies in which independence of the variables under test can be assessed statistically. These studies are usually based on food-frequency questionnaires, which probably allow cancer patients to recall their pre-illness diet reasonably accurately.

As already mentioned, there is strong evidence for a protective effect of

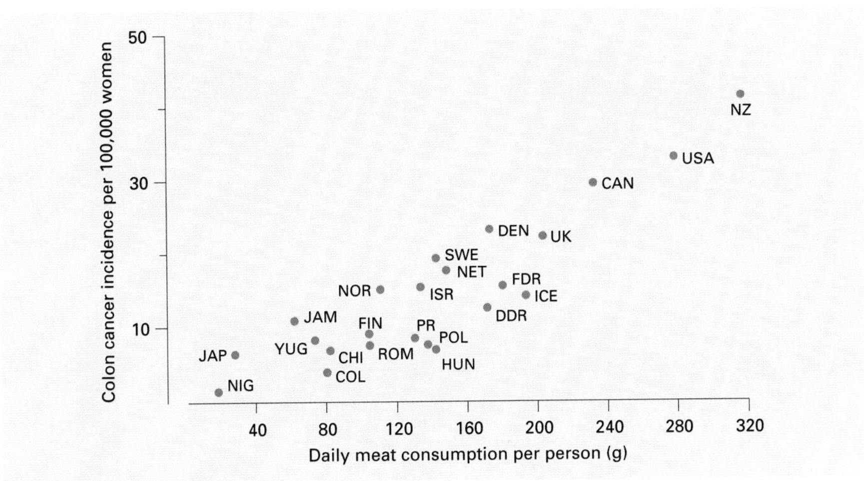

Fig. 5 Colon cancer incidence correlated with per capita meat consumption in different countries (from Ref [13] by permission of J Wiley & Sons Limited).

vegetables but an equivocal effect of cereal fibre, while 15 of 19 studies reported positive associations of colonic cancer with either animal fat or protein. Seventeen of 29 studies have shown an association between colon cancer and high red meat consumption, and the US Nurses Health Study found a significant dose-response for red meat consumption and even more strongly for the ratio of red meat to white meat [14] (Fig. 6). This remains a controversial area, as some studies – particularly from Europe – report no association between colon cancer risk and meat consumption; some Mediterranean countries such as Greece have high red meat intakes but low rates of colon cancer incidence. There is a possible pathophysiological basis for an effect of protein and particularly of fat. It is often forgotten that some fat and protein escape absorption and enter the colon, even in the absence of malabsorption, and there is evidence that an increased energy delivery here will increase the colon epithelial proliferation rate [15].

Significant associations have also been reported with obesity (Fig. 7) and lack of exercise, and it is not clear whether the dietary effects are related to any specific food components or simply to total energy intake.

Other reported associations with colon cancer – all weaker than those for energy intake, fat, meat and vegetables – include low intakes of calcium and vitamin D, folate, ascorbate and selenium. Selenium intake is very difficult to quantify as it is heavily dependent on the soil in which vegetables have been grown. Alcohol is also a risk factor but is difficult to distinguish from overall energy intake. Some but not all studies have shown a specific association with beer drinking, implying that a component of beer other than its alcohol content is responsible.

Further details of the relevant literature on colon cancer epidemiology can be found in the recent comprehensive review by Potter [5]. The possible roles of two specific dietary components – lectins and isothiocyanates – will be discussed here in more detail to illustrate the possible mechanisms involved.

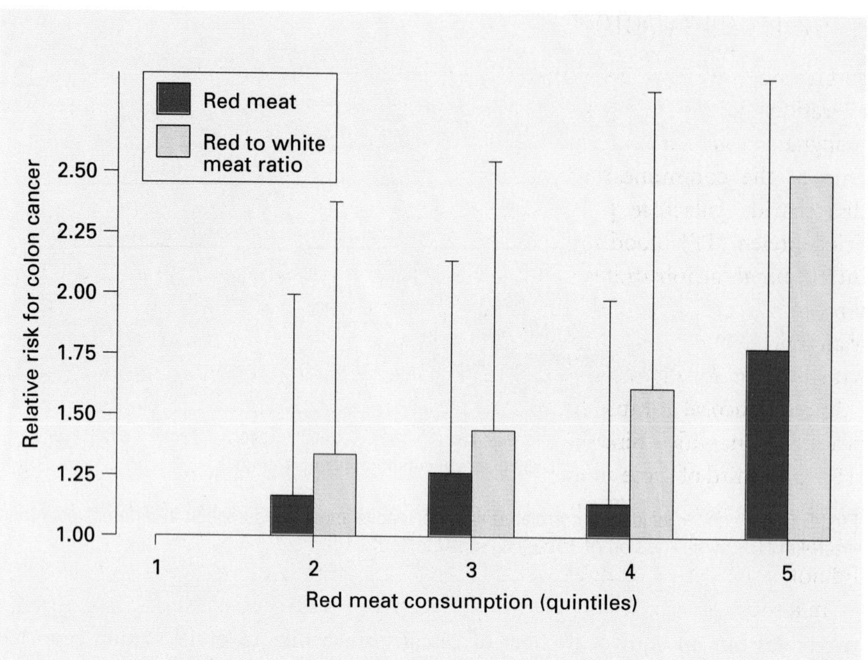

Fig. 6 Colon cancer risk correlated with quintiles for meat consumption, shown as relative risk and 95% CI (from Ref [14] by permission of the *N Engl J Med*).

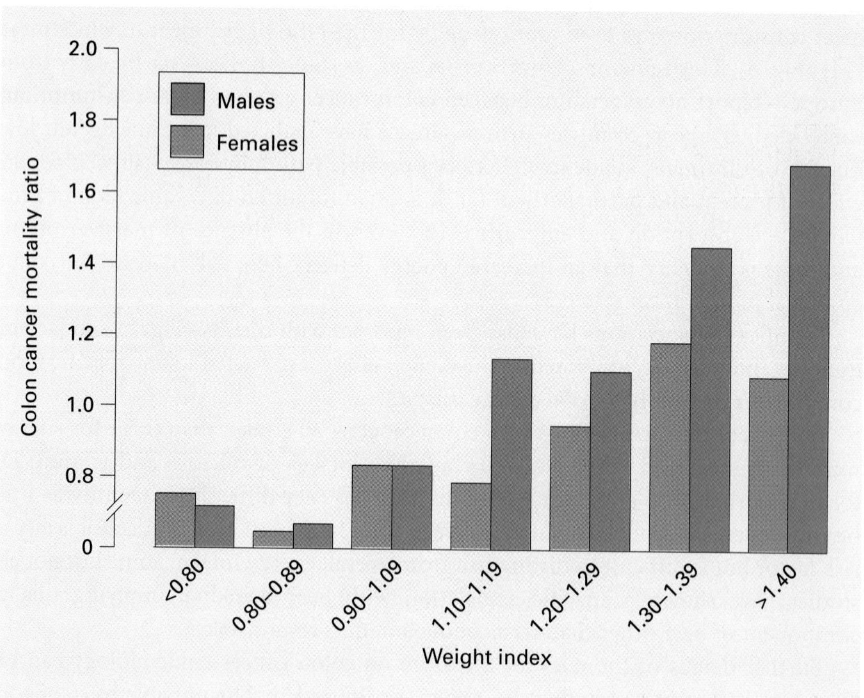

Fig. 7 Colon cancer risk versus body weight (the weight index is related to the subjects' 'ideal' body weight of 100%). (Drawn from data in Ref [16].)

☐ THE LECTIN-GALACTOSE STORY

In Liverpool, we have been interested in the possible functional significance of the alterations in mucosal glycosylation that are seen in colon cancer and in premalignant conditions such as adenomatous polyps and inflammatory bowel disease. One of the commonest abnormalities is increased mucosal expression of the disaccharide galactose β-1,3-N-acetylgalactosamine α-, which is the Thomsen Friedenreich (TF) blood group antigen [17]. We speculated that this might allow intraluminal carbohydrate-binding proteins (lectins) of dietary or bacterial origin to bind to mucosal cells and thus affect their proliferation and metabolism (Fig. 8). Many such lectins are tightly globular proteins which pass through the digestive tract with little or no digestion. In a series of studies – initially in cell lines, then on cultured mucosal samples and finally in human subjects – we have shown that peanut lectin, which binds the TF antigen, stimulates colon epithelial proliferation [18]. One-third of these subjects (patients with irritable bowel syndrome or sporadic polyps) expressed the TF antigen and, when they ate 100 g of peanuts per day for five days, the rectal mitotic index increased by about 40%; by contrast, subjects who did not express the TF antigen showed no significant response (Figs 9 and 10) [19].

In a subsequent case-control study of diet and colon cancer based in Merseyside,

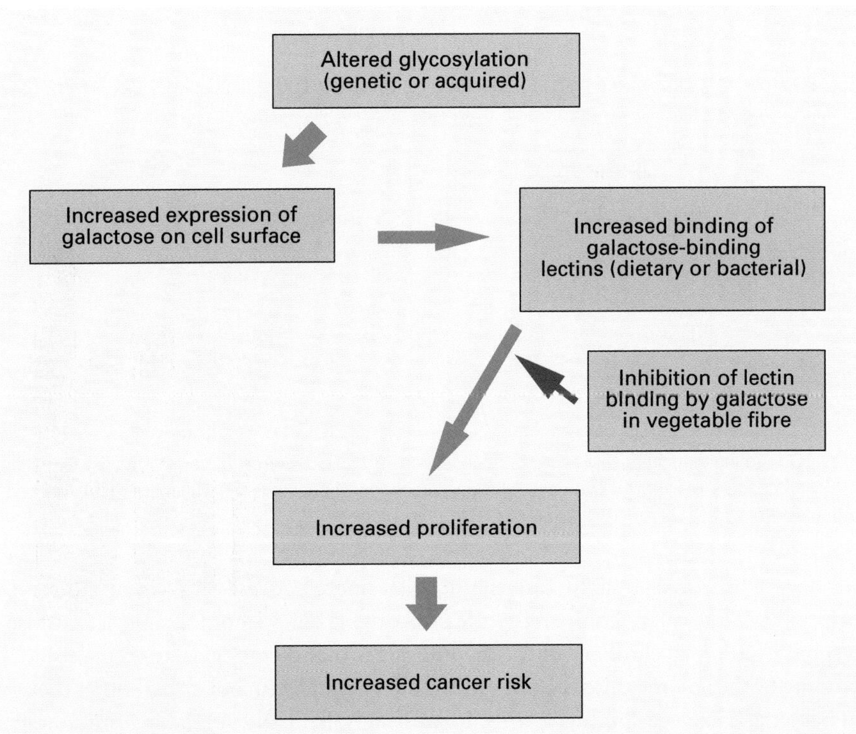

Fig. 8 Lectin/galactose hypothesis for interaction between altered mucosal glycosylation, either acquired or possibly genetically determined, and dietary galactose-binding lectins with inhibition by vegetable fibre containing galactose.

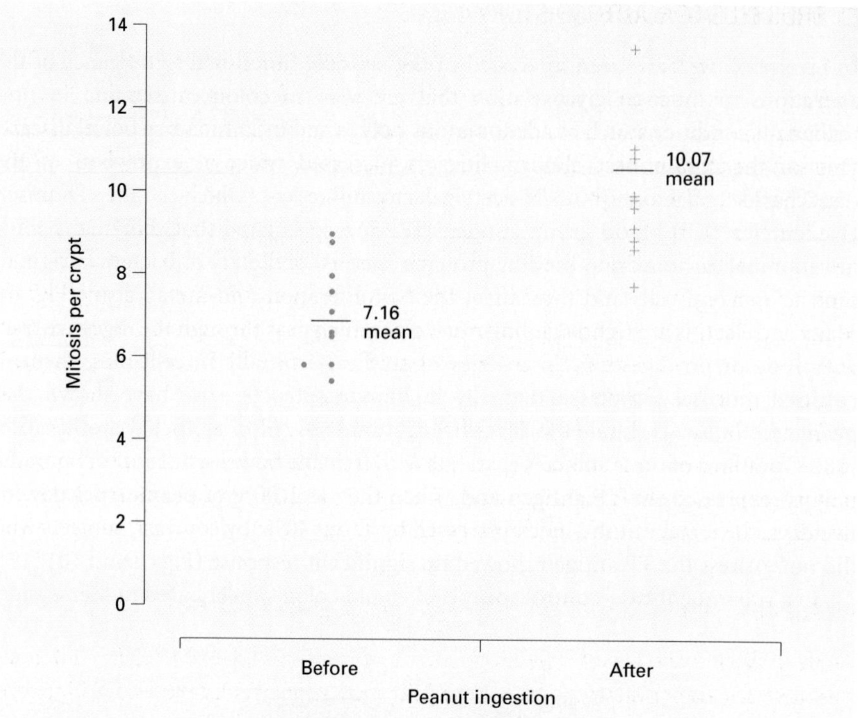

Fig. 9 Mitotic response of the human rectal mucosa to eating 100 g peanuts per day for five days (p=0.0009) (from Ref [18] by permission of *Gastroenterology*).

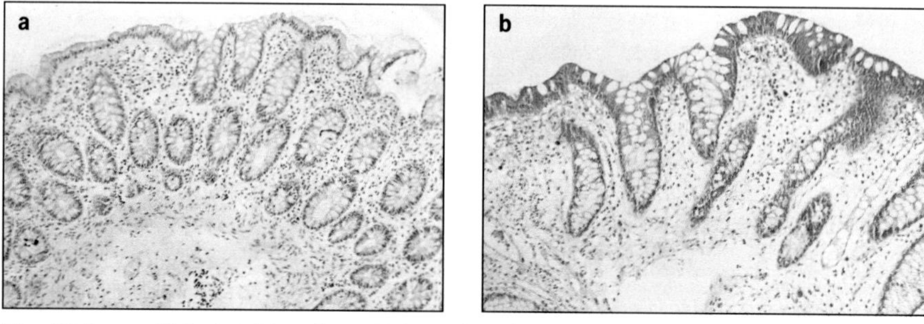

Fig. 10 Immunohistochemistry of rectal biopsy from a subject before **(a)** and after **(b)** ingesting 100 g of peanuts per day for five days, showing presence of peanut lectin within the rectal mucosa. (Adapted from Ref [18] by permission of *Gastroenterology*.)

we have confirmed a slight but significantly increased risk for colon cancer in habitual peanut eaters compared with non-eaters, but without a significant dose-response [20]. The corollary of this hypothesis is that dietary galactose might block binding to the colonic mucosa, not only of the peanut lectin but also of other dietary or bacterial galactose-binding lectins. Interestingly, fruit and vegetable fibre contains substantial amounts of galactose whereas cereal fibre does not, and our recent case-control study shows a trend towards a protective effect of vegetable fibre which becomes significant when assessed as fibre galactose content.

☐ BRUSSELS SPROUTS AND ISOTHIOCYANATES

It is possible that the apparent protective effect of vegetables might be attributable to a single species or group of species rather than a general effect of all vegetables. In 1978, Graham and colleagues [21] noted a particularly strong protective effect associated with consumption of brassicas (cabbage, Brussels sprouts and broccoli). These plants contain substantial amounts of isothiocyanates (R–N=C=S), the 'mustard oils' which give brassicas their pungent taste, and their glucosinolate precursors which can inhibit development of carcinogen-induced tumours in rodents. Subsequent studies have shown that the potent anticarcinogenic effects of these chemicals are probably the consequence of two complementary mechanisms, namely the suppression of carcinogen activation by cytochrome P-450 enzymes and the induction of 'Phase 2' enzymes such as glutathione transferases and NAD(P)H:quinone reductase which detoxify electrophilic metabolites generated by cytochrome activation [22]. Concentrations of the cancer-preventive substances are up to 100-fold higher in three-day-old sprouts than in mature plants – yet one more example of the complexities involved in attempting to formulate useful, evidence-based dietary advice [23].

☐ ASPIRIN AND COX-2: PREVENTION OF CANCER AND OTHER DISEASES?

There is now considerable evidence that chronic ingestion of aspirin and non-steroidal anti-inflammatory drugs (NSAIDs) such as piroxicam and sulindac is associated with reductions of up to 50% in colon cancer mortality, decreases in polyp growth and recurrence in man, and protection against chemically induced colon cancer in animal models [23]. This effect is probably mediated by inhibition of inducible cyclooxygenase (COX-2). COX-2 mRNA levels increase rapidly with mitotic stimulation of cells, and expression of the enzyme is increased in human colon cancers and in carcinogen-induced cancer in rodents; moreover, COX-2 over-expression results in resistance to apoptosis (Fig. 11). Cross-breeding between mice with polyposis due to a mutated APC (adenomatous polyposis coli) gene and COX-2 knockout mice has shown an 80–90% reduction in polyps in offspring that lack COX-2 (reviewed in [23]). A recent study in azoxymethane-induced colon cancer in rats showed that dietary supplementation with corn oil enhanced the carcinogen-induced increase in COX-2 expression and increased the number and size of tumours, whereas fish oil resulted in lower levels of COX-2 and in fewer and smaller tumours [24].

COX-2 inhibition, whether induced by fish oil or NSAIDs, also correlates with reduced risk for ischaemic heart disease. This strategy may therefore be coming close to our previously stated need for a dietary modification that could simultaneously protect against major killers of Western man, namely cancer and heart disease.

☐ THE FUTURE: INTERVENTION STUDIES

We are at last approaching the point where we have sufficient knowledge to test specific dietary interventions in controlled studies. As most colon cancers are thought to originate from adenomatous polyps, relatively short-term intervention

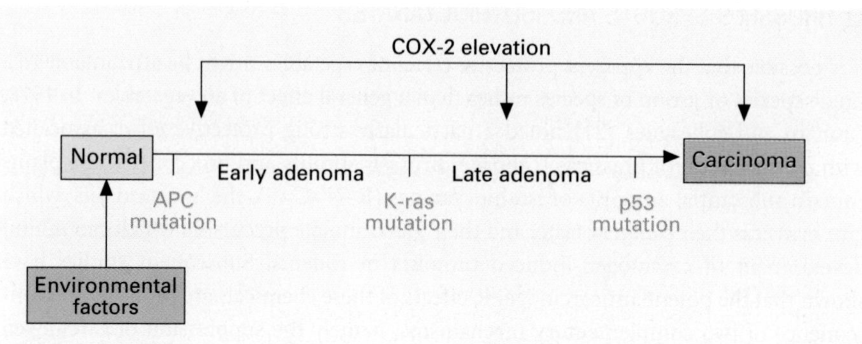

Fig. 11 Postulated sites of interaction for COX-2 in the Vogelstein model of colon cancer development (from Ref [21] by permission of the National Cancer Institute and Oxford University Press).

Table 2 Diet and colon cancer: questions that need answers

What foods should you eat? (eg which vegetables?)
Where should they be grown? (cf selenium)
How should they be harvested? (young sprouts)
How should they be cooked? (burnt meat)
How quickly should they be eaten? (is slowly, better?)
Which foods are good for which genes? (can slow acetylators eat roast beef?)
Does it matter what food you eat if you take an aspirin a day?

studies can be performed with polyp recurrence as the end-point. Some such studies have already been performed, though findings have so far been generally negative. They have, for example, shown a lack of significant benefit from supplementation with antioxidants [6] or from a combination of low fat, wheat bran and β-carotene [20]; however, the latter study demonstrated that the combination of low fat intake and added wheat bran significantly prevented the appearance of large adenomas.

To be successful, compliance with the recommended intervention would have to be high. It seems highly likely that weight loss in obese people would reduce their risk for colon cancer but, with the exception of gastric bypass or other surgical measures, predictably successful anti-obesity interventions have not yet been found. A more successful approach might be to exploit the impressive evidence regarding isothiocyanates and COX-2 inhibitors, in either of two ways: a trial of dietary modification with increased intake of fish and brassicas, or a placebo-controlled trial with purified or synthetic isothiocyanates and COX-2 inhibitors.

The latter approach might be regarded as defeatist by advocates of a natural healthy environment but might also achieve greater compliance amongst the sausage and chip eaters who are likely to be at greatest risk for colon cancer. Alternatively, there may still be a place for a herring or a plateful of young Brussels sprouts every day, rather than an aspirin.

REFERENCES

1 Doll R, Peto R. Avoidable risks of cancer in the US. *J Natl Cancer Inst* 1981; **66**: 1196–308.

2 Kolonel LN, Hinds MW, Hankin JH. Cancer patterns among migrant and native-born Japanese in Hawaii in relation to smoking, drinking and dietary habits. In: Gelboin HV, *et al* (Eds) *Genetic and Environmental Factors in Experimental and Human Cancer.* Tokyo, Japan Sci Soc Press, 1980: 327–40

3 World Cancer Research Fund/American Institute for Cancer Research. *Food, Nutrition and the Prevention of Cancer: a Global Perspective.* Washington: American Institute for Cancer Research, 1997: 216–51.

4 Cummings JH, Bingham SA, Heaton KW, *et al.* Fecal weight, colon cancer risk, and dietary intake of nonstarch polysaccharides (dietary fibre). *Gastroenterology* 1992; **103**: 1783–9.

5 Potter JD. Nutrition and colorectal cancer. *Cancer Causes and Control* 1996; **7**: 127–46.

6 Greenberg ER, Baron JA, Tosteson TD, *et al.* A clinical trial of antioxidant vitamins to prevent colorectal adenoma. Polyp prevention study group. *N Engl J Med* 1994; **331**: 141–7.

7 Hill MJ, Morson BC, Bussey HJR. Aetiology of adenoma-carcinoma sequence in large bowel. *Lancet* 1978; **i**: 245–7.

8 Vogelstein B, Fearon ER, Hamilton SR, *et al.* Genetic alterations during colorectal tumour development. *N Engl J Med* 1988; **319**: 525.

9 MacLennan R, Macrae F, Bain C, *et al.* Randomized trial of fat, fiber and beta carotene to prevent colorectal adenomas. The Australian polyp prevention project. *J Natl Cancer Inst* 1995; **87**: 1760–6.

10 Hill MJ. Bacterial metabolism and human carcinogenesis. *Br Med Bull* 1980; **36**: 89–94.

11 Morotomi M, Guillem JG, Lo Gerfo P, Weinstein IB. Production of diacylglycerol, an activator of protein kinase C, by human intestinal microflora. *Cancer Res* 1990; **50**: 3595–9.

12 Boland CR. Malignant tumours of the colon. In: Yamada T (Ed). *Textbook of Gastroenterology* 2nd edn. Philadelphia: JB Lippincott, 1995: 1967–2026.

13 Armstrong B, Doll R. Environmental factors and cancer incidence and mortality in different countries, with special reference to dietary practices. *Int J Cancer* 1975; **15**: 617–31.

14 Willet WC, Stampfer MJ, Colditz GA, *et al.* Relation of meat and fiber intake to the risk of colon cancer in a prospective study of colon cancer among women. *N Engl J Med* 1990; **323**: 1664–72.

15 Pell JD, Johnson IT, Goodlad RA. The effects of and the interactions between fermentable dietary fiber and lipid in germ-free and conventional rats. *Gastroenterology* 1995; **108**: 1745–52.

16 Lew EA, Garfinkel L. Variations in mortality by weight among 75,000 men and women. *J Chronic Dis* 1979; **32**: 563–76.

17 Campbell BJ, Hounsell E, Finnie IA, Rhodes JM. Direct demonstration of increased expression of Thomson-Friedenreich antigen (Galβ1-3GalNAc) by mucus in colon cancer and inflammatory bowel disease. *J Clin Invest* 1995; **95**: 571–6.

18 Ryder SD, Parker N, Eccleston D, *et al.* Peanut lectin (PNA) stimulates proliferation in colonic explants from patients with ulcerative colitis, Crohn's disease and colonic polyps. *Gastroenterology* 1994; **106**: 117–24.

19 Ryder SD, Jacyna MR, Levi AJ, *et al.* Eating peanuts increases rectal proliferation in individuals with mucosal expression of peanut lectin receptor. *Gastroenterology* 1998; **114**: 44–9.

20 Evans RC, Ashby D, Hackett A, *et al.* Consumption of peanuts, which contain a galactose-binding lectin, associates with increased risk for colorectal cancer whereas high non-starch polysaccharide galactose intake associates with reduced risk. *Gut* 1997; **41** (Suppl 3): A124.

21 Graham S, Dayal H, Swanson M, *et al.* Diet in the aetiology of cancer of the colon and rectum. *J Natl Cancer Inst* 1978; **61**: 709–14.

22 Verhoeven DT, Verhagen H, Goldbohm RA, *et al.* A review of mechanisms underlying anticarcinogenicity by brassica vegetables. *Chemico-Biological Interactions* 1997; **103**: 79–129.

23 Williams CS, Smalley W, DuBois RN. Aspirin use and potential mechanisms for colorectal cancer prevention. *J Clin Invest* 1997; **100**: 1325–9.

24 Singh J, Hamid R, Reddy BS. Dietary fat and colon cancer: modulation of cyclooxygenase-2 by types and amount of dietary fat during postinitiation stage of colon carcinogenesis. *Cancer Res* 1997; 57: 3465–70.

☐ MULTIPLE CHOICE QUESTIONS

1 The following are strongly associated with increased risk for colon cancer:
  (a) Low cereal fibre intake
  (b) Low vegetable intake
  (c) High fish intake
  (d) High fat intake
  (e) Obesity

2 Viable theories for explaining the protective effect of vegetables on colon cancer include:
  (a) Accelerated colon transit
  (b) Increased faecal pH
  (c) Cyclooxygenase (COX-2) inhibition
  (d) Isothiocyanate content
  (e) Galactose content

3 Which of the following statements concerning COX-2 inhibition and colon cancer are true?
  (a) Consumption of aspirin 300 mg/day has been associated with a 50% reduction in mortality from colon cancer
  (b) Corn oil feeding in experimental cancer increases COX-2 and increases risk for colon cancer
  (c) COX-2 expression is increased in colon cancer
  (d) Increased COX-2 expression inhibits apoptosis
  (e) Brussels sprouts only have significant COX-2 inhibitory activity when picked very young

4 Which of the following statements concerning isothiocyanates are true?
  (a) Brassicas are a rich source
  (b) Isothiocyanates suppress carcinogen activation by cytochrome p450 enzymes
  (c) Isothiocyanates induce glutathione transferase which detoxifies carcinogenic metabolites
  (d) Synthetic isothiocyanates have been shown in controlled trials to reduce colon cancer risk
  (e) Concentration of isothiocyanates in vegetables may vary up to 100 fold depending on their maturity when picked

5 Which of the following statements concerning the lectin/galactose hypothesis for diet and colon cancer are true?
  (a) Dietary lectins may survive transit through the gastrointestinal tract without digestion

(b) Dietary lectins may bind to blood group antigens expressed on the luminal surface of intestinal cells
(c) Cereal fibre is particularly rich in galactose
(d) Increased mucosal expression of unsubstituted galactose is a common feature in malignant and pre-malignant intestine
(e) Daily peanut consumption may increase rectal mitotic index by 40% in individuals who express mucosal galactose

ANSWERS

1a False	2a False	3a True	4a True	5a True
b True	b False	b True	b True	b True
c False	c False	c True	c True	c False
d True	d True	d True	d False	d True
e True	e True	e False	e True	e True

New prospects for the management of obesity: from molecular targets to novel drugs

Gareth Williams and Steven J McNulty

□ INTRODUCTION

If treatment imperatives relate to diseases that are common and dangerous to health, obesity should lie near the top of the list of priorities for most westernised countries. Obesity is already common in the developed world and rapidly becoming commoner, mainly because we fail to reduce our energy intake to compensate for the physical inactivity of the westernised lifestyle. In the UK, 15% of adults now have a body-mass index (BMI) that exceeds 30 kg/m^2, the threshold at which the risk of premature death begins to increase (Fig. 1) [1]. The prevalence of obesity in this country has doubled during the last decade and is set to continue rising; without a major preventive initiative in the next few years, Britons will soon catch up with present-day Americans, 25% of whom are overweight enough to shorten their life expectancy.

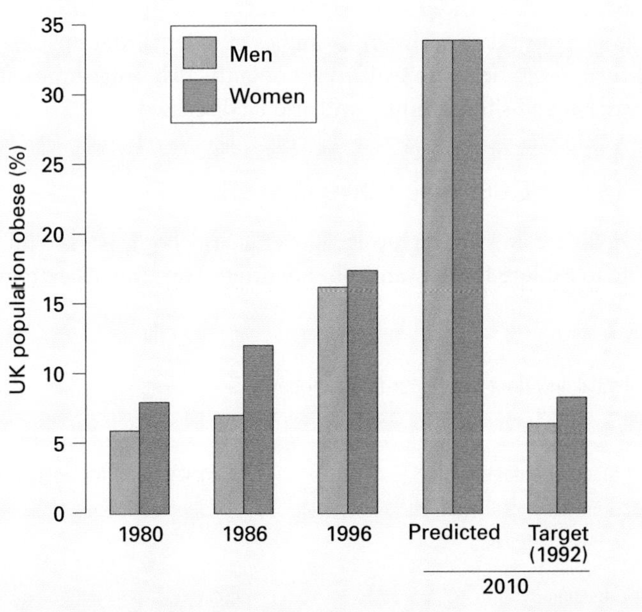

Fig. 1 Rising prevalence of obesity (body mass index >30 kg/m^2) in British men and women aged 16–64 years. The two far right columns show predicted prevalence in total adult population in 2010 compared with the target stated in *The health of the nation* (1992). Obesity has now been abandoned as a health target by the present UK Government.

Obesity can be mistaken for an essentially cosmetic issue, but only if its role as a powerful and independent risk factor for type 2 diabetes, hypertension, coronary heart disease and other serious conditions is ignored. The examples of rapid westernisation ('Cocacolonisation') in populations such as the Pima Indians of Arizona and the Nauruan Islanders of Micronesia suggest that the near-pandemic of obesity will soon be followed by dramatic increases in type 2 diabetes and ultimately premature cardiovascular death. It is unfortunate that influential voices, including the UK Government (Fig. 1) and authoritative medical journals [2], continue to underplay obesity's present and future threats to health.

Few doctors leap at the opportunity to manage obesity. Several factors are responsible, including the near-total neglect of the subject by undergraduate and postgraduate medical curricula; the persisting illusion that it is not a disease (and is the patient's fault anyway); and the absence of effective and safe anti-obesity drugs. Fortunately, times are changing. Obesity research has finally acquired scientific respectability, largely through the impact of molecular genetic techniques which have already answered several tantalising questions about the physiological control of energy balance in animals. Moreover, new understanding of several aspects of energy homeostasis has identified novel and potentially promising targets for the development of anti-obesity drugs (see Table 1). The key areas are: the central nervous system (CNS), which ultimately regulates both sides of the energy-balance equation; the thermogenic tissues; the gut, where energy enters the body; and the adipocyte, which has entered this arena with the discovery of leptin, a fat-derived hormone that acts on the CNS of rodents to inhibit feeding and stimulate thermogenesis.

This chapter will consider these options, concentrating on targets that appear promising now; most data derive from studies in rodents, and their extrapolation to man may turn out to be an unjustified act of faith. Two drugs now entering clinical service – orlistat and sibutramine – will also be discussed.

□ TARGETS IN THE CENTRAL NERVOUS SYSTEM

The CNS holds a commanding position over energy homeostasis and is therefore a rational site to explore for new anti-obesity drugs. However, its extreme complexity

Table 1 Potential new drug targets for treating obesity.

Central nervous system	Gut
• NPY Y5 receptor antagonists	• Inhibitors of triglyceride digestion (pancreatic lipase inhibitor: orlistat)
• Melanocortin-4 receptor agonists	
• Serotonin 5-HT$_{2c}$ agonists	
Thermogenic tissues	Leptin
• β_3 adrenoceptor agonists	• Recombinant human leptin
• Uncoupling agents	• Low-molecular weight leptin agonists

NPY, neuropeptide Y

demands accurate targeting, and therefore detailed understanding of the neural circuits and neurotransmitters that control feeding and energy expenditure. Previous centrally acting appetite suppressants were plagued with side effects ranging from addiction and dysphoria with dexamphetamine (an effective but unsafe weight-reducing drug) to the cardiovascular complications that led to the withdrawal of the fenfluramines. These problems have cast a long shadow, and future centrally acting drugs will be accepted only if they can demonstrate great selectivity and impeccable safety.

The hypothalamus plays a key role in coordinating energy balance and contains numerous neural pathways, some of which do not involve the classical 'feeding' and 'satiety' centres in the lateral hypothalamic area (LHA) and ventromedial nucleus, respectively (Fig. 2). Hypothalamic neurones contain a wealth of peptide and non-peptide neurotransmitters that affect feeding and/or energy expenditure when microinjected into specific hypothalamic sites or the adjacent cerebral ventricles. Some are more or less convincingly implicated in normal energy balance and in

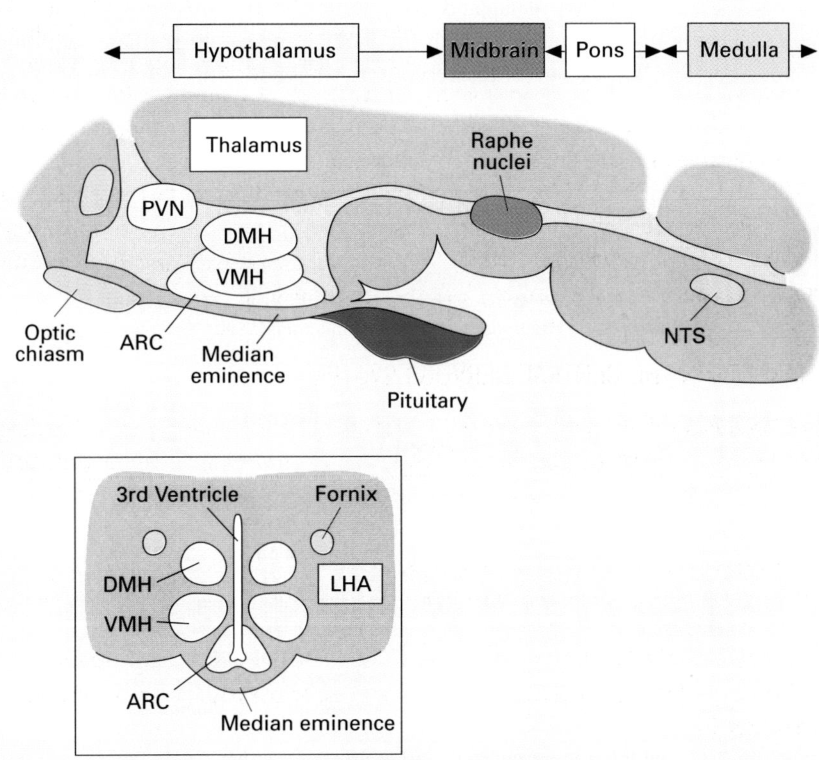

Fig. 2 The hypothalamus and some of the neural pathways involved in regulating energy balance in the rat: **top,** longitudinal section; **insert,** transverse section through mid-arcuate nucleus (ARC) (DMH, dorsomedial nucleus of the hypothalamus; LHA, lateral hypothalamic area; NTS, nucleus of the solitary tract; PVN, paraventricular nucleus; VMH, ventromedial nucleus).

causing obesity in animals (see Table 2), and various experimental approaches have been used to manipulate their availability or interactions with their receptors to decrease food intake and body weight (Fig. 3).

□ NEUROTRANSMITTERS THAT CAUSE WEIGHT LOSS

Serotonin

Serotonin (5-hydroxytryptamine, 5-HT) is synthesised by neurones of the raphe nucleus in the midbrain that project rostrally to various hypothalamic sites including the arcuate (ARC) and paraventricular nuclei (PVN) that are involved in controlling energy balance [3]. The ARC contains neuronal populations that produce neuropeptide Y (NPY) and melanocyte stimulating hormone (α-MSH), which respectively stimulate and inhibit feeding. The PVN is the site of convergence of many neural pathways involved in energy homeostasis (eg NPY and noradrenaline), and also contains neurones expressing corticotrophin-releasing factor (CRF), itself a potent hypophagic and thermogenic peptide.

Serotonin injected into the PVN and other sites inhibits feeding and stimulates thermogenesis, causing loss of fat and body weight. Numerous subtypes of 5-HT receptors have been identified, of which the 5-HT_{2c} appears to mediate serotonin's hypophagic action; 'knock-out' of this receptor in transgenic mice causes hyperphagia

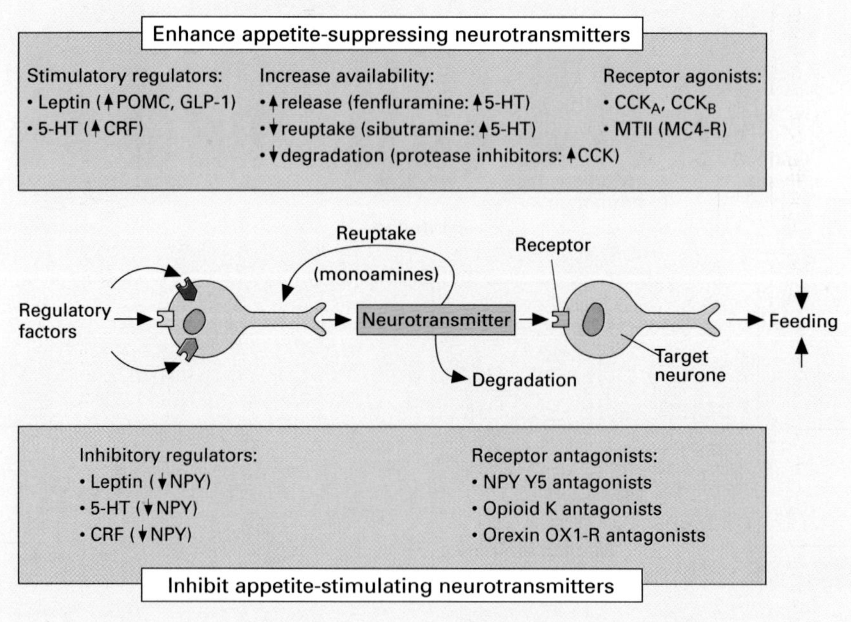

Fig. 3 Pharmacological approaches that manipulate appetite-regulating neurotransmitters to reduce food intake. Opposing strategies are used to target inhibitors (top) and stimulators (bottom) of feeding (CCK, cholecystokinin; CRF, corticotrophin-releasing factor; GLP, glucagon-like peptide; 5-HT, serotonin; MC4-R, melanocortin-4 receptor; NPY, neuropeptide Y; POMC, pro-opiomelanocortin).

Table 2 Some hypothalamic neurotransmitters implicated in the control of energy homeostasis.

	Neurones	Receptor	Other comments
Stimulate feeding			
NPY	ARC	Y5	• Most potent appetite stimulant known • ↓ thermogenesis, ↑ insulin secretion • Induces obesity with chronic administration
Galanin			• Transient stimulation of feeding only • Does not induce obesity
Orexin A	LHA	OX1-R	LHA most sensitive site
Noradrenaline	Medulla	$\alpha 2$	Potent Can induce obesity
Inhibit feeding			
Serotonin (5-HT)	Raphe nucleus	5-HT_{2c}	Potent
CCK	Periphery and CNS	• CCK_A (periphery) • CCK_B (brain)	• Combined peripheral (stomach) and central (NTS→PVN) actions
α-MSH	POMC in ARC	MC4-R	• MC4-R antagonised by agouti protein
CRF	PVN	CRF-2	• Inhibits NPY neurones in the ARC
GLP-1	Medulla	GLP-1	• Combined peripheral and central actions

ARC, arcuate nucleus; CCK, cholecystokinin; CNS, central nervous system; CRF, corticotrophin-releasing factor; GLP, glucagon-like peptide; LHA, lateral hypothalamic area; MC4-R, melanocortin-4 receptor; MSH, melanocyte stimulating hormone; NPY, neuropeptide Y; NTS, nucleus of the solitary tract; POMC, pro-opiomelanocortin; PVN, paraventricular nucleus.

and obesity. Interactions of 5-HT released in the hypothalamus with other neural pathways (eg inhibition of NPY, stimulation of CRF) may partly mediate its effects on energy balance.

Various serotonergic drugs have anti-obesity effects. The archetypes are fenfluramine (a racemate) and its D-isomer, dexfenfluramine, which enhance 5-HT action primarily by stimulating its release from nerve terminals; the fenfluramines also inhibit 5-HT reuptake and subsequent inactivation in the terminal. Both compounds cause weight loss in obese subjects (see Fig. 4), and about one-third of subjects lose more than the critical 10% of weight that is likely to confer definite clinical benefits [4]. As with all anti-obesity drugs tested to date, weight loss reaches a trough after several weeks, and weight is regained after stopping treatment.

Several concerns have been raised about the safety of the fenfluramines. Neurotoxicity (fall out of serotonin neurones) was seen in primates receiving high doses, and was attributed to the intense stimulation of 5-HT release. Rare, but potentially lethal, cardiovascular side effects, namely primary pulmonary hypertension (PPH) and valvular heart disease reminiscent of the carcinoid syndrome [5,6], led to withdrawal of the drugs in 1997. The cardiovascular complications have been attributed to raised 5-HT levels in plasma and/or platelets, favouring vasoconstriction, platelet aggregation and endothelial damage (see chapter 26).

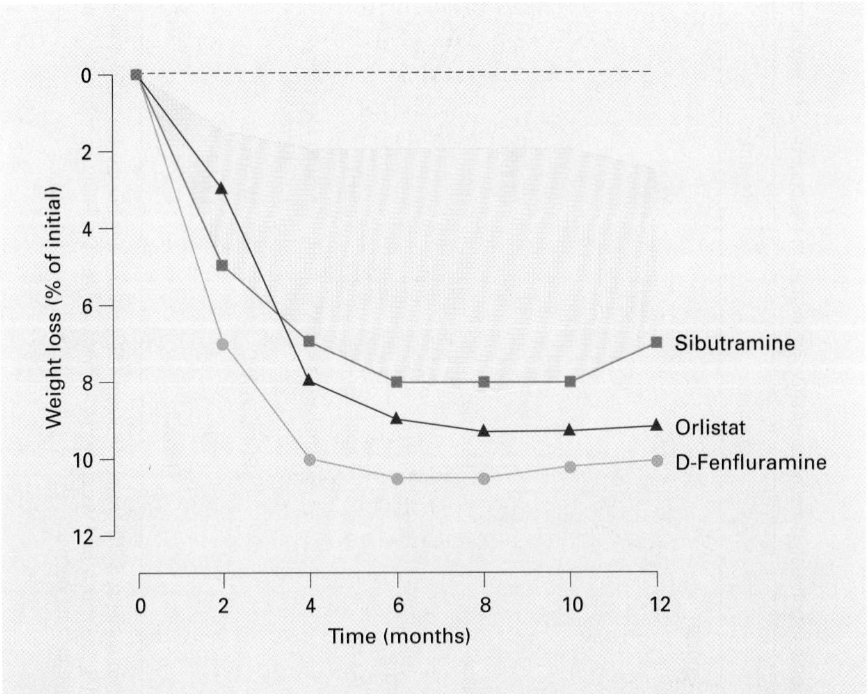

Fig. 4 Weight reduction achieved during clinical trials of sibutramine,[8] orlistat[26] and dexfenfluramine.[4] The yellow shaded area indicates the range of placebo responses in these trials: the upper limit is from the study of sibutramine and the lower limit from that of D-fenfluramine.

Sibutramine

Sibutramine is a centrally acting inhibitor of the reuptake of both 5-HT and noradrenaline. It is structurally distinct from the fenfluramines (see Fig. 5) and has a different mode of action: it does not stimulate 5-HT release, and does not apparently damage serotonergic neurones [7]. The significance of inhibiting noradrenaline reuptake is uncertain, but may confer central sympathomimetic activity; paradoxically, noradrenaline is a powerful feeding stimulant when injected into the PVN of the rat.

In humans, sibutramine inhibits appetite and may also have a mild thermogenic action. Clinical trials indicate that it is comparable to dexfenfluramine in its average weight-reducing effect (see Fig. 4) and in the percentage of treated patients (ca 30%) who lose more than the critical 10% of initial weight [8]. It appears to be well tolerated and there has been no evidence (including detailed prospective echocardiographic studies) of valvular damage or PPH; theoretically, these cardiovascular effects would not be anticipated, as inhibition of reuptake alone should not greatly elevate circulating 5-HT levels, and no causal link has been shown with other serotonin reuptake inhibitors such as fluoxetine. The main side effects are a mild tachycardia and a variable, but generally modest, elevation of blood pressure. These effects are presumably due to the central sympathomimetic action of sibutramine,

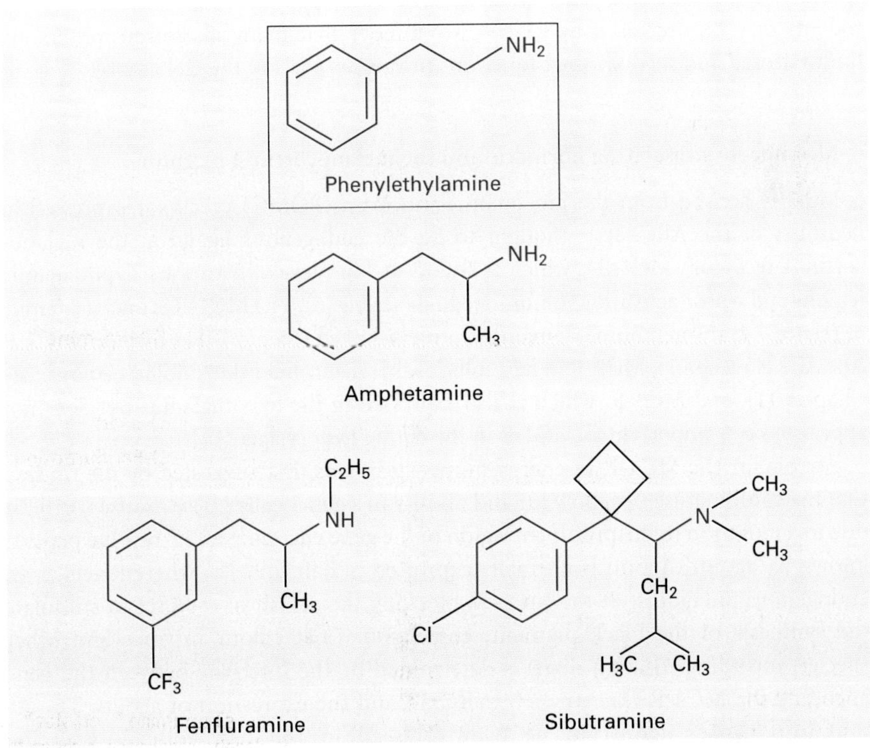

Fig. 5 Chemical structures of fenfluramine and sibutramine, contrasted with amphetamine.

and may be partly offset by the hypotensive effects of weight loss. However, caution will be required in patients with existing hypertension or heart disease.

Sibutramine is currently licensed for clinical use in North America, Latin America, Germany and Switzerland.

Cholecystokinin

Cholecystokinin (CCK) is a classical brain-gut peptide released from the intestine into the circulation after eating. As well as stimulating gall-bladder contraction, it may decrease food intake through both peripheral and central actions [9]. CCK apparently binds to specific CCK_A (peripheral-type) receptors expressed on vagal afferent (sensory) fibres in the stomach. The corresponding neurone cell bodies lie in the nucleus of the solitary tract (NTS) in the medulla, which projects to the PVN. This pathway involves the release of CCK, which here acts as a neurotransmitter that interacts with central-type (CCK_B) receptors.

Feeding is inhibited in rodents by giving a CCK_A agonist systemically or by injecting CCK into the PVN, implying that both receptor subtypes and both central and peripheral components are involved in mediating the satiety effects of CCK. In normal humans, hunger is decreased by infusing CCK intravenously to achieve the levels normally found after eating [10]. Various CCK analogues and agonists are under development, including some that can be given by nasal spray, but their efficacy, specificity and safety are yet to be determined. Intriguingly, short-term memory in rodents may be decreased by CCK – a reminder that many neurotransmitters are multitalented and serve distinct functions in various parts of the CNS.

α-Melanocyte stimulating hormone and the melanocortin-4 receptor

α-MSH is derived from the pro-opiomelanocortin (POMC) precursor expressed in neurones of the ARC. It is thought to be the endogenous ligand at the melanocortin-4 receptor (MC4-R), which is found at high levels in various hypothalamic regions and whose activation inhibits feeding (see Fig. 6). The MC4-R is one of a family of related 7-transmembrane domain, G-protein-linked receptors that includes MC1-R (the ACTH receptor), MC2-R in hair follicles that determines skin and hair colour (see Chapter 11), and MC3-R, which is also expressed in the hypothalamus but does not appear to be as important as MC4-R in mediating hypophagia [11].

A role for the MC4-R in energy homeostasis was first suggested by the finding that the combination of yellow fur and obesity in a genetically obese mouse (A^{vy}) was due to a mutation in the promoter region of the gene encoding a 132-residue peptide known as 'agouti'. Agouti is normally expressed in hair follicles, where it acts as an endogenous antagonist at the MC2-R, blocking the action of α-MSH to stimulate the synthesis of the black pigment, eumelanin. Coat colour in mice and other species, including Alsatian dogs, is determined by the interplay between the gene encoding the MC2-R (known as '*extension*') and the expression of agouti. The A^{vy} mutation causes agouti to be overexpressed in the hair follicles (causing predominance of the pale phaeomelanin pigment and therefore yellow fur) and in

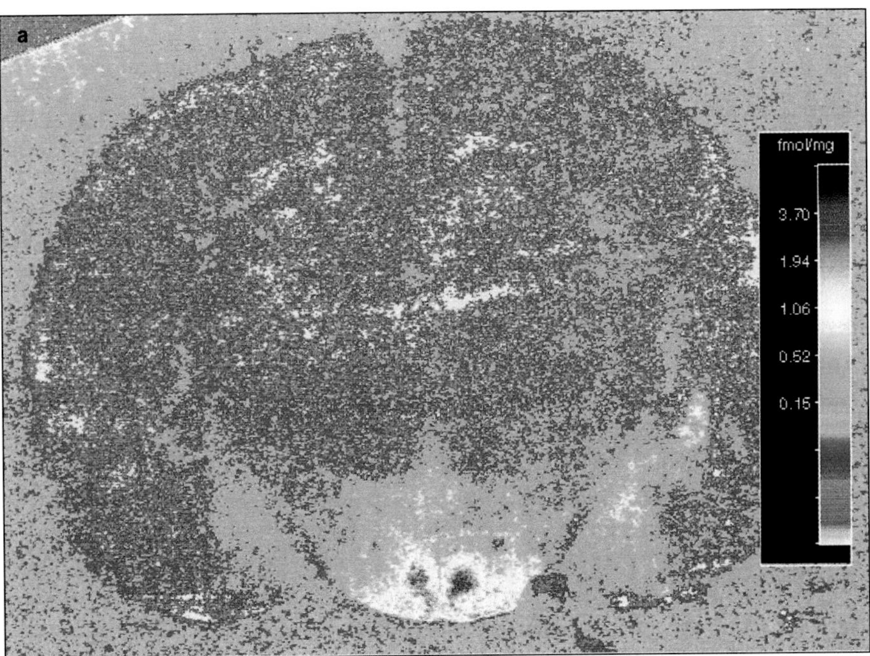

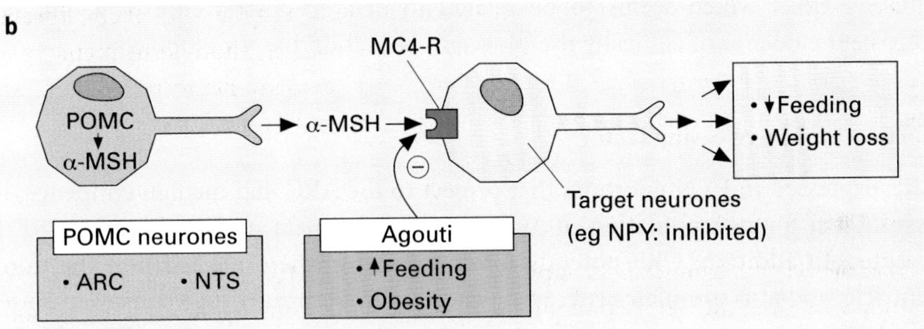

Fig. 6 The melanocortin-4 receptor (MC4-R): **(a)** distribution of MC4-R in the rat hypothalamus, visualised by ligand-binding autoradiography; **(b)** interactions between melanocyte-stimulating hormone (α-MSH), the derivative of pro-opiomelanocortin (POMC), believed to be the endogenous ligand, and the antagonist, agouti peptide (ARC, arcuate nucleus; NPY, neuropeptide Y; NTS, nucleus of the solitary tract).

other sites, including the hypothalamus [12]. Here, it antagonises the MC4 receptor, causing hyperphagia and obesity (see Fig. 6). Consistent with this, food intake and body weight are decreased by the MC4-R agonist MTII, whereas an MC4-R antagonist (SHU 9119) or 'knock-out' of the MC4-R gene stimulates feeding and causes obesity [13].

The MC4-R evidently plays a role in regulating food intake and body weight in humans, as a mutation analogous to *agouti* has recently been identified in a subject with childhood-onset morbid obesity [14]. However, it remains to be seen whether or not the MC4-R is relevant to the generality of human obesity, and whether

MC4-R agonists will prove useful in its treatment. Intriguingly, MTII causes penile erection and darkening of the skin as well as weight loss in rodents; unfortunately, mice are unlikely to benefit from the combination of thinness, tanned skin and priapism which appears to obsess many 20th century men.

Glucagon-like peptide-1 7-36 amide

Glucagon-like peptide (GLP-1) is another brain-gut peptide, derived by alternative processing of the pre-proglucagon gene. GLP-1 released into the gut after eating enhances insulin secretion by stimulating the islet beta cells (an 'incretin' effect, see chapter 18), and also delays gastric emptying by causing constriction of the pylorus.

This latter action may induce satiety, and (as with CCK) GLP-1 may also act within the CNS to decrease feeding. GLP-1 may enter parts of the brain that have a specifically modified blood-brain barrier, such as the median eminence/ARC and the area postrema in the floor of the fourth ventricle that overlies the NTS and vagal nuclei. Neurones expressing GLP-1 are found in the area postrema and project to the PVN and other sites where GLP-1 receptors are found. GLP-1 injected into the hypothalamus inhibits feeding and, more convincingly, central injection of the GLP-1 antagonist exendin stimulates feeding [15].

Some studies of GLP-1 in type 2 diabetes (see chapter 18) suggest a modest satiating effect which seems to be related to delayed gastric emptying, but no consistent evidence of clinically useful weight reduction has yet emerged.

Corticotrophin-releasing factor

CRF, expressed in PVN neurones that project to the ARC and median eminence, is best known for its stimulation of ACTH release, an effect mediated by the CRF-1 receptor. In addition, CRF potently inhibits feeding when injected into the third ventricle, and also stimulates energy expenditure by activating the sympathetic outflow to the thermogenic tissues. These weight-reducing actions are mediated by the CRF-2 receptor, and may be partly due to inhibition by CRF of the ARC NPY neurones [16]. Selective CRF-2 agonists, intended to decrease weight without affecting adrenocortical function, are under development.

□ NEUROTRANSMITTERS THAT CAUSE WEIGHT GAIN

Neuropeptide Y

NPY is a 36-residue, single-chain peptide belonging to the pancreatic polypeptide family. It is one of the most abundant neuropeptides in the mammalian CNS, and has an impressive list of putative physiological actions, mediated by several receptor subtypes (5 have been cloned so far).

NPY induces spectacular hyperphagia and obesity when injected into the hypothalamus of rats and other species, including primates (Fig. 7). NPY and related peptides are the most potent central appetite stimulants yet identified. Feeding is stimulated several-fold for some hours after a single injection and overrides normal

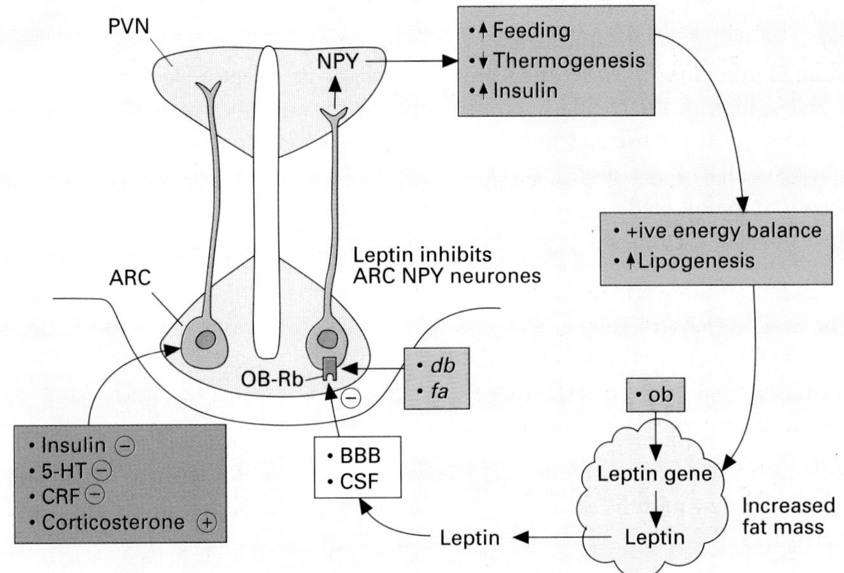

Fig. 7 Suggested role of neuropeptide Y (NPY) neurones in the hypothalamic arcuate nucleus (ARC) in regulating energy balance in rodents. Decreases in the inhibitory signals, insulin and leptin, are thought to stimulate these neurones during starvation, leading to hunger, hyperphagia and reduced thermogenesis – homeostatic changes to defend body weight. Interruption of the leptin signal by *ob*, *db* or *fa* mutations also causes activation of these neurones, which is inappropriate and leads to obesity (BBB, blood-brain barrier; CRF, corticotrophin-releasing factor; CSF, cerebrospinal fluid; 5-HT, serotonin; OB-R, leptin (OB) receptors; PVN, paraventricular nucleus).

satiety mechanisms, while chronic infusion of NPY causes sustained hyperphagia. The PVN and the adjacent perifornical area of the LHA are the most sensitive sites. NPY injection also inhibits the sympathetic outflow that stimulates heat production in thermogenic tissues, and reduces whole-body energy expenditure. Insulin secretion is stimulated, which promotes triglyceride deposition in fat. Overall, obesity can be induced, with a doubling of body-fat mass, within a few days. The obesity-inducing actions of NPY (hyperphagia and hypothermia) are apparently mediated by the Y5 receptor subtype, although this issue remains controversial [17].

Most hypothalamic NPY originates from neurones in the ARC that project to the PVN and related areas (Fig. 7). These neurones become overactive in food deprivation, suggesting that they may sense energy deficits and attempt to correct these by stimulating feeding and reducing energy expenditure [18]. These neurones express the fully functional long isoform (Ob-Rb) of the leptin receptor, and are inhibited by leptin. Other regulators include insulin (inhibitory) and glucocorticoids (stimulatory). NPY neuronal stimulation in food deprivation may be related to falls in leptin and/or insulin levels. Both these hormones can enter the ARC through the specially modified blood-brain barrier in the underlying median eminence (see Fig. 2). Inappropriate overactivity of the NPY neurones is found in, and may partly explain, the obesity syndromes of the *ob/ob* and *db/db* mice and *fa/fa* Zucker rat [19]; here, the neurones are stimulated by interruption of leptin's inhibitory influence, through mutations in either the leptin gene (*ob*) or its receptor (*fa* and *db*).

NPY appears a particularly promising target for anti-obesity drug development by virtue of its intense and unique obesity-inducing effects and the fact that these may be mediated by a specific receptor subtype. Prototype Y5 antagonists have been shown to inhibit feeding in certain leptin-dependent rodent models of obesity, but their possible usefulness in man remains entirely speculative.

The orexins (hypocretins)

Discovery of the orexins A and B was reported in early 1998 [20]. These peptides (33 and 28 residues, respectively) are structurally related (75% homology) and are both derived from prepro-orexin, expressed in specific neurones of the LHA. Their amino acid sequences are identical to those of the peptides termed 'hypocretins', described a few months earlier [21], and bear some relationship to the gut peptide secretin.

Orexin A stimulates feeding when injected intracerebroventricularly, although its hyperphagic effect is not as robust or as durable as with NPY, and obesity may not result with chronic administration; the LHA may be a more sensitive site. The OX1-R orexin receptor (also known as HFGAN 72) apparently mediates this action. Orexin B is also reported to stimulate feeding, though less powerfully. Prepro-orexin mRNA levels in the rat hypothalamus increase with starvation, suggesting an adaptive and possibly homeostatic response to energy depletion [20]. The role of the orexins in man is entirely unknown.

Other appetite-stimulating neurotransmitters

These include the peptides galanin and dynorphin (an opioid peptide), and noradrenaline. Galanin and dynorphin both stimulate feeding, via the GAL-1 and κ receptors, respectively, but do not induce obesity with chronic administration. Hypothalamic galanin levels are raised in the fatty Zucker rat and may contribute to obesity in this model, but its role in dietary-induced obesity (analogous to that in humans) is uncertain, and knock-out of the galanin gene does not affect energy balance. Noradrenaline injected into the PVN stimulates feeding, an effect blocked by α_2 adrenoceptor antagonists, and its continued administration can cause lasting hyperphagia and obesity in rats.

□ THERMOGENIC AGENTS

Heat is produced by various metabolic processes, including 'futile cycling' and the oxidation of fatty acids in mitochondria when this is 'uncoupled' from oxidative phosphorylation which normally produces ATP. ATP is generated by the flow of protons across the inner mitochondrial membrane (Fig. 8). Substances that interfere with this act as uncouplers and increase heat production; an example is dinitrophenol,

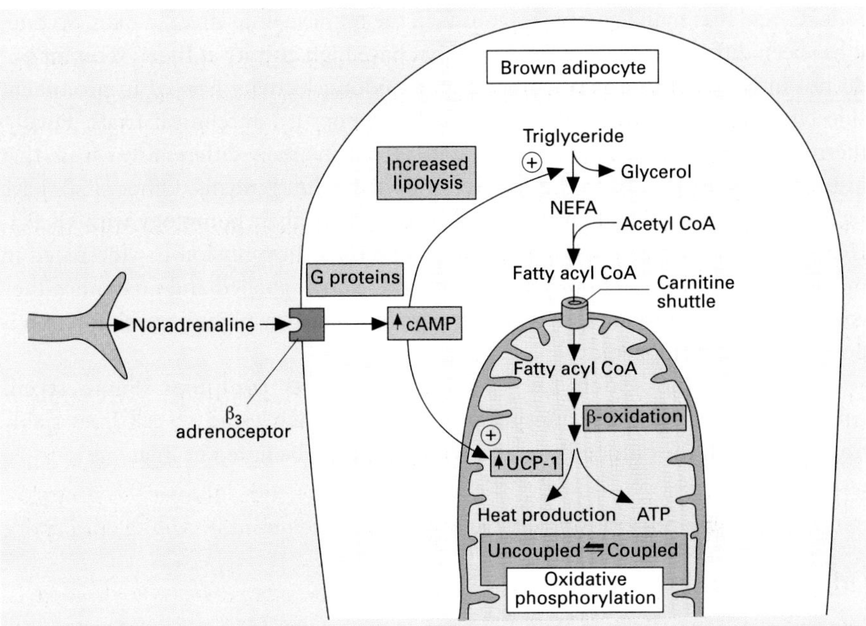

Fig. 8 Regulation of thermogenesis in brown adipose tissue. Noradrenaline released from sympathetic endings acts via the β_3 adrenoceptor to stimulate lipolysis and upregulate the synthesis and activity of uncoupling protein (UCP-1). Free fatty acids generated by lipolysis undergo β-oxidation in the mitochondria, where uncoupling of oxidative phosphorylation yields heat instead of ATP (CoA, co-enzyme A; NEFA, non-esterified fatty acid).

long used experimentally to uncouple oxidative phosphorylation and an effective but toxic weight-reducing agent.

The main heat-producing tissues in adult humans include muscle, the viscera and fat. Neonates also have depots of specialised mitochondria-rich fat (brown adipose tissue (BAT)) that disappear during infancy. Normal adults do not have discrete masses of BAT, although the 'brown' phenotype can be induced in white fat by the very high circulating catecholamine levels of phaeochromocytomas. In rodents, BAT persists into adulthood and is important in increasing thermogenesis in response to stimuli such as cold exposure and eating. Thermogenesis in rodent BAT is driven by sympathetic nerves releasing noradrenaline that interacts with a specific 'atypical' subtype (β_3) of adrenoceptor [22]. β_3 receptor activation is coupled through G-proteins to increase cyclic AMP production, and this in turn stimulates lipolysis of the triglyceride within the brown adipocyte, together with enhanced expression of a specific 32 kDa uncoupling protein now termed UCP-1 [23].

Sympathetic stimulation via the β_3 adrenoreceptor therefore increases heat production, and various catecholamine-like compounds (eg BRL 35135) were found to have potent thermogenic and anti-obesity effects in rodents. Some also have modest weight-reducing actions in man. Unfortunately, several problems have so far prevented their successful application to human obesity. First, it is now clear that the human β_3 receptor has quite different pharmacological properties from those in rodents, and that many potent β_3 agonists in the rat have little effect in man. Second, it has been difficult to design molecules that have high affinity at the β_3 receptor but do not interact with β_1 or β_2 adrenoceptors; poor selectivity has led to prominent side effects of tachycardia (β_1) and muscle tremor (β_2) in clinical trials. Finally, thermogenesis in man may be regulated in a fundamentally different way from that in rodents, even apart from the absence of BAT in adult humans. Other UCPs have recently been isolated and characterised by exploiting their homology with UCP-1. UCP-2 is found in white fat and muscle, while UCP-3 expression is widespread in many tissues [24,25]. It is not yet clear how these are regulated and how much they contribute to heat production; it is even possible that their physiological function is not primarily thermogenic.

Meanwhile, the search for selective β_3 agonists continues. Some recent compounds have shown promising properties in rodents and in cell lines stably transfected with the human β_3 receptor, but are yet to be tested in man.

☐ ANTI-OBESITY DRUGS ACTING ON THE GUT

Orlistat (tetrahydrolipstatin)

Decreasing the intestinal absorption of nutrients is a rational approach to the treatment of obesity, by decreasing energy intake. Fat is the most logical target, both because its energy content (9 kcal/g) is the highest of all the macronutrients and also because a high-fat diet *per se* appears to overcome satiety mechanisms and promote obesity. Over 95% of dietary fat is triglyceride, and its digestion depends critically on the pancreatic lipase which is secreted in pancreatic juice together with its activator, colipase, a 10 kDa protein.

Orlistat (tetrahydrolipstatin) is a semisynthetic derivative of a naturally occurring lipase inhibitor isolated from *Streptomyces* moulds [26]. Orlistat occupies and binds covalently to the active site of pancreatic lipase, permanently disabling the enzyme molecule (see Fig. 9). It is a highly potent inhibitor of all gut and several other lipases but, because very little (<1%) is absorbed systemically, its activity is confined to the gut lumen.

At therapeutic doses (120 mg thrice daily), orlistat decreases fat absorption by about 30%. This represents less than the calculated energy deficit achieved during clinical trials of orlistat. The drug may also encourage patients to avoid high-fat foods, possibly aided by the side effect of steatorrhoea that can follow a fat-rich meal. In placebo-controlled, randomised trials of up to two years' duration, orlistat produced consistently greater average weight loss than placebo (see Fig. 4), and about 30% of orlistat-treated patients lost more than 10% of their initial weight [27]. In terms of efficacy, therefore, orlistat is comparable to dexfenfluramine and sibutramine. In obese patients with type 2 diabetes, weight loss was accompanied by modest falls in blood glucose and Hb_{A1c} [28], and orlistat also reduced low-density lipoprotein cholesterol levels while raising high-density lipoprotein cholesterol.

The principal side effects of orlistat are the predictable consequences of fat malabsorption, and include loose fatty stools and, rarely, diarrhoea and faecal incontinence. These gastrointestinal side effects mostly resolve within a few weeks,

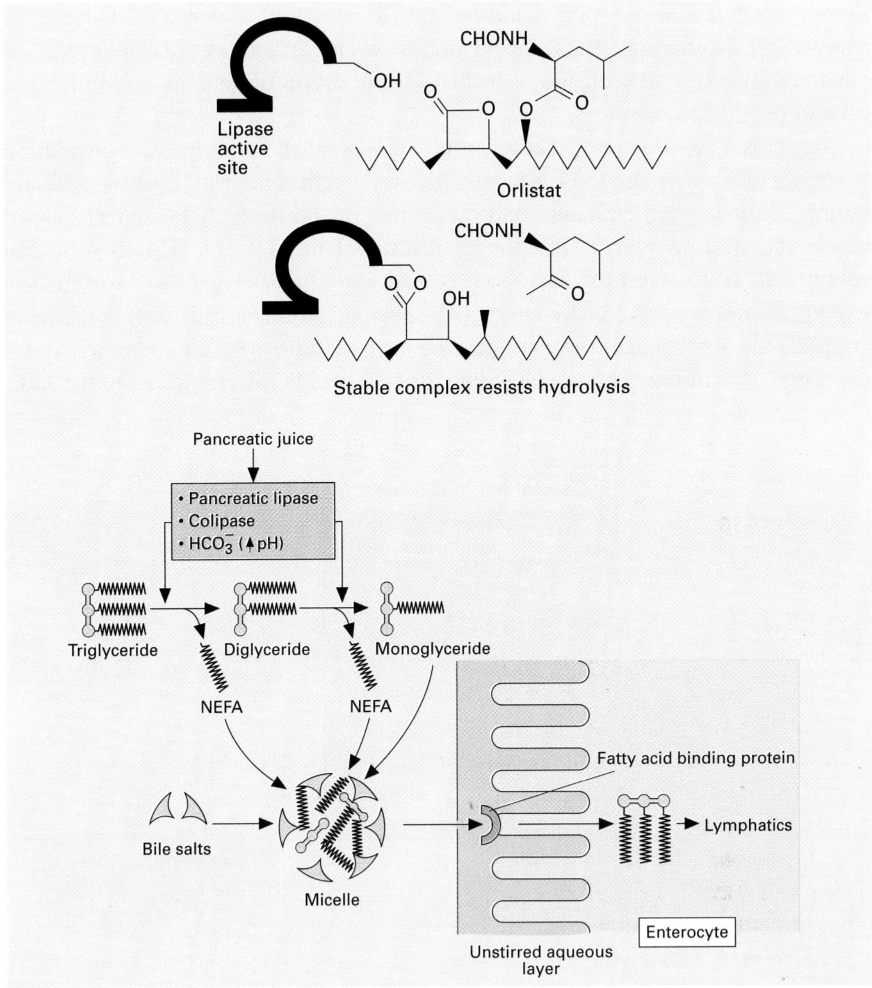

Fig. 9 Fat digestion and mode of action of orlistat (tetrahydrolipstatin). Orlistat inhibits pancreatic lipase, the key enzyme mediating the hydrolysis of triglyceride, which yields the products (free fatty acids, monoglyceride and glycerol) that are absorbed across the intestinal mucosa (NEFA, non-esterified fatty acid).

but may be precipitated by a fat-rich meal. Malabsorption of fat-soluble vitamins (A, D, E and K) and of β-carotene appears to be more a theoretical than a practical risk, but may emerge as a problem during long-term treatment of patients taking a nutritionally inadequate diet. A predicted tendency to gallstone formation has not been confirmed during clinical trials.

□ LEPTIN

Leptin is a hormone produced by adipose tissue that exerts concerted anti-obesity actions in rodents. It was discovered by positional cloning targeted at the *ob* gene, homozygosity for which causes morbid obesity and type 2 diabetes in the *ob/ob* mouse [29]. In the four years since its discovery, a vast amount of knowledge has been accumulated through the coordinated application of genetic, molecular and physiological approaches.

Leptin is a 16 kDa single-chain peptide. It is secreted by fat into the circulation from where it can enter the CNS, either directly across the modified blood-brain barrier of the median eminence and other sites, or indirectly by being transported across the choroid plexus into the cerebrospinal fluid (CSF) (Fig. 10). Several subtypes of leptin receptor have been cloned and characterised; they are derived from a common precursor by alternative splicing [30]. The fully functional form (OB-Rb) is a single-chain protein homologous to certain cytokine receptors, and is expressed by various neurones, including the NPY and POMC neurones of the ARC,

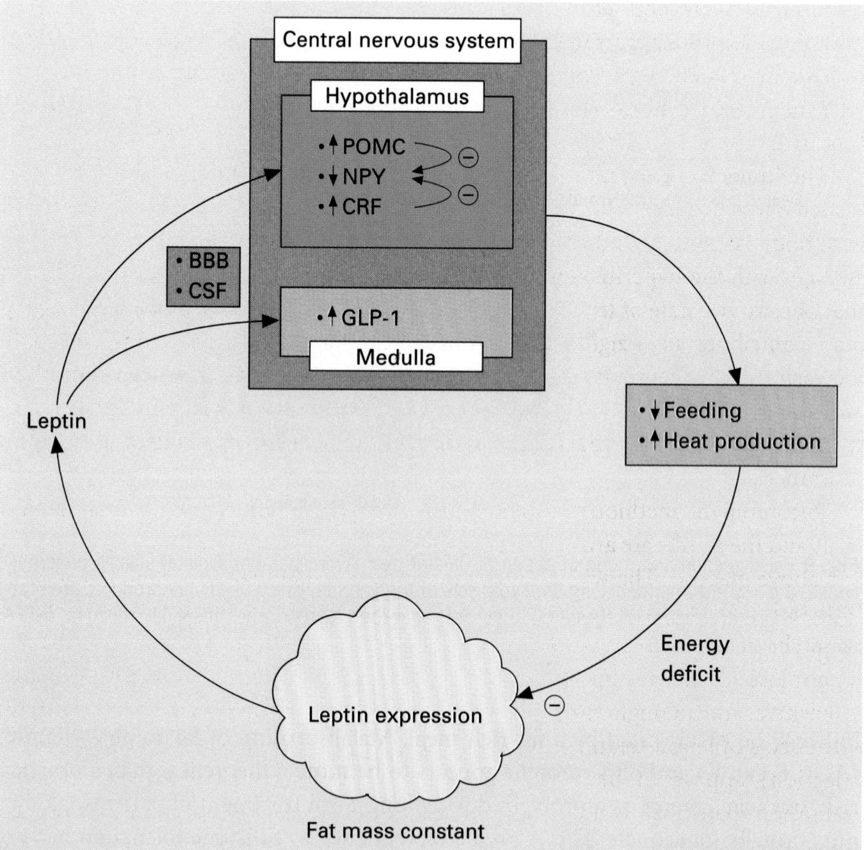

Fig. 10 Suggested role of leptin in regulating body fat mass in rodents. Leptin enters the central nervous system, either directly across modified regions of the blood-brain barrier (BBB) or by transport into the cerebrospinal fluid (CSF) across the choroid plexus (possibly mediated by the OB-Ra leptin receptor subtype). In the hypothalamus and other regions, leptin acts through OB-Rb receptors on various neurones, including neuropeptide Y (NPY) and pro-opiomelanocortin (POMC) in the arcuate nucleus, to decrease feeding and stimulate thermogenesis (CRF, corticotrophin-releasing factor; GLP, glucagon-like peptide; OB-R = leptin (OB) receptor).

and GLP-1 cells in the medulla. The long intracellular tail of the OB-Rb includes domains that interact with the JAK-STAT kinase system responsible for signal transduction within the target cell. A truncated form (OB-Ra) lacks the distal STAT-binding domain and cannot therefore signal binding of leptin to its extracellular part. The OB-Ra is expressed at high levels in the choroid plexus, where it may act to transport leptin from blood into the CSF.

The importance of leptin in rodents is emphasised by the obesity that develops in the *ob/ob* mouse, which lacks biologically active leptin, and in the *db/db* mouse and *fa/fa* Zucker rat, which have mutations in the leptin receptor (OB-R) gene [30]. Leptin given systemically, or intracerebroventricularly at much lower doses, dramatically reduces food intake in *ob/ob* mice, while increasing their thermogenesis (decreased energy expenditure is an important cause of fat gain in this model) [31]. Normal rodents require higher leptin dosages to suppress feeding, while *fa/fa* rats respond partially and *db/db* mice not at all, because of their leptin receptor mutations. Leptin appears to exert its central hypophagic and thermogenic effects in rodents by influencing several neuronal pathways, including inhibition of the ARC NPY neurones and stimulation of ARC POMC and medullary GLP-1 neurones (Fig. 10).

The importance of leptin in normal energy balance and in 'idiopathic' lifestyle-related obesity in man is not yet clear. In general, plasma leptin levels rise in parallel with body fat content and BMI, although there is wide variability (Fig. 11) [32]. By analogy with the hyperinsulinaemia of insulin-resistance states, it has been argued that obesity is a state of leptin insensitivity, and that attenuation of the leptin signal may contribute to weight gain. Human CSF leptin concentrations rise with increasing plasma leptin levels, except at high BMI values, where CSF concentrations are lower than predicted [34]. This may suggest that transport of leptin into the CNS is impaired in obesity, and such a defect could theoretically contribute to leptin resistance.

Recombinant methionyl human leptin is currently undergoing formal clinical trials and the results are awaited with interest; preliminary data indicate some weight loss above placebo. The wide population scatter of leptin concentrations at a given BMI (see Fig. 11) may suggest that those individuals with the lowest leptin levels might be relatively leptin-deficient, and that raising leptin may be rewarded by weight loss. Conversely, those with the highest leptin concentrations may be leptin-insensitive, and so might not respond well to leptin treatment. At present, the main side effects of leptin treatment (which has to be given by twice-daily subcutaneous injection) appear to be cutaneous reactions at injection sites. The growing realisation that leptin is not simply a regulator of body fat mass but also possesses many other peripheral and central activities (including reproduction, insulin secretion, immune function and direct effects in mobilising triglyceride) makes it possible that other unanticipated side effects will emerge.

Exceptions to the rule of human obesity are the vanishingly rare cases of hyperphagia and morbid obesity that are due to leptin mutations analogous to *ob* [35]. These patients have very low or undetectable plasma leptin concentrations, and display dramatic early-onset obesity with hypogonadotrophic hypogonadism. In

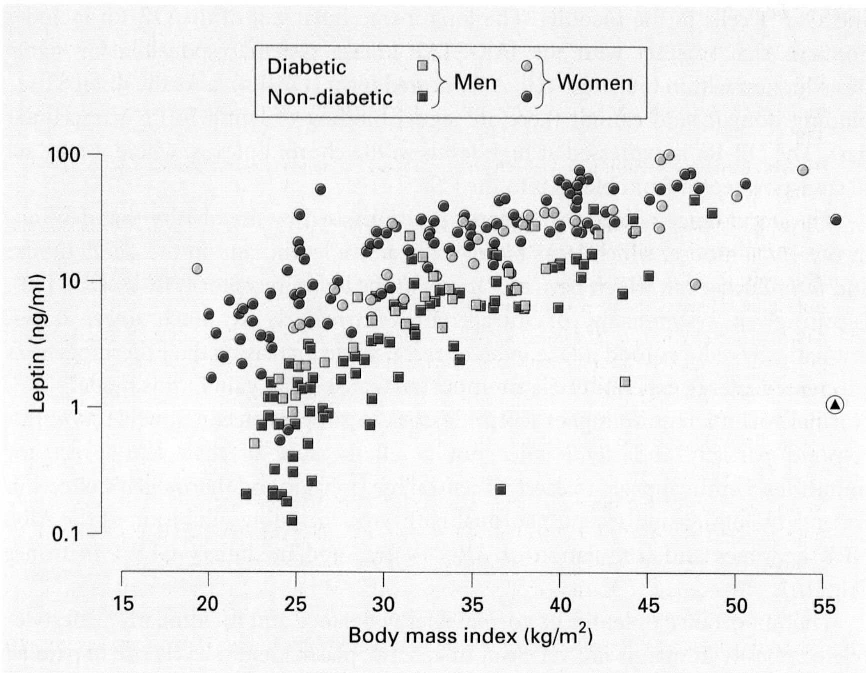

Fig. 11 Plasma leptin concentrations in man. Levels rise generally in proportion to body weight and fat-mass, but there is considerable individual variation. With the exception of extremely rare cases of leptin mutations, human obesity is not a condition of absolute leptin deficiency (▲ indicates a subject with a leptin missense mutation[33]).

one case, leptin treatment has reduced hyperphagia and decreased fat mass, but apparently has no thermogenic action.

The rare cases of leptin mutations are Nature's proof of the concept that leptin plays some part in regulating human feeding and body weight. However, the importance of leptin at 'physiological' levels (ie more than a total absence) is still controversial. Interestingly, the evolution and severity of obesity in the cases of leptin deficiency are similar to those of Prader-Willi and other genetic syndromes and even to some people with apparently idiopathic obesity, whose weight gain cannot be attributed to inherited defects in leptin or its receptors. This confirms that leptin is one of several factors that control body weight, and highlights how little is still known about the hierarchy in which the various environmental, neuroendocrine and behavioural determinants of body weight might operate.

☐ CONCLUSIONS

Obesity deserves to be taken seriously as a major threat to health, but the therapeutic cupboard of safe and effective anti-obesity drugs remains depressingly bare. Orlistat and sibutramine will undoubtedly fill useful niches in managing obesity, and we can be optimistic that other effective drugs will emerge within the next decade.

REFERENCES

1 Seidell JC, Flegal KM. Assessing obesity: classification and epediology. *Br Med Bull* 1997; **53**: 238–52.

2 Kassirer JP, Angell M. Losing weight – an ill-fated New Year's resolution. *N Engl J Med* 1998; **338**: 52–4.

3 Baez M, Kursa JD, Helton LA, *et al.* Molecular biology of serotonin receptors. *Obesity Res* 1995; **3**: 441–7.

4 Davis R, Faulds D. Dexfenfluramine – an updated review of its therapeutic use in the management of obesity. *Drugs* 1996; **52**: 696–724.

5 Abenheim L, Moride Y, Brenot F, *et al.* Appetite-suppressant drugs and the risk of primary pulmonary hypertension. *N Engl J Med* 1996; **335**: 609–16.

6 Khan MA, Herzog CA, St Peter JV, *et al.* The prevalence of cardiac valvular insufficiency assessed by transthoracic echocardiography in obese patients treated with appetite-suppressant drugs. *N Engl J Med* 1998; **339**: 713–8.

7 Stock MJ. Sibutramine: a review of the pharmacology of a novel anti-obesity agent. *Int J Obesity* 1997; **21**: S25–9.

8 Lean ME. Sibutramine – a review of clinical efficacy. *Int J Obesity* 1997; **21** (Suppl 1): S30–6.

9 Wank SA. Cholecystokinin receptors. *Am J Physiol* 1995; **32**: G628–46.

10 Ballinger AB, McLoughlin L, Medbak S, Clark ML. Cholecystokinin is a satiety hormone in humans at physiological post prandial concentrations. *Clin Sci* 1995; **89**: 375–81.

11 Griffon N, Mignon V, Facchinetti P, *et al.* Molecular cloning and characterization of the rat fifth melanocortin receptor. *Biochem Biophys Res Commun* 1994; **200**: 1007–14.

12 Fan W, Boston BA, Kesterson RA, *et al.* Role of melanocortinergic neurons in feeding and the agouti obesity syndrome. *Nature* 1997; **385**: 165–8.

13 Huszar D, Lynch CA, Fairchild-Huntress V, *et al.* Targeted disruption of the melanocortin-4 receptor results in obesity in mice. *Cell* 1997; **68**: 131–41.

14 Yeo GSH, Farooqi IS, Aminian S, *et al.* A frameshift mutation in *MC4R* associated with dominantly inherited human obesity. *Nat Genet* 1998; **20**: 111–2.

15 Turton MD, O'Shea D, Gunn I, *et al.* A role for glucagon-like peptide-1 in the central control of feeding. *Nature* 1996; **379**: 69–72.

16 Bray GA. Strategies for discovering drugs to treat obesity. In: Kopelman PG, Stock MJ (eds). *Clinical obesity.* Oxford: Blackwell Science, 1998: 508–44.

17 Gerald C, Walker MW, Criscione L, *et al.* A receptor subtype involved in neuropeptide Y-induced food intake. *Nature* 1996; **382**: 168–71.

18 Dryden S, Frankish H, Wang Q, Williams G. Neuropeptide Y and energy balance: one way ahead for the treatment of obesity? *Eur J Clin Invest* 1994; **24**: 293–308.

19 Dryden S, Pickavance L, Frankish HM, Williams G. Increased neuropeptide-Y secretion in the hypothalamic paraventricular nucleus of obese (*fa/fa*) Zucker rats. *Brain Res* 1995; **690**: 185–8.

20 Sakurai T, Amemiya A, Ishii M, *et al.* Orexins and orexin receptors: a family of hypothalamic neuropeptides and G protein-coupled receptors that regulate feeding behaviour. *Cell* 1998; **92**: 573–85.

21 De Lecea L, Kilduff TS, Peyron C, *et al.* The hypocretins: hypothalamus-specific peptides with neuroexcitatory activity. *Proc Natl Acad Sci USA* 1998; **95**: 322–7.

22 Himms-Hagen J, Ghorbani M. Reversal of obesity in *fa/fa* rats by treatment with a β_3-adrenoreceptor agonist, CL 316, 243: cellulary and biochemical characteristics of white and brown adipose tissues. *Obesity Res* 1995; **3**: 406–12.

23 Stock MJ. Energy balance and animal models of obesity. In: Kopelman PG, Stock MJ (eds). *Clinical obesity.* Oxford: Blackwell Science, 1998: 50–72.

24 Fleury C, Neverova M, Collins S, *et al.* Uncoupling protein-2: a novel gene linked to obesity and hyperinsulinemia. *Nat Genet* 1997; **15**: 269–72.

25 Boss O, Samec S, Paolini-Giacobino A, *et al.* Uncoupling protein-3: a new member of the mitochondrial carrier family with tissue-specific expression. *Fed Eur Biochem Soc Lett* 1997; **408**: 39–42.

26 Guerciolini R. Mode of action of orlistat. *Int J Obesity* 1997; **19** (Suppl 2): 41 (abstract).

27 Sjöstrom L, Rissanen A, Andersen T, *et al.* Randomised placebo-controlled trial of orlistat for weight loss and prevention of weight regain in obese patients. *Lancet* 1998; **352**: 168–72.

28 Hollander PA, Elbein SC, Hirsch IB, *et al.* Role of orlistat in the treatment of obese patients with type 2 diabetes: a 1-year randomized double-blind study. *Diabetes Care* 1998; **21**: 1288–94.

29 Zhang YY, Proenca R, Maffei M, *et al.* Positional cloning of the mouse obese gene and its human homolog. *Nature* 1994; **372**: 425–32.

30 Friedman JM, Halaas JL. Leptin and the regulation of body weight in mammals. *Nature* 1998; **395**: 763–70.

31 Campfield LA, Smith FJ, Guisez Y, *et al.* Recombinant mouse *ob* protein – evidence for a peripheral signal linking adiposity and central neural networks. *Science* 1995; **269**: 546–9.

32 Caro JF, Sinha MK, Kolaczynski JW, *et al.* Leptin – the tale of an obesity gene. *Diabetes* 1996; **45**: 1455–62.

33 Strobel A, Isaad T, Camoin L, *et al.* A leptin missense mutation associated with hypogonadism and morbid obesity. *Nat Genet* 1998; **18**: 213.

34 Koistinen HA, Karonen S-L, Iivanainen M, Koivisto VA. Circulating leptin has saturable transport into intrathecal space in humans. *Eur J Clin Invest* 1998; **28**: 894–7.

35 Montague CT, Farooqi IS, Whitehead JP, *et al.* Congenital leptin deficiency is associated with severe-early onset obesity in humans. *Nature* 1997; **387**: 903–8.

The Croonian Lecture
Bugs and guts: it's good to talk?

Michael J G Farthing

☐ INTRODUCTION

The human organism and its resident gastrointestinal microflora are inextricably linked, and have been since the earliest stages of our evolution. Indeed, in purely numerical terms, man is dominated by his bacteria; it has been estimated that about 10^{14} bacteria inhabit the human alimentary tract, about ten times more than the total number of host eukaryote cells in the body.

This association probably did not occur by chance and, from an evolutionary standpoint, is likely to be mutually advantageous. Symbiosis, the peaceful and profitable coexistence between two organisms, exists in the relationship between the human host and the commensal microflora of the gastrointestinal tract. Interestingly, symbiosis with prokaryotes may have played an even more fundamental role in the evolution of man, as all eukaryotic cells are thought to have evolved as add-on multiples of prokaryotes through the process of serial endosymbiosis [1]. The typical bacterial prokaryote has a nucleoid (or genophore) instead of a nucleus with nuclear membranes, and also lacks mitochondria, large ribosomes and endoplasmic reticulum; it has only a simple flagellum, unlike the more complex undulipodium of eukaryotes. There is now compelling evidence that the eukaryotic nucleus evolved from endosymbiotic fermenting thermophilic eubacteria, that mitochondria originated from aerobic eubacteria, and that internalised spirochaetes provided the motile cytoskeletal proteins that are vital for mitosis and meiosis, while other external spirochaetes formed the basis of the eukaryotic undulipodium [1].

However, not all bacteria in the alimentary tract are friendly. Closely related organisms can be either commensal or pathogen, the switch being initiated by the presence of genetic material commonly localised to a specific region of the bacterial chromosome or a plasmid, a so-called 'pathogenicity island' or 'locus', which encodes one or more virulence factors that are necessary for the expression of human disease. Overall, however, it would appear that virulent, disease-producing organisms are greatly outnumbered by their commensal cousins and that pathogenicity is a rare event.

Thus, the human organism is an eukaryote-prokaryote consortium with a high degree of interdependency. There is sophisticated 'cross-talk' between enteropathogens and the many cell systems that make up the gastrointestinal tract; enteropathogens have effectively learned to subvert the host's cytoskeletal machinery and signal transduction systems to colonise and create a favourable environment in the gut. The title of this article highlights the dilemma in communication that faces the human host, its commensals and its commensals turned pathogens. Communication is the name of the game; however, as in all human relationships, the messages transmitted and received are sometimes uninvited and undesirable.

□ GASTROINTESTINAL MICROFLORA

More than 500 species of bacteria colonise the adult human alimentary tract, with marked regional differences in both the type of bacteria and the numbers of organisms present [2]. Although countless bacteria are swallowed every day, the low intragastric pH restricts bacterial numbers in the stomach to about 10^3 per ml of gastric fluid; most of these are lactobacilli. The recently discovered *Helicobacter pylori* has probably resided in the human stomach for about 300 million years – and for even longer in some small mammals and other animals. However, it seems that peptic ulcer disease only began to appear during the last century, suggesting that *H. pylori* has been a commensal and possibly even a symbiont throughout the vast majority of our time together [3]; *H. pylori* might improve host defences against other pathogens, by stimulating gastric acid production and the inflammatory response in the gastric antrum (see chapter 7).

Bacterial counts rise in the duodenum to 10^4 per ml and, as in the stomach, these are predominantly lactobacilli. There is a sharp increase in the distal ileum to 10^6 organisms/ml, with streptococci appearing in addition to the lactobacilli. In the caecum, bacterial counts rise markedly to 10^{12} per gram of faeces, with the emergence of large numbers of anaerobic organisms such as *Bacteroides*, clostridia and methanogenic bacteria [4].

The gastrointestinal tract of the neonate is sterile, but within hours it gradually becomes colonised by bacteria acquired from the mother and other environmental sources. The neonatal intestine contains predominantly lactobacilli and bifidobacteria but, as the infant is weaned, the microflora begins to resemble that of the adult.

Influence of the microflora on gut structure and function

An important symbiotic element in the relationship between man and his intestinal microflora is the maintenance of mucosal structure, in which bacteria apparently play a major role [4]. Studies in germ-free animals have shown that introduction of normal microflora results in increased mucosal mass, an expanded intestinal surface area and enhanced epithelial cell turnover. These structural alterations almost certainly have functional implications with respect to nutrient, fluid and electrolyte absorption, and also to regeneration and repair.

Microflora and host defence

The intestine of germ-free animals contains relatively few immunocytes and other inflammatory cells, a situation that can be reversed by introducing a normal microflora. The population of immune competent cells within the epithelium and lamina propria represents the front line of the host's immune defences against invading enteropathogens, and it therefore seems likely that the resident microflora is important in maintaining this non-specific background protective mechanism. There is also increasing evidence that the commensal microflora plays a direct role in suppressing the colonisation and proliferation of the gut by enteropathogens [5]. Lactobacilli produce lactic acid and short-chain fatty acids, which reduce intraluminal pH and inhibit the growth of acid-tolerance organisms *in vitro*; clinical data also suggest that certain strains of lactobacilli can reduce the risks of acquiring intestinal bacterial infections. Moreover, bifidobacteria, a major commensal of the neonate, have been shown to reduce dramatically the risk of rotavirus infection in this age group [6].

Nutrition

The rumen of some herbivores contains a highly specialised microflora, which is able to digest cellulose and other plant materials, making them available to the host as energy substrates. In the human colon, many bacterial species metabolise fibre and other unabsorbed carbohydrates to produce short-chain fatty acids, thus liberating and allowing the retrieval of energy substrates (up to 300 kcal each day) which would otherwise be lost in the faeces. Butyrate is of particular interest: as well as being an important fuel for the colonocyte, it may also have preventive effects against neoplasia (see chapter 8). Bacteria may also contribute directly to the host's nutritional status by synthesising vitamins such as vitamin K and vitamin B_{12}.

Factors that modify the gastrointestinal microflora

Many factors can influence the gut microflora, both qualitatively and quantitatively [7]. Gastric acid presents a formidable barrier to organisms entering the gut, although bacteria nonetheless exist in the upper gastrointestinal tract in reasonable numbers. There is evidence that reductions in gastric acid secretion – whether due to the development of gastric atrophy or the use of acid-inhibitory drugs – increase bacterial counts within the stomach and upper small intestine and enhance the risk of acquiring intestinal infections.

Bacterial counts in the proximal small intestine also rise markedly in intestinal motility disorders, particularly those associated with diabetes mellitus, systemic sclerosis and chronic idiopathic intestinal pseudo-obstruction due to either a visceral myopathy or neuropathy. In these conditions, normal peristalsis is impaired, which enables higher numbers of bacteria to proliferate in and colonise the proximal small intestine.

Dietary influences are also important in modifying the intestinal microflora. Poorly absorbed carbohydrates such as fibre and digestion-resistant starches increase the numbers of some species of colonic bacteria (*Bacteroides* and bifidobacteria). It has been suggested that certain dietary manipulations might be important in modulating the risk of colorectal cancer (see chapter 8), and it is possible that some of these effects may be mediated by alterations in the flora of the large intestine, perhaps operating through their production of metabolites that influence colonic epithelial turnover and proliferation (see above).

Administration of broad-spectrum antimicrobial agents is an obvious way to disturb the normal human intestinal microflora. Diarrhoea is commonly associated with antibiotic therapy; at least 70% of cases can be attributed to the emergence of *Clostridium difficile*. It is presumed that this organism is present in many healthy adults but is normally kept in check by other components of the resident microflora; when this 'host defence' is disturbed, *C. difficile* proliferates, and its toxin causes diarrhoea and pseudomembranous colitis. Despite the acute, clinically dramatic effects of short-term broad-spectrum antibiotic therapy, it is virtually impossible to make any long-term impact since the microflora rapidly returns to baseline once antibiotics are discontinued.

□ COMMENSAL TURNS PATHOGEN: WHAT MAKES THE DIFFERENCE?

One of the most common bacterial species in the human alimentary tract is *Escherichia coli*, which in healthy subjects is almost invariably a harmless commensal. However, during the past 50 years several sub-types have been characterised that are pathogenic to humans and animals, producing an extensive spectrum of clinical disease, including acute watery diarrhoea, dysentery and persistent diarrhoea, sometimes with nutrient malabsorption (see Table 1). The various pathogenic sub-types possess virulence factors that directly determine the nature of the intestinal disease. Enterotoxigenic *E. coli* (ETEC) possess two major virulence factors, both plasmid-encoded. First, they have highly specialised attachment

Table 1 Enterovirulent *Escherichia coli:* clinical syndromes and virulence factors.

Type	Major clinical syndrome	Virulence factors
Enteropathogenic (EPEC)	Persistent diarrhoea	Bundle-forming pili Esp A, B, D Intimin Tir
Enterotoxigenic (ETEC)	Acute watery diarrhoea	Pili LT-I, LT-II STa
Enterohaemorrhagic (EHEC)	Dysentery	As for EPEC Also SLT-I, SLT-II
Enteroinvasive (EIEC)	Dysentery	Ipa ShET II
Enteroaggregative (EaggEC)	Persistent diarrhoea	Bundle-forming pili EAST I

Esp, EPEC secreted protein; Tir, translocated intimin receptor; LT, heat labile toxin; STa, heat stable toxin; SLT, Shiga-like toxin; Ipa, invasion plasmid antigen; ShET, Shigella enterotoxin; EAST, enteroaggregative *E. coli* heat stable toxin.

organelles called pili (or fimbriae) which mediate adherence to host epithelium; mutants in which the pilus gene is deleted are unable to colonise the gut and cannot produce clinical disease. Second, ETEC possess genes that encode secretory enterotoxins.

Enteropathogenic *E. coli* (EPEC) and enterohaemorrhagic *E. coli* (EHEC) have a pathogenicity locus carrying several genes that enable these organisms to attach to and penetrate the intestinal epithelium. EHEC also release proinflammatory cytotoxins, particularly IL-8, which contribute to the pathogenesis of the colitis by promoting the entry of inflammatory cells such as neutrophils into the mucosa.

Thus, the difference between *E. coli* as a commensal and a pathogen depends entirely on the presence of additional genetic material encoding one or more virulence factors [8,9]. These virulence factors are often located close together on the bacterial chromosome or plasmid, suggesting that over time they have moved together to endow previous commensals with a complete 'pathogenicity package' or virulence cassette.

It's good to talk? Establishing the lines of communication.

Enteric pathogens use a variety of lines of communication to secure a colonisation niche within the intestine, exploiting techniques that often involve subversion of host intracellular signalling pathways and the utilisation of certain structural components of the host epithelial cell, particularly the cytoskeleton [10]. Bacterial communication strategies can be classified into four major types depending on the locations of the bacterium and its target site, namely:

- The intestinal lumen
- The apical membrane of the enterocyte
- Invasion into the epithelium and sub-epithelial structures
- Systemic effects either by direct penetration into the circulation or through the distant actions of signalling molecules such as cytokines.

Although enteric pathogens have their primary interactions with the intestinal epithelial cell or its specialised relative, the M cell (which covers the dome of Peyer's patches), it is now increasingly clear that these bacteria also engage in cross-talk with the host through additional endogenous lines of communication such as the mucosal immune system, other inflammatory cells involved in host defence (including polymorphonuclear neutrophils and mast cells), and the enteric nervous system.

'Communication' from the intestinal lumen

Bacterial enteropathogens such as *Vibrio cholerae* and ETEC colonise the small intestine following pilus-mediated adherence to the enterocyte and then cause acute watery diarrhoea by the liberation of enterotoxins. Cholera toxin and *E. coli* heat-labile toxin (LT) are closely related, both structurally and immunogenically. They have a molecular weight of 84 kDa, share about 85% sequence homology and possess the same A-B subunit substructure that comprises one 'active' A subunit and five 'binding' B subunits; both interact with the same GM1 ganglioside receptor on the enterocyte apical membrane, which activates adenylate cyclase located on the basolateral membrane of the enterocyte. This raises intracellular levels of cyclic adenosine monophosphate (cAMP), which ultimately results in phosphorylation of the cystic fibrosis transmembrane regulator (CFTR). This is a chloride channel in the cell membrane (see chapter 27), and its opening leads to active chloride ion secretion into the gut lumen, and concomitant obligatory losses of cations, resulting in the characteristic watery diarrhoea.

E. coli heat-stable toxin (STa) is a much smaller molecule (about 2,000 kDa) which binds to an apical membrane receptor that is linked to guanylate cyclase, and whose activation stimulates production of cyclic guanosine monophosphate (cGMP).

These mechanisms have been well characterised at a molecular level, but there are as yet no drugs available that reliably interfere with these pathways and that could be used therapeutically to inhibit chloride secretion and thus to treat the diarrhoea.

It has recently become evident that the classic adenylate cyclase-cAMP pathway is not the only secretory mechanism mediating the effects of cholera toxin, and that a neural reflex within the intestine may account for up to 50–60% of cholera toxin-induced fluid and electrolyte losses [11] (see Fig. 1). Cholera toxin is thought to release the potent intestinal secretagogue, 5-hydroxytryptamine (5-HT; serotonin) from enterochromaffin cells situated within the intestinal epithelium; these cells are abundant in the intestinal tract and constitute the major reservoir of 5-HT in humans. 5-HT apparently activates 5-HT_3 receptors on a sensory afferent nerve which, through an uncharacterised interneurone in the myenteric plexus, activates a VIPergic secretomotor afferent which releases the secretory neurotransmitter vasoactive intestinal peptide (VIP) at the basolateral membrane of the enterocyte. VIP is the product of the neuroendocrine gut tumours that produce the VIPoma ('WDHA') syndrome of watery diarrhoea, hypokalaemia (due to enhanced intestinal K^+ losses) and achlorhydria (inhibition of gastric acid secretion is another of VIP's actions). Cholera toxin-induced VIP release similarly activates specific receptors and initiates intestinal secretion of chloride- and potassium-rich fluid. 5-HT may also activate 5-HT_2 receptors in the lamina propria and on the enterocyte to promote the synthesis and release of prostaglandins, in particular PGE_2 which also powerfully stimulates intestinal secretion.

Recent human studies have demonstrated that the 5-HT_3 receptor antagonist granisetron can inhibit cholera toxin-induced intestinal secretion in humans [12]. 5-HT_3 antagonists may act not only by blocking 5-HT receptors on target neurones but also by antagonising autoreceptors on the enterochromaffin cell, thereby preventing further 5-HT release (see Fig. 1).

'Communication' at the enterocyte apical membrane

Some enteropathogens adhere intimately to the enterocyte microvillus membrane at

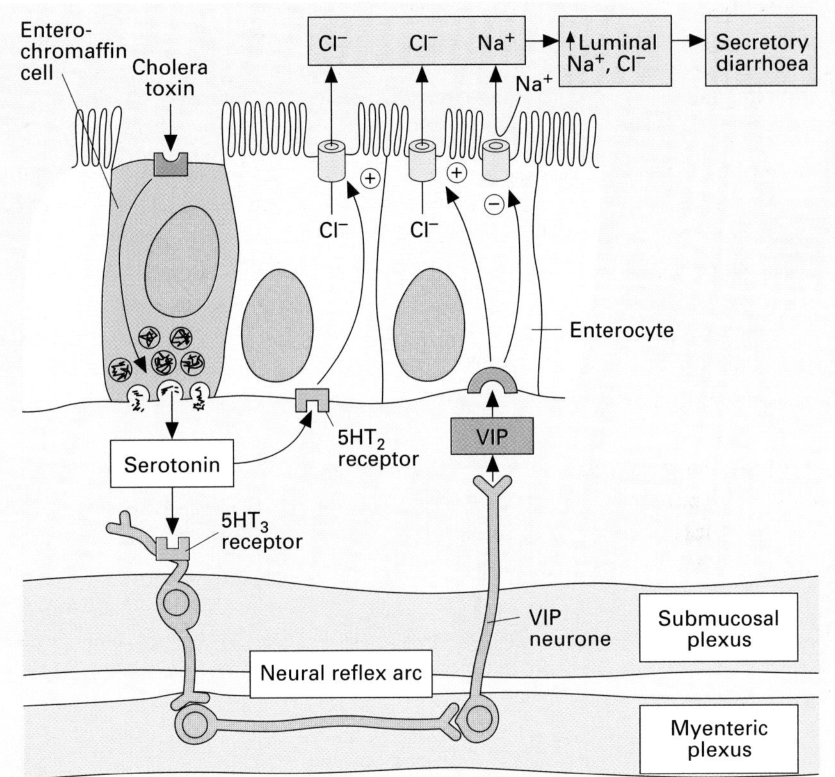

Fig. 1 Role of the enteric nervous system in cholera toxin-induced intestinal hypersecretion. This is in addition to the 'classical' direct effects of cholera toxin on the enterocyte. Current evidence suggests that cholera toxin releases 5-HT from enterochromaffin cells (EC) which acts on 5-HT_2 receptors on enterocytes to promote chloride ion channel (Cl^-) secretion. In addition, 5-HT is thought to bind to neural 5-HT_3 receptors activating a neural reflex involving a substance P/cholinergic interneurone and a VIPergic secretory efferent neurone with activation of VIP (vasoactive intestinal polypeptide) receptors on the enterocyte basolateral membrane; this neural reflex results in Cl^- secretion and impaired Na^+ and Cl^- absorption.

the apical (luminal) surface of the cell, and activate host intracellular signalling pathways. EPEC produces an 'attaching and effacing' lesion; a three-stage model has been developed to describe the process (Fig. 2) [13,14]. The first stage comprises 'non-intimate' attachment, which is mediated by a filamentous organelle containing an EPEC-secreted protein, EspA, that is exported by a type III secretion system. The second stage involves signal transduction and cytoskeletal rearrangement in the host cell, initiated by other proteins (EspB and EspD) which are secreted by the bacteria and translocated into the infected host cell. The final stage, intimate bacterial adhesion, accompanied by actin accumulation in the host cell beneath the organism, is followed by pedestal formation. This requires an outer membrane protein adhesion 'intimin' which binds to a specific receptor formerly termed Hp90; this receptor was originally thought to originate from the host, but is now confirmed to

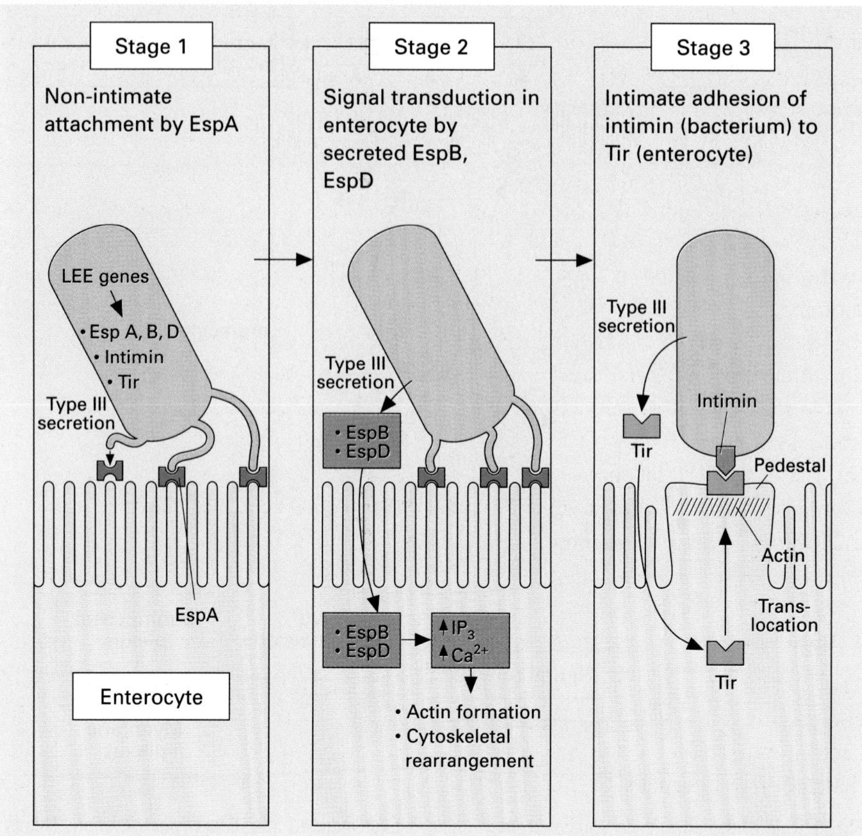

Fig. 2 Interactions between enteropathogenic *E. coli* (EPEC) and the enterocyte. Following *non-intimate attachment* which is mediated by a filamentous organelle containing EPEC secreted protein (EspA), signal transduction and cytoskeletal rearrangements occur in the host cell initiated by EspB and EspD. *Intimate attachment* follows binding of the bacterial ligand, intimin, to Tir (translocated intimin receptor) formerly called Hp90 (host protein 90).

be an EPEC-secreted protein and is thus known as the translocated intimin receptor (Tir). The EPEC genes encoding EspA, EspB and EspD, intimin and Tir are contained in a chromosomal pathogenicity island, designated the 'locus for enterocyte effacement' (LEE). EHEC produces a similar 'attaching and effacing' lesion, and has the same pathogenicity locus. Thus, these organisms are able to rearrange the host cytoskeleton, presumably to create an effective environment for colonisation, and have evolved the extraordinary strategy of synthesising an attachment ligand together with its specific receptor, which is then secreted and inserted into the host cell membrane.

Intestinal protozoa are also able to signal to host cells, again presumably to create a more advantageous environment. *Cryptosporidium parvum* secretes a phospholipase which appears to be essential in the attachment process and may also be involved in initiating intracellular signals that lead to cytoskeletal rearrangements

[15]. *Giardia intestinalis*, an exclusively extracellular protozoan, also appears to be able to signal to the host cell purely through cell-cell surface contact and – by an as yet unidentified pathway – stimulates the enzyme ornithine decarboxylase, which is a marker of cell proliferation [16].

Although *Entamoeba histolytica* produces ulceration and inflammation in the colon, it is not primarily an invasive organism. It produces its cytolethal effects through cell-cell contact; initial engagement depends on a galactose-binding lectin which is associated with its cell membrane and which mediates adherence to the host epithelial cell; following this, a variety of hydrolytic enzymes and pore-forming proteins are released. One protein of particular interest, amoebapore, is inserted into the host cell membrane where it produces high-conductance ion channels that allow the influx of extracellular calcium ions; this results in a rapid increase in intracellular calcium which causes cell death [17]. *E. histolytica* has also been shown to contain and release 5-HT, which theoretically could activate neural reflexes that promote chloride loss from the enterocytes as described above for cholera toxin. As yet, there is no evidence that this is an important mechanism of diarrhoea in human amoebic dysentery.

'Communication' by invasion

The mechanisms by which invasive organisms such as *Salmonella*, *Shigella* and enteroinvasive *E. coli* (EIEC) enter the host epithelial cell depend on the ability of the bacterium to trigger a signalling cascade which leads to cytoskeletal rearrangements that promote internalisation of the organisms in an endocytotic vacuole. Following contact of the organism with the host surface membrane, the latter shows localised ruffling, rearrangement of underlying actin filaments, and capping of its surface proteins [9].

Salmonella invade rapidly, being internalised in vacuoles within minutes. Invasion is associated with calcium influx and activation of the inositol phosphate transduction pathways. The cytoskeletal rearrangement appears to be regulated by CDC42, one of the *ras*-related superfamilies of small GTPases [9]. *Salmonella* has a chromosomal pathogenicity island (SPI 1) that contains several invasion operons, including *inv/spa* which is homologous with the invasion genes of other invasive bacteria.

Shigella invades by mechanisms that are similar to those used by *Salmonella* and involve actin polymerisation, which in this case is dependent on the small GTPase, Rho. Invasion is mediated by three surface proteins (IpaB, IpaC and IpaD), which trigger endocytosis of the bacterium by the enterocytes; IpaB then mediates release of *Shigella* from the vacuole into the cytosol of the host cell [9]. These invasion mechanisms again exemplify the stealth of enteropathogenic bacteria in using their own surface or secreted proteins to subvert host-cell structures into advancing the process of colonisation.

Intimate attachment and invasion of enteropathogens into the host epithelial cell can also stimulate the synthesis and release of pro-inflammatory cytokines. Many organisms – such as EHEC, *Shigella*, *Salmonella* and *Cryptosporidium parvum* –

stimulate intestinal epithelial cells to produce interleukin-8 (IL-8), a potent chemoattractant which promotes a rapid influx of neutrophils into the lamina propria of the infected intestine [18] (Fig. 3). Although this is an appropriate host response that can potentially limit the spread of infection, the presence of large numbers of neutrophils enhances the inflammatory cascade and ultimately leads to increased tissue damage and a secretory response by the epithelium. Experimental inhibition of neutrophil influx by administration of an antibody against the cell adhesion molecule CD18 not only reduces the mucosal inflammatory response and the associated structural damage but also decreases the epithelial secretion of fluid and electrolytes [19].

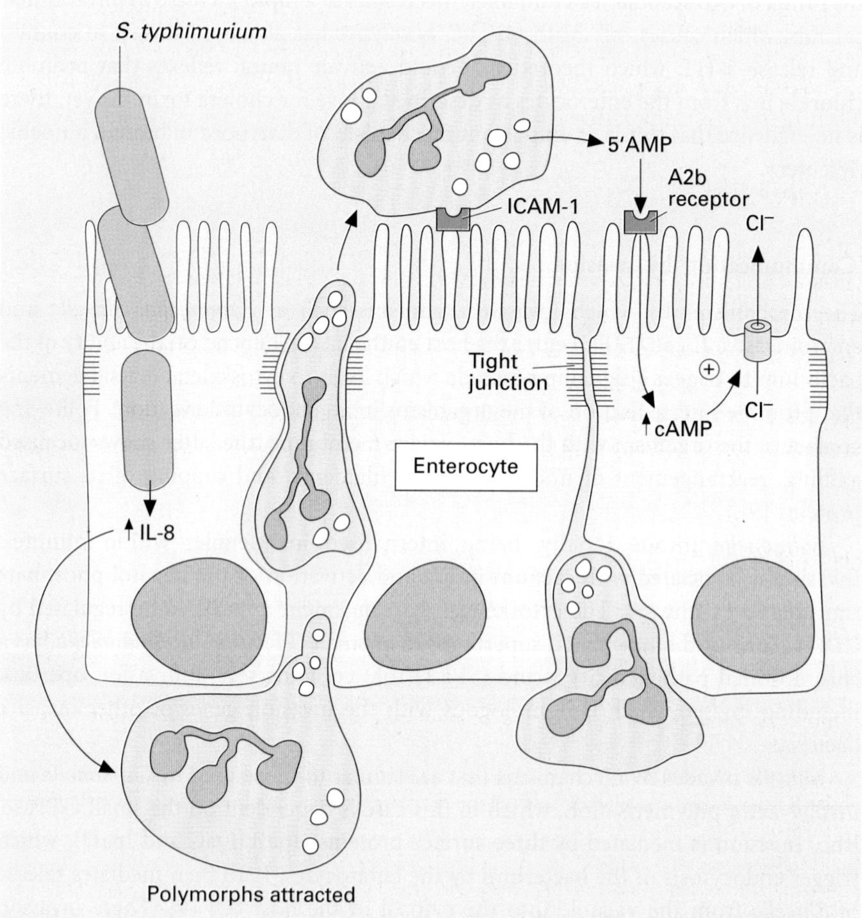

Fig. 3 *Salmonella* invades enterocytes by subverting the host cytoskeleton with associated actin polymerisation which is dependent on the GTPase, Rho. Invasion results in secretion of the potent chemoattractant IL-8 which leads to entry of neutrophil polymorphs into the lamina propria which penetrate the zonula occludens ('tight junction') and enter the intestinal lumen; this process is facilitated by binding to the cell adhesion molecule ICAM-I expressed on the enterocyte apical membrane. Neutrophils release the secretagogue 5'-adenosine monophosphate (5'-AMP) which binds to adenosine 2b receptors to produce Cl^- secretion.

'Communication' by distant signalling molecules

Micro-organisms that invade the epithelium and even penetrate the systemic circulation can have far-reaching effects that extend beyond the local structural and functional derangements in the intestine. Organisms that produce a chronic inflammatory process within the intestine cause additional sequelae such as fever, anorexia and – if infection is prolonged – undernutrition. Increasing evidence indicates that these infections result in the release of pro-inflammatory cytokines such as interleukins IL-1 and IL-6 and tumour necrosis factor-α (TNF-α) These cytokines mediate the effects of systemic immune activation and are probably the prime effectors of anorexia and undernutrition. In models of chronic intestinal inflammation associated with anorexia and weight loss, it is now established that these cytokines (particularly IL-1 and IL-6) have central effects on key hypothalamic pathways and neurotransmitters responsible for the control of feeding behaviour (see chapter 9). Thus, the inflammatory responses in the intestine can affect host nutrition through central nervous system pathways.

□ CONCLUSIONS

The lines of communication between micro-organisms within the gastrointestinal tract and host epithelial cells, enteric nerves and a variety of inflammatory cells are varied and complex. Enteropathogens utilise host intracellular machinery to their own ends, to optimise the colonisation process, and probably to ensure wider dissemination and survival of the species. Identification and elucidation of these pathways has already offered new possibilities for the treatment of bacterial gastrointestinal infections, and is likely to continue to provide new therapeutic targets in the future.

REFERENCES

1. Margulis L. Serial endosymbiosis theory. In: *Symbiosis in Cell Evolution.* 2nd edn. New York: Freeman and Co, 1993: 1–18.
2. Tannock GW. *Normal Microflora. An introduction to microbes inhabiting the human body.* London: Chapman and Hall, 1995.
3. Blaser MJ. Not all *Helicobacter pylori* strains are created equal: should all be eliminated? *Lancet* 1997; **349**: 1020–2.
4. Heneghan JB. Alimentary tract physiology: interactions between the host and its microflora. In: Rowland IR (Ed). *Role of the Gut Flora in Toxicity and Cancer.* London: Academic Press, 1988: 39–77.
5. Bengmark S. Ecological control of the gastrointestinal tract. *Gut* 1998; **42**: 2–7.
6. Saavedra JM, Bauman NA, Oung I, *et al.* Feeding of bifidobacterium bifidum and *Streptococcus thermophilus* to infants in hospital for prevention of diarrhoea and shedding of rotavirus. *Lancet* 1994: **344**: 1046–9.
7. Mallett AK, Rowland IR. Factors affecting the gut microflora. In: Rowland IR (Ed). *Role of the Gut Flora in Toxicity and Cancer.* London: Academic Press, 1988: 347–82.
8. Strauss EJ, Falkow S. Microbial pathogenesis: genomics and beyond. *Science* 1997; **2276**: 707–12.
9. Finley BB, Falkow S. Common themes in microbial pathogenicity revisited. *Microbiol Mol Biol Rev* 1997; **61**: 136–69.

10 Cossart P. Subversion of the mammalian cell cytoskeleton by invasive bacteria. *J Clin Invest* 1997; **99**: 2307–11.

11 Turvill JL, Mourad FH, Farthing MJG. Crucial role for 5-HT in cholera toxin but not *Escherichia coli* heat labile enterotoxin-intestinal secretion in rats. *Gastroenterology* 1998; **115**: 883–90.

12 Turvill JL, Farthing MJG. Effect of granisetron on cholera toxin-induced enteric secretion. *Lancet* 1997; **349**: 11293.

13 Kenny B, DeVinney R, Stein M, *et al.* Enteropathogenic *E. coli* (EPEC) transfers its receptor for intimate adherence into mammalian cells. *Cell* 1997; **91**: 511–20.

14 Knutton S, Rosenshine I, Pallen MJ, *et al.* A novel EspA-associated surface organelle of enteropathogenic *Escherichia coli* involved in protein translocation into epithelial cells. *EMBO J* 1998; **17**: 2166–76.

15 Pollok RCG, Farthing MJG. The role of *Cryptosporidium parvum* derived phospholipase in mediating enteric host cell invasion *in vitro*. *Gut* 1998; **42** (Suppl 1): A84.

16 Cevallos AM, Scott-Russell AM, Katelaris PH, *et al.* Mechanisms of ornithine decarboxylase activity stimulation *in vitro* by *Giardia lamblia*. *Gastroenterology* 1995; **108**: A794.

17 Leippe M, Ebel S, Schoenberger OL, *et al.* Pore-forming peptide of pathogenic *Entamoeba histolytica*. *Proc Natl Acad Sci USA* 1991; **88**: 7659–63.

18 Eckmann L, Kagnoff MF, Fierer J. Epithelial cells secrete the chemokine interleukin-8 in response to bacterial entry. *Infect Immun* 1993; **61**: 4569–74.

19 Elliott EJ, Zhi Li, Bell C, *et al.* A monoclonal antibody against the CD18 adhesion molecule inhibits colonic structural and ion transport abnormalities caused by enterohaemorrhagic *E. coli* 0157:H7 in rabbits. *Gastroenterology* 1994; **106**: 1554–61.

Sun, skin and cancer: from oncogenes to red-hair genes

Jonathan L Rees

□ INTRODUCTION

The ready accessibility of the skin provides unparalleled opportunities to characterise the early stages and natural history of neoplasia in humans, and we have already built up an impressive knowledge of skin cancers. The primary aim of this chapter is to highlight the contributions made by genetic approaches to our understanding of the pathogenesis of skin cancers and the factors that predict their behaviour and prognosis. I shall first review the various types of skin cancer and the arguments for and against genetic factors playing an important role in their development, including evidence implicating specific mutations in oncogenes and tumour suppressor genes. The final section will deal with the genetic basis for one of the longest-recognised associations with skin cancer, namely a pale complexion and red hair.

Skin cancers, like cancers elsewhere, develop through the unlucky interaction between a genetic predisposition and environmental triggers. In the case of skin cancers, the main environmental villain is sunlight, and specifically its ultraviolet component. The well known ability of both skin pigmentation and hair to protect the skin from sunlight is a theme that will recur as this story unfolds.

Professors of dermatology, like everyone else, should not need to be reminded that hair is nature's best sunblock, although those who are balding are destined to rediscover this fact for themselves. Bald heads are an appropriate starting point for this chapter, as they highlight the fact that loss of the hair's protection against ultraviolet radiation can lead to dysplasia and neoplasia in the skin (Fig. 1). The biological significance of skin pigmentation is less certain. Most hairy mammals have pale skin under their fur; exceptions include rodents' tails, whose sparse covering of hair may have encouraged the spread of melanocytes from hair follicles into the interfollicular skin. The major biological purposes of skin pigmentation appear to have been camouflage and sexual behaviour (see Fig. 2), and any protective function against ultraviolet radiation was perhaps an evolutionary afterthought. Loss of hair during human evolution might be expected to exert selection pressure in favour of dark skin, to protect against the development of skin cancers; as evolution has also led to loss of pigmentation, other pressures have evidently sometimes operated, perhaps including the capacity of a fair skin to promote vitamin D synthesis and thus protect against rickets.

It has been argued that there is not a strong case for selection pressure operating against skin cancers, as both melanoma and non-melanoma skin cancers tend to occur after the reproductive period has finished, at least in developed countries.

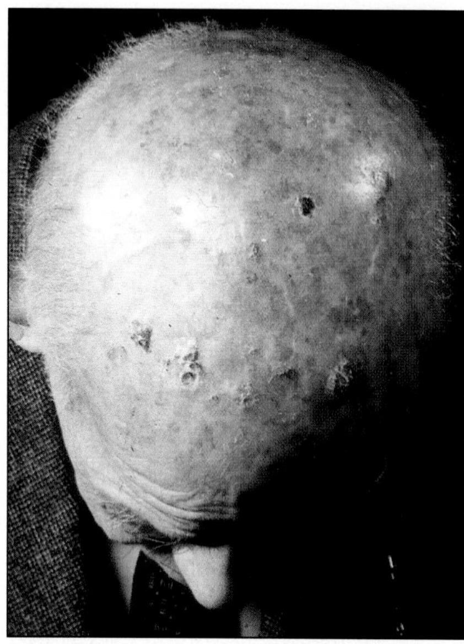

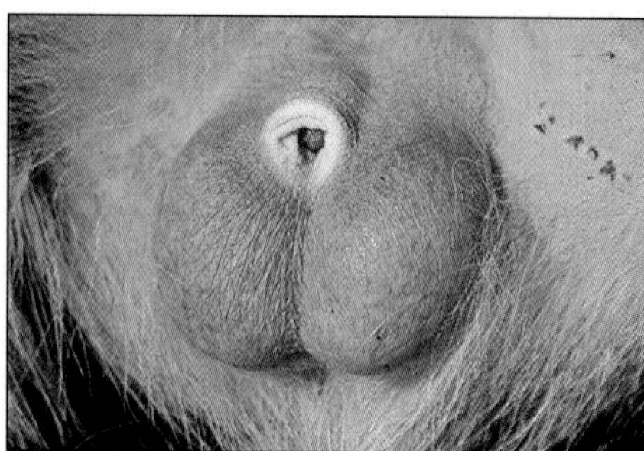

Fig. 2 The scrotum of the blue vervet monkey. The scrotal colour is due to pigment which lies deep within the dermis and thus appears blue instead of brown (much as in a Mongolian spot in newborn babies, and in blue naevi). The major purpose of pigmentation in many animals is sexual behaviour and camouflage.

Fig. 1 Hair is an effective sunblock. Bald scalps show a greatly increased risk of neoplasia and dysplasia, and also pigmentary abnormalities; in this case, the latter are pathological, but serve as a reminder that pigmentation is a mechanism for protecting interfollicular skin against ultraviolet radiation.

However, this may be a rather parochial view. Albinos in equatorial Africa develop non-melanoma skin cancers that carry significant morbidity and mortality. Moreover, individuals with xeroderma pigmentosa – a defect in DNA repair mechanisms that selectively interferes with the nucleotide excision pathways used to repair ultraviolet radiation-induced damage – develop skin cancers that, untreated, cause death in early adolescence in many cases. By contrast, the propensity to rickets in individuals with dark skin and with limited exposure to sunlight is a matter of recent clinical record.

☐ A CLASSIFICATION OF SKIN CANCERS

Based on the cell of origin, skin cancers can be usefully classified into those derived from keratinocytes (non-melanoma skin cancer) and melanoma (see Table 1) [1,2]. This subdivision also reflects differences in clinical behaviour and prognosis.

Non-melanoma skin cancer comprises a range of tumours, including basal cell carcinomas, squamous cell carcinomas, keratoacanthomas and the premalignant condition of actinic keratoses. In general, the diagnosis of these tumours is straightforward and is based primarily on the clinical appearance (Fig. 3), together with histological confirmation [1]. The therapeutic principles of destroying the tumour have remained unchanged for around a century; treatment is remarkably effective, and these tumours generally have low mortality and morbidity [1]. Non-melanoma tumours are extremely common: basal cell carcinoma is the most frequent malignancy in Caucasian populations, and indeed is commoner than all other solid tumours put together.

Table 1 Classification of skin cancers.

Non-melanoma (keratinocyte-derived)	Malignant melanoma
• Basal cell carcinoma (including Gorlin's syndrome) • Squamous cell carcinoma • Keratoacanthoma • Actinic keratoses (premalignant)	• Sporadic • Familial

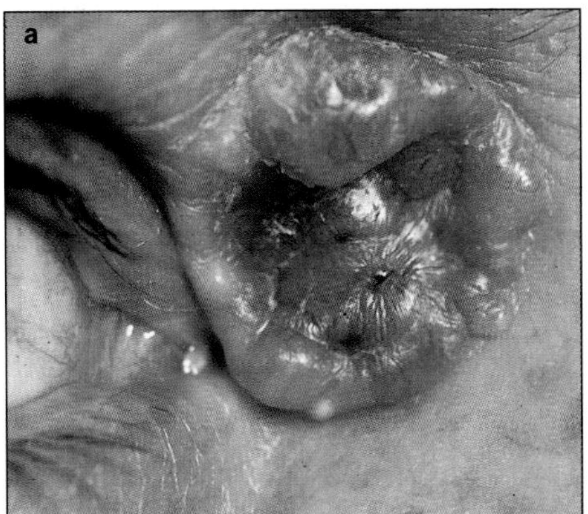

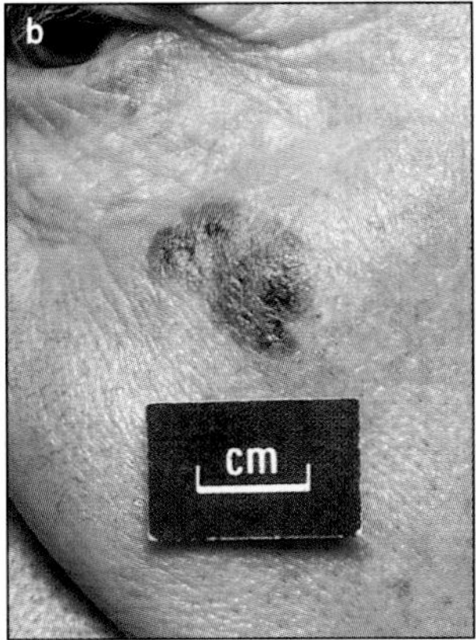

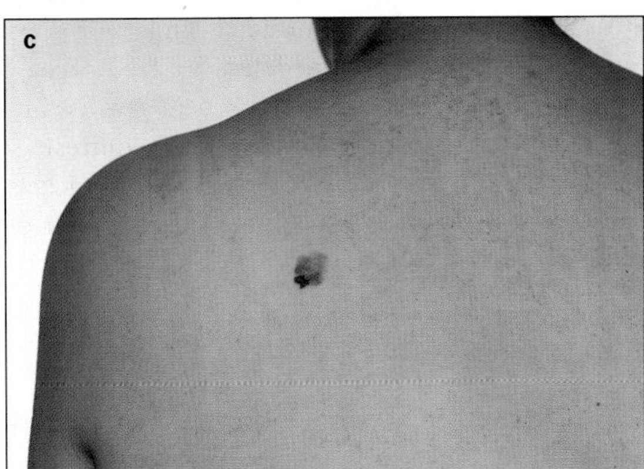

Fig. 3 Examples of common skin cancers. **(a)** A basal cell carcinoma adjacent to the eye. **(b)** Lentigo malignant melanoma. **(c)** A malignant melanoma developing in a pre-existing melanocytic naevus.

By contrast, melanoma is much rarer, with an annual incidence in the UK of about 10:100,000. Its recorded frequency has increased, partly due to a genuine increase in incidence and perhaps because earlier screening may have yielded a population of lesions that might not have reached medical attention 30 or 40 years ago (an interpretation disputed by some authorities) [1,3]. Treatment for melanoma is effective if the patient presents early, but for tumours that have metastasised at presentation there has been little significant clinical advance in the past 30 years; overall case fatality remains about 20% [1].

□ SKIN CANCERS AS GENETIC DISEASES

Cancer can be viewed as genetic disease in which the accumulation of genetic abnormalities – the activation of oncogenes and/or the inactivation of tumour suppressor genes – leads to a neoplastic clone whose phenotype allows it to expand [4]. These two processes, the generation of genetic diversity and the selection of the mutated phenotype, are the same that operate in macro-evolution. It is now clear, based on the pioneering work of Knudson on retinoblastoma, that the same genes are often involved in sporadic cancers as in familial cancer syndromes [4,5].

There is convincing evidence that genetic factors predispose to the development of skin cancers in at least some cases. About 3–5% of melanomas occur in individuals with a family history of the tumour (see Fig. 4) [6,7]. Another familial skin cancer is the naevus basal cell carcinoma syndrome (NBCCS), or Gorlin's syndrome, characterised by multiple basal cell carcinomas, medulloblastomas and dysmorphic facies (Fig. 5) [2]. The specific mutations now implicated in these syndromes are discussed below.

Various skin cancers show signs of genetic change, including relatively gross abnormalities such as loss of parts of specific chromosomes, as well as the point

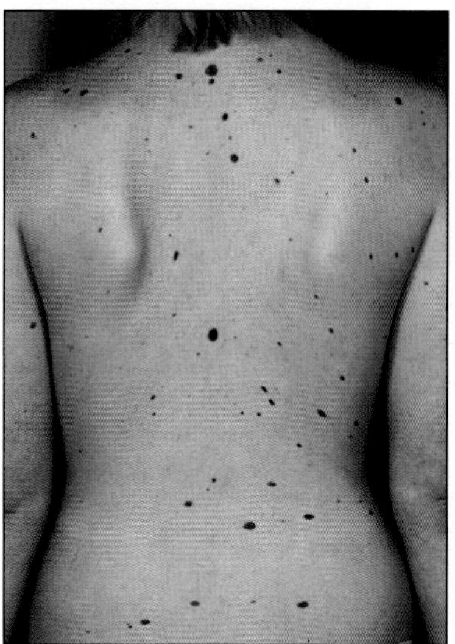

Fig. 4 A patient with a history of familial melanoma, in this case due to a mutation of p16. (Courtesy of Dr Wilma Bergman and Dr Nelleke Gruis, University of Leiden.)

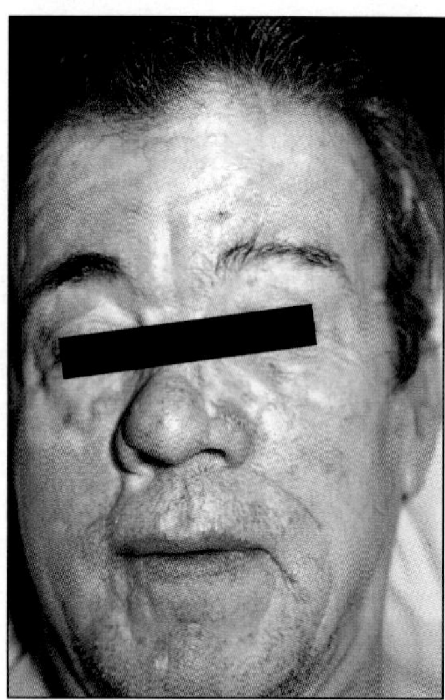

Fig. 5 A patient with a naevoid basal cell carcinoma (Gorlin's syndrome). This syndrome is inherited as an autosomal dominant and is characterised by multiple (sometimes hundreds) of basal cell carcinomas, medulloblastomas, dysmorphic facies, and other abnormalities. These patients' basal cell carcinomas should be treated surgically, as ionising radiation therapy is often followed by further tumour development.

mutations in regulatory genes described later. If there were a causal relationship between genotype and phenotype, genetic change should predict the tumour's clinical behaviour. Examination of a range of non-melanoma skin cancers does indeed show that such correlations exist, at least at the descriptive level of correlations between clinical behaviour and the extent and pattern of genetic change [2]. For example, the pattern of chromosome loss is more limited in basal cell carcinomas than in squamous cell carcinomas, and this may partly explain the more aggressive course of the latter of these two keratinocyte-derived tumours (Fig. 6) [8]. Moreover, keratoacanthoma, a spontaneously regressing form of squamous cell carcinoma, shows far less genetic change than the usual squamous cell carcinoma (Fig. 7) [2,9]. Similarly, melanomas that show loss of chromosome arms 10q or 6p (which presumably reflects loss of specific tumour suppressor genes at these sites) are more likely to metastasise than tumours in which these chromosomes are intact (see Fig. 8) [10].

By contrast, other aspects of the relationship between genetic change and behaviour are less clear. Actinic keratoses are small red scaly lesions characterised histologically by focal areas of dysplasia (Fig. 9) [1]. Although most run a banal clinical course, they are thought to be precursors of squamous cell carcinomas. Surprisingly, we showed that there is a high rate of mutation in actinic keratoses, even higher than that in cutaneous squamous cell carcinomas (Fig. 10) [11,12]. Interpretation of these experiments is difficult, as inevitably one group of lesions is compared with another group; it is not possible to follow individual lesions with sequential biopsies. Nevertheless, actinic keratoses may be a distinct entity, rather than a simple precursor of squamous cell carcinomas. This failure to reconcile genetic changes with clinical observations of tumour behaviour may reflect the limitations of our current genetic techniques, or the influence of other genetic and/or environmental factors. A final conceptual difficulty with the classical model of multistage carcinogenesis, requiring a critical number of 'hits' on the genome before neoplasia develops, is that the relationship between genetic change and tumour evolution is not always straightforward. The obvious example is basal cell carcinoma, which can show multiple genetic defects but has no apparent precursor lesion. The enigmatic relationship between actinic keratoses and squamous cell carcinoma has already been discussed.

The clinical impact of our present state of genetic knowledge is so far limited. Despite the convincing association between genetic changes and the clinical evolution of melanomas (including their crucial tendency to metastasise), genetic analyses add little to a robust and familiar measurement of tumour aggressiveness, namely its 'Breslow thickness' (the tumour's depth from the granular layer of the epidermis down to the lowest tumour cell in the dermis) [10]. Similarly, once the clinical diagnosis of sporadic non-melanoma skin cancer is made, there is little convincing evidence that genetic studies currently contribute anything useful to the clinical perspective.

□ SPECIFIC MUTATIONS IN SKIN CANCERS

Melanoma

Mutations of the p16 tumour suppressor gene have been identified in kindreds with familial melanoma. However, even in these families, about one-quarter of the

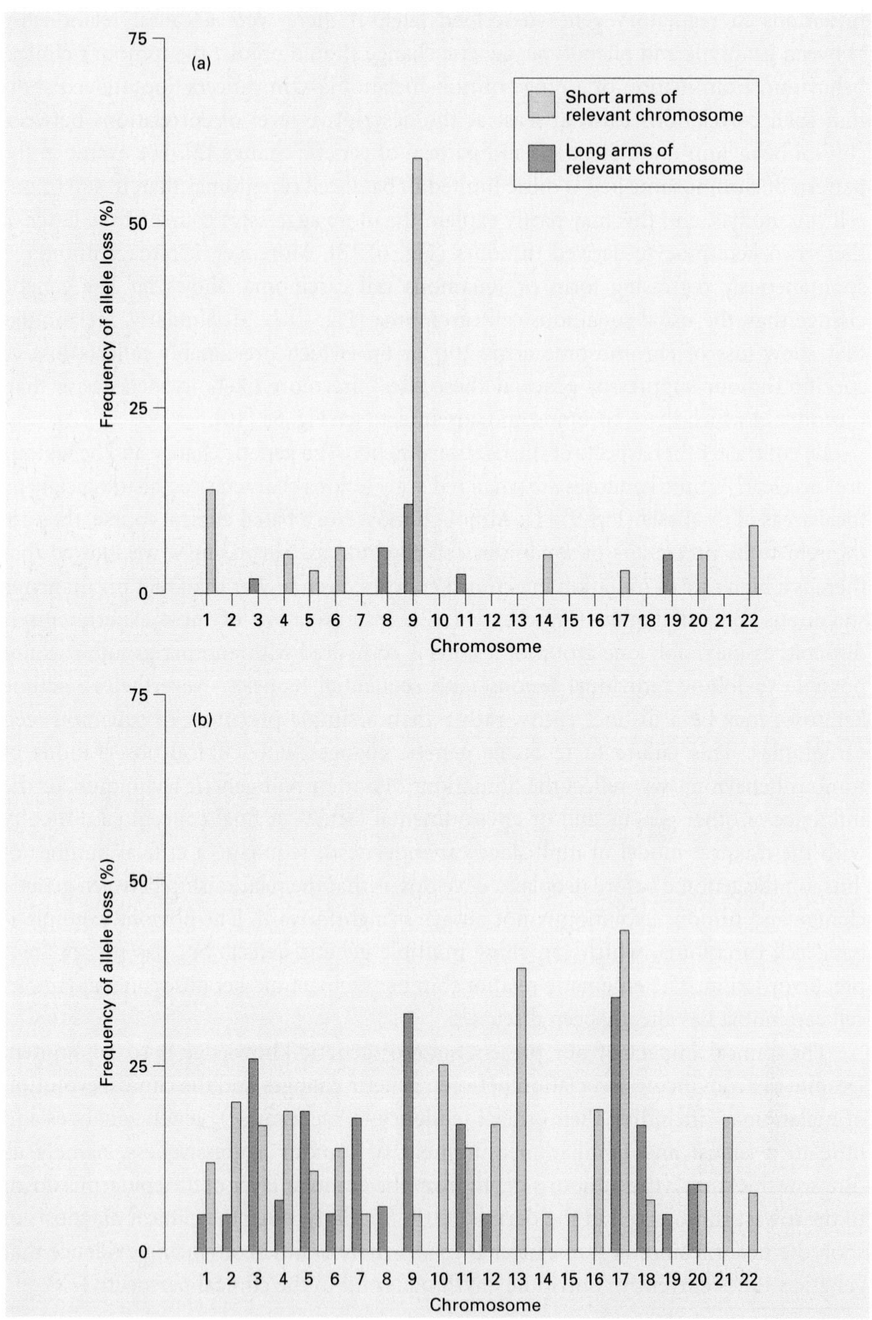

Fig. 6 The commonest mechanism of inactivation of tumour suppressor genes in cancer is by loss of the relevant area of the chromosome. This can be detected by 'loss of heterozygosity' analysis using PCR-based assays which can be performed on routine paraffin-embedded histological material. A comparison is shown between **(a)** the pattern of loss in basal cell carcinomas and **(b)** squamous cell carcinomas for each of the autosomes. Significant differences are present; in basal cell carcinomas most of the loss is confined to 9q whereas in squamous cell carcinomas of the skin the loss is more widespread.

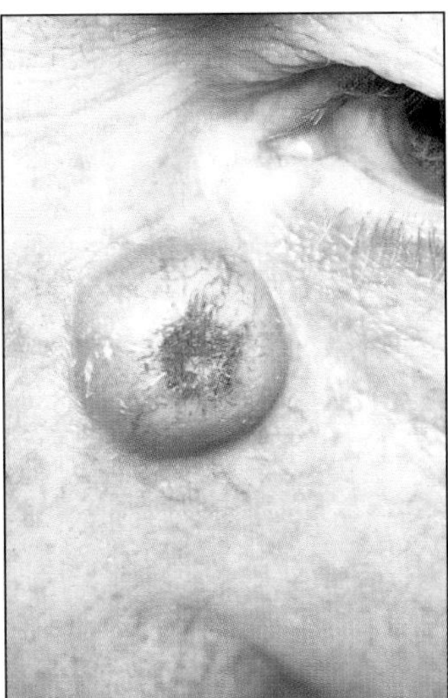

Fig. 7 Typical keratoacanthoma. These intriguing tumours have many histological and sometimes clinical similarities to cutaneous squamous cell carcinomas, but are characterised by spontaneous regression. Genetic analysis of these tumours shows multiple differences from squamous cell carcinomas.

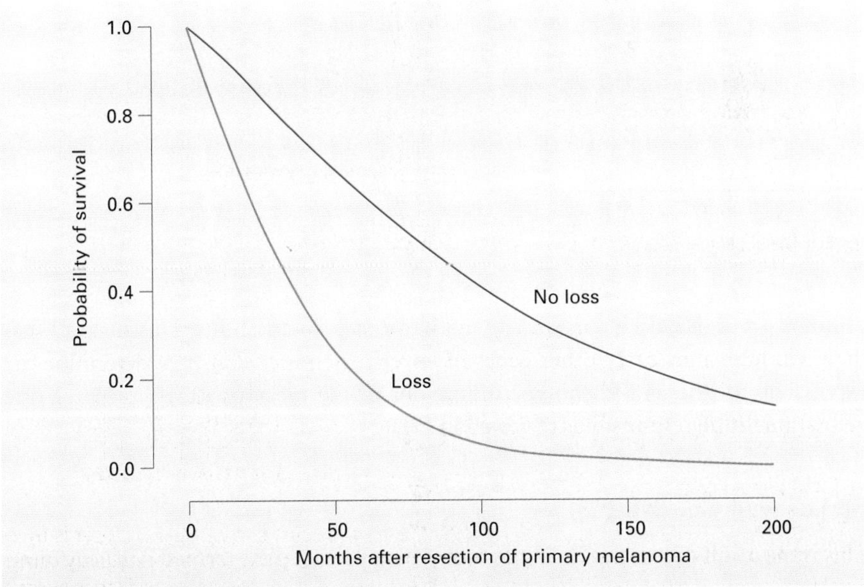

Fig. 8 Effects of genetic damage on survival in cutaneous melanoma. Loss-of-heterozygosity analysis can usefully predict the subsequent course of disease in patients who present with primary melanoma. Loss of chromosome 10q, a chromosomal region that presumably includes a key tumour suppressor gene, predicts a poor prognosis.

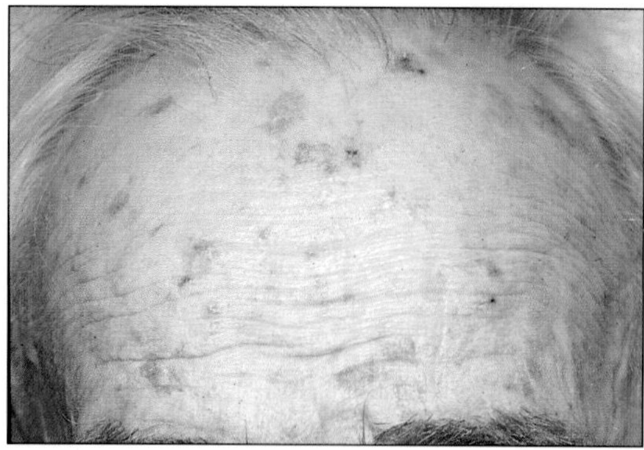

Fig. 9 Actinic keratoses are red scaly areas characterised by dysplasia histologically. They are very common, particularly in Caucasian populations in Australia. They are often multiple; clinically, it may be difficult to determine which area of the skin is normal.

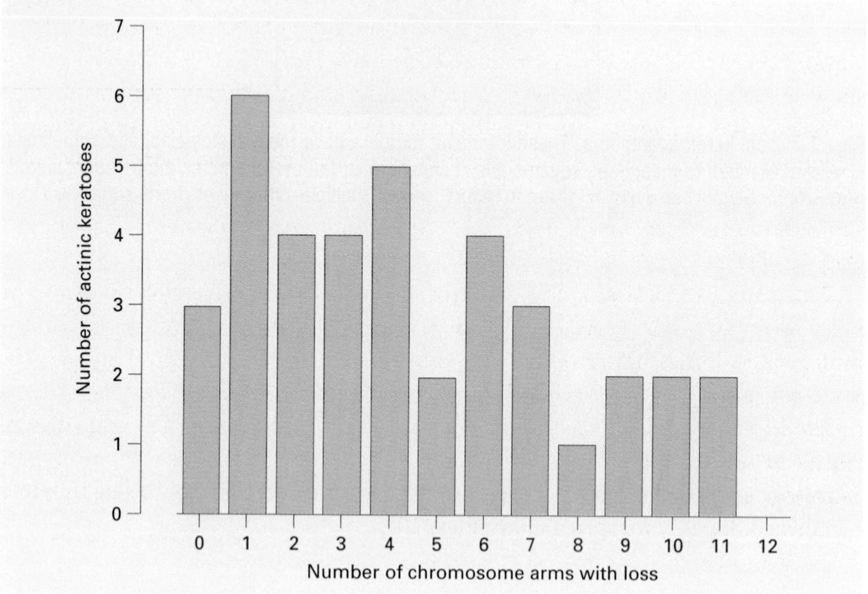

Fig. 10 Loss of chromosomal regions in actinic keratoses. This is surprisingly marked, in contrast to their banal clinical course.

tumours occur in individuals who do not harbour p16 mutations. This suggests that these kindreds may carry other genes of lower penetrance that may determine the expressivity of the p16 phenotype; mutations of the melanocortin-1 receptor (see below) might be responsible (reviewed in [7]).

Gorlin's syndrome (NBCCS)

This is the result of a mutation in the tumour suppressor gene termed *patched*, found on the short arm of chromosome 9. Loss or mutation of *patched* is also common in sporadic basal cell carcinomas. Recently, mutations in *smoothened* (*SMO*), an oncogene complementary to *patched* in the same signalling pathway, have been identified in some sporadic basal cell carcinomas (reviewed by Rees [13]).

□ SUNSHINE AND SKIN CANCER

The final part of this chapter will consider the molecular mechanisms through which ultraviolet radiation leads to the development of skin cancer, and the ways in which genetic factors might modulate this effect by influencing skin colour.

Ultraviolet radiation, molecular footprints and p53 clones

Ultraviolet radiation is carcinogenic and experimental models suggest that it is a complete carcinogen: it is mutagenic, can act as a tumour promoter, and can also depress the function of the cutaneous immune system which many believe to be important in protecting against skin cancer. Nevertheless, despite the convincing epidemiological evidence that ultraviolet radiation causes cutaneous neoplasia, direct proof of its role as a mutagen in human non-melanoma skin cancer (with or without other mechanisms) has only recently been established. Brash *et al* [14–16] showed that the 'footprint' pattern of mutations of the p53 tumour suppressor gene in cutaneous squamous cell carcinomas strongly suggested that ultraviolet B radiation was the causative mutagenic agent (Fig. 11). Brash's group have also shown, using whole mount p53 immunostaining of skin, that skin exposed to sun can harbour up to 40 clones/cm^2 of keratinocytes containing mutated p53 (Fig. 12) [17].

Early studies examining the mutational spectra in psoralen and ultraviolet A induced tumours (PUVA therapy) suggest that these are not the result of psoralen mutagenesis, but rather relate to some other aspect of PUVA on the skin, perhaps involving tumour promotion or immunosuppression [18,19]. Application of a similar logic to that for Bowen's disease has shown that some cases of Bowen's disease (intraepithelial carcinoma) on the trunk are probably not due to ultraviolet radiation, as the p53 mutational spectrum is very different from that of skin tumours or Bowen's disease on exposed body sites [20].

Skin cancer, red-hair genes and the melanocortin-1 receptor

People with red hair and pale skin have a greatly elevated risk of most forms of skin cancer, including melanoma and basal and squamous cell carcinomas. The genetic control of skin pigmentation is complex in man and other mammals; over 30 genes may influence coat colour in the mouse. Five years ago the genetic basis of one axis determining murine coat colour was elucidated. The *extension* locus was cloned and found to encode a seven-domain, G-protein coupled transmembrane receptor, termed the melanocortin-1 receptor, which belongs to a family of receptors including the ACTH receptors (reviewed in [21,22]); (see chapter 9). Melanocyte stimulating hormone (MSH), a cleavage product of propiomelanocortin (POMC) or possibly another ligand, acts through this receptor to increase the ratio of black (eumelanin) to red (phaeomelanin) pigment in the melanocytes of the hair follicle. The 133-residue peptide termed 'agouti' is produced within the follicle and antagonises the action of α-MSH, thus inhibiting the production of black pigment and lightening the coat colour (Fig. 13) [23]. Because both α-MSH and agouti also

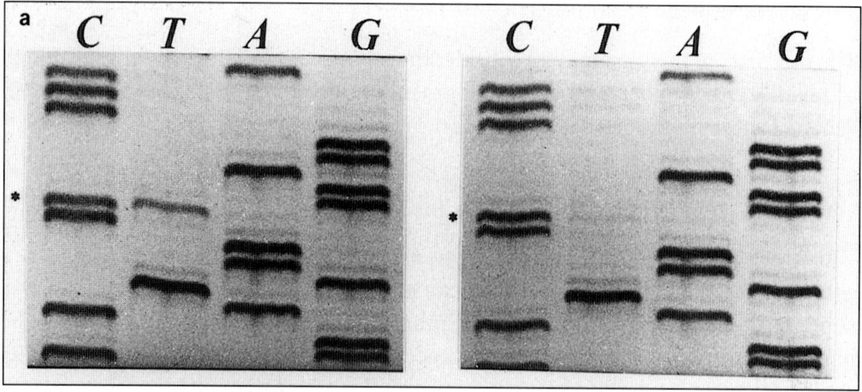

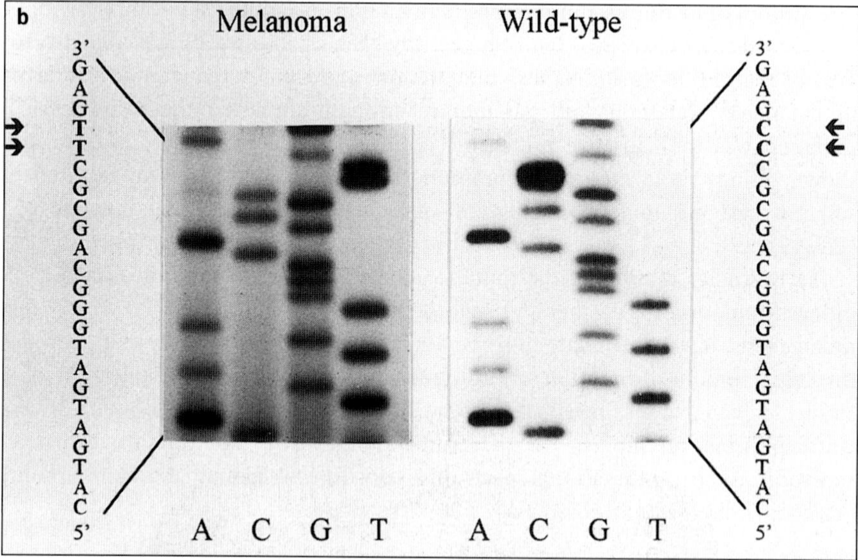

Fig. 11 Ultraviolet radiation induces a characteristic spectrum of mutation. The pattern of mutations, or 'molecular footprints', of ultraviolet radiation gives a clue to the causative mutagenic role of ultraviolet radiation in the pathogenesis of cutaneous tumours. **(a)** Left: * shows a mutation (C→T transition) at codon 248 of the p53 gene in a case of Bowen's disease. Right: * shows normal sequence at codon 248. **(b)** a CC→TT transition in the p16 gene in a case of cutaneous melanoma.

act at other melanocortin receptors, mouse mutants that express agouti inappropriately in various sites can show a range of phenotypes [23]. These include a yellow coat (the mouse equivalent of red) due to the effects of agouti blockade at the follicle's melanocortin-1 receptor, and obesity because agouti also inhibits the melanocortin-4 receptors which are expressed in the hypothalamus where they mediate the appetite-suppressing effects of α-MSH.

This brings us back to the control of human skin pigmentation. We have shown that the melanocortin-1 receptor is a key control point in the determination of skin colour in humans [24,25]. Sequence variants of this gene are common and most

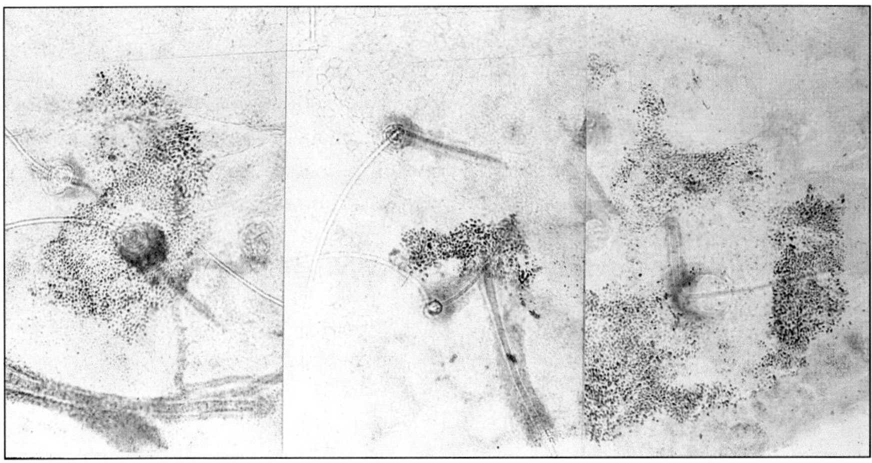

Fig. 12 Whole mount of sun-exposed human epidermis, immunostained for p53. Three different fields are shown, stained with an antibody against either wild-type or mutant p53. There are numerous clones of cells, many of which harbour p53 mutations. Such clones can be found at a density of up to 20–30 per cm^2.

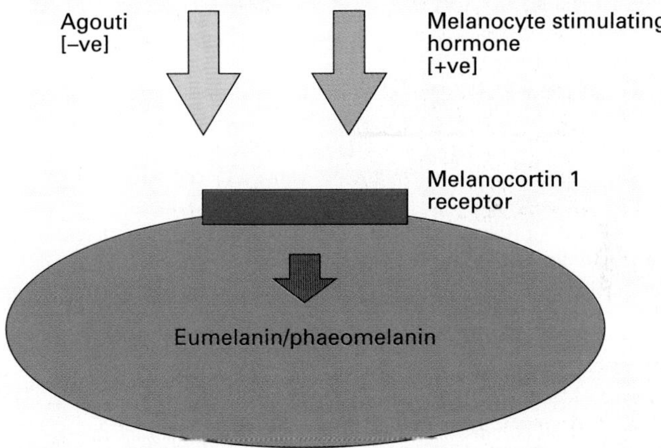

Fig. 13 Schematic model of the role of the melanocortin-1 receptor in the control of pigmentation. α-Melanocyte stimulating hormone acts as an agonist, possibly with other as yet uncharacterised ligands; agouti acts as a competitive antagonist or an inverse agonist. Acting through the melanocortin-1 receptor which is a 7-domain, G-protein coupled transmembrane receptor, α-MSH acts to increase the amount of eumelanin compared with phaeomelanin synthesis in the hair follicle, resulting in a darker coat colour.

individuals with red hair appear to be either compound heterozygotes or homozygous for two out of three crucial changes; together with early family studies, these data suggest that the trait is approximating to a Mendelian recessive. Perhaps not surprisingly, in individuals with skin cancer there is an over-representation of receptor mutations [24,26].

☐ CONCLUSIONS

Genetic approaches have already made an important contribution to the science of skin cancer, but few direct changes in clinical practice have so far flowed from these discoveries. New mechanistic insights could be particularly valuable for melanoma, where our understanding of the pathogenesis is less secure, treatment remains unsatisfactory, and the prognosis of patients with metastases is still poor. Whether further elucidation of the genetic abnormalities in melanoma, or alternative strategies more directly concerned with therapy, will be fruitful remains to be seen.

REFERENCES

1 Rees JL. Skin cancer (CME Dermatology-1). *J R Coll Physicians Lond* 1997; **31**: 246–50.

2 Rees JL. Non-melanoma skin cancer. In: Vogelstein B, Kinzler K (Eds). *The Genetics of Cancer.* New York: McGraw-Hill, 1997.

3 Rees JL. The melanoma epidemic: reality and artefact. *Br Med J* 1996; **312**: 137–8.

4 Kinzler KW, Vogelstein B. Lessons from hereditary colorectal cancer. *Cell* 1996; **87**: 159–70.

5 Knudson A. Genetic events in human carcinogenesis. In: Brugge J, Curran T, Harlow E, McCormick F (Eds). *Origins of Human Cancer.* New York: Cold Spring Harbor Laboratory Press, 1991: 17–26.

6 Marks R. An overview of skin cancers: incidence and causation. *Cancer* 1995; **75** (Suppl): 607–12.

7 Rees JL, Healy E. Molecular genetic approaches to non-melanoma and melanoma skin cancer. *Clin Exp Dermatol* 1996; **21**: 253–62.

8 Quinn AG, Sikkink S, Rees JL. Basal cell carcinomas and squamous cell carcinomas of human skin show distinct patterns of chromosome loss. *Cancer Res* 1994; **54**: 4756–9.

9 Waring AJ, Takata M, Rehman I, Rees JL. Loss of heterozygosity analysis of keratoacanthoma reveals multiple differences from cutaneous squamous cell carcinoma. *Br J Cancer* 1996; **73**: 649–53.

10 Healy E, Belgaid C, Takata M, *et al.* Prognostic significance of allelic losses in primary melanoma. *Oncogene* 1998; **16**: 2213–8.

11 Rehman I, Takata M, Wu YY, Rees JL. Genetic change in actinic keratoses. *Oncogene* 1996; **12**: 2483–90.

12 Rehman I, Quinn AG, Healy E, Rees JL. High frequency of loss of heterozygosity in actinic keratoses, a usually benign disease. *Lancet* 1994; **344**: 788–9.

13 Rees JL. Skin cancer. In: Scriver CR, Beaudet AL, Sly WS, Valle D, Vogelstein B (Eds). *Metabolic and Molecular Basis of Inherited Diseases*, 8th edn. New York: McGraw-Hill, in press.

14 Brash DE, Ziegler A, Jonason AS, *et al.* Sunlight and sunburn in human skin cancer:p53, apoptosis, and tumour promotion. *J Invest Dermatol Symp Proc* 1996; **1**(**S**): S136–42.

15 Brash DE. Sunlight and the onset of skin cancer. *Trends Genet* 1997; **13**: 410–4.

16 Leffel DJ, Brash DE. Sunlight and skin cancer. *Scientific American* 1996; **275**: 52–9.

17 Jonason AS, Kunala S, Price GJ, *et al.* Frequent clones of p53-mutated keratinocytes in normal human skin. *Proc Natl Acad Sci USA* 1996; **93**: 14025–9.

18 Nataraj AJ, Wolf P, Cerroni L, Ananthaswamy HN. p53 mutation in squamous cell carcinomas from psoriasis patients treated with psoralen plus UVA (PUVA). *J Invest Dermatol* 1997; **109**: 238–43.

19 Gasparro FP. p53 in dermatology. *Arch Dermatol* 1998; **134**: 1029–32.

20 Takata M, Rehman I, Rees JL. p53 mutation spectrum in Japanese Bowen's disease suggests a role for mutagens other than ultraviolet light. *Int J Cancer* 1997; **71**: 370–2.

21 Cone RD, Lu D, Koppula S, *et al.* The melanocortin receptors: agonists, antagonists, and the hormonal control of pigmentation. *Recent Progr Hormone Res* 1996; **51**: 287–317.

22 Rees JL, Healy E. Melanocortin receptors, red hair, and skin cancer. *J Invest Dermatol Symp Proc* 1997; **2**: 94–8.

23 Barsh GS. The genetics of pigmentation: from fancy genes to complex traits. *Trends Genet* 1996; **12**: 299–305.

24 Smith R, Healy E, Siddiqui S, *et al.* Melanocortin 1 receptor variants in an Irish population. *J Invest Dermatol* 1998; **111**: 119–22.

25 Valverde P, Healy E, Jackson I, *et al.* Variants of the melanocyte-stimulating hormone receptor gene are associated with red hair and fair skin in humans. *Nature Genet* 1995; **11**: 328–30.

26 Valverde P, Healy E, Sikkink S, *et al.* The AspGlu variant of the melanocortin 1 receptor (MC1R) is associated with melanoma. *Hum Mol Genet* 1996; **5**: 1663–6.

Atopic eczema

Peter Friedmann

☐ INTRODUCTION

The atopic state is a genetic predisposition to altered function of the immune system, which results in allergic reactions to environmental allergens. This immune dysfunction underlies the clinical syndromes, including allergic rhinitis, asthma and atopic eczema.

The defining characteristic of atopic individuals, which results from the immune dysregulation, is the capacity to form antibodies of the IgE class in response to antigens that enter the body through mucosal routes. IgE antibodies can be detected *in vivo* by immediate weal and flare responses to prick-test challenge with a wide range of allergens, including pollens, animal furs and danders and the house dust mite. *In vitro*, antigen-specific IgE is detected by RAST (radio-allergo-sorbent test).

☐ CLINICAL FEATURES OF ATOPIC ECZEMA

Atopic eczema begins most commonly in infancy. The rash of erythematous areas comprises tiny papules, sometimes with an urticaria-like component, which may join to form confluent red sheets. In infants, it commonly affects the whole body, including the head and face; on the limbs, predominantly extensor surfaces are affected. When the baby begins to crawl, the eczema tends to localise to extensor surfaces of the hands, wrists, knees and ankles. These changes in distribution are probably related to changes in exposure or contact with exogenous triggers, including friction from dusty floor surfaces. Once the upright toddling stage is reached, the eczema moves to flexural sites such as the popliteal and antecubital fossae (Fig. 1). The intensity of the rash may range from mild and limited in extent to severe, with extensive angrily inflamed involvement of most of the body surface. During acute exacerbations, lesions may be weepy and crusted, which usually signifies superinfection with staphylococci (Fig. 2). Chronic excoriated lesions are often thickened and lichenified.

Individuals with atopic eczema are prone to certain infective complications, because their immune resistance to various microbial pathogens is reduced. In particular, viral warts and lesions of molluscum contagiosum (Fig. 3) can be numerous and slow to clear. 'Eczema herpeticum' (Fig. 4) is infection with herpes simplex viruses, which may be extensive and aggressive.

☐ PREVALENCE OF ATOPIC ECZEMA

The prevalence of atopic diseases of all types has risen steadily over the past 30 years [2]. Data extracted from population-based surveys indicate that the percentage of

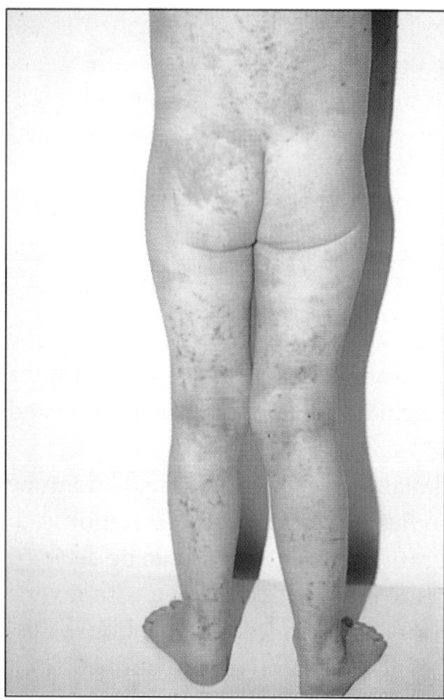

Fig. 1 Typical childhood atopic eczema involving trunk and flexures.

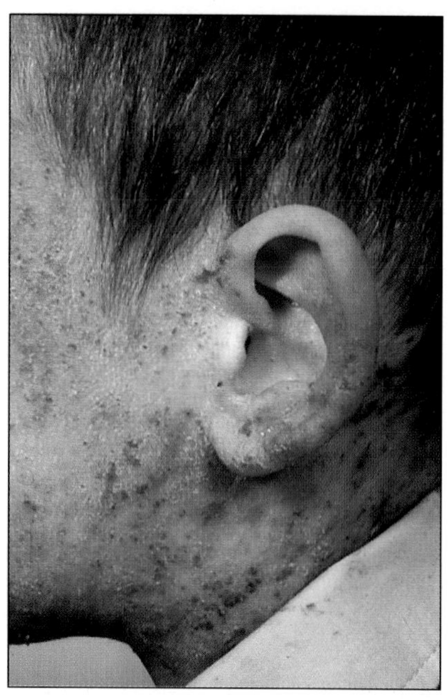

Fig. 2 'Impetiginised' eczema with staphylococcal superinfection.

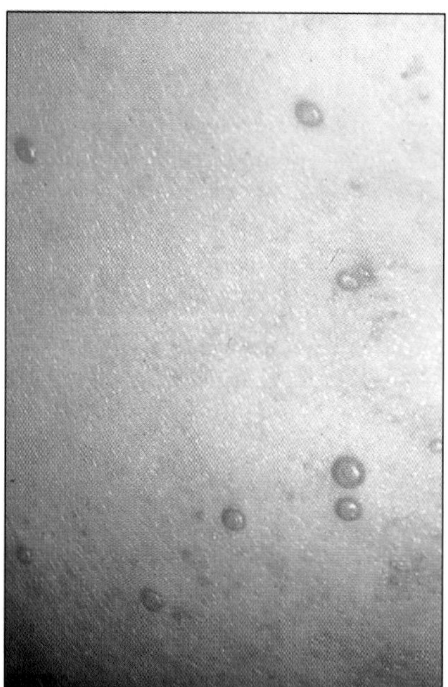

Fig. 3 Typical lesions of molluscum contagiosum. Note the depressed 'umbilicated' centre with altered appearance.

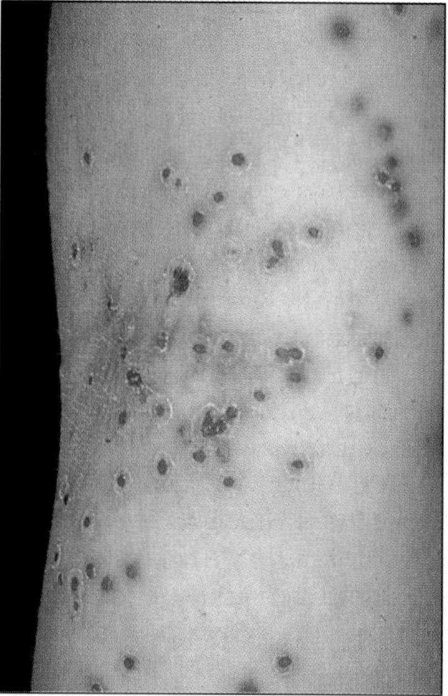

Fig. 4 Eczema herpeticum: infection with *Herpes simplex* virus. Note rather uniform size of erosions. (Figs 1–4 Reproduced by permission of the *British Medical Journal* from [1]).

children affected by atopic eczema was 4–8% in the 1960s, 9–12% in the 1970s and 15–20% in the 1980s. Epidemiological studies undertaken in the 1990s showed, for example, a lifetime prevalence of 24% in Austrian children up to the age of 8 years, a total prevalence of 22% in Danish children up to age 15, a total in England of 20%, and 15% of primary school children in Germany. It is not yet clear what is driving this change, but possible causes include changing rates of infection with measles, whooping cough and other microbes, as well as differences in atmospheric pollution levels and nutritional factors in the antenatal period.

□ CAUSES OF ATOPY

Genetic basis

The genetic base of the atopic state is the subject of intensive study. Atopy appears to be dominantly inherited; when both parents are atopic, their children have a 70% chance of being affected. A gene(s) that apparently determines the capacity to produce IgE has been reported on chromosome 11q13 and has been found to be linked with atopic asthma; however, linkage of this locus with eczema has not been confirmed [3]. It appears that the maternal genes at this site are more strongly linked than the paternal genes to the development of atopy in the offspring. Linkage has also been found at 5q31-33, a region where genes include those encoding interleukin (IL)-4, IL-12 and the β_2 adrenergic receptor. Most recently, a mutation in the α subunit of the IL-4 receptor resulting in 'gain of function' has been found strongly associated with atopy [4]. It is clear that the genetic basis of the atopic syndromes is complex and is likely to be determined by several genes.

Immune dysregulation in atopy

Immune dysregulation that favours IgE production appears to depend upon the selective activation of allergen-specific $CD4^+$ helper T cells of the Th2 phenotype in preference to the Th1 type [5]. Th2 cells produce IL-4 and IL-5 which stimulate IgE production by B lymphocytes, whereas Th1 cells produce interferon gamma (IFN-γ) which suppresses IgE synthesis (Fig. 5).

The mechanisms by which Th2 lymphocytes are produced in response to allergens are not completely understood. During the initiation of immune sensitisation, antigen-presenting cells (APC) process the antigen, cleaving it into small peptides which combine with HLA Class 2 molecules on the APC surface. The complexes of HLA Class 2 and associated peptides are 'inspected' by $CD4^+$ T helper cells, presumed to be so-called Th0 precursor cells. If the T cell receptor recognises the HLA Class 2/peptide complex, the T cell then receives activation signals from the APC through the binding of various ligands and their partners and through the actions of particular cytokines. Examples include the adhesion molecules, intercellular adhesion molecule (ICAM)-1 on the APC, and lymphocyte function associated molecule (LFA)-1 on the T cell. One of the critically important activation signals is through the interaction of CD28 on the T cell with its ligands B7.1 or B7.2 on the APC surface. It appears that if the T cell interacts with B7.1 it matures into

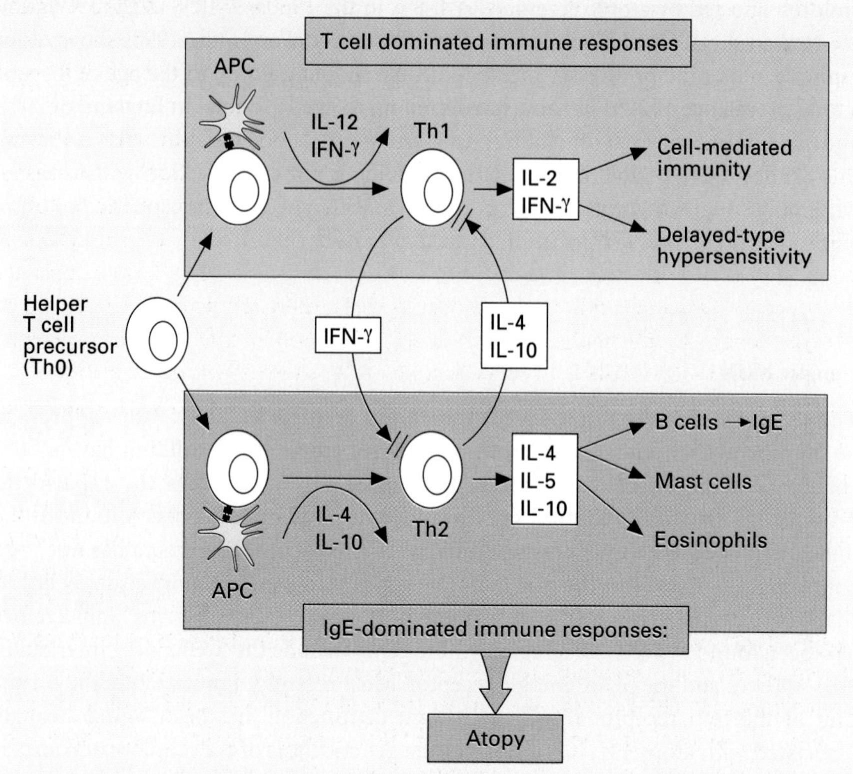

Fig. 5 Regulation of differentiation of T helper lymphocytes. Antigen presenting cells (APC) communicate with precursor Th0 cells via various surface ligands and cytokines. The balance between these determines differentiation towards either the Th1 or Th2 phenotype. In atopic individuals, there is probably preferential contact of APC and Th0 cell via B7.2, together with a relative deficiency of interferon-γ (IFN-γ) and the presence of interleukin 4 (IL-4). This results in predominant generation of Th2 cells, which in turn stimulate growth and differentiation of mast cells and encourage B cells to synthesise IgE. These immune alterations lay the foundation for the development of atopy.

the Th1 phenotype, whereas binding with B7.2 favours development into a Th2 type. In addition, the cytokines interacting with the T cell during this activation are also critical to its subsequent maturation. Interleukin-1 (IL-1) is probably always produced by APC, but other interleukins may play crucial roles: Th1 differentiation is favoured by IL-12, while Th2 maturation is promoted by IL-4 and possibly IL-6. In atopic individuals, it is presumed that the various signals from the APC to a Th0 cell have the overall effect of inducing it to mature into a Th2 type of cell.

Atopic responses are also determined by the type of antigen being processed, as demonstrated by studies of peripheral blood T cells from atopic patients which were stimulated with atopy-related allergens such as DerP1 from the house dust mite (HDM) *Dermatophagoides pteronyssinus* or antigens such as tetanus toxoid or *Candida albicans.* When cloned, T cells stimulated with allergens – but not those stimulated with tetanus toxoid or *C. albicans* – were predominantly of the Th2 type, producing high amounts of IL-4 and IL-5 and little or no IFN-γ. Moreover, these allergen-specific Th2 cells could induce IgE production by normal B cells *in vitro*. By contrast, allergen-specific clones from non-atopic control subjects were of Th1 type, producing IFN-γ and little or no IL-4 or IL-5.

Another component of immune regulation that appears significantly disturbed in atopy is the production of IFN-γ, as demonstrated in peripheral blood mononuclear leucocytes from atopic donors [6]. This altered balance of cytokine production appears to be one of the critical factors underlying the IgE production in atopy. IgE-class antibodies are produced against a wide range of environmental allergens, including aeroallergens such as pollens, animal fur, HDM excreta, and various foods. Interestingly, reduced levels of IFN-γ are found in cord-blood mononuclear cells of babies born to families with a history of atopic allergies [7]. Moreover, when these babies were followed for the first year of life, there appeared to be a good correlation between the presence of decreased cord-blood IFN-γ concentrations and the subsequent development of atopic dermatitis. This suggests that the imbalance of cytokine production is an early and possibly primary event.

The reduced production of IFN-γ in atopy appears to result from increased activity of cyclic AMP (cAMP) phosphodiesterase. This defect can be demonstrated in all leucocytes (including T cells) from atopic dermatitis patients, although it is most evident in blood monocytes. The increased phosphodiesterase activity blunts the cAMP responses to stimulation [8], which in turn results in overproduction of prostaglandin E_2 (PGE_2) by mononuclear leucocytes. The increased PGE_2 appears to be responsible for the reduced generation of IFN-γ, as IFN-γ release was significantly augmented by indomethacin, an inhibitor of prostaglandin synthesis.

These findings suggest that the dysregulation between Th1 and Th2 cells and their cytokines may be determined at the level of their interaction with APC [9]. This is consistent with the observation that Langerhans cells (the APC in the skin) from patients with atopic dermatitis carry IgE on their surface. The IgE is bound by both the high-affinity receptor (FceRI) [9] and the low-affinity receptor CD23 (FceRII), and apparently participates in the presentation of allergens [10] (see below). It therefore appears possible that T cells stimulated by Langerhans cells under the appropriate conditions can develop into IL-4 producing Th2 cells.

Pathogenesis of atopic eczema

Histological examination of eczematous skin reveals an inflammatory infiltrate of mononuclear cells including $CD4^+$ T lymphocytes, similar to that seen in classical contact dermatitis evoked by sensitisers such as nickel. This suggests that T cell-mediated allergic responses may also be involved.

Allergy and atopic eczema

Most subjects with atopic eczema exhibit immediate hypersensitivity reactions to both prick test challenge and intradermal inoculation of antigens. Prick tests, which are the standard test for detection of immediate or 'Type 1' hypersensitivity, involve assisting the penetration of allergens through the skin surface with a tiny point. Intradermal tests involve inoculation of antigen with a hypodermic syringe to a slightly deeper level in the dermis. The relevance of immediate hypersensitivity to eczema is unclear. Moreover, delayed-type hypersensitivity to a variety of antigens, including HDM, has also been shown by many workers. For example, we challenged a group of patients with atopic eczema intradermally with extracts of HDM and monitored the reactions clinically and by increases in skin thickness [11]. There was a weal and flare, maximal at 15–30 min, followed by an erythematous, palpable reaction that was present at 6 hours and persisted for 48–72 hours (Fig. 6). This sequence of events indicates a complex response, with initial immediate hypersensitivity succeeded by a late-phase reaction which continues into a form of delayed hypersensitivity. Furthermore, *in vitro* lymphocyte proliferative responses can be elicited with allergens, including HDM and grasses, also indicating the presence of delayed-type hypersensitivity [12].

Several groups have examined the responses to topical patch-test challenge, the standard method for demonstrating allergic contact hypersensitivity to chemicals such as nickel in jewellery. An example was our study of 31 adults and 24 children with atopic dermatitis, all investigated when the eczema was quiescent (partly reported in [13]). Antigens were applied by epicutaneous patches to skin on the back that had been stripped with adhesive tape, and included HDM, *Dermatophagoides farinae*, cat fur and mixed grasses. Patches were applied for 48 hours and read as for standard contact allergy patch tests. Eczematous responses were obtained with at least one antigen in most atopic subjects but none was observed in 13 non-atopic

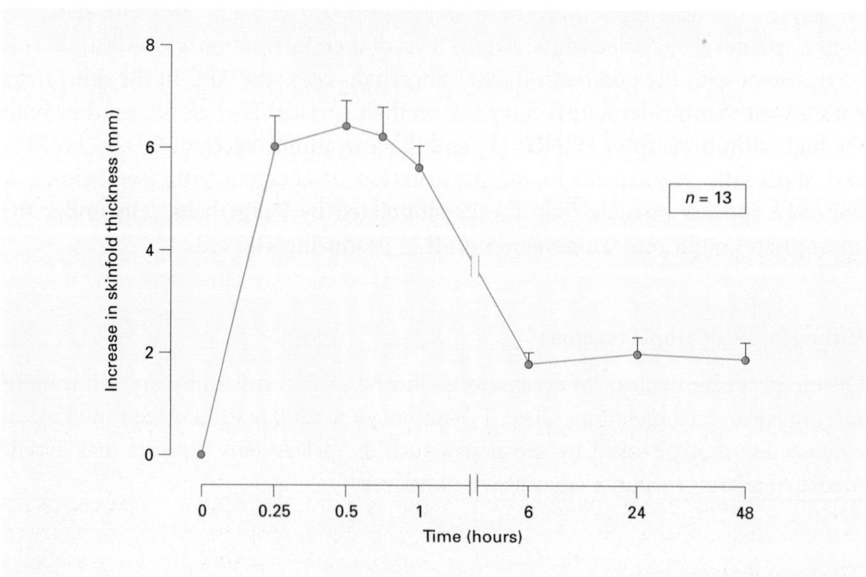

Fig. 6 Response to intradermal challenge with house dust mite antigen (DerP1). Following inoculation of 50 μl containing DerP1 30 Biological Units, oedema was measured with callipers as skinfold thickness. There is a weal and flare between 15 and 60 minutes, a 6 hour late phase response and a 24–48 hour delayed response. Note the non-linear x-axis.

controls (Table 1). Seventy per cent gave positive patch test responses to HDM, which were dose-related both in terms of number of times that the skin had been stripped and the antigen concentration. There was a strong correlation between the presence of positive patch tests and positive immediate prick tests, but these were dissociable; occasional subjects gave positive patch tests but negative prick tests, while 25% gave positive prick tests and negative patch tests (Table 2).

The natural history of inflammatory changes following epicutaneous patch-test challenge may mimic those in naturally occurring eczema. Immunocytochemical studies of skin biopsies eight hours after challenge show increased expression of adhesion molecules ICAM-1 and E-selectin on dermal microvascular endothelium and upregulated ICAM-1 on epidermal keratinocytes. There is also degranulation of mast cells which progresses up to 48 hours post-challenge, infiltration with activated eosinophils between 24 and 48 hours, infiltration with IL-4 expressing T cells (Th2 type) at 24 hours, and a progressive accumulation of T cells expressing IFN-γ up to 72 hours. The different time-courses of infiltration with Th2 and Th1 cells have been shown by cloning cells from sequential biopsies. These and other studies suggest overall that the response to challenge with allergen initially involves

Table 1 Patch tests with different allergens in atopic eczema; data are from sites stripped 7 times with cellophane tape.

	D. pteronyssinus	*D. farinae*	Cat fur	Grass pollen
Atopic adults				
Number tested	31	21	31	22
Number positive	21	9	16	11
% positive	68%	43%	54%	50%
Atopic children				
Number tested	24	15	20	24
Number positive	14	2	8	6
% positive	58%	13%	40%	25%
Healthy controls				
Number tested	13	13	13	13
Number positive	0	0	0	0

Table 2 Responses to prick/patch challenge with different allergens in patients with atopic eczema. No positive responses were obtained in 13 healthy, non-atopic controls.

Prick	Patch	*D. pteronyssinus*	*D. farinae*	Cat fur	Grass pollen
+	+	31/50	10/33	14/48	18/39
–	+	4/50	1/33	6/48	0/39
+	–	12/50	14.33	14/48	15/39
–	–	5/50	8/33	9/48	6/39

recruitment of Th2 type T cells, followed by infiltration with Th1 type cells [14,15]; apparently Th1 cytokines somehow convert the early inflammation into eczema.

Causal relevance of allergy: house dust mites cause eczema

Although allergic reactions can be elicited by skin prick or patch tests, it is still uncertain whether responses truly identify clinically significant provoking factors. One way to ascertain the role of a particular allergen in an individual is to observe the effects of removing it from the subject's environment; for aeroallergens this is not easy to achieve.

House dust mites (*D. pteronyssinus*) and the antigens found in their faecal pellets (DerP1) have long been suspected to be important, and this has recently been confirmed by a study that we performed to answer two critical questions [16]: first, how effectively could a combination of commercially available anti-HDM measures reduce the load of DerP1 in the bedroom and living-room; and second, would these measures produce any clinical benefit in patients with severe atopic eczema. Forty-eight patients (including 24 children aged 6–16) completed a double-blind, placebo-controlled trial of 6 months duration. Active treatment comprised extremely fine-mesh (Goretex®) bags applied to the mattress, top covers and pillows of all beds in the patient's bedroom; the application of a spray containing benzyl alcohol and tannic acid (Allersearch DMS) which claimed to kill mites and denature their allergens; and a high-powered vacuum cleaner. Placebo treatment was light cotton bags, water spray and a standard domestic vacuum cleaner. The anti-mite measures were applied by a trained nurse. Dust was sampled in a standard fashion with a vacuum cleaner and filter chamber, before and during the study, and was weighed and its DerP1 content determined by ELISA (ALK). We found that the Goretex® bed bags were highly effective at containing the dust within the bedding (Fig. 7), and that the resulting fall in DerP1 load resulted in highly significant improvements in the clinical scores of eczema severity in both children and adults (Fig. 8); those with the most severe eczema showed the greatest benefit. There were no differences in the final dust content or in the irreducible minimal load of DerP1 in the carpets of either group, showing that the ordinary domestic vacuum cleaner was as effective as the expensive one combined with an acaricidal spray.

Thus, it is possible to eliminate dust mite antigens from beds (but not carpets), with considerable clinical improvements. These findings demonstrate clearly that allergy to dust mites is a major provoking factor in a substantial proportion of people with atopic eczema, and also highlight the need for improved methods to identify those who will benefit from such anti-HDM measures.

□ TREATMENT OF ATOPIC ECZEMA

An approach to management is outlined in Fig. 9. The major components of treatment include regular use of moisturisers such as emulsifying ointment or aqueous cream which can control many symptoms, and also topical steroids. The latter range from weak (eg 1% hydrocortisone) to moderately strong (eg clobetasone butyrate) – which should be used when eczema is not too active – to potent (betamethasone

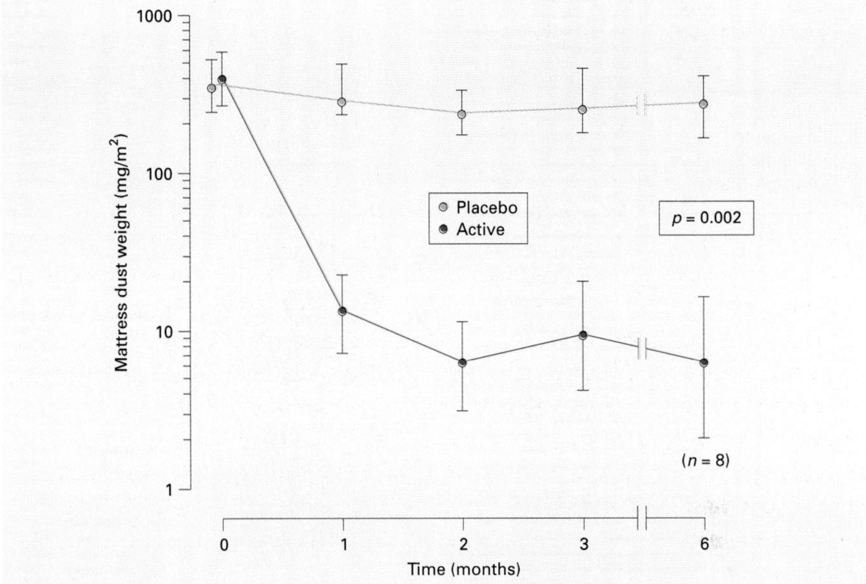

Fig. 7 Effect of ultrafine mesh Goretex® bed bags on the weight of dust on the mattress surface. Dust was collected over two minutes from the whole upper surface of the mattress with a standard dust sampler filter. The active treatment reduced dust quantity so greatly that there was insufficient dust to extract for DerP1 assay. For this reason, only eight beds were sampled at six months. (Reproduced from [16] by permission of the *Lancet*.)

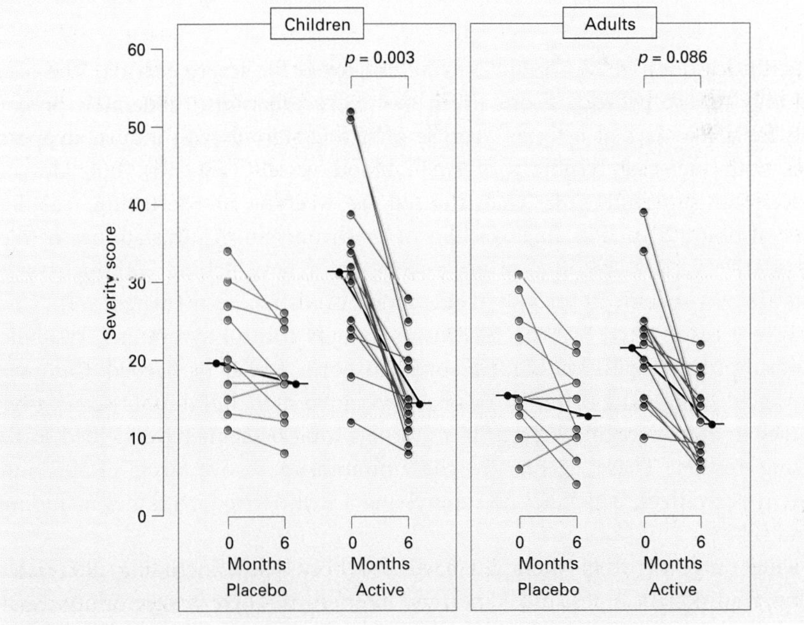

Fig. 8 Clinical effects of house dust mite avoidance on severity of atopic eczema. Eczema severity scores for each individual before and after six months of dust mite avoidance are connected by coloured lines. Medians in each group are joined by black lines.

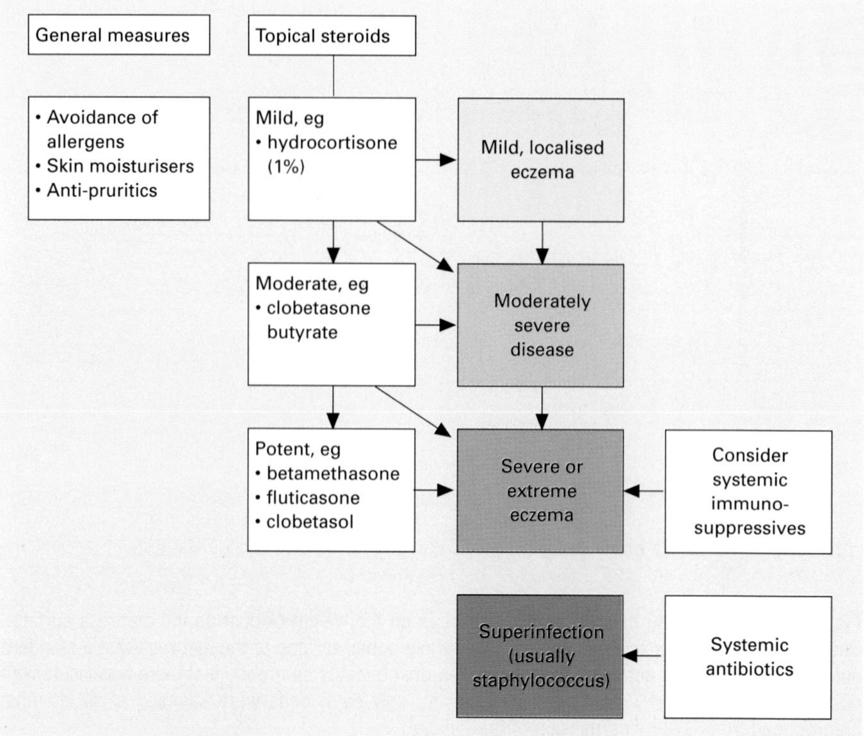

Fig. 9 Scheme for management of atopic eczema.

valerate, fluticasone) which should only be employed for severe eczema. The face should only receive hydrocortisone or, in severe exacerbations, moderately potent steroids for a few days at a time. Overuse of strong steroids will induce atrophic changes with increased visibility of small blood vessels (Fig. 10). Episodes of staphylococcal superinfection, characterised by weeping and crusting, require systemic antibiotics such as flucloxacillin or erythromycin. Antihistamines of the older, sedative variety are often given, as they can relieve itching, although their benefits are non-specific as the itch of eczema is not histamine-mediated.

In severe cases where topical treatments cannot control symptoms, systemic immunosuppression with azathioprine or cyclosporin A may be needed. Gamma-linolenic acid (in evening primrose oil) has been advocated, but doubts persist over its efficacy in atopic eczema. Recent trials of new topical agents have yielded some promising results. These agents are the immunosuppressive drug FK506 and ascomycin derivatives, which act by suppressing T cell-derived cytokines including IL-2 and IFN-γ.

A wide range of other therapies have also been used, including ultraviolet radiation, traditional Chinese medicines, and interferons. There is uncertainty about the reliability of some of these therapies.

More detailed consideration of management of atopic eczema is provided in a recent review [13].

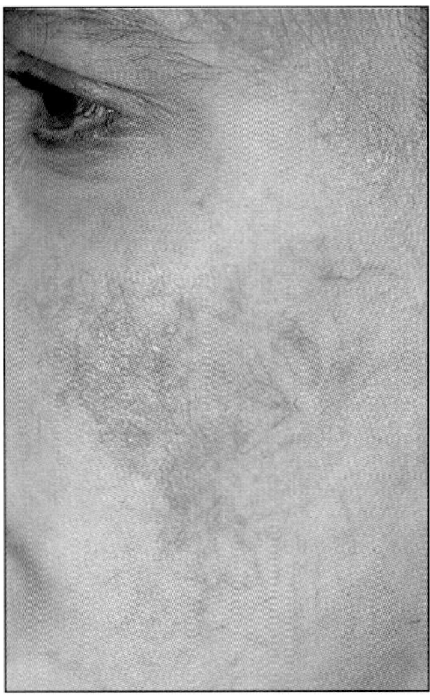

Fig. 10 Chronic eczema sufferer with steroid-induced telangiectasia following long-term topical application.

REFERENCES

1 Friedmann PS. Allergy and the skin. II. Contact and Atopic Eczema. *Brit Med J* 1998; **316**: 1226–9.

2 Williams HC. Is the prevalence of atopic dermatitis increasing? *Clin Exp Dermatol* 1992; **17**: 385–91.

3 Coleman R, Trembath RC, Harper JI. Chromosome 11q13 and atopy underlying atopic eczema. *Lancet* 1993; **341**: 1121–2.

4 Hershey GKK, Friedrich MF, Esswein LA, *et al.* The association of atopy with a gain-of-function mutation in the alpha subunit of the interleukin-4 receptor. *N Engl J Med* 1997; **337**: 1720–5.

5 Romagnani S. Biology of human Th1 and Th2 cells. *J Clin Immunol* 1995; **15**: 121–9.

6 Renz H, Jujo K, Bradley KL, *et al.* Enhanced IL-4 production and IL-4 receptor expression in atopic dermatitis and their modulation by interferon-gamma. *J Invest Dermatol* 1992; **99**: 403–8.

7 Warner JA, Miles EA, Jones AC, *et al.* Is deficiency of interferon gamma production by allergen-triggered cord blood cells a predictor of atopic eczema? *Clin Exp Allergy* 1994; **24**: 423–30.

8 Holden CA. Atopic dermatitis: messengers, second messengers and cytokines. *Clin Exp Dermatol* 1993; **18**: 201–7.

9 Chan SC, Li SH, Hanifin JM. Increased interleukin-4 production by atopic mononuclear leukocytes correlates with increased cyclic adenosine monophosphate-phosphodiesterase activity and is reversible by phosphodiesterase inhibition. *J Invest Dermatol* 1993; **100**: 681–4.

10 Mudde GC, van Reijsen FC, Boland GJ, *et al.* Allergen presentation by epidermal Langerhans cells from patients with atopic dermatitis is mediated by IgE. *Immunology* 1990; **69**: 335–41.

11 Munro CS, Higgins EM, Marks JM, *et al.* Cyclosporin A in atopic dermatitis: therapeutic response is dissociated from effects on allergic reactions. *Br J Dermatol* 1991; **124**: 43–8.

12 Ramb Lindhauer C, Feldmann A, Rotte M, Neumann C. Characterization of grass pollen reactive T-cell lines derived from lesional atopic skin. *Arch Dermatol Res* 1991; **283**: 71–6.

13 Friedmann PS, Tan BB, Musaba E, Strickland I. Pathogenesis and management of atopic dermatitis. *Clin Exp Allergy* 1995; **25**: 799–806.

14 Thepen T, Langeveldwildschut EG, Bihari IC, *et al.* Bi-phasic response against aeroallergen in atopic eczema, showing an in-situ switch from a Th2 into a Th1 response. *J Allergy Clin Immunol* 1995; **95**: 365.

15 Krutmann J, Grewe M. Sequential activation of Th1 and Th2 cells in the immunopathogenesis of atopic eczema: the 2-phase model. *Allergologie* 1996; **19**: 449–51.

16 Tan BB, Weald D, Strickland I, Friedmann PS. Double-blind controlled trial of effect of housedust-mite allergen avoidance on atopic dermatitis. *Lancet* 1996; **347**: 15–8.

☐ MULTIPLE CHOICE QUESTIONS

1 Typical features of atopic eczema are:
(a) Distribution over extensor surfaces
(b) Elevated total IgE
(c) Family history of atopic allergies (asthma or hayfever)
(d) Provocation of skin lesions by contact with nickel
(e) Good clinical response to non-sedating antihistamines

2 Characteristic features of the atopic state are:
(a) Low production of interferon gamma by peripheral blood mononuclear leucocytes
(b) Elevated plasma IgA concentration
(c) Positive weal and flare responses to aero-allergens
(d) An infiltrate of $CD4^+$ T lymphocytes in the skin
(e) Increased susceptibility to severe herpes simplex 1 infection

3 Atopic eczema is characterised by:
(a) Autosomal dominant inheritance pattern
(b) Itching made worse by sweating
(c) Delayed blanche reaction to stroking the skin
(d) Cholinergic urticaria
(e) Delayed hypersentivity response to dust mites
(f) Increased susceptibility to irritation by soaps
(g) Increased susceptibility to viral warts

4 Atopic eczema is:
(a) More common in postmature babies
(b) Characteristically distributed over the extensor surfaces in pre-walking babies
(c) Associtaed with lymphocyte responses of the Th2 type
(d) Responds well to desensitisation therapy
(e) Diagnosed by the presence of positive patch test responses to house dust mites

ANSWERS

1		2		3		4	
1a	False	2a	True	3a	True	4a	True
b	True	b	False	b	True	b	True
c	True	c	True	c	True	c	True
d	False	d	True	d	False	d	False
e	False	e	True	e	True	e	False
				f	True		
				g	True		

Management of psoriasis: recent developments in phototherapy

James Ferguson

☐ INTRODUCTION

Psoriasis is a generally benign non-life-threatening skin disease that affects approximately 2% of the Caucasian population. It has a remarkable range of presentations, from a non-pustular variant of early onset to a generalised late-onset pustulosis form with many variants between. In its mildest form, it is merely inconvenient, but when severe and chronic it may destroy a patient's quality of life.

☐ AETIOLOGY OF PSORIASIS

Strong evidence of a genetic basis for psoriasis has been recognised for many years, particularly from epidemiological [1] and twin studies, but the precise mode of inheritance is still unknown.

Early-onset psoriasis appears to be associated with specific Class 1 and 2 HLA antigen loci (B13, B17, B39, B57, Cw6, Cw7, DR4, DR7) on chromosome 6 and as such represents a potential target for the application of genomic technology [2]. Further study has revealed other possible linkages with chromosomes 2, 8 and 20 [3].

There is evidence for T lymphocyte involvement in the pathogenesis of psoriasis, with a wide range of abnormally expressed cytokines and growth factors; psoriasis has common features with other relapsing T cell mediated diseases, such as rheumatoid arthritis and Crohn's disease [4]. Multiple environmental factors including drugs (eg lithium, beta-blockers), injury, infection and superantigens, particularly streptococcal, are known to interact with the genetic predisposition and precipitate or aggravate the disease. This wide span of inheritable and environmental factors suggests that – despite current enthusiasm – gene therapy may be some way off.

☐ MANAGEMENT OF PSORIASIS

Present therapy for mild localised disease includes topical tars, dithranol and vitamin D analogues. These have the attraction of being relatively cheap and suitable for use at home. However, for those with moderate to severe psoriasis, topical therapy is inadequate because of its slow progress, inconvenience, tendency to stain skin and clothing and the need for prolonged application times. These patients ultimately require the use of ultraviolet-B (UVB) phototherapy or photochemotherapy (PUVA), ie the combination of ultraviolet-A (UVA) with a 'psoralen' agent. If these are not available, systemic cytotoxic therapies such as methotrexate, cyclosporin, hydroxyurea and acitretin must be considered (Fig. 1).

The rest of this chapter will concentrate on the various forms of phototherapy.

Phototherapy: principles and history

Sunlight has long been recognised to be of value to psoriasis sufferers. It is, however, an unpredictable commodity in northern latitudes, with the additional problem in industrial countries that most of the population works indoors, even in summer months. The development of artificial light sources at the start of this century provided the opportunity for controlled phototherapy, initially with electric discharge lamps and, more recently, with fluorescent tubes. In 1903, Niels Finsen (Fig. 2) was awarded the Nobel Prize for Medicine 'in recognition of his contribution to the treatment of skin diseases, particularly lupus vulgaris, with concentrated light irradiation, whereby he has opened a new avenue for medical science'. Thus began a technology-led process whose subsequent refinements (notably the invention of fluorescent sources with specific phosphors designed to emit therapeutic wavelengths) have brought so much relief to many psoriasis sufferers. Within the United Kingdom, the current move away from inpatient to outpatient management, together with increased awareness of the carcinogenic risks of PUVA, has led to the increasing use of UVB phototherapy for psoriasis. PUVA involves oral ingestion or bath exposure to a psoralen (purified plant extract, eg 5-methoxypsoralen extracted from the oil of bergamot orange) which is followed by UVA irradiation, usually delivered in a stand-up cubicle. This is a remarkably effective therapy that can clear extensive psoriasis in 12–18 treatments when given twice weekly. However, it has significant long-term risks. Since its introduction for the treatment of psoriasis in 1973, it has become apparent that multiple courses result in chronic damage to the skin, notably leading to an 83-fold increased risk of squamous-cell carcinoma in

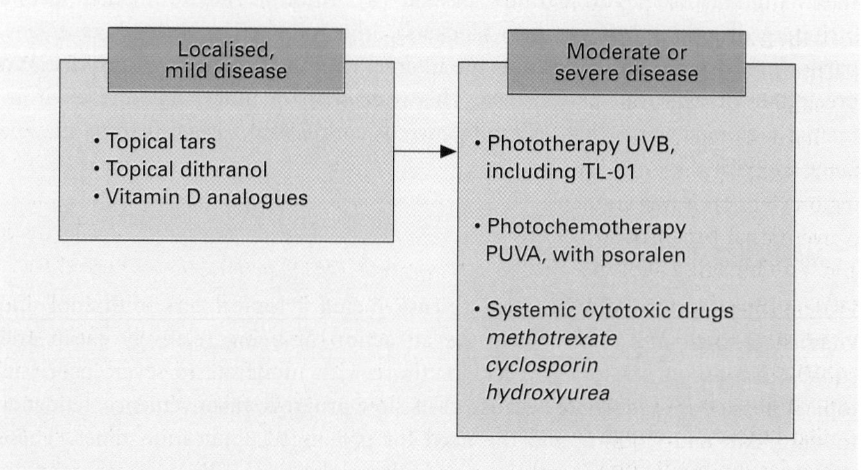

Fig. 1 Management of psoriasis.

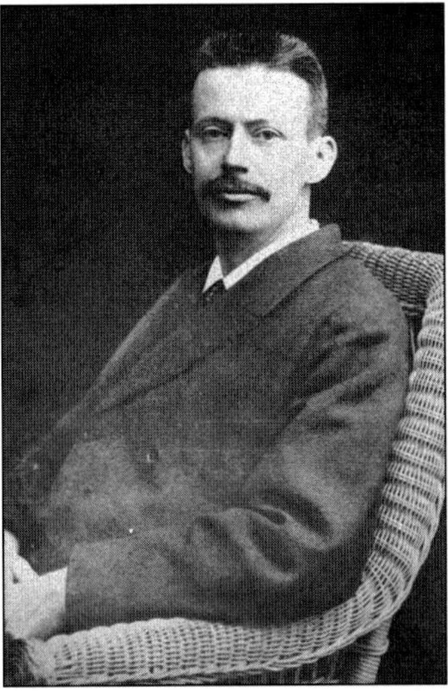

Fig. 2 Niels Ryberg Finsen (1860–1904), discoverer of phototherapy.

those patients who have received more than 300 treatments. There is good evidence that carcinogenesis is significantly less of a problem with UVB than PUVA, and this in part explains the surge in use of UVB phototherapy [5].

Optimising phototherapy

The central theme in the development of new therapeutic light sources to treat skin diseases is that of 'therapeutic action spectroscopy', namely the precise determination of the optimal wavelengths and irradiation dose relationships of the therapeutically active part of the electromagnetic spectrum. Much work strongly suggests that psoriasis has its own particular waveband responsible for disease clearance, lying within the UVB region (295–320 nm) (Fig. 3). As some evidence suggests that the shortest of these wavelengths are the most capable of inducing cancer, attention has focused on finding a suitable fluorescent light source that emits UVB of mainly longer wavelengths.

Ten years ago, a Dutch group [6] persuaded Philips Lighting to manufacture a fluorescent tube lamp (TL-01) that emitted a narrow peak at 312 nm within the UVB region (Fig. 4). It was argued that the omission of the shorter wavelengths present in conventional broad-band UVB sources would provide more therapeutically active and less damaging light treatment for psoriasis. The key questions about the efficacy, safety, optimal usage and performance compared with other therapies are only now being answered. Over the past 10 years, several clinical studies have consistently reported greater therapeutic effect of the TL-01 source in psoriasis, compared with conventional broad-band sources [7] (Fig. 5). Comparisons with PUVA show a similar efficacy, although it is clear that some patients still require PUVA to achieve a long-lasting remission.

Combination therapy with tars, dithranol or oral retinoids reduces the total

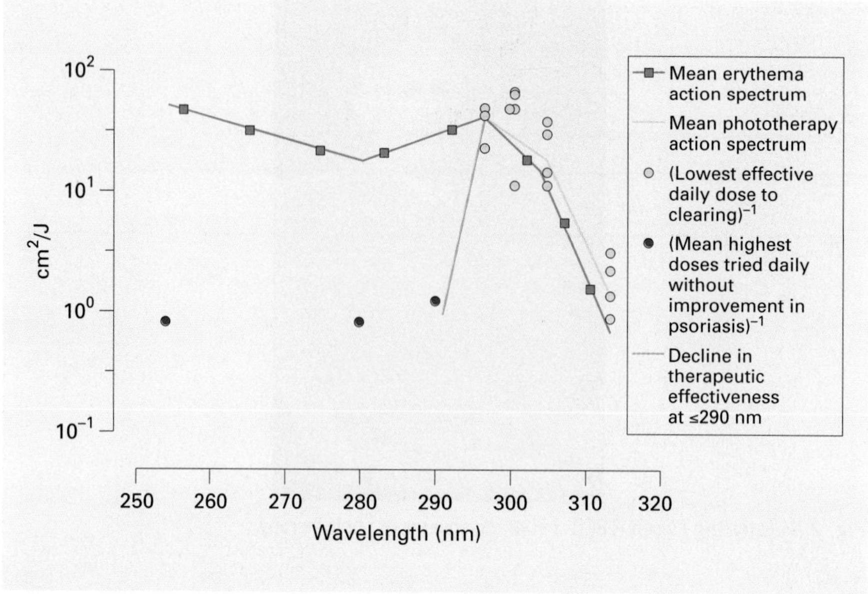

Fig. 3 Action spectra for the phototherapy of psoriasis.

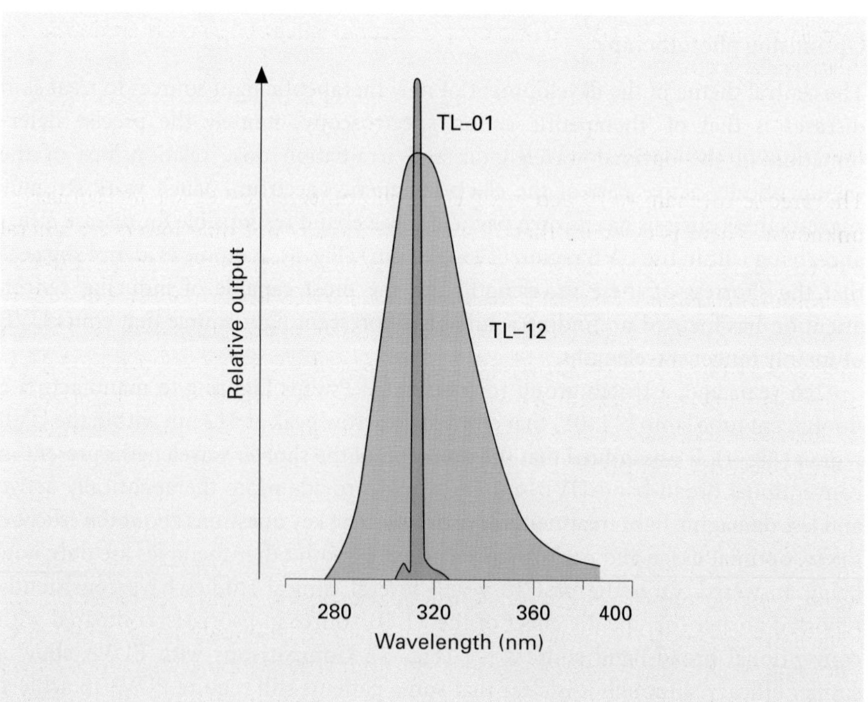

Fig. 4 Action spectra for the TL-01 fluorescent tube, compared with a conventional broad-band tube (TL-12).

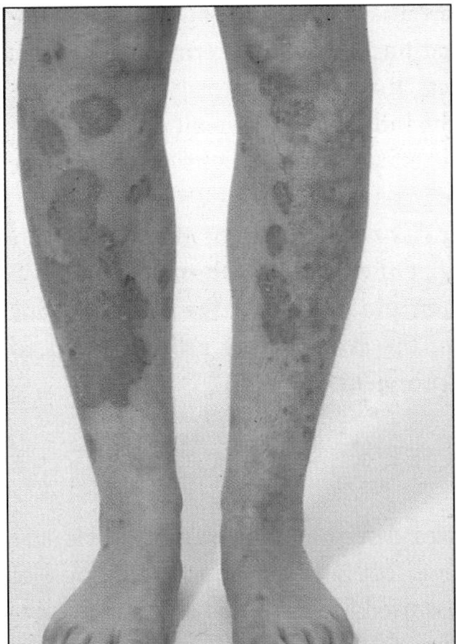
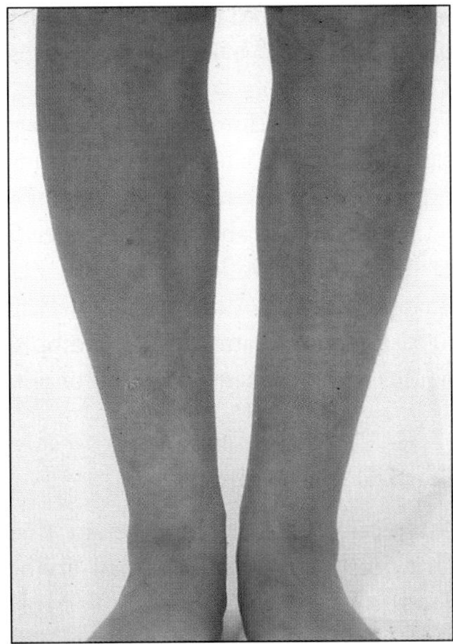

Fig. 5 Clearing of psoriatic lesions following a course of UBV phototherapy. Fifty percent of treated patients remain disease-free 6 months after stopping therapy.

cumulative number of UVB treatments to clearance, although such additions are unattractive for many.

How does phototherapy work?

The precise mechanism of action of UVB phototherapy or PUVA in psoriasis is unknown. There is evidence that TL-01 phototherapy not only lowers peripheral natural killer cell activity, but also inhibits lymphoproliferation and the production of immunoregulatory cytokines by both Th_1 and Th_2 T cell populations. Other actions may include enhanced degradation of inflammatory mediators and direct effects on the DNA of keratinocytes. The ability of TL-01 irradiation to depress major components of cell-mediated immune function may ultimately be linked to its beneficial effect in other inflammatory skin diseases (eg atopic dermatitis, polymorphic light eruption).

Risks of phototherapy

As with any new therapy involving chronic exposure to ultraviolet radiation, the long-term risks of skin malignancy with TL-01 must be quantified [8]. Studies in mice suggest that biologically-equivalent radiation doses with the TL-01 source have twice the potential of broad-band UVB sources to induce tumours [9]. However, these data cannot be directly extrapolated to humans without considering the context of clinical use. Significantly fewer minimal erythema doses (MEDs; defined below) are required to achieve clearance of psoriasis when using narrow-band compared with broad-band sources, suggesting that the overall long-term cancer risk of TL-01 is probably comparable to or even less than that of broad-band sources. Furthermore, preliminary data indicate that the individual treatment dose of TL-01 can be reduced without loss of therapeutic effect, which might reasonably be expected to reduce further the potential cancer risk.

As mentioned above, the long-term cancer risk with UVB phototherapy appears to be significantly less than with PUVA [5]. Other general advantages of UVB therapy over PUVA include its safety in children and pregnancy, the absence of any need for post-treatment eye photoprotection, the avoidance of psoralen-induced nausea and the financial savings of not using psoralens.

Practical considerations

A typical course of phototherapy first involves determination of the individual's ultraviolet sensitivity (minimal erythema dose, MED) using a separate bank of TL-01 tubes. Usually, 70% of this MED value is used for the initial exposure; thereafter treatment is given three times weekly with 10–20% increments depending on patient tolerance. The use of this new light source allows each therapy dose to remain well below the levels that induce erythema. Patients can expect to be clear of psoriasis after between 12 and 20 treatments, with 50% remaining disease-free 6 months after stopping therapy.

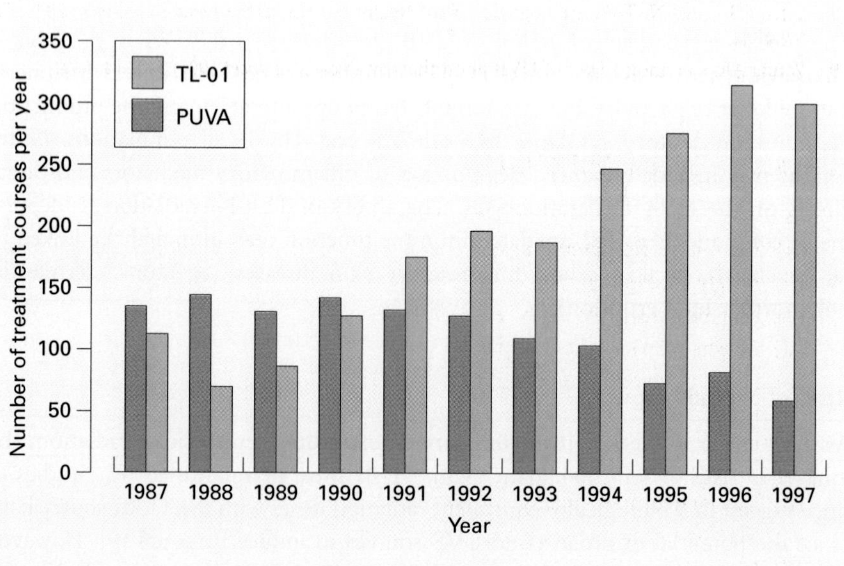

Fig. 6 Psoriasis treatment in Tayside, Scotland 1987–1997.

☐ CONCLUSION

Controlled study data support the theoretical view that TL-01 UVB is in practice more effective, and probably has no greater risk, compared with conventional UVB phototherapy in the treatment of psoriasis. Recent sales figures show the lamp to have an increasing share of the therapeutic UVB market within Europe. Early indications suggest that it will not only replace broad-band phototherapy, but will also significantly reduce PUVA use (Fig. 6). This trend seems rational on current published evidence.

The need remains to target treatment to psoriasis lesions while sparing nearby normal skin. New light sources should be developed, using photodiode or perhaps laser technology to provide safer, faster and cheaper therapy for psoriasis.

REFERENCES

1 Lomholt G. *Psoriasis: Prevalence, Spontaneous Course, and Genetics.* Copenhagen, Denmark: GEC GAD, 1963.
2 Elder JT, Nair RP, Guo S, *et al.* The genetics of psoriasis. *Arch Dermatol* 1994; **130**: 216–24.
3 Trembath RC, Clough RL, Rosbotham JL, *et al.* Identification of a major susceptibility locus on chromosome 6p and evidence for further disease loci revealed by a two stage genome-wide search in psoriasis. *Hum Mol Genet* 1997; **6**: 813–20.
4 Griffiths CEM, Voorhees JJ. Psoriasis, T cells and autoimmunity. *J R Soc Med* 1996; **89**: 315–9.
5 de Gruijl FR. Long-term side effects and carcinogenesis risk in UVB therapy. In: Honigsmann H, Jori G, Young AR (Eds). *The Fundamental Bases of Phototherapy.* Milan: OEMF spa, 1996: 153–67.
6 van Weelden H, Baart de la Faille H, Young E, van der Leun JC. A new development in UVB phototherapy of psoriasis. *Br J Dermatol* 1988; **119**: 11–9.
7 British Photodermatology Group. An appraisal of narrowband (TL-01) UVB phototherapy. Workshop report (April 1996). *Br J Dermatol* 1997; **137**: 327–30.
8 Stern RS, Laird N. The carcinogenic risk of treatments for severe psoriasis. *Cancer* 1994; **73**: 2759–64.
9 Young AR. Carcinogenicity of UVB phototherapy assessed. *Lancet* 1995; **345**: 1431–2.

☐ MULTIPLE CHOICE QUESTIONS

1 Psoriasis:
(a) Is a T-cell mediated disease
(b) Rarely causes distress
(c) May be associated with severe arthritis
(d) Affects 0.2% of the population
(e) Has a polygenic inheritance

2 Psoriasis:
(a) Is purely cutaneous
(b) Has a chronic relapsing course
(c) May be precipitated by drugs
(d) Presents in many forms
(e) Is associated with internal malignancy

3 Ultraviolet phototherapy for psoriasis:
   (a) Is the treatment of choice for moderate/severe disease
   (b) Requires UVA (sunbed) wavelengths
   (c) Is an expensive form of treatment
   (d) Usually does not require addition of topical treatment
   (e) Has less cancer risk than PUVA

ANSWERS

1a True	2a False	3a True
b False	b True	b False
c True	c True	c False
d False	d True	d True
e True	e False	e True

Genetic skin disorders

Celia Moss

□ INTRODUCTION

The skin is the perfect subject for those interested in genetic disease. Precise diagnoses can be made on simple inspection: rashes that differ subtly in the colour, size, scaliness or distribution of the spots can be distinguished, whereas such differences are rarely detectable in internal organs. Patients can even make the diagnosis in their relatives, so historical pedigrees show unusual accuracy. The skin can be biopsied, cultured, genetically altered and transplanted. Because of the unique accessibility of the skin, dozens of genes related to dermatological function and disease have been identified in the past 10 years [1].

The most accessible part of the skin is the epidermis. This is a relatively simple tissue, the main components being keratinocytes which move outwards from the basal layer to desquamate from the stratum corneum, and melanocytes which manufacture and distribute pigment. Accordingly, epidermal disorders are either structural (scaly or blistering) or pigmentary.

Genes responsible for epidermal disorders are the subject of this chapter. All these conditions are congenital, lifelong, and incurable.

□ PIGMENTARY DISORDERS

The genetic control of pigmentation is complex; in the mouse, at least 50 genes are involved. Table 1 shows some of the steps in normal human pigmentation, and some of the errors that lead to genetic disorders of pigmentation [2]. Disorders where the pathogenesis is known are discussed below. We are a long way from matching up all the known disorders of pigmentation with the candidate genes identified to date. In the case of two conditions, neurofibromatosis type 1 and tuberous sclerosis, a great deal is known about the genes responsible for the disorders but nothing at all about the pathogenesis of the hyper- and hypo-pigmented patches that characterise them.

Human piebaldism

This autosomal dominant trait is characterised by congenital patches of depigmented skin and hair on the forehead (white forelock), distal limbs, and belly (Fig. 1). The white patches contain irregular brown spots. Piebaldism is due to mutations in the c-KIT oncogene which encodes a cell-surface growth factor receptor expressed on the primitive melanoblast and other cell types [3]. The ventral and distal pattern of hypopigmentation in humans and in mice with mutations in the homologous gene (*dominant white spotting*) suggests that melanoblasts destined for the sites furthest from the neural crest fail to migrate normally.

Table 1 Some steps in normal human pigmentation, and some errors leading to genetic disorders.

Step in pigmentation	Genetic disorder
Melanoblasts differentiate in the neural crest	
Melanoblasts migrate along Blaschko's lines	Piebaldism
Melanoblasts differentiate into melanocytes	
Melanocytes colonise the epidermis	
Melanosomes are organised	Hermansky–Pudlak syndrome
Materials for synthesising melanin are imported	Oculocutaneous albinism type 2 (p-gene)
Melanin is synthesised	Oculocutaneous albinism type 1 (tyrosinase negative)
	McCune-Albright syndrome
Melanin is distributed to keratinocytes	

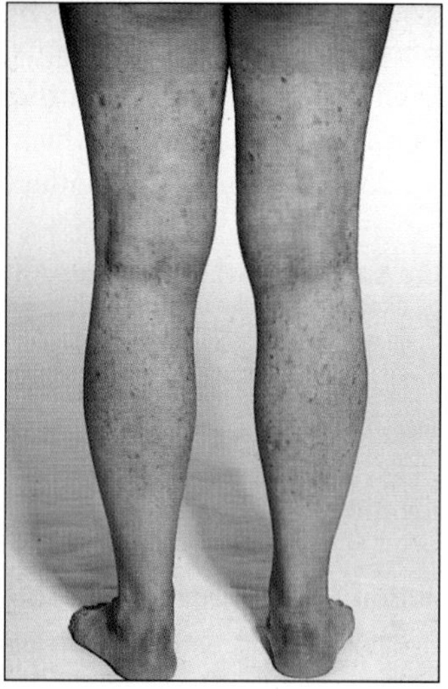

Fig. 1 Abnormal pigmentation in human piebaldism.

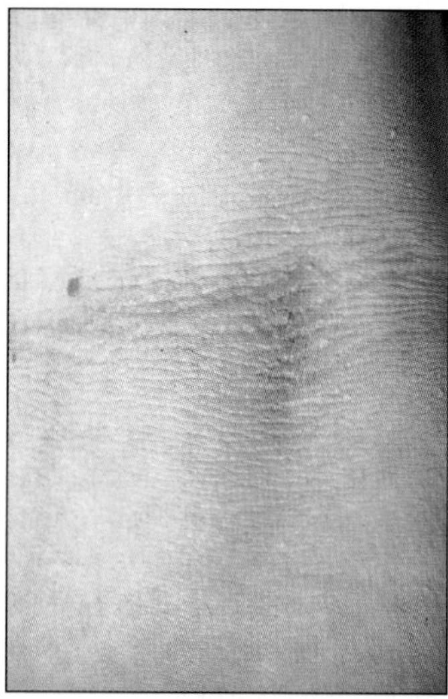

Fig. 2 Acanthosis nigricans of the antecubital fossa in a patient with Crouzon syndrome due to FGFR3 mutation.

Waardenburg syndrome

The pattern of skin hypopigmentation in Waardenburg syndrome is similar to that in piebaldism but there are additional defects, suggesting a more profound disorder of development. These include facial dysmorphism and abnormalities in other neural-crest derivatives (nerves as well as melanocytes) causing deafness and aganglionosis of the colon (Hirschsprung's disease). This autosomal dominant syndrome is due to mutations in an important organisational gene, HUP-2 (corresponding to PAX-3 in the mouse).

Oculocutaneous albinism type 1 (tyrosinase negative)

Patients with the autosomal recessive condition, oculocutaneous albinism (OCA) type 1, are completely devoid of melanin because of mutations in the gene encoding tyrosinase, the enzyme essential for melanin production. Many different mutations have been reported. Patients also suffer from visual impairment due to misrouting of optic nerve fibres, and from photosensitivity with accelerated skin ageing and increased risk of skin cancer.

Oculocutaneous albinism type 2 (tyrosinase positive)

This is a heterogeneous group of disorders, all of which are recessively inherited. Patients with OCA type 2 are not as blond as patients with OCA type 1, and have some pigment in hair and eyes. The offspring of two people with OCA type 2 will be normally pigmented if the parents have a different genotype. The tyrosinase gene itself is not affected, and the phenotype is due to mutations in other cellular components related to pigmentation. Some patients have a defective 'p-gene' (also responsible for the *pink-eyed* mutation in mice). The function of the p-gene may be to transport tyrosinase across intracellular membranes.

Hermansky-Pudlak syndrome

This autosomal recessive disorder, characterised by a type 2 (tyrosinase positive) OCA, bleeding tendency and lysosomal storage disorder, is due to mutations in a gene coding for a transmembrane polypeptide that is important in the development of subcellular organelles. The pigmentary abnormality is related to defective melanosomes [4].

McCune-Albright syndrome

The sporadic occurrence and patchy manifestations of McCune-Albright syndrome suggest that it is a mosaic disorder (see below). The hyperpigmentation, endocrine hyperactivity (particularly precocious puberty in girls) and polyostotic fibrous dysplasia of bones are all due to activating mutations in the GNAS-1 gene which stimulates hormone-sensitive c-AMP in endocrine cells and melanocytes.

□ STRUCTURAL DISORDERS OF THE EPIDERMIS

These include overgrowth of the epidermis (acanthosis), thickening of the stratum corneum (ichthyosis and keratoderma) and blistering. Splitting of the epidermis and hyperkeratosis often coexist and may be functionally related. Most of these conditions affect the whole skin surface but may be modified by site; for example, acanthosis nigricans predominantly affects the flexures, while others specifically affect or spare palmoplantar skin.

Acanthosis nigricans

Despite its dark appearance, acanthosis nigricans is a disorder of epidermal cell (acanthocyte) turnover, not of pigmentation. Onset in an adult usually signifies advanced upper gastrointestinal carcinoma; the tumours apparently produce epidermal growth-promoting factors. Acanthosis nigricans in childhood is not related to malignancy and is usually caused by massively raised circulating insulin levels, due to mutations in the insulin receptor gene or other disorders that cause severe insulin resistance. The epidermal overgrowth is probably mediated by insulin acting on insulin-like growth factor receptors in the epidermis. Some patients with autosomal dominant craniosynostosis (Crouzon syndrome) also have acanthosis nigricans [5]. The condition is very extensive, affecting perioral, periorbital, popliteal and antecubital skin as well as axillae, groins and neck (Fig. 2). These subjects do not have hyperinsulinism, and the causative mutation is in the fibroblast growth factor receptor gene, FGFR3 (not the FGFR2 gene responsible for most cases of Crouzon syndrome). FGFR3 is expressed on epidermal cells as well as fibroblasts, and can be alternatively spliced to code for a growth factor receptor on keratinocytes rather than on fibroblasts.

Ichthyosis and palmoplantar keratoderma (tylosis)

Ichthyosis denotes scaling of the skin due to thickening of the stratum corneum and reflects a failure in the normal process of epidermal cell maturation and desquamation. The same process affecting palms and soles is termed 'keratoderma' or 'tylosis'. These conditions are congenital, lifelong, and disabling. The abnormality may involve intercellular cement, corneocyte membranes, or the internal structure of keratinocytes (Table 2). The major structural components of the epidermis are keratin filaments. Keratin proteins are either acidic or basic and one of each combine to form a heterodimer, two of which align to form a tetramer. There are more than 5,000 tetramers in

Table 2 Genetic causes of ichthyosis and keratoderma.

Disorder	Gene
Lipid defects	
X-linked ichthyosis	Steroid sulphatase
Sjögren-Larsson syndrome	Fatty aldehyde dehydrogenase
Corneocyte membrane defects	
Non-bullous ichthyosiform erythroderma	Transglutaminase
Vohwinkel mutilating palmoplantar keratoderma	Loricrin
Keratin defects	
Bullous ichthyosiform erythroderma	Keratins 1 and 10
Palmoplantar keratoderma	Keratin 9
Pachyonychia congenita type 2	Keratin 17

a single keratin filament. The keratin genes lie in two clusters on chromosomes 12 and 17. Pathogenic mutations affect the highly conserved regions at the ends of the rod domains, which are critical for normal keratin filament assembly. Keratin gene mutations cause several hyperkeratotic disorders, as well as blisters [6]. The phenotype depends on which keratin is affected: keratins 5 and 14 are expressed in basal epidermal cells; 1, 2e and 10 in suprabasal cells; 6, 16 and 17 in other keratinising tissues, for example nails and hair; and 9 in palmoplantar epidermis (Table 3).

X-linked ichthyosis

This disorder is illustrated in Fig. 3. It affects 1 in 6,000 males and is due to mutations and deletions of the gene for steroid sulphatase. The precise function of this enzyme in maintaining normal desquamation is not known, but presumably involves the regulation of lipids in corneocyte membranes and/or intercellular substances. The only associated abnormality is hypogonadotrophic hypogonadism which occurs if the deletion extends to the Kalman locus that lies next to the steroid sulphatase gene (an example of the 'contiguous gene syndrome'). Female carriers have normal skin.

Sjögren-Larsson syndrome

This recessively inherited triad of congenital ichthyosis, developmental delay and spastic paraparesis is due to mutations in the gene for fatty aldehyde dehydrogenase [7]. Again, the precise pathogenesis is unknown, but this enzyme presumably affects lipids in the central nervous system as well as in the skin.

Non-bullous ichthyosiform erythroderma

This is probably a heterogeneous disorder. It is recessively inherited and usually presents as a collodion membrane in the neonate; later the skin appears red and scaly. Some patients have mutations in the gene for transglutaminase, an enzyme involved in crosslinking keratin filaments and other precursors of the cornified envelope of the epidermal cell [8]. These precursors (loricrin, involucrin, elafin and filaggrin) are other candidate genes for ichthyoses.

Table 3 Summary of skin disorders due to known keratin gene defects.

Gene	Disorder
Keratins 5 and 14	Epidermolysis bullosa simplex
Keratins 1 and 10	Non-bullous ichthyosiform erythroderma
Keratin 2e	Ichthyosis bullosa of Siemens
Keratin 9	Epidermolytic palmoplantar keratoderma
Keratin 6	Focal non-epidermolytic palmoplantar keratoderma
Keratin 16	Pachyonychia congenita type 1
Keratin 17	Pachyonychia congenita type 2

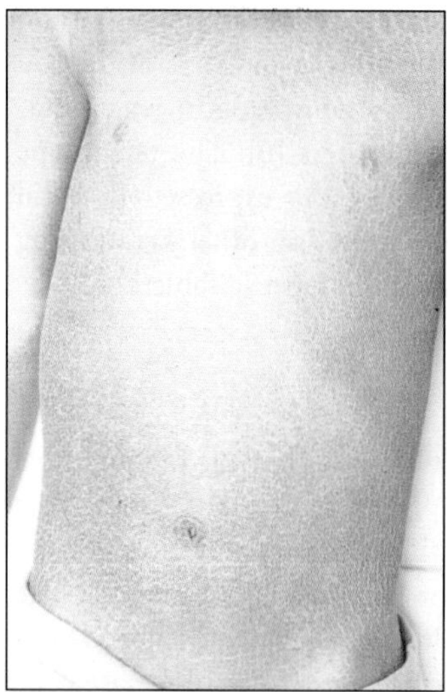

Fig. 3 X-linked recessive ichthyosis due to steroid sulphatase deficiency.

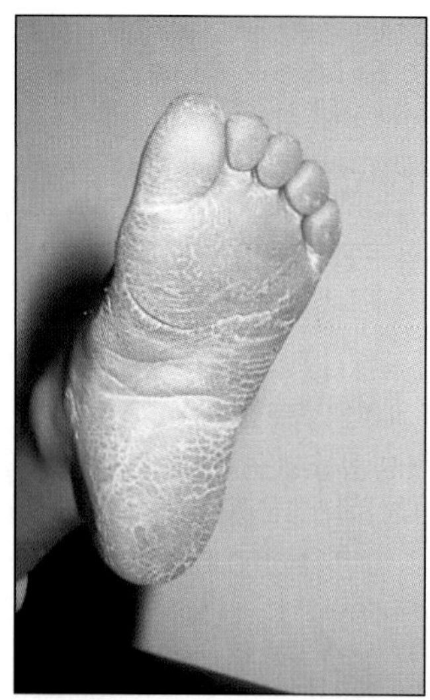

Fig. 4 Palmoplantar keratoderma (tylosis).

Bullous ichthyosiform erythroderma

The early severe blistering of this dominantly inherited disorder gives way later to extensive hyperkeratosis. Histologically, there is splitting of the epidermis (epidermolysis) and hyperkeratosis, with clumping of the abnormal keratin filaments. It is due to mutations in the genes for keratins 1 and 10. Patients have been described who are mosaic for such mutations, and whose ichthyosis is confined to linear streaks (see below). Such patients may also have gonadal mosaicism, in which case they may pass on the full-blown disorder to their children.

Palmoplantar keratoderma (tylosis)

This denotes thick yellow callus affecting the palms and soles (Fig. 4), with normal skin elsewhere. Several clinical subtypes have been differentiated according to the pattern of callus and associated features [9]. Diffuse palmoplantar keratoderma with histological epidermolysis and no other associated features is due to keratin 9 mutations, and diffuse mutilating palmoplantar keratoderma to mutations affecting the loricrin gene. Focal palmoplantar keratoderma is associated with blistering, nail dystrophy and other ectodermal features in pachyonychia congenita types 1 and 2, due to mutations in keratins 16 and 17, respectively. The cause of the rare but well known syndrome of palmoplantar keratoderma and oesophageal cancer is not known.

Epidermolysis bullosa

Genetically determined congenital blistering is called epidermolysis bullosa. There are several types varying in severity from mild to lethal in infancy (Table 4) [10]. The

Table 4 Main types of epidermolysis bullosa, and associated gene defects.

Type of epidermolysis bullosa	Gene defect
Epidermolysis bullosa simplex	
Weber-Cockayne type (palms and sole)	Keratins 5 and 14
Dowling-Meara type (generalised)	Keratins 5 and 14
Associated with muscular dystrophy	Plectin
Junctional epidermolysis bullosa	
Lethal (Herlitz) type	Laminin 5
Generalised atrophic benign	Collagen XVII (bullous pemphigoid antigen)
Non-lethal, with pyloric atresia	Alpha-6,beta-4 integrin
Non-lethal	Linear IgA disease (LAD-1) antigen
Dystrophic epidermolysis bullosa	
Recessive	Collagen VII
Dominant	Collagen VII

skin defect produces a plane of cleavage in the skin, along which blisters spread. Parents soon learn to burst new blisters to prevent this. Three main types can be distinguished according to the level of blister formation (Fig. 5). Advances in our understanding of the genetic basis of epidermolysis bullosa have made first-trimester diagnosis possible.

Recently, it has been recognised that some of the skin components genetically absent in epidermolysis bullosa are also the targets of autoimmune attack in certain acquired bullous disorders. For example, one form of junctional epidermolysis bullosa is due to absence of collagen XVII, now identified as the autoantigen in bullous pemphigoid, and another to absence of LAD-1, the antigen for linear immunoglobulin (Ig)A disease. Similarly, the acquired immune disorder epidermolysis bullosa aquisita is due to antibodies to collagen VII, the component of anchoring fibrils which is missing in patients with dystrophic epidermolysis bullosa. This has led to new directions of research: immunologists are now looking for antibodies to other components of the basement membrane zone identified by the geneticists, and vice versa.

Epidermolysis bullosa simplex

This is characterised by epidermal blisters which do not scar. It is usually due to mutations in keratins 5 or 14, which constitute the epidermal cytoskeleton. Like other keratin gene defects described above, epidermolysis bullosa simplex is usually dominantly inherited and not associated with systemic abnormalities. Different mutations give rise to different phenotypes. The commonest is the Weber-Cockayne variant, in which blisters occur at sites of maximum friction and may be confined to the soles. Much more serious is the Dowling-Meara type (Fig. 6), characterised by

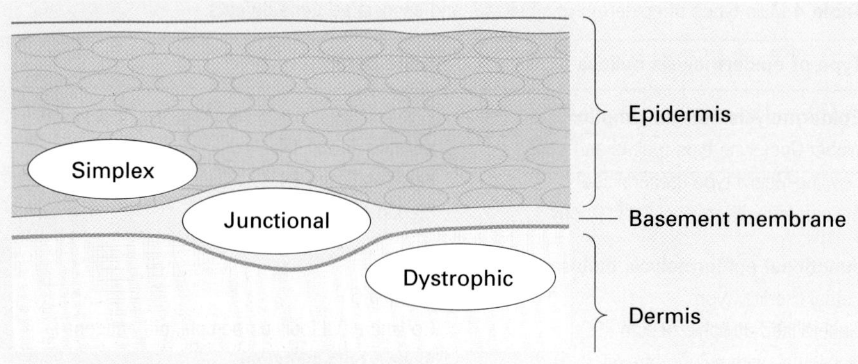

Fig. 5 Levels of blistering in epidermolysis bullosa.

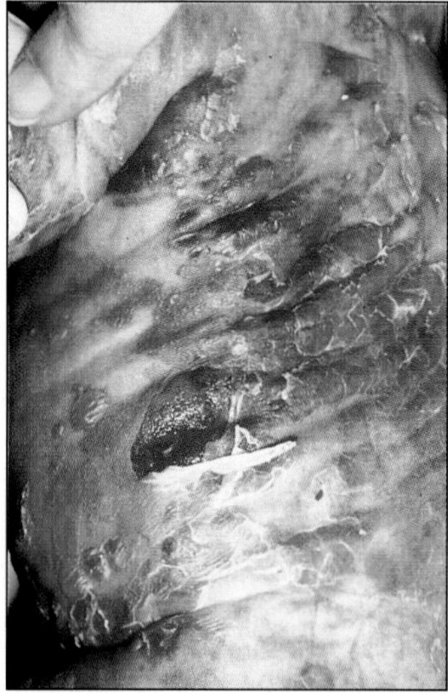

Fig. 6 Severe neonatal blistering in epidermolysis bullosa simplex (Dowling-Meara).

generalised blistering particularly in the neonatal period, and later by palmoplantar keratoderma and nail hypertrophy.

Rare cases of dominant epidermolysis bullosa simplex associated with muscular dystrophy are due to mutations in the gene encoding plectin, which is expressed in muscle as well as epidermis.

Junctional epidermolysis bullosa

In junctional epidermolysis bullosa, blisters occur in the basement membrane zone of the epidermis (Fig. 7). All types are recessively inherited. Scarring is minimal, but nails are usually shed. The lethal Herlitz form should be suspected in a neonate with blistering, a hoarse cry and periungual inflammation; death in infancy is usually due to laryngeal involvement. This disorder is due to mutations in genes encoding the laminins, which constitute the anchoring filaments that attach the basal cells of the

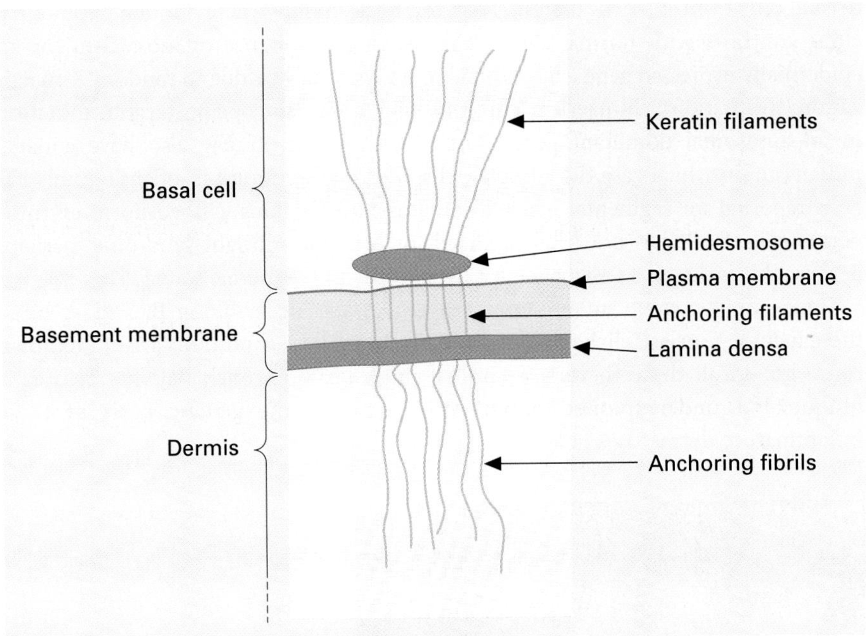

Fig. 7 Ultrastructure of epidermolysis bullosa.

epidermis to the basement membrane. The non-lethal generalised atrophic benign form is due to mutations in collagen type XVII (bullous pemphigoid antigen) which is found in the hemidesmosomes in the basal epidermal cells. Other non-lethal types are due to mutations in LAD-1 (linear IgA disease antigen, localised to the superior aspect of anchoring filaments) and α6,β4 integrin (a component of hemidesmosomes). The latter is associated with pyloric atresia.

Dystrophic epidermolysis bullosa

This is due to mutations in the gene for collagen type VII, which forms the anchoring fibrils that attach the basement membrane to the dermis. The recessively inherited Hallopeau-Siemens variant causes severe scarring and nail loss with cocooning of the hands and feet. Dominantly inherited and mild sporadic cases are due to heterozygous mutations; the phenotype is much milder, with minimal blistering on frictional areas, and nail dystrophy.

□ EPIDERMAL MOSAICISM

The epidermis is the only part of the body in which genetic mosaicism can easily be visualised. Patients mosaic for mutations in epidermal genes show streaks of scaliness or dyspigmentation that conform to Blaschko's lines (named after the German dermatologist who drew attention 100 years ago to the constant pattern followed by epidermal birthmarks). These lines are now thought to reflect the migratory paths of epidermal cells from the neural crest. They can be seen only where a mutant epidermal clone contrasts with normal skin – that is, in the presence of mosaicism for an epidermally expressed gene (Fig. 8). The mosaicism may be due to random X-inactivation (lyonisation), chimaerism, chromosomal mosaicism, or a postzygotic mutation in an autosomal dominant gene (Table 5). The patient may also have gonadal mosaicism, in which case the complete disorder may be found in offspring; this has been reported for segmental neurofibromatosis and bullous ichthyosiform erythroderma (Fig. 8). It has not been reported for McCune-Albright syndrome, perhaps because this is due to a lethal gene survivable only in the mosaic state [11].

Occasionally, some inflammatory disorders also occur along Blaschko's lines; these include psoriasis, lichen planus and eczema. These conditions are of unknown cause but in all three there is a familial predisposition. Such patients provide a unique and underexploited opportunity to study the genetic basis of these inflammatory dermatoses [12].

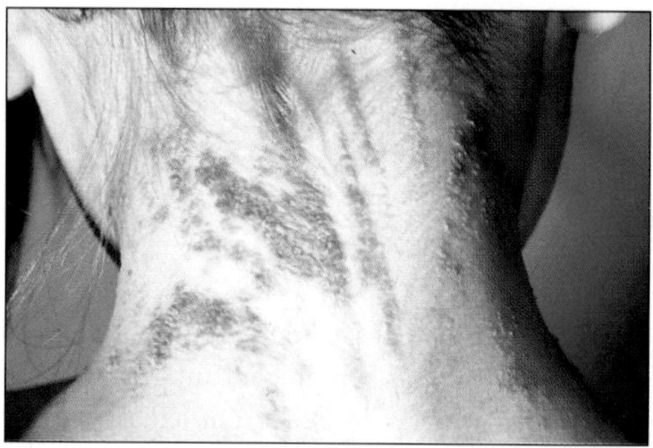

Fig. 8 Hyperkeratosis following Blaschko's lines in a child showing mosaicism for a keratin 10 mutation.

Table 5 Mosaic skin disorders classified according to cause of mosaicism.

X-linked disorders
Incontinentia pigmenti
Goltz focal dermal hypoplasia
X-linked chondrodysplasia punctata
Carrier state of hypohidrotic ectodermal dysplasia

Chimaerism

Chromosomal mosaicism
Hypomelanosis of Ito
Mosaic dyspigmentation

Postzygotic mutations in autosomal dominant genes
Segmental neurofibromatosis
Linear bullous ichthyosiform erythroderma
Linear Darier's disease
Linear psoriasis
McCune-Albright syndrome

REFERENCES

1 Moss C, Savin J. *Dermatology and the New Genetics*. Oxford: Blackwell Science, 1995.
2 Hearing VJ. Unraveling the melanocyte (Editorial). *Am J Hum Genet* 1193; **52**: 1–7.
3 Ward KA, Moss C, Sanders DSA. Human piebaldism: relationship between phenotype and site of *kit* gene mutation. *Br J Dermatol* 1995; **132**: 929–35.
4 Bailin T, Oh J, Feng GH, *et al.* Organization and nucleotide sequence of the human Hermansky-Pudlak syndrome (HPS) gene. *J Invest Dermatol* 1997; **108**: 923–7.
5 Wilkes D, Rutland P, Pulleyn LJ, *et al.* A recurrent mutation, ala391glu, in the transmembrane region of FGFR3 causes Crouzon syndrome and acanthosis nigricans. *J Med Genet* 1996; **33**: 744–8.
6 Fuchs E. Genetic skin disorders of keratin. *J Invest Dermatol* 1992; **99**: 671–4.
7 Laurenzini V, Rogers GR, Tarcsa E, *et al.* Sjögren-Larsson syndrome is caused by a common mutation in northern European and Swedish patients. *J Invest Dermatol* 1997; **109**: 79–83.
8 Huber M, Rettler I, Bernasconi K, *et al.* Mutations of keratinocyte transglutaminase in lamellar ichthyosis. *Science* 1995; **267**: 525–8.
9 Ratnavel RC, Griffiths WAD. The inherited palmoplantar keratodermas. *Br J Dermatol* 1997; **137**: 485–90.
10 Moss C. Hereditary bullous disorders. *Curr Paediatr* 1995; **5**: 252–7.
11 Happle R. Lethal genes surviving by mosaicism: a possible explanation for sporadic birth defects involving the skin. *J Am Acad Dermatol* 1987; **16**: 899–906.
12 Moss C, Jones DO, Blight A, Bowden PE. A birthmark due to cutaneous mosaicism for a keratin 10 mutation. *Lancet* 1995; **345**: 596.

☐ MULTIPLE CHOICE QUESTIONS

1 Acanthosis nigricans is:
(a) An abnormality of melanin production
(b) An early sign of gastrointestinal malignancy
(c) Sometimes associated with hyperinsulinism
(d) Most marked in axillae and groins
(e) Only seen in obese individuals

2 Patients with oculocutaneous albinism:
(a) Have associated deafness
(b) Are at increased risk of skin cancer
(c) Always have pink eyes
(d) Never have normally pigmented children if both parents are albino
(e) Have no melanocytes

3 Ichthyosis:
(a) Is usually associated with mental retardation
(b) Affects at least 1 in 6,000 males
(c) Persists into adult life
(d) Is so called after the Greek word for a fish
(e) Is a variant of psoriasis

4 Palmoplantar keratoderma (tylosis) is:
(a) Dominantly inherited

(b) Usually associated with abnormal nails and teeth
(c) Usually a marker of underlying malignancy
(d) Often associated with oesophageal tumours
(e) Associated with oesophageal web

5 Epidermolysis bullosa:
(a) Is associated with mental retardation
(b) Can be diagnosed antenatally
(c) Is always recessively inherited
(d) Should be treated by bursting the blisters
(e) Can be lethal

ANSWERS

1a False	2a False	3a False	4a True	5a False
b False	b True	b True	b False	b True
c True	c False	c True	c False	c False
d True	d False	d True	d False	d True
e False	e False	e False	e False	e True

Acromegaly: a fresh look at its outcome and management

Richard N Clayton

☐ INTRODUCTION

Acromegaly is uncommon, having a prevalence in European populations of about 40/million and an annual incidence of 4–6 new cases per million. It is a condition of middle age, with its peak incidence between 30 and 60 years in both men and women; there is no sex predilection. About 99% of cases of acromegaly are due to a pituitary somatotrophinoma secreting growth hormone (GH), with exceedingly rare cases caused by ectopic production of growth hormone releasing hormone by neuroendocrine tumours of the lung (bronchial carcinoids), pancreas or hypothalamus, which give rise to somatotroph hyperplasia. The onset of the condition is often insidious, especially in older patients; retrospectively, photographic evidence of acral expansion may be apparent 5–10 years before biochemical confirmation of the diagnosis (see Fig. 1). This may explain why 60–70% of somatotrophinomas are relatively large 'macroadenomas' (ie >1 cm in diameter) at diagnosis. Moreover, the prolonged exposure of tissues to excessive growth levels before treatment may be relevant to the long-term outcome and mortality (see below).

The presentation of acromegaly is very variable. The commonest features are the consequences of GH excess, such as enlargement of the hands, feet, jaw and face, excessive sweating and greasy skin, and the carpal tunnel syndrome. On the other hand, associated diabetes mellitus, hypertension and renal calculus formation may be the initial clue to the diagnosis. Other patients have symptoms directly attributable to an expanded pituitary gland, particularly headache and visual impairment, or to hypopituitarism. Some cases are diagnosed coincidentally from the patient's characteristic appearance when presenting with unrelated problems. The varied presentation and rarity of acromegaly often means that it goes unrecognised by the non-specialist, so the endocrinologist frequently encounters the patient when complications have developed. The long-term care of acromegaly is demanding, because of its serious complications and substantial morbidity and mortality; this is not a condition to be managed by generalists.

☐ DIAGNOSIS OF ACROMEGALY

Table 1 shows the key questions to be answered by the investigation and assessment of a patient with suspected acromegaly. The diagnosis of acromegaly is usually obvious to the trained observer from the clinical appearance of acral enlargement, although the features may be subtle early in the disease (see Fig. 1). Thus, any clinical suspicion must be verified biochemically, by confirming elevated levels of GH and insulin-like growth factor 1 (IGF-1).

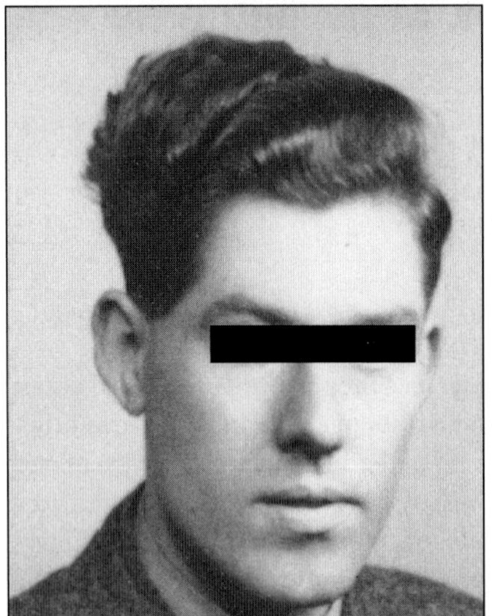
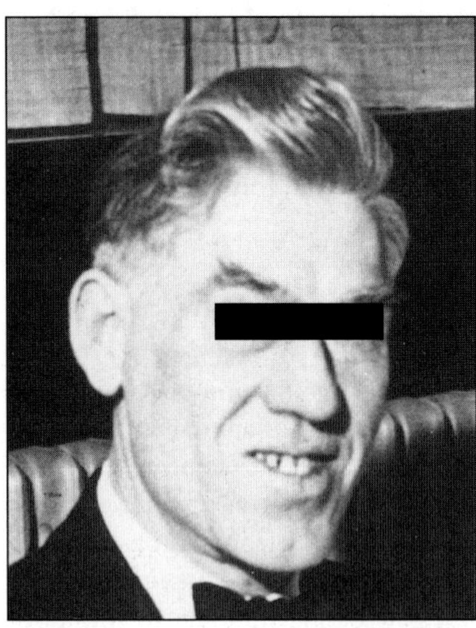

Fig. 1 Photographs of an acromegalic patient at 31 years of age (left) and at 46 years of age (right). At 46 years of age the prognathisan, frontal skull bossing, and prominent nose are obvious. At 31 years of age there are no obvious signs of acromegaly.

Table 1 Investigation and diagnosis of acromegaly.

1 Is GH secretion excessive?
- GH levels >2 mU/l during OGTT
- Raised IGF-1 levels (above age-related range)

2 What is the anatomy of the tumour?
- Contrast-enhanced MRI scan of pituitary
- Visual field testing by perimetry

3 Is pituitary function compromised?
- Cortisol: short synacthen or hypoglycaemia stress test
- Gonadotrophins: basal levels and responses to GnRH; gonadal steroids
- Prolactin
- Thyroid hormones and thyroid-stimulating hormone
- Consider water deprivation test if symptoms of diabetes insipidus

4 Are complications of acromegaly present?
- Diabetes mellitus: blood glucose (OGTT)
- Hypercalciuria: urinary calcium, abdominal X-ray
- Hypertension, vascular disease: ECG; echocardiography; consider exercise stress test

GH = growth hormone
GnRH = gonadotrophin-releasing hormone
IGF = insulin-like growth factor
MRI = magnetic resonance imaging
OGTT = oral glucose tolerance test

The secretion of GH is pulsatile, in a few short-lived bursts that mostly occur during the night in both children and adults. In adults, serum GH levels (as measured by conventional radioimmunoassays or the more sensitive immunofluorometric assays) are undetectable (<1 mU/l) throughout much of the day [1]. Spontaneous peaks may occur and may be detected by a random blood sample. It follows that random samples are often uninformative, though an undetectable GH level (<1 mU/l), accompanied by a normal age-related IGF-1 concentration, excludes active acromegaly.

The most reliable diagnostic criterion is the degree of GH suppression during a 75-g oral glucose tolerance test (OGTT). The diagnosis is confirmed if GH remains above 2 mU/l during the test (together with an elevated IGF-1 level), and virtually excluded if GH suppresses to <2 mU/l at any time. Active acromegaly, with raised serum IGF-1 levels, may be present when the average of several GH levels lies between 2 and 5 mU/l, especially if there is no pulsatile secretion. Some patients show a paradoxical rise in GH after glucose loading. Other tests of GH secretion, such as GH responses to thyrotrophin-releasing hormone (TRH) or gonadotrophin-releasing hormone (GnRH), are not useful for diagnostic purposes.

IGF-1, produced by the liver in response to GH, mediates GH's growth-promoting effects and is a reliable biological marker of GH action. However, its absolute levels vary widely with age and are also influenced by serum IGF binding proteins (see Fig. 2). Serum IGF-1 is maximal at the time of the pubertal growth spurt, remains high in young adults and then falls slowly with age; a subject's value must therefore be compared with an age-related reference range. The relationship between GH and serum IGF-1 is asymptotic; IGF-1 levels rise approximately linearly in proportion to GH levels between 2 and 30 mU/l, but reach a plateau above GH concentrations of 30–40 mU/l, as IGF-1 synthesis is maximal.

Tests of other anterior pituitary hormone reserve should be performed to uncover occult or obvious hypopituitarism. About 30% of acromegalic patients have mild elevations of serum prolactin, as some adenomas are mixed 'somatolactotrophs', reflecting dedifferentiation of the tumour cells to earlier stages in their lineage. Large pure somatotroph tumours may also compress the pituitary stalk, causing prolactin secretion to rise through loss of the inhibitory factor dopamine, secreted by hypothalamic neurones into the hypothalamo-hypophyseal portal vessels that run down the stalk.

Adenoma size and anatomy are best assessed by contrast-enhanced MRI scanning. Contrast is required to identify microadenomas, and precise definition of any extrasellar extension of macroadenomas is an essential prerequisite for surgical intervention (see Fig. 3).

□ MORBIDITY AND MORTALITY IN ACROMEGALY

Over the past 25 years, several retrospective studies have reported that acromegalic patients have a 2–3-fold excess mortality compared with age- and sex-matched controls (Table 2). Overall, there appears to be no sex difference in the increased mortality, although one London-based study [2] reported significantly higher rates

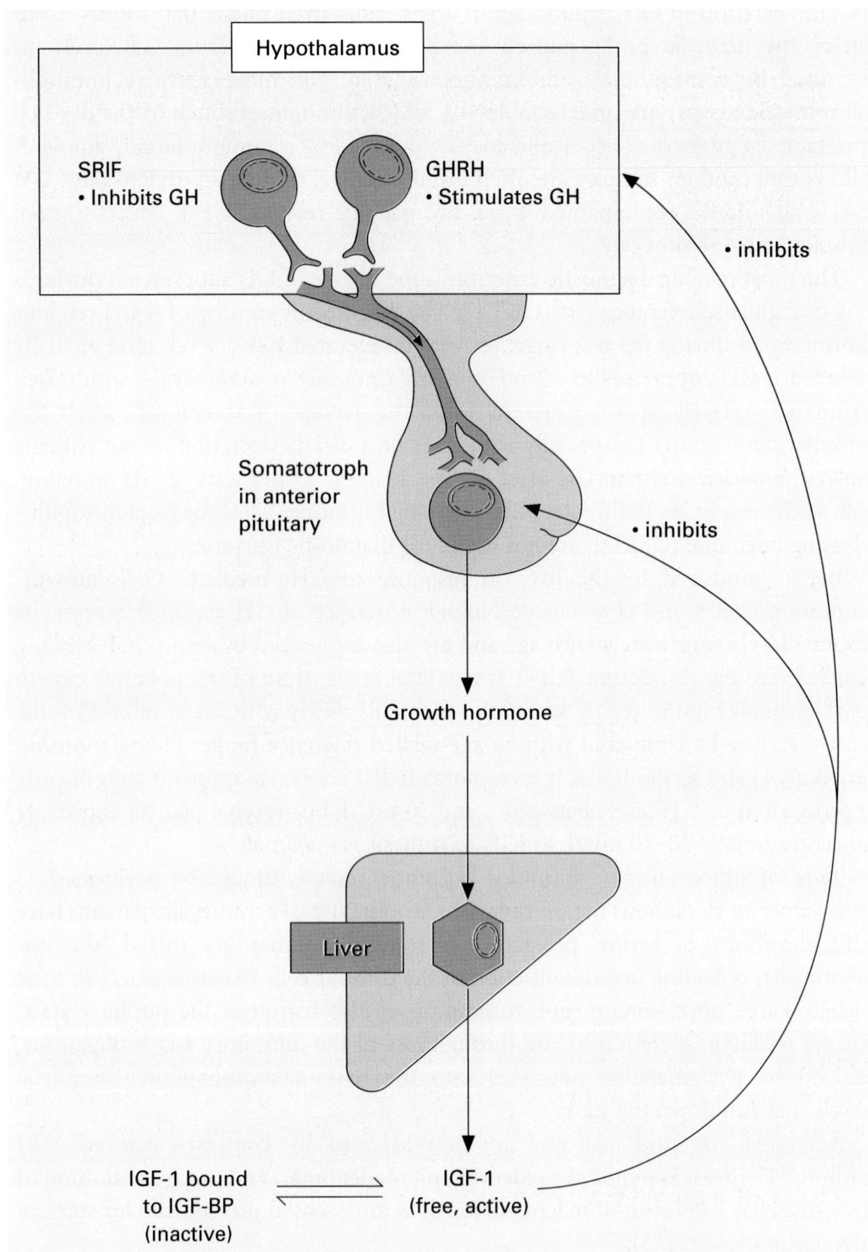

Fig. 2 Regulation of growth hormone (GH) secretion and action.

in men under the age of 55 and in women (Table 2). The increased death rate lowers the average age of death to around 60 years (Table 2), and probably represents a 5–10 year reduction in life expectancy.

Most of the cases were treated in various ways for symptomatic relief, decompression of the sella or management of complications; accordingly, there are

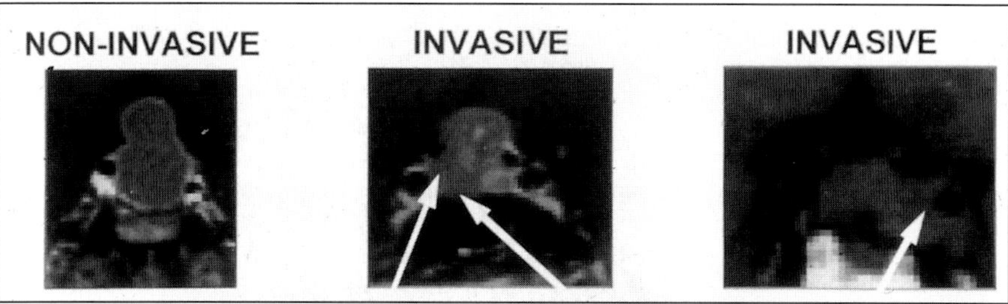

Fig. 3 Contrast enhanced pituitary MRI scans of patients with acromegaly. Left panel shows a macroadenoma with suprasellar extension but no lateral or infrasellar extension. Middle panel shows early invasion into the right cavernous sinus (left arrow) and breach of the sellar floor (right arrow). Right panel shows lateral invasion (arrow) into the left cavernous sinus with tumour surrounding the carotid artery.

Table 2 Mortality in acromegaly.

Series	Number of patients	Observed/ expected death ratio	Significance value	Median†/or mean* age of death (years)
Wright *et al.* [14]	194	1.9	<0.002	not given
Alexander *et al.* [3]	164	3.3	<0.001	57*
Nabarro *et al.* [2]	256 (overall)	1.3	NS	not given
	Male <55 y	1.9	<0.05	
	Female all ages	1.7	<0.05	
Bengtsson *et al.* [15]	166	3.2	<0.01	64*
Bates *et al.* [4]	79	2.7	<0.001	63†
Rajasoorya *et al.* [5]	151	not reported	not reported	57†
Orme *et al.* [6]	1362	1.6	<0.001	not given

NS = not significant

no systematic comparisons to determine whether treatment itself influences mortality, although Alexander *et al.* [3] comment that overall mortality in their treated cases was 22% compared with 40% in the untreated group. These retrospective surveys demonstrate excess mortality, but this does not necessarily imply that treatment does not improve the long-term outcome. Indeed, more recent studies [4–6] suggest that treatment is beneficial (see below).

Causes of death in acromegaly

The causes of excess deaths in acromegalics generally reflect those in the general population (Table 3), with cardiovascular disease being a major contributor. A series from New Zealand reported significantly increased mortality ratios for cardiovascular (3:1) and cerebrovascular disease (3.3:1) [5]. Recently, a large retrospective UK study of over 1,200 patients, with >16,000 person-years of follow-up, confirmed a 2.5-fold excess mortality from cardiovascular and cerebrovascular disease [6].

Table 3 Causes of death in acromegalic subjects, showing the percentages of deaths attributable to vascular, respiratory and malignant disease.

		Major causes of death (%)		
	Country	**Vascular**	**Respiratory**	**Malignant**
Wright *et al.* [14]	UK	38.5	18	18
Alexander *et al.* [3]	UK	60	15.5	15.5
Bengtsson *et al.* [15]	Sweden	47	–	24
Bates *et al.* [4]	UK	57	25	11
Nabarro *et al.* [2]	UK	55	6	23
Orme *et al.* [6]	UK	49	12	23
Rajasoorya *et al.* [5]	New Zealand	62.5	–	9

Death from malignancy deserves discussion because of the suggested association between acromegaly and colonic polyps, which may progress to malignancy [7–13]. The UK retrospective survey [6] showed a non-significant 70% increase in overall colon cancer incidence compared with the normal population, but mortality from this cause was 2.5 times greater than expected ($p < 0.01$). Few studies have directly determined the prevalence of colonic neoplasms in acromegalic and control populations. The colonoscopic study by Vasen *et al.* [12] was the first to show an increased incidence of polyps in an acromegalic cohort compared with age- and sex-matched controls (the latter had mild abdominal complaints and underwent colonoscopy to exclude serious pathology). Eleven of 49 (22%) acromegalics had histologically proven colonic adenomas, compared with 5/57 (9%) of the control population, and low-grade dysplasia (thought to be premalignant) was found in 9 of the 11 adenomas in the acromegalics and 3/5 of the controls. This study clearly indicates that subjects with acromegaly are at increased risk. In the study by Jenkins *et al.* [13] of 129 patients, the overall odds ratio for colorectal cancer was 13.5, but the confidence interval was wide (3.1–75) and was age-dependent with an odds ratio of 4.2 for those aged over 49 years. Overall, these data indicate that acromegalic patients must be actively screened for colonic neoplasms, and Jenkins *et al.* [13] have suggested colonoscopic surveillance of all acromegalics every 3 years, beginning at age 40.

Acromegaly is known to predispose to various forms of respiratory disease, including upper airways obstruction and sleep apnoea, and several studies report excess mortality from respiratory disorders (Table 3).

Predictors of increased mortality in acromegaly

Various clinical features, either present at diagnosis or developing subsequently, may determine long-term outcome. As might be predicted from their known associations with vascular mortality, some studies reported that diabetes and hypertension were significantly more frequent in acromegalic subjects who had died than in survivors [5,14]; however, others did not confirm this [4,15].

A younger age at diagnosis carries a worse prognosis. For example, Orme *et al.* [6] showed that all-cause mortality and cerebrovascular death rates were twice as high in those diagnosed before the age of 34 than in those diagnosed over 60 years. This may be because younger patients have more aggressive disease; their serum GH levels are usually higher.

Although difficult to estimate accurately, the duration of acromegaly before diagnosis may influence mortality. Wright *et al.* [14] found no difference in estimated duration of acromegaly before diagnosis between survivors and those who had died, while Rajasoorya *et al.* [5] found that the duration of disease before diagnosis was significantly longer (10 years) in those who had died than in those alive and with minor symptoms (5 years). However, neither the total duration of acromegaly [5] nor its duration since diagnosis influenced long-term outcome. As discussed below, early diagnosis and effective treatment are essential if long-term outcome is to be improved.

Relationship of growth hormone and IGF-1 levels to long-term outcome in acromegaly

Accurate GH assays have been widely used since the mid- to late 1960s, while IGF-1 measurements were introduced during the late 1980s. Various studies have examined the relationship between serum GH and IGF-1 levels and the morbidity and mortality in acromegaly, and its response to treatment. However, only three have attempted to relate serum GH levels at diagnosis and during follow-up to long-term morbidity and mortality [4–6].

Bates *et al.* [4] examined retrospectively the case records of 79 patients studied at Stoke-on-Trent between 1967 and 1991, with a median follow-up of 10 years; 28 patients (35%) died during this period. GH levels, assessed annually by the mean of 4 or 5 measurements taken between 0800 and 1800 hours, were significantly higher in those who had died than in those who were still alive (Fig. 4). Moreover, mortality in patients whose lowest post-treatment GH levels were <5 mU/l was not significantly different from healthy controls, but was twice as high in those with GH levels >10 mU/l; this latter threshold has been used in several previous studies to define a 'cure', and is clearly not sufficiently rigorous. Similarly, Orme *et al.* [6] reported that GH levels of <5 mU/l were not associated with a significant excess of deaths, but that all-cause mortality increased stepwise with GH levels lying within the ranges 5–20 and >20 mU/l (see Fig. 5).

Rajasoorya *et al.* [5] also confirmed the association of increased mortality with high GH levels, at presentation and following treatment. Patients who died or suffered major complications (diabetes or visual impairment) had initial GH levels twice as high (mean values ~200 mU/l) as those with clinically milder disease. The product of GH level at diagnosis and the estimated duration of symptoms before this – a surrogate for total exposure to GH – showed a striking relationship with disease severity and mortality (see Fig. 5). The last recorded GH was found to be the strongest predictor of clinical outcome on multivariate analysis, and was significantly higher in those who died than in those who

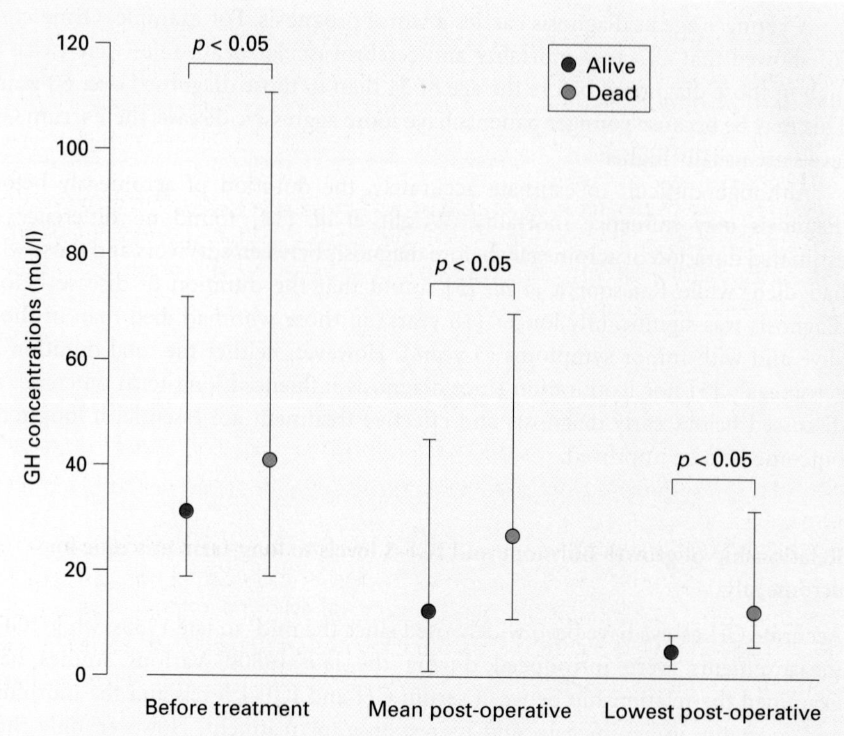

Fig. 4 Growth hormone (GH) levels (median and interquartile range) in acromegalic patients who had died and in those who remained alive. Data are shown for before treatment (left); throughout follow-up (middle; expressed as the mean of all GH values obtained and the lowest 24-h GH values obtained); and the lowest 24-h GH values observed during annual review postoperatively (right). (Adapted from Bates *et al.* [4].)

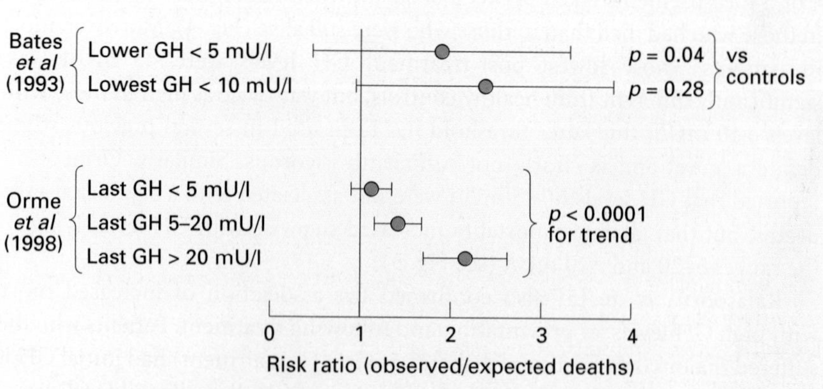

Fig. 5 Mortality in acromegaly, expressed as the risk ratio (observed deaths compared with expected numbers of deaths in matched non-acromegalic subjects), related to growth hormone (GH) levels, in the studies of Bates *et al.* [4] and Orme *et al.* [6]. Bates *et al.* used mean GH values derived from a 5-point 24-h profile, while Orme *et al.* employed either the most recent random GH value or the average of the last 5 samples. Data are means and 95% confidence intervals.

survived with major or minor complications (mean values of 66 and 10 mU/l, respectively). Similarly, Wrightson *et al.* [16] found that 10-year survival after treatment was significantly better if the last serum GH was <10 mU/l than if it was >10 mU/l (93% vs 87%); moreover, the chances of 'good' clinical status at last follow-up were greater if the latest GH values were <4 mU/l compared with >10 mU/l.

Many of the available data are retrospective and imprecise, and many studies were small. These issues must be investigated rigorously in a large, prospective multicentre study which accurately ascertains the onset of symptoms; such a study has now been initiated in the UK.

☐ BIOCHEMICAL 'CURE' OF ACROMEGALY: A VALID AND USEFUL CONCEPT?

In attempting to define a biochemical 'cure', it is necessary to consider normal GH secretory dynamics and GH responses to provocative stimuli in normal and acromegalic adults.

As already discussed, about 95% of GH in normal adults is secreted in a few brief pulses in any 24-hour period, and is undetectable the rest of the time (see Fig. 6). The amplitude of GH pulses is both age- and sex-dependent, falling with age and being greater in women [1]. In acromegaly, GH pulse frequency is increased and about 50% of GH is secreted in a non-pulsatile fashion [17–19]. Persistent basal non-pulsatile GH secretion may contribute to high IGF-1 levels. Other abnormalities of GH secretion in acromegaly include the paradoxical increase following glucose challenge, and GH release evoked by TRH and sometimes GnRH.

In 'absolute' terms, a biological cure would imply restoration of normal GH secretory dynamics including: undetectable interpulse GH values; lowering of basal GH and IGF-1 values to within age- and sex-related normal ranges; and abolition of any paradoxical responses. The pertinent issues are how often these stringent criteria are achieved after treatment, and whether these targets must be met to achieve clinical remission and to normalise life expectancy.

Two recent studies have addressed GH secretory dynamics after trans-sphenoidal removal of somatotrophinomas. In 14 patients studied 9–10 days after successful surgery (defined by normalisation of basal GH levels, GH responses to oral glucose, and IGF-1 values), van den Berg *et al.* [17] reported that GH pulse frequency, quantity of GH secreted per pulse, and nadir GH levels all also returned to normal; moreover, as has been shown previously in several studies, paradoxical responses to TRH were abolished. By contrast, Ho *et al.* [18] failed to show any change in GH pulse frequency 2 months after successful surgery, although mean GH levels, inter-pulse GH values, GH pulse amplitudes and paradoxical GH responses to glucose and TRH were normalised, as were IGF-1 levels.

Detailed dynamic testing may confirm restoration of physiological patterns of GH secretion after surgery, but probably does not offer any practical advantage over basal GH and IGF-1 values in the routine management of acromegaly; biochemical 'cure' is still generally defined in terms of these latter measurements. Indeed, it may be more useful and pragmatic to define target basal GH and IGF-1 levels which

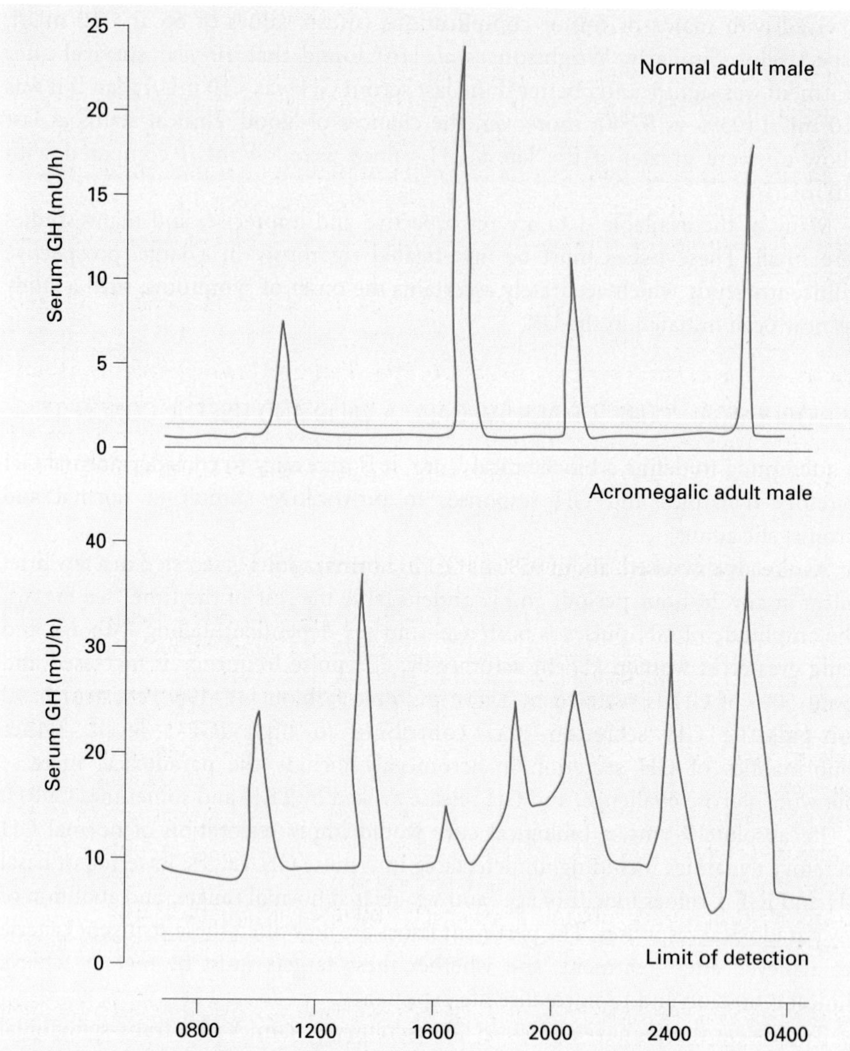

Fig. 6 Schematic representation of growth hormone (GH) secretory profiles in a normal adult male and in an acromegalic male. For most of the 24-hour period GH is undetectable (<1 mU/l, blue line) with occasional bursts of GH secretion. In contrast, in acromegaly nadir GH values never become undetectable, GH bursts are more frequent, and amplitude of GH bursts is higher than in normal adults.

reliably predict clinical remission and survival; these values do not strictly define a cure, but rather a safe range. Current evidence suggests that 'safe' basal or random GH levels are <5 mU/l (2.5 ng/ml), together with normal age-related IGF-1 levels. The general use of these simple criteria would make it possible easily to compare the outcome of surgical and other treatments between centres; this has previously been impossible because of the variable and non-standardised criteria used to define a cure.

Outcome of trans-sphenoidal surgery: cured or safe?

Until the early 1990s, when 'cure' was defined as basal GH levels <10 mU/l [20], several authorities reported overall success rates of 60–80% (Table 4). Surgical outcome is related to tumour size (which in turn is directly related to preoperative serum GH levels) and to the direction and extent of tumour extension, being worst for tumours that invade the cavernous sinus [23,24]. The success rate reported in a series is therefore highly dependent on the proportion of large tumours (>1 cm) that it includes.

Series using the criterion of GH <5 mU/l are few and small (Table 5). Overall, 30–60% of subjects achieve postoperative basal GH levels of <5 mU/l, and probably only 30–40% would have basal levels of <2 mU/l. Thus, the results of selective trans-sphenoidal adenomectomy for treatment of acromegaly are not particularly good, and it follows that at least 50% of patients will need additional therapy following surgery. Interestingly, Osman *et al.* [25] reported that 95% of patients with a basal

Table 4 Some recent results of trans-sphenoidal surgery for acromegaly.

		Percentage of cases achieving postoperative GH levels of:	
Study	**Number of subjects**	**<10 mU/l (5 ng/ml)**	**<5 mU/l (2.5 ng/ml)**
Fahlbusch *et al.* [23]	224	71%	not reported
Laws [24]	100	74%	not reported
Tindall *et al.* [21]	103	81%	not reported
Wrightson *et al.* [16]	38	61%	32%
Osman *et al.* [25]	79	not reported	59%
Jenkins *et al.* [22]	89	not reported	33%

Table 5 Outcomes in acromegaly following trans-sphenoidal surgery, based on early postoperative GH levels, expressed as the mean of several random values.

	Likely outcome at GH levels of:		
Outcome	**<5 mU/l**	**5–10 mU/l**	**>10 mU/l**
Symptomatic and metabolic control	Likely	Possible	Unlikely
Normal IGF-1 levels	Likely	Possible	Unlikely
Recurrence of symptoms and tumour	Unlikely	Possible	Likely
Long-term mortality/morbidity outlook	Excellent	Fair	Poor
Need for further therapy	Unlikely; careful follow-up required	Consider sooner rather than later	Definitely required

GH concentrations: 1 mU/l = 0.5 ng/ml

GH of <5 mU/l and suppression of GH to <2 mU/l during an OGTT 6–8 weeks after surgery had similar values when tested an average of 7 years later, without any additional interim treatment. A 'safe' early outcome therefore seems to predict that this will be maintained in the long term.

Table 5 summarises the likely outcomes of surgery, stratified according to early postoperative basal serum GH levels. The degree to which the physician should strive to achieve the lowest GH target (<5 mU/l) should be individualised for each patient, but in general should be greater for younger patients who have more to gain in the long term.

☐ TREATMENT OPTIONS IN ACROMEGALY

These are summarised in Table 6 and Fig. 7. Acromegaly is generally more aggressive (both symptomatically and biochemically) with younger ages of onset, and also carries worse long-term morbidity and mortality. Management decisions should therefore include age as an important factor. The scheme suggested in Fig. 6 is based upon facts that have emerged in the past few years, as discussed above.

Surgery

Despite its somewhat disappointing failure to achieve a target GH of <5 mU/l, trans-sphenoidal adenomectomy remains the initial treatment of choice, on several counts. It is the most rapidly effective form of therapy for alleviating symptoms and lowering serum GH, and is safe and cost-effective. Moreover, even if the tumour cannot be removed in its entirety, it is likely that initial debulking will render adjuvant therapy (external radiotherapy or drugs) more effective.

Table 6 Treatment options in acromegaly.

Surgery

- *Treatment of choice*
  - Trans-sphenoidal adenomectomy
  - Trans-frontal hypophysectomy (large tumour)

External beam radiotherapy (DXT)

- *Adjuvant therapy after surgery*
- *Primary therapy in patients unfit for surgery*

Drug treatment

- *Adjuvant therapy after surgery or DXT*
- *Primary therapy in patients unfit for or awaiting surgery*
  - Dopamine agonists: bromocriptine
    cabergoline } long-acting
    quinagolide } long-acting
  - Somatostatin analogues: octreotide
    octreotide LAR } long-acting
    lanreotide } long-acting

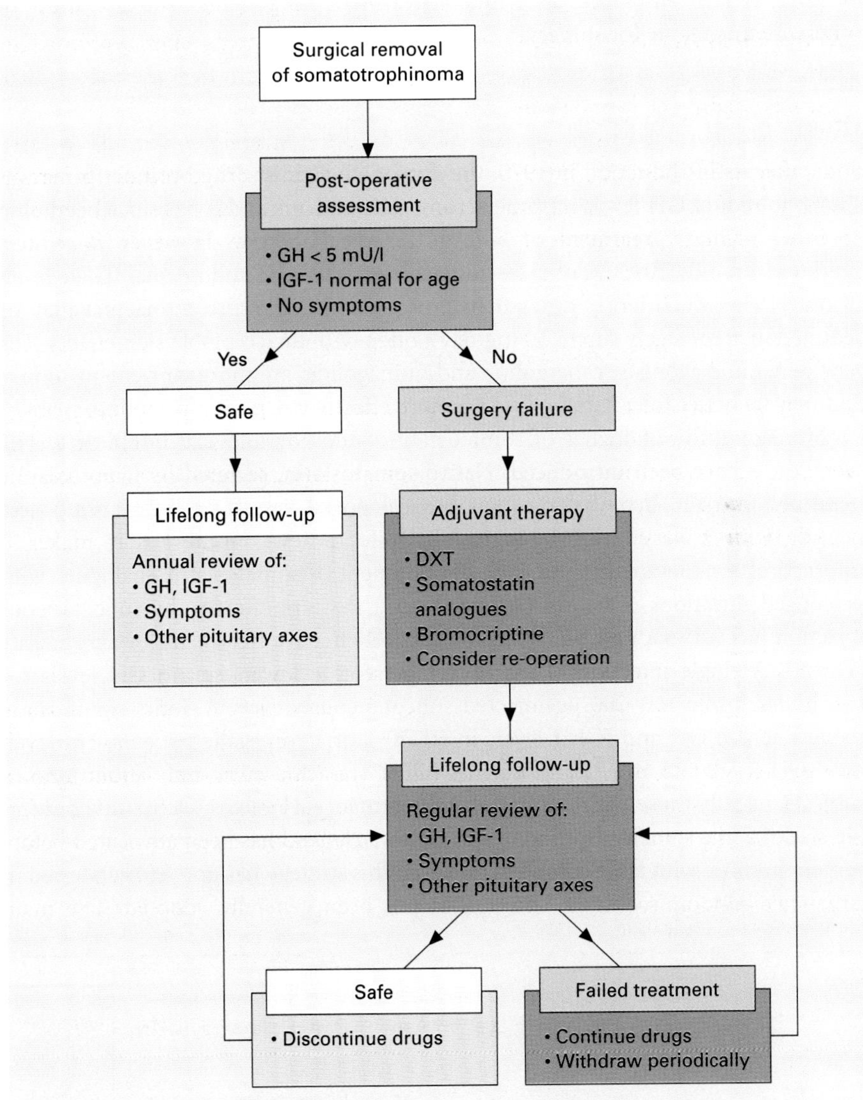

Fig. 7 Algorithm for the management of acromegalic patients aged <65 years who are suitable for pituitary surgery.

External radiotherapy

Additional treatment to achieve satisfactory GH and IGF-1 levels is usually first undertaken with external radiotherapy (DXT). This is undoubtedly simple, safe and effective but has the disadvantages of a slow onset of action and the subsequent development of hypopituitarism. The greatest fall in GH occurs within the first 2 years and further gradual decreases follow. The risk of some degree of hypopituitarism increases with time, reaching about 50% after 20 years; all patients who have received pituitary DXT therefore require lifelong surveillance.

DXT is also employed as primary treatment in patients who are unfit or otherwise unsuitable for surgery.

Drugs

Soon after its introduction in 1970, the dopamine agonist drug bromocriptine was shown to reduce GH levels in some acromegalic patients and it has since been used as either primary treatment or adjuvant medical therapy. However, it reduces symptoms in only 20–30% of cases and achieves 'safe' GH and normal IGF-1 levels in only 10%. Much larger doses than those used in hyperprolactinaemia may be required in acromegaly (up to 30 mg/day), often with unacceptable side-effects. The new dopamine agonists, cabergoline and quinagolide, are more convenient to take and may be better tolerated, but are no more effective than bromocriptine.

More recently, analogues of somatostatin – the physiological inhibitor of GH secretion – have been introduced. Native somatostatin, secreted by hypothalamic neurones into the hypothalamo-hypophyseal portal vessels, is a 14 amino acid peptide with a very short biological half-life (a few minutes) that makes it impractical for therapeutic use. The development of somatostatin analogues with prolonged durations of action (several hours) that are effective by subcutaneous injection has led to a new pharmacological and effective treatment for acromegaly (Fig. 8). A single injection of 100 μg of octreotide lowers serum GH levels for 6–8 hours, while 100–200 μg injected subcutaneously every 8 hours significantly reduces serum GH and IGF-1 levels in 60–70% of acromegalic patients. However, 'safe' GH levels (<5 mU/l) and normal IGF-1 are achieved in only about 40% of subjects, usually those with the lowest pretreatment GH values. Octreotide reduces the size of some somatotrophinomas by up to 50%, and has been advocated before surgery in those with large tumours; however, this strategy has not yet been tested in large-scale randomised trials and so has not been generally adopted. The main

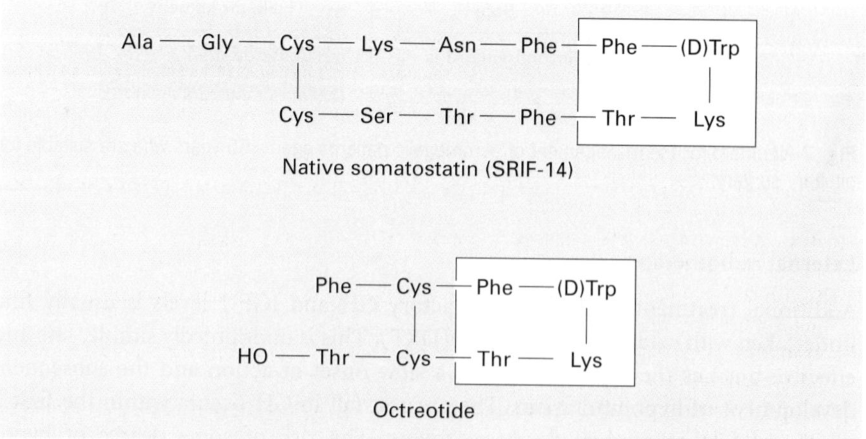

Fig. 8 Structures of native somatostatin (SRIF-14) and the synthetic octapeptide analogue (white area: biologically active portion of the molecules).

side-effects of octreotide are gastrointestinal, particularly abdominal discomfort and flatulence, which usually resolve spontaneously. The incidences of gallstone and biliary sludge formation are probably increased due to biliary stasis from inhibition of cholecystokinin release. Although this is frequently asymptomatic, it is prudent to perform a gall bladder ultrasound scan before starting a somatostatin analogue, and to repeat this if abdominal symptoms develop.

The drawbacks of octreotide include the inconvenience of 8-hourly subcutaneous injections and its high cost, currently £6–12,000 per annum depending on dosage. The pharmacokinetic problems have been circumvented by the development of slow-release formulations, namely lanreotide and octreotide LAR, which are given every 2 and 4 weeks, respectively. Each is effective, and continuous therapy can lower GH and IGF-1 levels for up to 3 years, with no evidence of 'escape' from effective suppression; these preparations are thus highly suitable for long-term treatment. The impressive biochemical responses to somatostatin analogues are accompanied by symptomatic and metabolic improvement, often within the first few weeks of treatment.

When should somatostatin analogues be used to treat acromegaly? Some have advocated their use as primary treatment, especially in those unfit for pituitary surgery. The decision will depend upon the severity of symptoms and the likely benefits for the patient's symptomatic improvement and long-term outcome. Given the high cost of this treatment and its potentially long duration, rigorous cost-benefit analysis is clearly required.

A more logical use of somatostatin analogues is to produce rapid biochemical and symptomatic control during the 2–3 years after DXT, while waiting for the latter to become effective. It is reasonable to employ somatostatin analogues in this context, interrupting treatment every 6–12 months to assess serum GH and IGF-1 levels; if these remain acceptably low and the patient is asymptomatic, the somatostatin analogue can be discontinued.

REFERENCES

1. Van den Berg G, Veldhuis JD, Frolich M, Roelfsma F. An amplitude-specific divergence in the pulsatile mode of growth hormone (GH) secretion underlies the gender difference in mean GH concentrations in men and postmenopausal women. *J Clin Endocrinol Metab* 1996; **81**: 2460–7.
2. Nabarro JDN. Acromegaly. *Clin Endocrinol* 1987; **26**: 481–512.
3. Alexander L, Appleton D, Hall R, *et al.* Epidemiology of acromegaly in the Newcastle region. *Clin Endocrinol* 1980; **12**: 71–9.
4. Bates AS, Van't Hoff W, Jones JM, Clayton RN. An audit of outcome of treatment in acromegaly. *Q J Med* 1993; **86**: 293–9.
5. Rajasoorya C, Holdaway IM, Wrightson P, *et al.* Determinants of clinical outcome and survival in acromegaly. *Clin Endocrinol* 1994; **41**: 95–102.
6. Orme SM, McNally R, Cartwright RA, *et al.* Mortality and cancer incidence in acromegaly: a retrospective cohort study. *J Clin Endocrinol Metab* 1998; **83**: 2730–4.
7. Klein I, Parveen G, Gavoeler JS, Vanthiel DH. Colonic polyps in patients with acromegaly. *Ann Intern Med* 1982; **97**: 27–30.
8. Ituarte EA, Pebnni J, Hershman JM. Acromegaly and colon cancer. *Ann Intern Med* 1984; **101**: 627–8.

9 Brunner JE, Johnson CC, Zafar S, *et al.* Colon cancer and polyps in acromegaly: increased risk associated with family history of colon cancer. *Clin Endocrinol* 1990; **32**: 65–71.
10 Ezzat S, Melmed S. Are patients with acromegaly at increased risk for neoplasia? *J Clin Endocrinol Metab* 1991; **72**: 245–9.
11 Ron S, Gridley G, Hrubec H, *et al.* Acromegaly and gastrointestinal cancer. *Cancer* 1991; **68**: 1673–7.
12 Vasen HFA, van Erpeaum KJ, Roelfsma F, *et al.* Increased prevalence of colonic adenomas in patients with acromegaly. *Eur J Endocrinol* 1994; **131**: 235–7.
13 Jenkins PJ, Fairclough PD, Richards T, *et al.* Acromegaly, colonic polyps and carcinoma. *Clin Endocrinol* 1997; **47**: 17–22.
14 Wright AD, Hill DM, Lowy C, *et al.* Mortality in acromegaly. *Q J Med* 1970; **39**: 1–16.
15 Bengtsson B-A, Eden S, Ernest I, *et al.* Epidemiology and long-term survival in acromegaly. *Acta Med Scand* 1988; **223**: 327–35.
16 Wrightson P, Rajasoorya C, Holdaway IM, Scott J. Acromegaly: factors affecting the long-term outcome after surgical treatment. *J Clin Neurosci* 1994; **1**: 164–72.
17 van den Berg G, Frolich M, Veldhuis JD, Roelfsma F. Growth hormone secretion in recently operated acromegalic patients. *J Clin Endocrinol Metab* 1994; **79**: 1706–15.
18 Ho PJ, Jaffe CA, Friberg RD, *et al.* Persistence of rapid growth hormone pulsatility after successful removal of GH producing pituitary tumours. *J Clin Endocrinol Metab* 1994; **78**: 1403–10.
19 Hartman ML, Veldhuis JD, Vance ML, *et al.* Somatotrophin pulse frequency basal concentrations are increased in acromegaly and are reduced by successful therapy. *J Clin Endocrinol Metab* 1990; **79**: 1375–84.
20 Klibanski A, Zervas NT. Diagnosis and management of hormone secreting pituitary adenomas. *N Engl J Med* 1991; **324**: 822–31.
21 Tindall GT, Oyesiku NM, Watts NB, *et al.* Trans-sphenoidal adenomectomy for growth hormone secreting pituitary adenomas in acromegaly: outcome analysis and determinants of failure. *J Neurosurg* 1993; **78**: 205–17.
22 Jenkins D, O'Brien I, Johnson A, *et al.* The Birmingham pituitary database: auditing the outcome of treatment of acromegaly. *Clin Endocrinol* 1995; **43**: 517–22.
23 Fahlbusch R, Honegger J, Scholt W, Buchfelder M. Results of surgery in acromegaly. In: Wass JAH (ed). *Treating Acromegaly.* Bristol: Journal of Endocrinology Ltd, 1994: 49–57.
24 Laws ER. Results of trans-sphenoidal microsurgical management of acromegaly. In: Wass JAH (ed). *Treating Acromegaly.* Bristol: Journal of Endocrinology Ltd, 1994: 59–63.
25 Osman IA, James RA, Chatterjee S, Mathias D, Kendall-Taylor P. Factors determining the long-term outcome of surgery for acromegaly. *Q J Med* 1994; **87**: 617–23.

□ MULTIPLE CHOICE QUESTIONS

1 Which of the following statements is true with respect to acromegaly?
   (a) Hypertension and diabetes mellitus are more prevalent compared with age- and sex-matched normal subjects.
   (b) The observed to expected mortality rate from all causes is decreased in acromegaly.
   (c) There is an increased rate of cardiovascular deaths in acromegalics.
   (d) There is an increased incidence of colonic polyps in acromegalics.
   (e) In retrospective analyses mortality decreases the lower the serum GH level.

2 Which of the following statements about the biochemical diagnosis of active acromegaly is true?
   (a) An undetectable random serum GH and normal age-related IGF-1 excludes the diagnosis of active acromegaly.

(b) An elevated random serum GH and IGF-1 confirms the diagnosis of acromegaly.
(c) Failure of serum GH to suppress to <2 mU/l during OGTT confirms the diagnosis of acromegaly.
(d) Serum GH may be increased by TRH in acromegalics.
(e) Serum prolactin may be raised in patients with acromegaly.

3 In acromegaly which of the following statements is true?
(a) The serum levels of GH and IGF-1 are linearly related.
(b) The serum levels of GH and IGF-1 are asymptotically related.
(c) Serum levels of IGF-1 are likely to be normal if random basal serum GH levels are <5 mU/l.
(d) A 'safe' level of serum GH with respect to long-term mortality is <10 mU/l.
(e) Treatment objectives should be to reduce serum GH to <5 mU/l and normalise serum IGF-1 levels.

4 Which of the following statements is true concerning the treatment of acromegaly?
(a) Trans-sphenoidal hypophysectomy is the initial treatment of choice for most patients.
(b) The outcome of hypophysectomy, in terms of serum GH achieved, is unrelated to size of tumour and preoperative GH levels.
(c) Not all patients with acromegaly necessarily require treatment.
(d) External pituitary irradiation reduces serum GH levels rapidly (<6 months).
(e) The incidence of some degree of hypopituitarism 20 years after external pituitary irradiation is 10%.

5 Which of the following drugs may be used to suppress serum GH levels in acromegaly?
(a) Bromocriptine
(b) Cabergoline
(c) Ethinyl oestradiol
(d) Octreotide
(e) Lanreotide

ANSWERS

1a True	2a True	3a False	4a True	5a True
b False	b False	b True	b False	b True
c True	c True	c True	c True	c False
d True	d True	d False	d False	d True
e True	e True	e True	e False	e True

Hyponatraemia

Peter H Baylis

□ INTRODUCTION

Serum sodium concentration is normally maintained between the tight limits of about 136–144 mmol/l, dependent on individual laboratory reference ranges. In clinical practice, significant hyponatraemia may be defined by a serum sodium concentration less than 130 mmol/l (Fig. 1). It is the most common electrolyte disorder recognised in hospital practice, with an annual incidence of 1–2% and a prevalence of 2–4%. Mild degrees of hyponatraemia (serum sodium concentrations of 120–130 mmol/l) often cause no symptoms and have little clinical significance, but the condition becomes increasingly life-threatening as serum sodium falls towards 100 mmol/l. Indeed, the mortality of patients with a serum sodium of 106 mmol/l or below is 30–40%, and approaches 85% if the patient is cachetic or

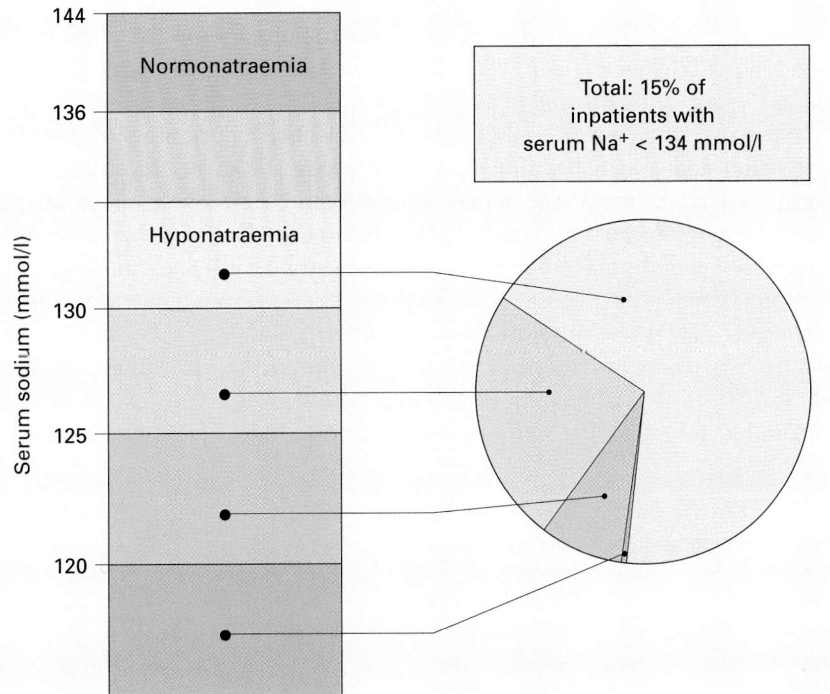

Fig. 1 Grades of hyponatraemia and prevalence amongst unselected hospital inpatients in Newcastle, UK (data from Ref 1).

alcoholic. Therefore, severe hyponatraemia presents the clinician with major challenges in both diagnosis and management.

The pathophysiology, complications and management of hyponatraemia have recently been reviewed in detail [2–4]. This chapter presents a pragmatic approach to the patient with hyponatraemia. Its various causes will be discussed, with particular emphasis on the syndrome of inappropriate antidiuresis, cerebral salt wasting and the 'sick cell' concept. Treatment options will be reviewed, with a specific focus on patients with severe hyponatraemia (serum sodium concentration <120 mmol/l) and on the importance of the rate of correction of serum sodium. 'Pseudohyponatraemia', for example due to high plasma levels of glucose, triglycerides or paraprotein, will not be considered.

□ AETIOLOGY AND CLASSIFICATION

Hyponatraemia develops when water intake exceeds renal water excretion. All cases therefore have a relative excess of body water, even though the total body sodium content of the hyponatraemic patient is variable. The maintenance of salt and water homeostasis in man is regulated by a series of complex neuro-endocrine and renal factors (Table 1). The inability to excrete water adequately is generally due to impaired renal diluting capacity, frequently a consequence of excessive non-osmotic secretion of vasopressin – the release of which is normally inhibited by a fall in plasma osmolality [5]. Indeed, over 97% of all hyponatraemic patients have detectable or elevated plasma vasopressin concentrations, irrespective of the underlying cause of hyponatraemia. The regulation and biological renal actions of vasopressin are summarised in Fig. 2.

Hyponatraemia has many causes and can be classified in various ways. One of the most useful and pragmatic approaches is to group the causes according to the patient's extracellular volume status: hypovolaemic, normovolaemic or hypervolaemic hyponatraemia [5]. Figure 3 presents this classification of hyponatraemia, with a selection of the commonest causes in each category [6]. The commonest type of hyponatraemia is normovolaemic, with the syndrome of inappropriate antidiuresis (SIAD) as its most frequent underlying cause [5].

Most hyponatraemic patients can readily be allocated to one of these classes on the basis of clinical examination and routine biochemical measurements in blood and urine. This method of classification will direct the clinician's thinking to

Table 1 Some of the major factors involved in salt and water homeostasis.

Thirst	Natriuretic peptides
Sympathetic nerves	Renin-angiotensin-aldosterone axis
Catecholamines	Nitric oxide
Vasopressin	Prostaglandins
Endothelins	Kallikreins
Substance P	Bradykinins

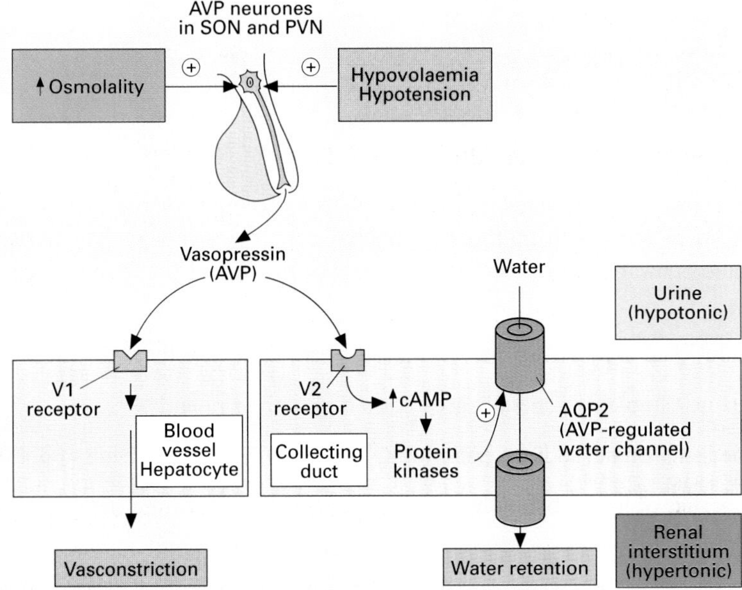

Fig. 2 Regulation and biological actions of vasopressin (AVP). V1 receptors mediate vasoconstriction, while activation of V2 receptors in the collecting ducts stimulates the expression of the water-channel protein (aquaporin; AQP2). This renders the collecting duct permeable to water, which then passes from the hypotonic urine into the hypertonic renal interstitium, causing net water retention.

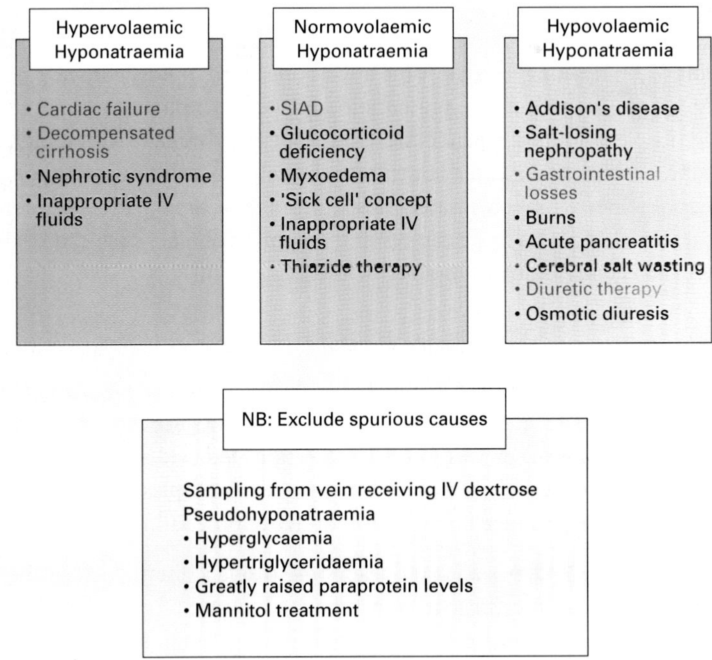

Fig. 3 Common causes of hyponatraemia classified by the extracellular volume status.

determine the underlying diagnosis and the general and specific measures to treat the patient.

□ SPECIFIC CAUSES OF HYPONATRAEMIA

Syndrome of inappropriate antidiuresis

This syndrome was first suggested in the 1920s to account for the hyponatraemia observed in patients with pulmonary tuberculosis. It was finally characterised by Bartter and Schwartz [7] in 1967 and can now be defined by the following cardinal features:

- □ dilutional hyponatraemia, with plasma osmolality less than 270 mOsmol/kg
- □ urine osmolality generally greater than plasma osmolality
- □ persistent renal sodium excretion (>30 mmol/l in a 'spot' urine sample)
- □ absence of hypotension, hypovolaemia or oedema-forming states
- □ normal renal and adrenal function.

In addition, there is often hypouricaemia. The persistent urinary excretion of salt is due principally to inhibition of the renin-angiotensin-aldosterone system and the increase in circulating atrial natriuretic peptides, which both follow expansion of total body water. Circulating vasopressin levels are raised in most hyponatraemic patients (see Fig. 4), so measurements of vasopressin are not helpful in confirming the diagnosis.

The syndrome has a wide variety of causes (Fig. 5), with drugs being particularly important and frequent. The syndrome affects one-third of hospitalised patients with AIDS. An increasingly common presentation of acute symptomatic hyponatraemia is in young people who have taken 'ecstasy' in a hot environment with a high water or beer intake. Although the latter contributes by causing a dilutional hyponatraemia, vasopressin levels are inappropriately raised in some of these patients. Neurosurgery and subarachnoid haemorrhage can result in hyponatraemia, which can be due either to SIAD or to cerebral salt wasting (see below).

Vasopressin secretion in the syndrome of inappropriate antidiuresis

Vasopressin release is normally stimulated by increases in plasma osmolality, rising exponentially above a threshold of 280–290 mOsmol/kg (see Figs. 2 and 4). Studies on the osmoregulation of vasopressin secretion have identified four different patterns of relationship between plasma vasopressin and plasma osmolality during osmotic stimulation produced by infusion of hypertonic saline [8] (Fig. 4):

- □ *Type A* pattern shows an erratic response displaced to the left of the normal reference area. Intermittent, non-regulated release of vasopressin from a tumour can account for this pattern. It is also seen in some patients with non-malignant disease, suggesting erratic non-osmotic vasopressin release from the posterior pituitary.

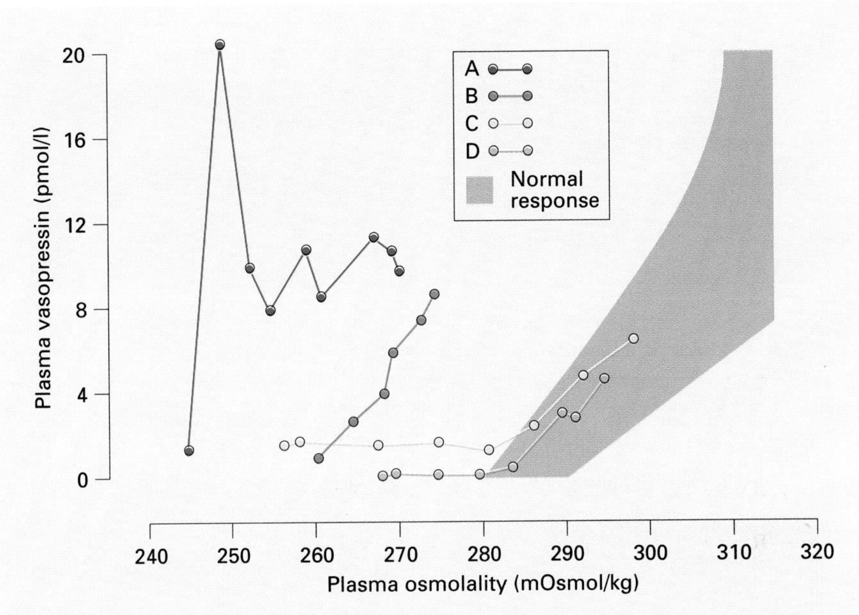

Fig. 4 Patterns of vasopressin secretion as a function of plasma osmolality in different subsets of patients with the syndrome of inappropriate antidiuresis. The shaded area represents the normal reference range (type A: erratic release; type B: reset osmostat; type C: 'persistent leak'; type D: normal pattern of osmoregulation).

- *Type B*, the 'reset osmostat' pattern, shows a close linear relationship between plasma vasopressin and osmolality but is shifted to the left of normal. Possible explanations for this pattern include loss of normal baroregulatory inhibition, increased sensitivity of the posterior pituitary due to hypovolaemia, or the sick cell concept (see below). Types A and B account for about 75–80% of all patients with SIAD.
- *Type C*, in which it appears that vasopressin secretion cannot be completely inhibited near the normal osmolality threshold but there is normal osmoregulation at higher plasma osmolality values.
- *Type D* pattern, displayed by a few patients, represents normal osmoregulation. This implies enhanced sensitivity to vasopressin, perhaps due to a highly sensitive V2-receptor in the kidney, to other influences such as abnormal renal prostaglandin function, or another antidiuretic factor.

It is now recognised that no particular disease is associated with a specific type of vasopressin pattern of release, and that investigating the osmoregulation of vasopressin release is unhelpful in identifying the cause. There have been no formal studies on osmoregulation of thirst in SIAD but these hyponatraemic and hypotonic patients continue to drink and their thirst appears not to be completely inhibited.

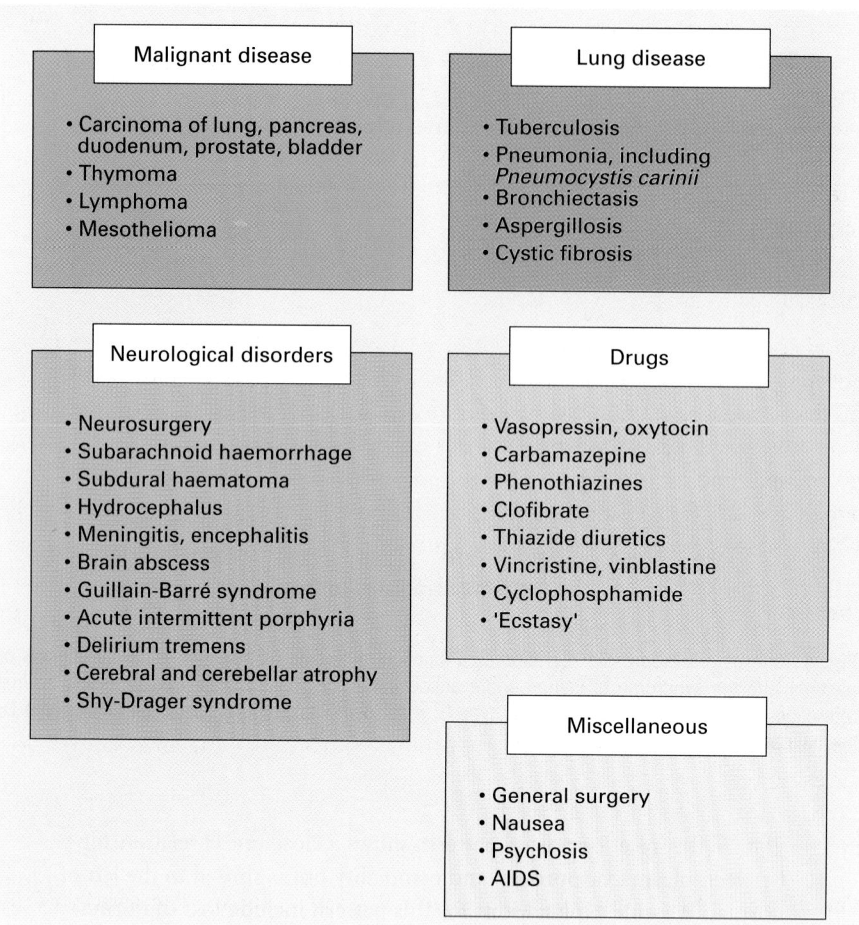

Fig. 5 Some causes of the syndrome of inappropriate antidiuresis.

One physiological state that leads to mild hyponatraemia due to resetting of the vasopressin and thirst osmostats (type B pattern) is pregnancy. Pregnant women continue to concentrate and dilute urine, but do so around a lower set point; serum sodium falls by about 5 mmol/l. Hyponatraemia corrects spontaneously after delivery.

Cerebral salt wasting

The disorder of cerebral salt wasting is defined by the association of excessive renal salt loss (>30 mmol/l) with intracranial disease, resulting in hyponatraemia and hypovolaemia. It is most commonly observed after acute events, particularly subarachnoid haemorrhage and/or related neurosurgery. First described in the 1950s, it subsequently became an unfashionable diagnosis and then controversial when SIAD was fully recognised. Now, however, it is appreciated that it is a distinct entity [9]. The pathogenesis of cerebral salt wasting is not clearly understood but probably involves enhanced release of cerebral natriuretic factors (atrial and brain natriuretic peptides, oubain-like substances and bradykinins), and possibly neural mechanisms including sympathetic hyperactivity (proximal tubule).

Both cerebral salt wasting and SIAD may occur with subarachnoid haemorrhage, the two being differentiated by the low and normal extracellular volumes, respectively.

'Sick cell' concept

Another controversial syndrome was described by Flear [1] to account for hyponatraemia in severely ill patients. He postulated that various pathogenic mechanisms, all leading to cell-membrane dysfunction, might be responsible. This type of hyponatraemia involves the loss of intracellular osmolytes (organic solutes, potassium) and transiently, is recognised by a normal plasma osmolality with hyponatraemia (ie an osmolar gap). These osmolytes are ultimately excreted by the kidney, thus leading to hypo-osmolar hyponatraemia and resetting of the osmostat – which is similar to the type B pattern of vasopressin release in SIAD (Fig. 4). An alternative explanation is the leakage of extracellular sodium into the cell in exchange for anions that are then excreted by the kidney.

Although there are clear data from acute animal experiments to support the sick cell concept, there is little evidence that it operates in humans. Indeed, many in the field believe that it does not exist in man and that these hyponatraemic patients have SIAD, type B.

☐ CLINICAL FEATURES OF HYPONATRAEMIA

The clinical features of hyponatraemia are well known (Fig. 6). The severity of the symptoms is related both to the degree of hyponatraemia and to the rate of fall of the serum sodium concentration. Symptoms are particularly prominent in patients who become hyponatraemic within 48 hours; these subjects are also most likely to suffer permanent neurological damage.

Most of the central nervous system features of hyponatraemia are due to brain oedema, particularly in acute hyponatraemia (developing in <3 days), in which the brain cells have failed to adapt to osmotic shifts. The brain is able to swell by

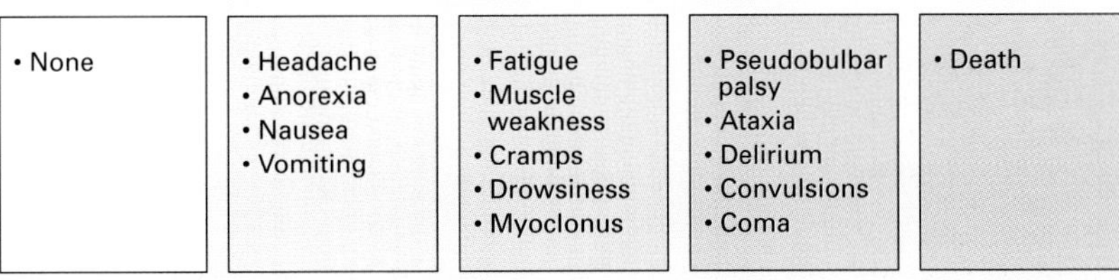

Fig. 6 Clinical manifestations of hyponatraemia. The pattern and severity of the symptoms are variable and influenced both by the level of serum sodium and by its rate of fall.

approximately 8% before it is confined by the skull and symptoms become prominent. This degree of brain swelling is recognised when serum sodium falls by 8% (ie to about 125 mmol/l), and it is therefore unusual for significant neurological symptoms to develop with mild hyponatraemia above this level. Below 125 mmol/l, symptoms develop progressively with further acute falls in serum sodium, but may be minimal if the decline in sodium is slow. As serum sodium approaches 105 mmol/l or below, virtually all patients become severely symptomatic, irrespective of the rate of serum sodium fall.

Ultimately, death may occur, often from the effects of 'coning', with compression of the cardiovascular and respiratory centres in the medulla by the cerebellar tonsils herniating through the foramen magnum.

☐ INVESTIGATION AND EVALUATION OF THE HYPONATRAEMIC PATIENT

The first step in the evaluation of the hyponatraemic patient is to define, if possible, the extracellular volume status (see Fig. 7).

Hypovolaemia is suggested by orthostatic hypotension, tachycardia, dry mucous membranes, poor skin turgor and a low central venous pressure.

Hypervolaemia (ie an oedematous state) is recognised by dependent oedema, ascites, increased central venous pressure (sometimes with other signs of cardiac failure). There may also be other features of the nephrotic syndrome, renal failure or decompensated cirrhosis. It is frequently difficult to distinguish between mild degrees of volume depletion and normovolaemia (eg SIAD).

Signs of underlying causes such as Addison's disease may also be present.

Laboratory investigations

The laboratory investigations are indicated in Fig. 7, and a diagnostic algorithm is

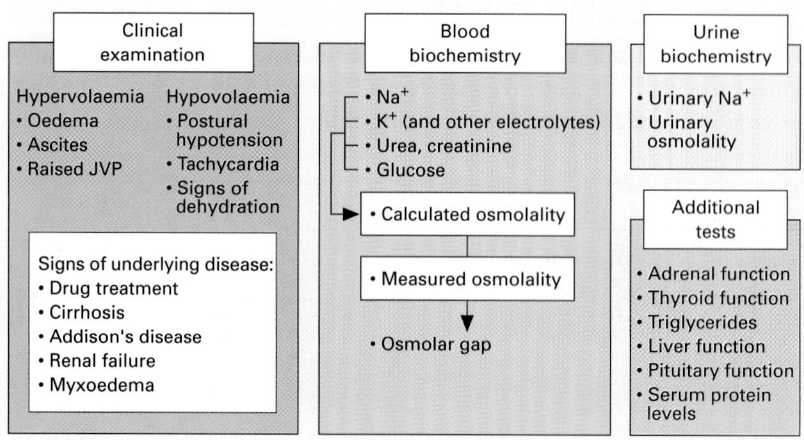

Fig. 7 Investigation of hyponatraemia.

shown in Fig. 8. Plasma osmolality should be measured to exclude spurious or pseudohyponatraemia due to excessive concentrations of substances such as glucose, triglycerides, protein or mannitol. The presence of these substances is indicated by an 'osmolar gap' of >10 mOsmol/kg. The formula for calculating the gap reflects the major contribution usually made to plasma osmolality by sodium ions:

- Osmolar gap = Measured osmolality – calculated osmolality
- Calculated osmolality = 2 × ([Na^+] + [K^+]) + [urea] + [glucose] (where all concentrations are mmol/l or mOsmol/kg).

Estimation of urinary sodium concentration in a 'spot' sample is useful and easier than a 24-hour collection, and provides important information. In SIAD and cerebral or renal salt wasting states, urinary sodium is greater than 30 mmol/l. Hypovolaemic patients have low urinary sodium concentration (<20 mmol/l) unless they also have a renal or cerebral salt wasting disorder (>30 mmol/l). In general, oedematous states have low urinary sodium concentrations. Urine osmolality measurements may not be particularly helpful, although low values of about 100 mOsmol/kg suggest water intoxication (eg due to compulsive drinking), and levels of more than 300 mOsmol/kg are generally present in SIAD.

Assessment of adrenal and thyroid function is advisable.

TREATMENT

Treatment is guided by the extracellular volume status, and by the severity of hyponatraemia and the speed with which it developed. Acute-onset hyponatraemia developing within 48 hours should be treated more urgently because of the risk of permanent neurological sequelae. By contrast, chronic hyponatraemia (present for over 72 hours) should not be corrected too rapidly because this may precipitate the osmotic demyelination syndrome which can also cause severe neurological damage, including spastic tetraparesis (discussed further below). Some of the therapeutic points of intervention are shown in Fig. 9.

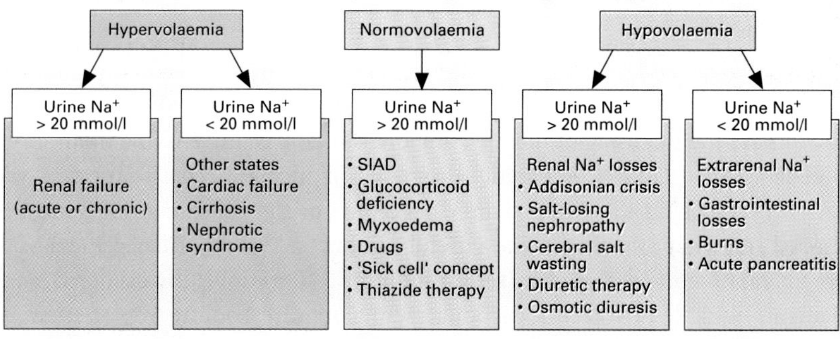

Fig. 8 Diagnostic algorithm for hyponatraemia, based on the patient's extracellular volume and urinary sodium excretion (modified from Ref 10).

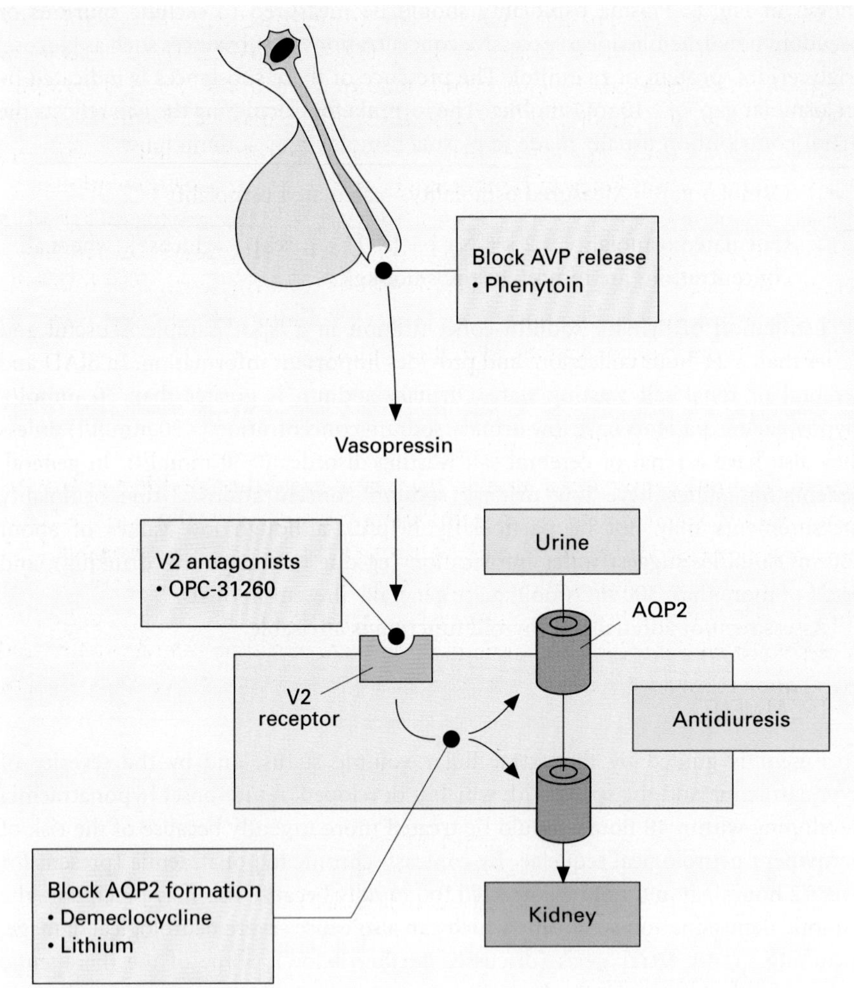

Fig. 9 Some specific therapeutic measures to treat the syndrome of inappropriate antidiuresis. The aquaretic OPC-31260 remains experimental and is not in clinical use.

In hypervolaemic hyponatraemia, the aim is to remove both sodium and water, while managing the underlying cause and maintaining nutrition. Diuretics with fluid restriction are the mainstay of therapy; angiotensin-converting enzyme inhibitors are helpful in cardiac failure. 'Aquaretic' drugs which increase renal solute-free water excretion by blocking the vasopressin V2 receptor in the collecting ducts are being developed and will probably provide a useful adjunct (see below). Management of very severe hyponatraemia of this type (serum sodium <110 mmol/l) is considered below.

Patients with hypovolaemic hyponatraemia require sodium replacement and correction of blood and extracellular volume depletion. Isotonic saline infusion and colloidal solutions are necessary if hypotension is present. Management of the underlying disorder (eg Addison's disease) is also essential.

Most hyponatraemic patients, however, are normovolaemic and frequently have SIAD. Figure 10 presents the therapeutic options available for these patients. In general, if hyponatraemia is mild (serum sodium >125 mmol/l) and is asymptomatic, active treatment of the hyponatraemia *per se* may not be necessary. In asymptomatic chronic hyponatraemia, the safest approach is fluid restriction. Abnormal vasopressin function is fundamental to the syndrome, so inhibition of its secretion (eg with phenytoin) or antagonism of its renal action is a logical approach (see below). Demeclocycline (300–900 mg/day) can be given, and acts beyond the V2 receptor to inhibit the action of vasopressin on the collecting duct. Nephrotoxicity and skin reactions are the main side effects. Lithium acts similarly, but its neurotoxicity has made it unpopular in this context.

Rate of correction of serum sodium

One of the most controversial areas in the treatment of profound hyponatraemia concerns the rate of correction of serum sodium. Since the mortality and morbidity of these patients is so high, there have been strong advocates of rapid correction [11]. There are, however, clear data indicating that in certain circumstances, notably chronic (>3 days' duration asymptomatic hyponatraemia), rapid sodium correction is associated with significant neurological sequelae, including central pontine and extrapontine myelinolysis (osmotic demyelination syndrome) (see Fig. 11). The

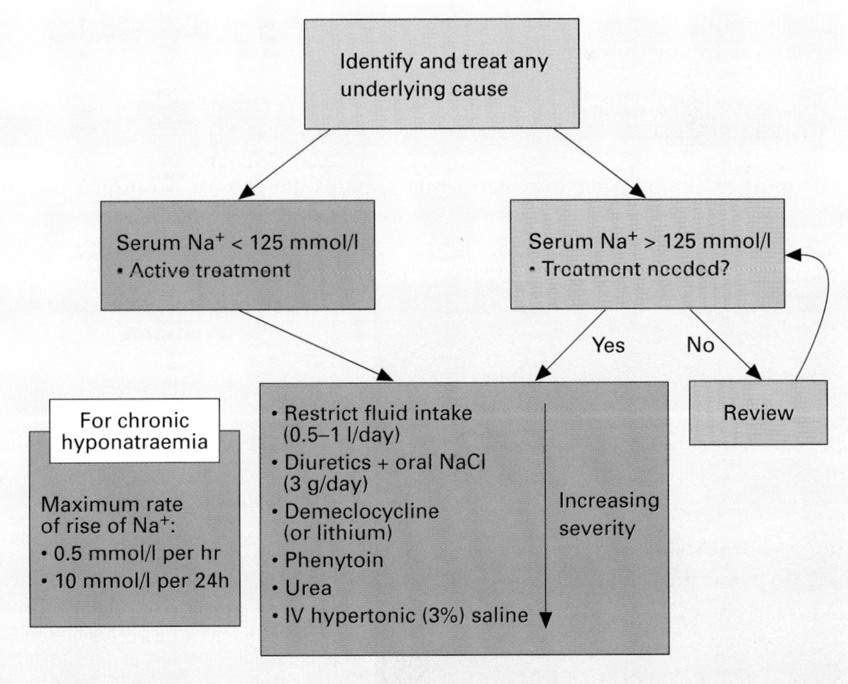

Fig. 10 Algorithm for the practical management of the syndrome of inappropriate diuresis.

precise pathogenesis is unknown, but manifestations include spastic tetraparesis and mutism.

Careful evaluation of data by Sterns [13] has led to the conclusion that in chronic asymptomatic hyponatraemia, the rate of rise of serum sodium should be no more than 0.5 mmol/l/h and less than 10 mmol/l in 24 hours (Table 6). Acute symptomatic hyponatraemia may correct more quickly, but no faster than 2.0 mmol/l/h and no more than 25 mmol/l during the initial 24–48 h [11].

These guidelines are independent of the method of correction, but infusion of hypertonic (3%) saline (compare 'normal' isotonic saline, 0.9%) poses the greatest danger because there is considerable room for error. Serum sodium should therefore be checked 2–4 hourly during saline infusion. Furthermore, it is essential to calculate the sodium load required and the rate of correction using either the principles developed by Arieff [11] or the following empirical formula:

- □ Rate of infusion of 3% saline (ml/hr) = body weight (kg) × desired rate of correction of serum sodium (mmol/l/h).

Experimental treatments for the syndrome of inappropriate antidiuresis

Antagonism to the action of vasopressin at its V2 receptor in the collecting duct is a theoretically attractive option for managing SIAD. Various prototype peptide antagonists have been developed; initial studies have shown efficacy in animals, but they are less successful in man. By contrast, linear non-peptide vasopressin antagonists such as OPC-31260 appear to be more efficacious. These drugs, termed aquaretic agents, increase renal solute-free water excretion, and preliminary data on effectiveness appear very promising [14].

□ CONCLUSIONS

In its most extreme forms, hyponatraemia remains dangerous. A rational plan of

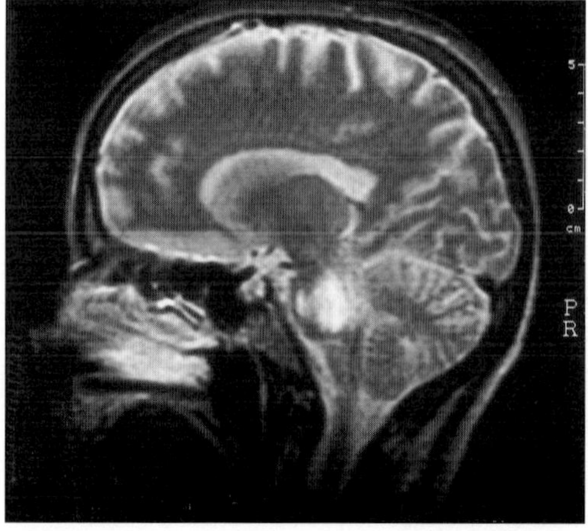

Osmotic demyelination syndrome

- Spastic tetraparesis
- Mutism
- Pseudobulbar palsy

Fig. 11 Osmotic demyelination syndrome (pontine myelinolysis): clinical features and appearances on computed tomography (magnetic resonance imaging) scanning.

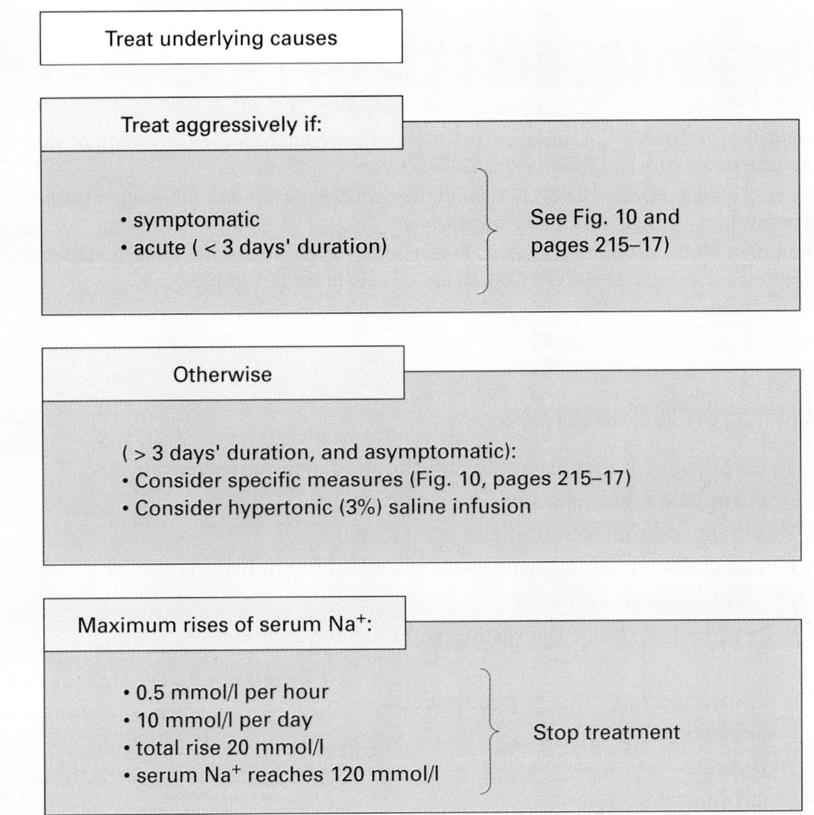

Fig. 12 Recommendations for management of severe hyponatraemia (serum sodium <120 mmol/l).

investigation and treatment should help to reduce the hazards both of the condition itself, and of inappropriate medical management.

REFERENCES

1 Flear CTG, Gill GV, Burn J. Hyponatraemia: mechanisms and management. *Lancet* 1981; **ii**: 26–31.

2 Fried LF, Palevsky PM. Hyponatremia and hypernatremia. *Med Clin N Am* 1997; **81**: 585–609.

3 Ellis SJ. Severe hyponatraemia: complications and treatment. *Q J Med* 1995; **88**: 905–9.

4 Gill G, Leese G. Hyponatraemia: biochemical and clinical perspectives. *Postgrad Med J* 1988; **74**: 516–23.

5 Anderson RJ, Chung H-M, Kluge R, Schrier RW. Hyponatraemia: a prospective analysis of its epidemiology and the pathogenetic role of vasopressin. *Ann Intern Med* 1985; **102**: 164–8.

6 Berl T, Anderson RJ, McDonald KM, Schrier RW. Clinical disorders of water balance. *Kidney Intern* 1976; **10**: 117–32.

7 Bartter FC, Schwartz WB. The syndrome of inappropriate secretion of antidiuretic hormone. *Am J Med* 1967; **42**: 790–806.

8 Zerbe R, Stropes L, Robertson GL. Vasopressin function in the syndrome of inappropriate antidiuresis. *Annu Rev Med* 1980; **31**: 315–27.

9 Harrigan MR. Cerebral salt wasting: does it exist? *Neurosurgery* 1996; **38**: 152–60.

10 Kumar S, Berl T. Sodium. *Lancet* 1998; **352**: 220–8.

11 Arieff AI. Management of hyponatraemia. *Br Med J* 1993; **307**: 305–8.

12 Lundboom N, Laurila O, Laurila S. Central pontine myelinolysis after correction of chronic hyponatraemia (letter). *Lancet* 1993; **342**: 247–8.

13 Sterns RH, Riggs JE, Schochet SS Jr. Osmotic demyelination syndrome following correction of hyponatremia. *N Engl J Med* 1986; **314**: 1535–42.

14 Ohnishi A, Orita Y, Okahara R, *et al.* Potent aquaretic agent: a novel nonpeptide selective vasopressin 2 antagonist (OPC-31260) in men. *J Clin Invest* 1993; **92**: 2653–9.

☐ MULTIPLE CHOICE QUESTIONS

1 In the syndrome of inappropriate antidiuretic hormone secretion:
- (a) Serum uric acid is elevated
- (b) Urinary sodium excretion rate is increased
- (c) Plasma vasopressin measurement is helpful in confirming the diagnosis
- (d) Total body water is raised
- (e) Treatment of choice is a vasopressin receptor-2 agonist

2 The following drugs cause hyponatraemia:
- (a) Vinblastine
- (b) Oxytocin
- (c) Carbimazole
- (d) Chlorpromazine
- (e) Angiotensin-converting enzyme inhibitors

3 Cerebral salt wasting:
- (a) Causes normovolaemic hyponatraemia
- (b) Is treated with fluid restriction and oral salt
- (c) Is a recognised complication of subarachnoid haemorrhage
- (d) Is caused by intracellular solute loss due to the sick cell syndrome
- (e) Results in dilute urine (urine osmolality <200 mOsmol/kg)

4 In the treatment of severe hyponatraemia (sodium<120 mmol/l):
- (a) Rapid correction of serum sodium is recommended for acute symptomatic hyponatraemia
- (b) If due to the syndrome of inappropriate antidiuretic hormone secretion, lithium is recommended
- (c) Hypertonic saline infusion is contraindicated
- (d) If associated with hypervolaemia, the purpose of therapy is to raise extracellular and intravascular sodium content
- (e) If chronic (developing over more than 3 days), the optimal rate of serum sodium rise should be 1–2 mmol/l/h

5 Central pontine myelinolysis:
(a) Causes neurological sequelae within 2 days of starting treatment of hyponatraemia
(b) Will not occur if there is a slow correction of hyponatraemia
(c) Causes transient neurological features
(d) Is associated with plaques of demyelination within the brainstem
(e) Will not occur after rapid correction of hyponatraemia by methods other than hypertonic or normal saline infusion

ANSWERS

1a False	2a True	3a False	4a True	5a False
b True	b True	b False	b False	b False
c False	c False	c True	c False	c False
d True	d True	d False	d False	d True
e False	e True	e False	e False	e False

Diabetic retinopathy: what goes wrong in the retina?

John V Forrester and Rachel M Knott

□ INTRODUCTION

Diabetic retinopathy is a major complication of the disease; its importance is highlighted by the fact that it remains the leading cause of blindness and severe visual impairment in British people of working age. The two forms of retinopathy that are a risk to vision are well recognised, namely diabetic maculopathy and proliferative diabetic retinopathy (Figs 1 and 2). Diabetic maculopathy, now the main cause of diabetes related blindness, affects central vision, while proliferative retinopathy can cause profound loss of vision owing to vitreous haemorrhage and traction retinal detachment.

Technical refinements in laser photocoagulation and vitreo-retinal surgery have considerably improved the outlook for patients with various stages of sight-threatening retinopathy, and the landmark Diabetes Control and Complications Trial (DCCT) has confirmed that the imposition of tight glycaemic control can significantly reduce the risk of retinopathy developing in patients with insulin-dependent (type 1) diabetes [1] (see Fig. 3). Nonetheless, diabetic retinopathy remains an important clinical problem and a scientific challenge. It is undoubtedly a microvascular disease – perhaps more accurately an 'endotheliopathy' since it is primarily effects on the endothelial cells of the retinal vessels that lead to damage in the retina – and is caused by prolonged exposure to high glucose levels. Certain pathophysiological features of diabetic retinopathy are well described; these include increased vascular permeability, raised retinal blood flow, microaneurysms, thickening and altered composition of the basement membrane, loss of pericytes (the contractile supporting cells that surround the endothelial cells) and, ultimately, the angiogenesis that identifies the stage of neovascularisation or proliferative retinopathy. Yet, apart from the links with hyperglycaemia and possibly other factors such as blood pressure, we still do not have a clear idea of the pathogenesis of diabetic retinopathy and, in particular, why it presents in the way it does. For instance, how do microaneurysms form and what is their natural history? Why do some patients develop exudative maculopathy, while others have few exudates and a macula that does not appear particularly abnormal, yet lose central vision because of macular oedema or ischaemia? What causes retinal ischaemia, which is thought to be the proximate cause of new vessel growth? Also, what are the molecular and cellular mechanisms through which raised glucose levels damage the retinal vasculature?

To try to answer these questions, it is necessary to investigate systematically the changes occurring in the diabetic retina, starting as early as possible in the evolution of retinopathy. This chapter will focus on specific pathological processes that are currently thought to lead to the two clinically important end-points – increased

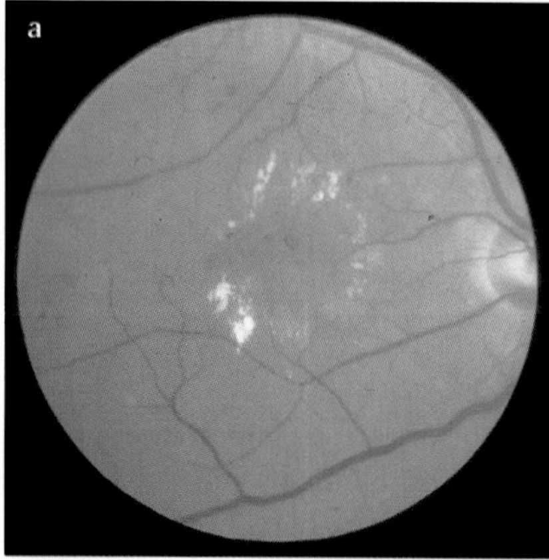

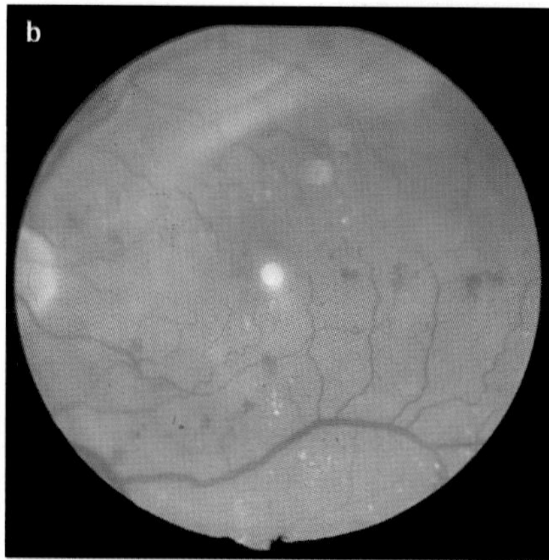

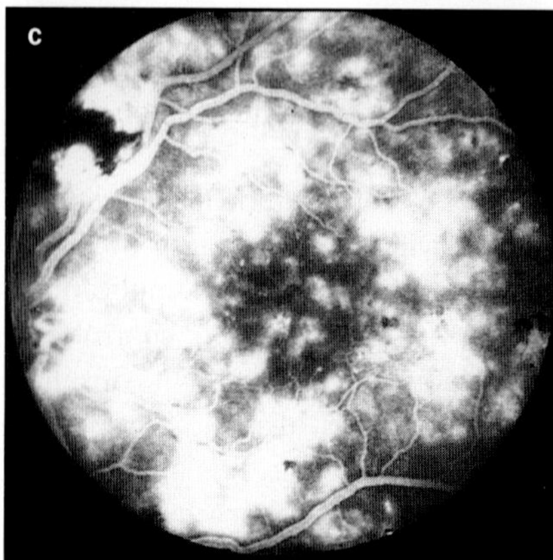

Fig. 1 Diabetic maculopathy. **(a)** Focal exudate formation at the macula. **(b)** Ischaemic maculopathy, showing unremarkable appearance of the fundus. **(c)** The same fundus, showing extensive vascular leakage demonstrated by fluorescein angiography. Reproduced with permission of the Royal College of Ophthalmologists.

vascular permeability (causing maculopathy) and neovascularisation. In particular, we shall review the roles of high glucose levels and the various growth factors that might enhance vascular permeability and stimulate angiogenesis, and finally discuss the possibility that activated white blood cells are crucially important, both by blocking capillaries and by generating growth factors. The overall scheme of events is summarised in Fig. 4, which highlights the central role that vascular endothelial growth factor (VEGF; also known as vascular permeability factor, VPF) seems to play in both capillary leakage and the development of new vessels. These effects are mediated by the interaction of VEGF with specific receptors which are expressed by the retinal endothelium, and whose expression is enhanced under hyperglycaemic conditions.

First, it is useful to consider how the retina handles glucose, and the ways in which high glucose levels may damage the retinal vessels.

□ GLUCOSE AND THE RETINA

The retina is highly glucose dependent, and has high rates of both anaerobic and

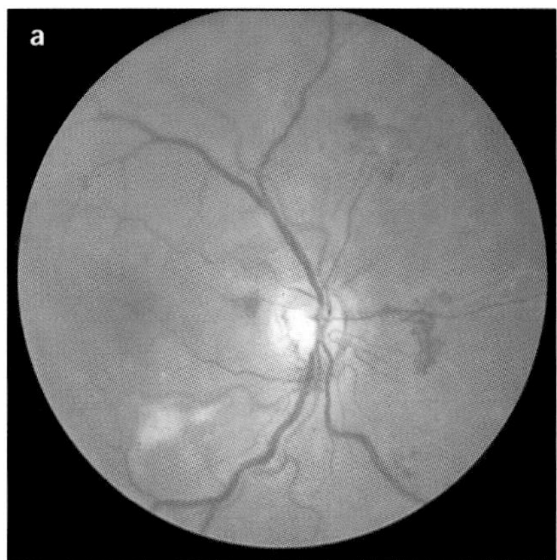

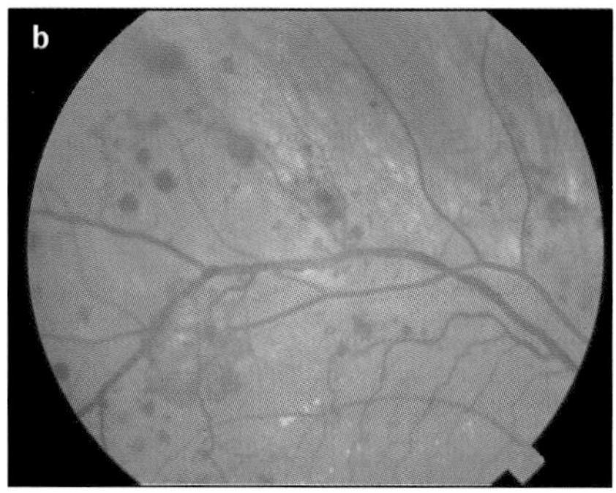

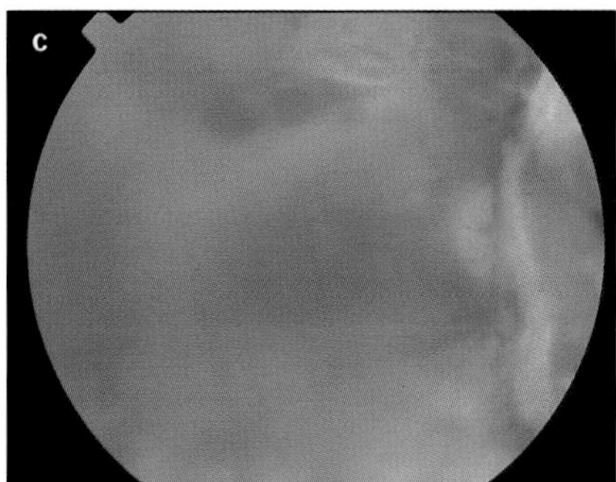

Fig. 2 Proliferative diabetic retinopathy, showing: **(a)** new vessel formation on the disc (NVD); **(b)** new vessel formation elsewhere in the retina (NVE); and **(c)** extensive sight-threatening changes, including retinal detachment and vitreous haemorrhage. Reproduced with permission of the Royal College of Ophthalmologists.

aerobic glycolysis, largely owing to the intense metabolic activity of the photoreceptors. This results in abundant production of free radicals; the retina contains appropriate scavenging systems to minimise potential tissue damage from these.

Glucose enters the retina by being transported across the blood-retina barrier (the retinal capillary endothelium and the retinal pigment epithelium) and thus into the neural cells and photoreceptors. Glucose transport is mediated by a series of integral membrane proteins that act as facilitative glucose carriers [2]. Retinal endothelial cells express two glucose transporters, GLUT-1 and GLUT-3 [3], while neural tissue utilises only GLUT-3 (Fig. 5). Previous studies suggested that retinal damage due to high blood glucose was due to the production of sorbitol via the aldose reductase (polyol) pathway, effectively representing an attempt by the cells to shunt off excess intracellular glucose via this normally quiescent metabolic pathway. However, we have shown that the expression of GLUT-3 and aldose reductase in endothelial cells is differentially regulated in response to high concentrations of glucose [4], suggesting that this pathway is unlikely to be a significant player in determining how the retina and its endothelial cells deal with hyperglycaemia.

High glucose levels have a number of potentially damaging effects on retinal cells and especially the endothelium, which could contribute both to enhanced permeability and to angiogenesis. These effects include:

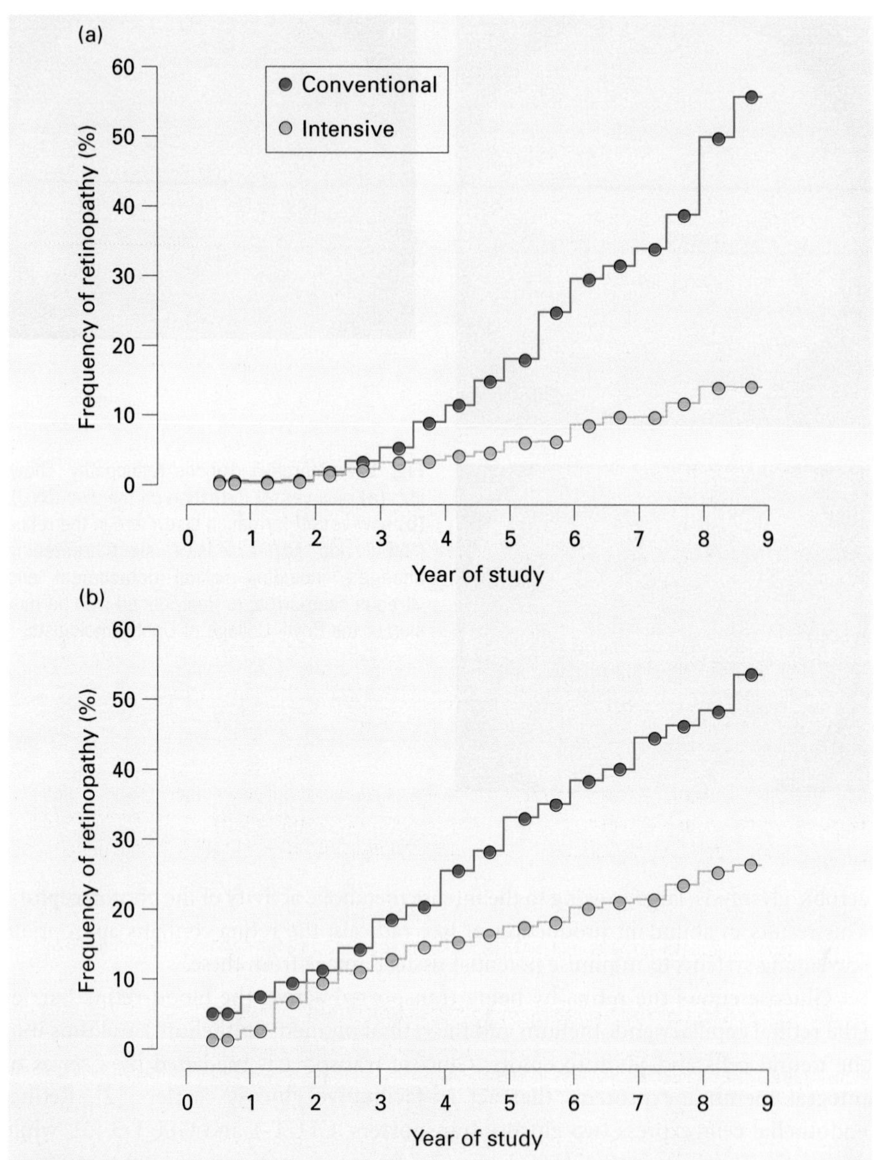

Fig. 3 Significant reductions in the cumulative incidence of retinopathy in patients who received intensified insulin treatment, compared with others who received a conventional insulin regimen. **(a)** Development of background retinopathy in patients with no retinopathy at entry. **(b)** Development of advanced retinopathy in subjects who had background changes at entry. Data from the DCCT [1].

- Altered sensitivity of endothelial cells to growth factors [5]. In particular, sensitivity to the actions of VEGF is enhanced because hyperglycaemia induces overexpression of VEGF receptors. This in turn amplifies one of the actions of VEGF within endothelial cells, namely the phosphorylation of specific proteins in the tight junction complexes that are critical for preserving

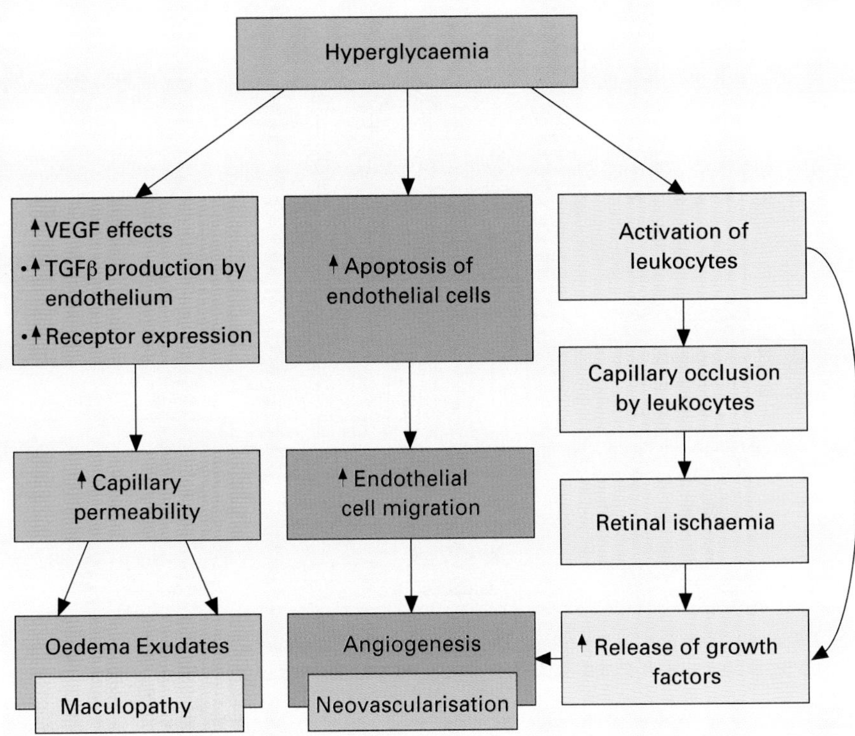

Fig. 4 Overall scheme of proposed pathophysiological events in causing the two sight-threatening features of diabetic retinopathy – maculopathy and neovascularisation. Note the central roles of growth factors, particularly VEGF, and leukocyte activation. TGFB; transforming growth factor.

the permeability barrier of the endothelium. Increased phosphorylation of these proteins (cingulin and occludin) by the tyrosine kinase that is activated by VEGF-receptor binding allows the tight junctions to separate, thus increasing endothelial permeability (Fig. 6). Another consequence of altered sensitivity to growth factors such as EGF, VEGF and PDGF is the induction of protein kinase C (PKC); this is of considerable interest, because a specific PKC isoform (PKCβ) has recently been implicated in the ability of VEGF to induce retinal endothelial cell proliferation in diabetic retinopathy [6] (see below).

- Increased rates of apoptosis in endothelial cells [7], which may be an early trigger for endothelial cell migration and ultimately angiogenesis.
- Enhanced release of the growth factor, transforming growth factor-β (TGF-β), by retinal endothelial cells [8]. TGF-β stimulates endothelial cells to form tubular structures, a fundamental step in the generation of new vessels.
- Activation of leukocytes (polymorphs and monocytes) which then occlude retinal capillaries (causing local ischaemia) and also release large amounts of growth factors with angiogenic properties. This is discussed further below.

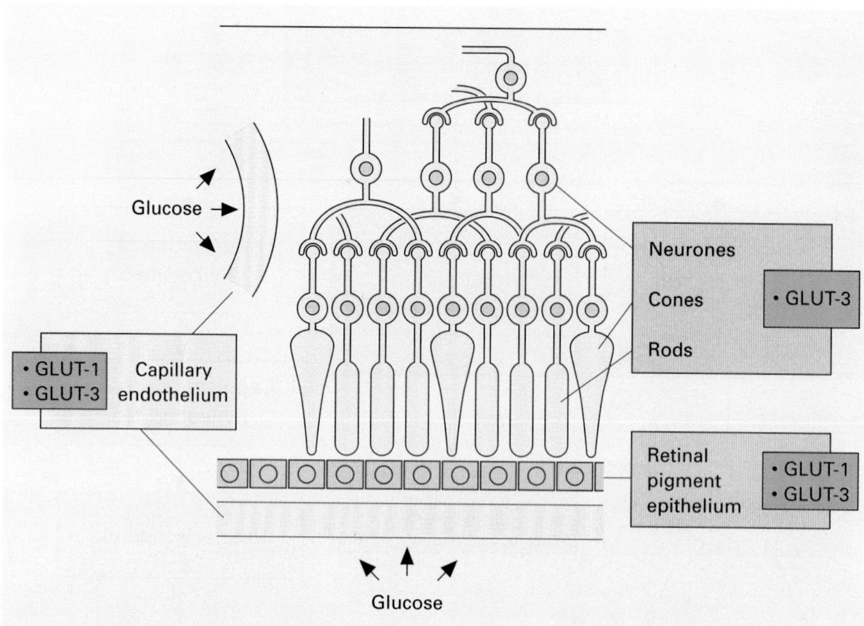

Fig. 5 Glucose transport in the retina. The retinal capillary endothelial cells express the glucose transporter proteins GLUT-1 and GLUT-3, while the retinal neurones express GLUT-3 only.

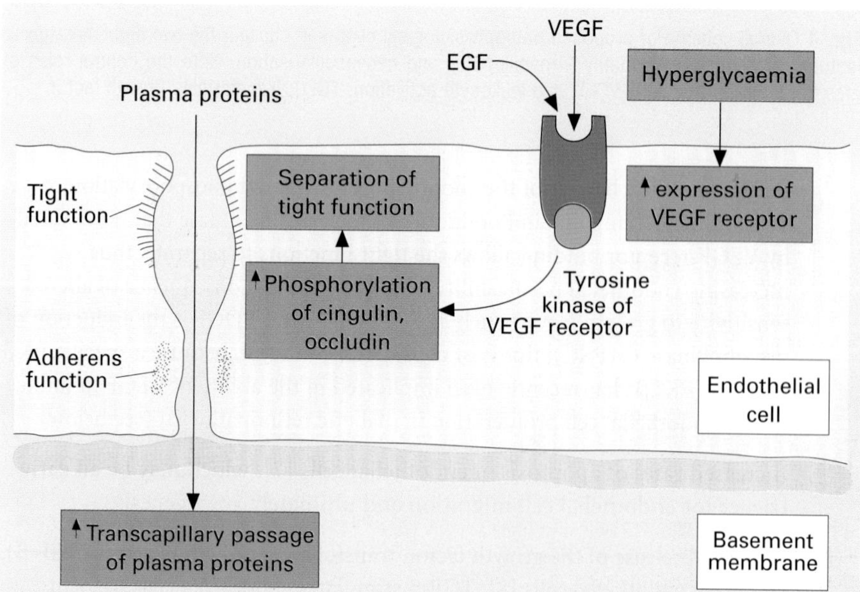

Fig. 6 Role of VEGF in increasing capillary permeability in diabetes, the cause of macular oedema and exudate formation. Hyperglycaemia enhances expression of the VEGF receptor, which can also be activated by epidermal growth factor, EGF. Increased activity of the receptor's tyrosine kinase phosphorylates the tight-junction proteins, cingulin and occludin. This leads to separation of the tight junctions between the capillary endothelial cells, the main component of the blood-retina barrier.

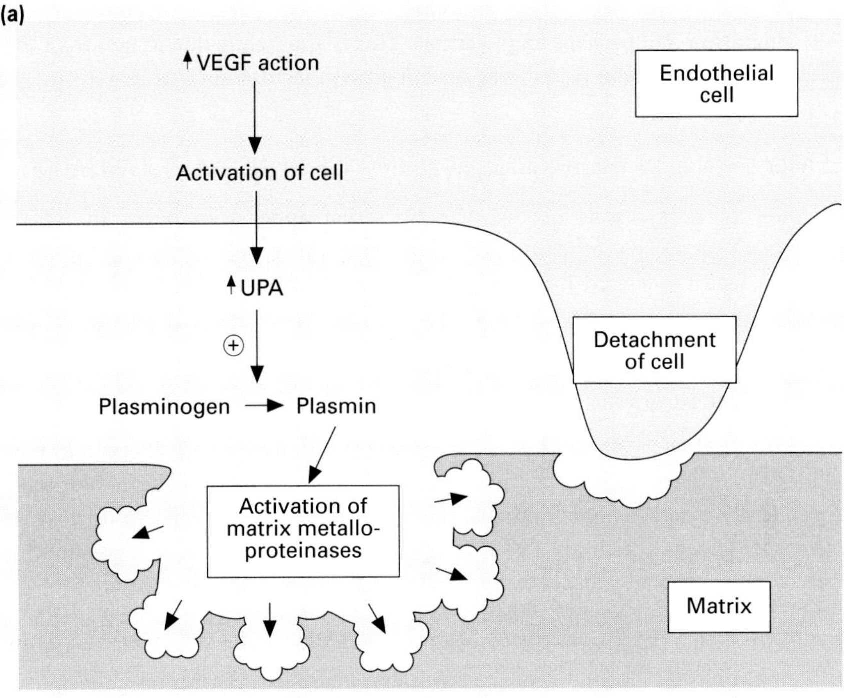

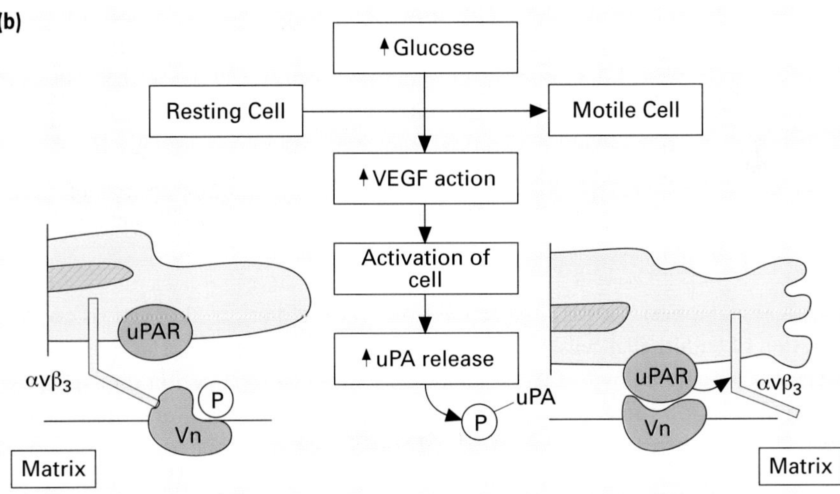

Fig. 7 Suggested roles of urokinase-plasminogen activator (uPA) in cell migration. **(a)** uPA may act both by generating plasmin, which could break down the underlying matrix and cause separation of focal adhesion points, and **(b)** by acting as a 'molecular switch' that regulates the binding of the integrin receptor $\alpha_v\beta_3$ on the cell surface to vitronectin in the matrix (right). In the resting state (left side), P (PAI-1) is bound to matrix molecules such as Vn (vitronectin) preventing attachment of the uPA receptor (uPAR) to the matrix – so the cell cannot move because it is firmly bound. When the cell is activated (right side), uPA is released and it competitively dislodges P from Vn and allows uPAR to bind to Vn. This provides a looser attachment of the cell to $\alpha_v\beta_3$ and acts as a lever for forward movement of the cell, through linkage of the uPAR-Vn complex to $\alpha_v\beta_3$ integrin and second messenger activator.

- ☐ Impaired capacity of retinal endothelial cells to proliferate, again favouring migration and perhaps angiogenesis. This is apparently due to failure of the endothelial cells to respond to certain growth factors, such as IGF-1.

☐ EARLY EVENTS IN THE ANGIOGENIC RESPONSE OF NEOVASCULARISATION

Formation of new vessels in the diabetic retina appears to begin in foci of ischaemia, where the endothelium is damaged and where angiogenesis is stimulated by growth factors secreted by various cell types in response to ischaemia and/or hyperglycaemia [9].

Endothelial cell turnover

Failure of endothelial cells to respond to certain growth factors in diabetes may have considerable implications for turnover and integrity of the endothelium. Normally, the proliferative capacity of endothelial cells is low, but there is sufficient turnover to replace ageing cells which are lost through apoptosis. Replacement is assumed to occur by activation of adjacent endothelial cells around the dying cell; the surrounding cells become motile, slide laterally to cover the defect, and then divide to restore endothelial continuity.

In conditions of chronic exposure to high glucose concentrations, the rate of apoptosis is increased [7], while the overall proliferative capacity of the cell population is reduced; it might therefore be expected that cell activation and motility at sites of cell death would increase. As a result, foci of actively motile endothelial cells would develop around patches of cell injury or death. Activation and cell migration are known to be the initiating events in the angiogenic response [8]; it therefore seems likely that retinal neovascularisation is initially induced in areas of glucose-mediated damage, as outlined here.

Role of endothelial cell migration

Angiogenesis appears to be triggered by abnormalities in the activation and migration of endothelial cells. Cells migrate by crawling across a surface; directional movement is achieved by the leading lamellipodium gaining traction on the surface by the formation of focal adhesions, while the rearward foci of adhesion progressively detach from the surface. This process of coordinated cell attachment and detachment is mediated by proteolytic enzymes associated with the cell surface, particularly urokinase-plasminogen activator (uPA) which is released by the cell. Previous studies have shown that plasmin generated by uPA activates metalloproteinases in the underlying matrix, and may thus permit the migrating cells to invade dense extracellular material. In addition, plasmin produced in the pericellular space probably acts to detach focal adhesion sites in an advancing cell.

Recent studies [10] suggest that pericellular uPA may also promote cell migration through a non-proteolytic mechanism in which the uPA receptor behaves as a molecular switch (Fig. 7). Cells normally attach themselves to the substrate by their 'integrin' receptors which bind to specific extracellular matrix proteins, notably fibronectin and vitronectin in the case of endothelial cells. In the resting state, vitronectin binds to its receptor on the cell, $\alpha_v\beta_3$ integrin, thus anchoring the cell. However, vitronectin also binds the uPA receptor (uPAR), an interaction that causes a looser attachment of the cell to the matrix (Fig. 7b); up-regulation of uPAR expression, for instance when the cell is activated by growth factors such as VEGF, therefore leads to competition for binding of vitronectin to the $\alpha_v\beta_3$ receptor, favouring detachment of the cell. Binding of uPA to its receptors is also regulated by plasminogen activator inhibitor-1 (PAI-1) which is abundant in the pericellular matrix. However, when uPA is released in quantity following activation of the cell, it binds avidly to PAI-1 thus freeing uPAR binding sites for vitronectin.

Cell motility may be regulated by differential expression of uPAR on the cell membrane between the leading and trailing edges of the cell, with fine tuning by several regulatory components including the activating growth factors, the level of expression of uPAR, the balance between pericellular uPA and PAI-1 and the competition between uPAR and $\alpha_v\beta_3$.

Retinal endothelial cells presumably utilise such mechanisms, as they express the uPAR and $\alpha_v\beta_3$ receptors, and secrete uPA (and tissue type PA, tPA) together with large quantities of PAI-1. In addition, a further level of control of cell movement and angiogenic responses is exerted by the different types of growth factor that may act on the cell. For instance, VEGF and basic fibroblast growth factor (bFGF) both promote endothelial cell migration, while transforming growth factor beta (TGF-β) inhibits migration and growth but encourages differentiation of cells into vessel structures (tube formation). These growth factors also have differential effects on PAI-1 and uPA production, in that TGF-β stimulates PAI-1 production and inhibits uPA release, while the converse applies to VEGF and bFGF.

The precise abnormalities that occur at the cellular and molecular levels in the diabetic retina, and that alter endothelial cell behaviour so as to encourage angiogenesis, are still unknown. However, hyperglycaemia affects numerous aspects of these processes, including endothelial cell turnover, the production of various growth factors and the sensitivity of the endothelial cells to them. Some of these points have been discussed above. We have also shown that high glucose levels stimulate the release of TGF-β, but that this adaptive response is lost when the glucose concentration becomes too high.

Overall, the persisting insult of chronic hyperglycaemia probably induces a state of continuing activation of the endothelial cells, which predisposes to the angiogenic response of neovascularisation.

☐ RETINAL ISCHAEMIA: A ROLE FOR LEUKOCYTES?

Most authorities agree that the proximal cause of retinal neovascularisation is retinal ischaemia. How retinal ischaemia induces new vessel growth is less clear. It is thought that ischaemic signals cause release of endogenous retinal growth factors, either from dead or dying cells (eg FGF from photoreceptors and neurones) or by stress-induced responses in cells that can act as a source of growth factors, such as retinal pigment epithelial cells. There are many known angiogenic factors, of which VEGF is currently regarded as particularly important; it seems most likely to be the best initiator of vascular growth, as well as having an important role in the early stages of vessel leakiness (see Fig. 4). The properties of some key growth factors and mediators are summarised in Table 1.

A crucial mechanistic question in proliferative diabetic retinopathy is how retinal ischaemia is induced. Retinal ischaemia is the direct result of capillary closure and is evident as areas of non-perfusion on fluorescein angiograms in patients with pre-proliferative retinopathy as well as in the presence of new vessels; smaller patches of capillary occlusion occur early in diabetic retinopathy and are associated with the formation of microaneurysms, which would appear to be an abortive attempt by the blood vessels to revascularise the retina (Fig. 8). With prolonged uncontrolled hyperglycaemia, areas of ischaemia expand progressively. Other consequences of widespread ischaemia include extensive venous beading (due to shunting of blood

Table 1 Growth factors and adhesion molecules implicated in the pathogenesis of diabetic retinopathy.

Class and name	Source	Targets	Actions
Growth factors			
VEGF (VPF)	Neural retina Circulating leukocytes	Retinal endothelium	↑ Capillary permeability • phosphorylates tight-junction proteins Angiogenic • ↑ endothelial cell migration • ↑ endothelial cell proliferation
EGF	Neural retina	Retinal endothelium	↑ Capillary permeability Angiogenic • 'cross-talk' with VEGF receptor
IFG-1	Photoreceptor cells		
TGF-β	Neural retina	Retinal endothelium	Angiogenic • ↓ endothelial cell migration • endothelial tube formation
bFGF	Vascular endothelium	Retinal endothelium	Angiogenic • ↑ endothelial cell migration
Adhesion molecules			
E-selectin	Endothelium	Retinal endothelium	Angiogenic • ↑ endothelial cell migration
VCAM-1	Endothelium	Retinal endothelium	Angiogenic • ↑ endothelial cell migration

VEGF, vascular endothelial growth factor (VPF, vascular permeability factor); EGF, epidermal growth factor; IGF-1, insulin-like growth factor-1; TGF-β, transforming growth factor-β; bFGF, basic fibroblast growth factor; VCAM-1, vascular cell adhesion molecule-1.

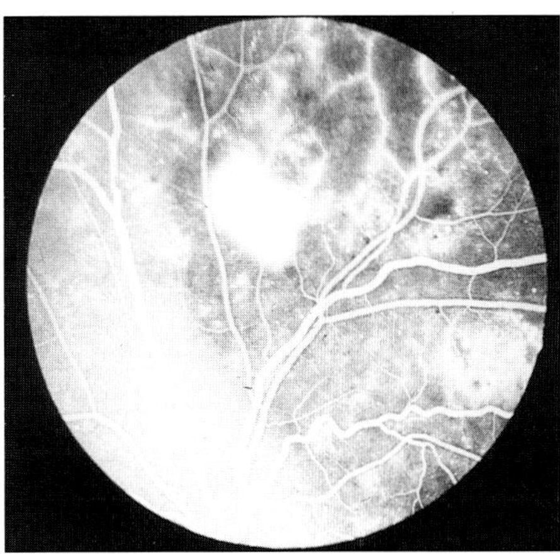

Fig. 8 Areas of capillary occlusion and non-perfusion. Non-perfused areas appear dark in these fluorescein angiograms.

away from non-perfused areas) and, eventually, the development of new vessels arising from the post-capillary venule.

The causes of capillary occlusion and the sources of the angiogenic growth factors have been controversial, but recent studies suggest that leukocytes may be involved in both of these aspects of angiogenesis. The fact that new vessels continue to grow from ischaemic areas implies that there is a renewable supply of growth factors. The most likely source is circulating blood cells, particularly leukocytes; activated leukocytes may directly cause capillary occlusion by adhering to the damaged endothelial surface. Recent studies in experimental alloxan-induced diabetes in the rat [11] support the hypothesis that retinal capillary occlusion is caused by activated leukocytes. Polymorphonuclear leukocytes and monocytes were found to be directly activated by high glucose levels. In addition, leukocytes were found occluding small retinal vessels and, in the reparative phase of clot resolution, trapped monocytes migrated through the walls of the damaged vessels and proliferated as macrophages in the perivascular tissue. Macrophages, neutrophils and platelets are known to be rich sources of angiogenic factors, although only proliferating cells will provide these in a sustained fashion.

A number of studies have shown that several aspects of leukocyte activity (eg free radical release, protease production and shedding of adhesion molecules) are up-regulated in diabetic patients, and are correlated with glycaemic control, measured as either glucose levels or glycosylated haemoglobin (HbA1c) levels. Thus, glucose-mediated activation of leukocytes and the induction of leukocyte-endothelial cell interactions could contribute to many if not all of the phases of diabetic retinopathy from the early phases of damage to the endothelial cells that result in vascular leakage, and the formation of microaneurysms and exudates, to the later stages of retinal neovascularisation.

□ INVOLVEMENT OF ADHESION MOLECULES

Serum concentrations of the adhesion molecules E-selectin and vascular cell adhesion molecule-1 (VCAM-1) are elevated in patients with diabetic retinopathy, and the levels correlate with the severity of retinopathy; E-selectin levels peak at the stage of pre-proliferative retinopathy while VCAM-1 levels are highest in patients with active neovascularisation [12]. Interestingly, intercellular adhesion molecule-1 (ICAM-1) levels show no correlation with retinopathy, although they have previously been shown to be elevated in diabetic patients generally.

Both E-selectin and VCAM-1 are endothelial cell surface proteins and are normally shed into the circulation at low levels; raised serum concentrations indicate endothelial cell activation and/or increased leukocyte-endothelial cell interaction. E-selectin and VCAM-1 are themselves angiogenic factors, and exposure to antibodies against these adhesion molecules can inhibit retinal endothelial cell migration *in vitro* [12].

There is also some evidence for leukocyte activation, consistent with the proposed model that centres on diabetes-enhanced leukocyte-endothelial cell interactions. We have shown that circulating leukocytes from patients with proliferative retinopathy appear to express high levels of TGF-β mRNA, while VEGF mRNA is raised in diabetic patients before the onset of retinopathy; these abnormalities are related to the level of diabetic control. This differential regulation of growth factor expression by circulating leukocytes may have implications for the development of macular oedema and new vessels in the later stages of the disease.

□ CONCLUSIONS

These findings suggest that diabetes-induced damage to the retina evolves through several stages. High glucose levels cause early direct damage to the endothelium, and also favour adhesion of platelets and leukocytes which cause capillary occlusion and retinal ischaemia. Initially, levels of injury are low, resulting in limited formation of microaneurysms. With time, progressively more capillaries become occluded by activated leukocytes, producing wider areas of retinal ischameia and eventually providing a sufficient and sustained stimulus for new vessel growth. It is likely that synergism occurs between the several growth factors released by the activated leukocytes.

However, this model should not be viewed rigidly as the only version of events occurring in diabetic retinopathy. There are substantial changes in retinal blood flow, but they are probably secondary to many of the changes described above; it is unlikely that they are directly involved in, for example, the induction of growth factor expression by retinal cells. In addition, the recent interesting findings regarding the protective effects of angiotensin converting enzyme inhibitors on the development of retinopathy [13] suggest a role for endothelial cell-derived angiotensin in the early stages of endothelial cell activation. Finally, it is also likely that various advanced glycation end-product (AGE) derivatives of proteins have direct effects on endothelial cells and leukocytes, in addition to the actions of glucose. Nonetheless, activated leukocytes seem likely candidates in the basic pathogenic mechanisms causing capillary occlusion and the retinal angiogenic response – key stages in the evolution of proliferative retinopathy.

REFERENCES

1 The Diabetes Control and Complications Trial. The effect of intensive treatment of diabetes on the development and progression of long-term complications in insulin-dependent diabetes mellitus. *N Engl J Med* 1993; **329:** 977–86.

2 Bell GI, Kayano T, Buse JB, *et al.* Molecular biology of mammalian glucose transporters. *Diabetes Care* 1990; **13:** 198–208.

3 Knott RM, Robertson M, Muckersie E, *et al.* Regulation of glucose transporters (GLUT-1 and GLUT-3) in human retinal endothelial cells. *Biochem J* 1996; **318:** 313–7.

4 Knott RM, Robertson M, Forrester JV. Regulation of glucose transporter (GLUT-3) and aldose reductase mRNA in bovine retinal endothelial cells and retinal pericytes in high glucose and high galactose culture. *Diabetologia* 1993; **36:** 808–12.

5 Merrall NW, Plevin R, Gould GW. Growth factors, mitogens, oncogenes and the regulation of glucose transport. *Cell Sig* 1993; **5:** 667–75.

6 Aiello LP, Bursell S, Clermont A, *et al.* Vascular endothelial growth factor-induced retinal permeability is mediated by protein kinase C *in vivo* and suppressed by an orally effective b-isoform-selective inhibitor. *Diabetes* 1997; **46:** 1473–80.

7 Baumgartner-Parzer SM, Wagner L, Petterman M, *et al.* High-glucose-triggered apoptosis in cultured endothelial cells. *Diabetes* 1995; **44:** 1323–7.

8 Pascal MM, Knott RM, Forrester JV. Glucose-mediated regulation of transforming growth factor beta in human retinal endothelial cells. *Biochem Soc Trans* 1996; 657th meeting: 228. (Submitted to *Current Eye Research.*)

9 Forrester JV, Knott RM, Olson J, *et al.* Growth factors and diabetic retinopathy. *Diabetes Rev Int* 1997; **6:** 9–12.

10 Stefansson S, Lawrence DA. The serpin PAI-1 inhibits cell migration by blocking integrin alpha(v)beta3 binding to vitronectin. *Nature* 1996; **383:** 441–3.

11 Schroder S, Palinski W, Schmid-Schonbein GW. Activated monocytes and granulocytes, capillary nonperfusion and neovascularization in diabetic retinopathy. *Am J Pathol* 1991; **139:** 81–100.

12 Olson JA, Whitelaw CM, McHardy KC, *et al.* Soluble leucocyte adhesion molecules in diabetic retinopathy stimulate retinal capillary endothelial cell migration. *Diabetologia* 1997; **40:** 1166–71.

13 The Euclid Study Group. Randomised placebo-controlled trial of lisinopril in normotensive patients with insulin-dependent diabetes and normalbuminuria or microalbuminuria. *Lancet* 1997; **349:** 1787–91.

☐ MULTIPLE CHOICE QUESTIONS

1 Proliferative diabetic retinopathy:
(a) Is caused by capillary occlusion
(b) Is associated with hypertension
(c) Is worsened by tight glucose control
(d) Is more common in young diabetics
(e) Is worsened by hyperlipidaemia

2 Ischaemic maculopathy:
(a) Is the major cause of visual loss
(b) Is characterised by exudates
(c) Is treatable with focal laser
(d) Can be reversible
(e) Is detectable by ophthalmoscopy

3 Microaneurysms in diabetic retinopathy:
   (a) Are a consistent feature
   (b) Are the cause of exudates
   (c) Are a sign of ischaemia
   (d) Are short-lived
   (e) Are a cause of visual loss

4 Diabetic macular oedema:
   (a) Causes blindness in young diabetics
   (b) Causes blindness in diabetic children
   (c) Reflects changes in the outer retina
   (d) Treatment with laser leads to better vision
   (e) Is characteristic of proliferative retinopathy

5 Advanced glycation end-products:
   (a) Are the results of sorbitol accumulation
   (b) Cause microaneurysms
   (c) Correlate with HbA1c
   (d) Are the results of collagen crosslinking
   (e) Bind to receptors on endothelial cells

ANSWERS

1a True	2a False	3a True	4a True	5a False
b False	b False	b False	b False	b False
c False	c False	c True	c True	c False
d True	d True	d False	d False	d False
e False	e True	e True	e False	e True

New drugs for the treatment of diabetes and its complications

John Wilding

☐ INTRODUCTION

Considering the huge burden that diabetes places on health care resources worldwide, it is perhaps surprising that the introduction of new anti-diabetic agents has been so slow. The discovery of insulin in 1922 by Banting and Best has benefited many millions of patients with diabetes, but it is widely recognised that even the most sophisticated insulin replacement regimens are imperfect. Moreover, it has become clear that most cases of diabetes are not due to absolute insulin deficiency, and that insulin resistance, relative insulin deficiency and other complex metabolic abnormalities conspire to produce the group of diseases now recognised as type 2 (non-insulin dependent) diabetes. Several novel approaches to the treatment of diabetes are beginning to emerge, particularly for type 2 diabetes, although the precise role of many of the new agents is yet to be defined [1,2] (Fig. 1).

This review will concentrate on three main areas:

- ☐ new treatments for type 1 (insulin-dependent) diabetes, specifically the new 'designer' insulins with improved pharmacokinetic profiles and analogues of the β-cell peptide, amylin;

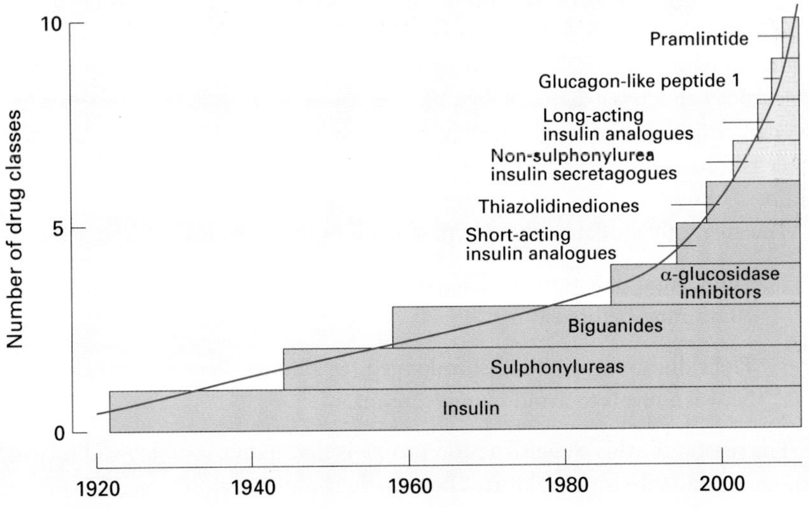

Fig. 1 The exponential rise in new treatments for diabetes since the discovery of insulin (1922), showing the various classes of glucose-lowering drugs and their actual (blue) or projected (green) dates for introduction into clinical practice.

- ☐ prospects for the treatment of type 2 diabetes; and
- ☐ the use of specific therapy to reduce diabetic complications.

☐ NEW DRUGS FOR TYPE 1 DIABETES

Important problems and shortcomings of current insulin replacement regimens, whether conventional or more sophisticated, were clearly demonstrated in the Diabetes Control and Complications Trial (DCCT) [3]. The DCCT compared conventional insulin treatment (once- or twice-daily injections) with intensive regimens that used the best available techniques, including multiple daily injections of short- and long-acting insulin and continuous insulin infusion given by portable pumps. The aim was to achieve near normoglycaemia in the intensively-treated group and to determine its impact on chronic diabetic complications. In fact, normoglycaemia was achieved in only a minority of patients; the mean haemoglobin (Hb)A_{1c} level in intensively- and conventionally-treated patients was 7% and 9%, respectively – substantially above the non-diabetic range of less than 6.1%. Intensive control significantly reduced the progression of some microvascular complications (notably nephropathy and retinopathy), but at the expense of a weight gain of 3–5 kg and a threefold increase in the incidence of severe hypoglycaemia, despite intensive education and careful attention to diet and exercise to avoid these two effects. These problems, together with the relatively poor record of success in restoring normoglycaemia, make it essential to consider alternative strategies for insulin replacement therapy.

Insulin analogues: improving on nature

Ideally, insulin treatment regimens would mimic the normal profile of insulin secretion in the non-diabetic person: meal-related peaks superimposed on a background of basal release. The closest approximations to this physiological pattern are achieved by the 'basal-bolus' subcutaneous injection regimens comprising one or two daily injections of long-acting insulin together with short-acting insulin given either before main meals or by continuous subcutaneous infusions via an insulin pump.

The currently available 'short-acting' insulins have two main drawbacks:

- ☐ Their onset of action is relatively slow, so they have to be given about 30 minutes before eating.
- ☐ Their duration of action is prolonged (6–8 hours), so patients have to snack between meals to avoid hypoglycaemia.

The reason for this sluggish action profile is that native soluble insulin (whether human- or animal-sequence) forms hexameric complexes at the injection site, which have to dissociate into monomers before being absorbed into the bloodstream.

Several attempts have been made to produce monomeric insulin analogues that resist hexamerisation and are therefore more rapidly absorbed and have a faster onset of action. Early analogues (eg Asp B28 insulin) ran into problems because of cross-reactivity with the insulin-like growth factor-1 receptor which could potentially promote neoplasia. Newer compounds avoid this interaction, yet remain fully active at the insulin receptor; they include insulin lispro (Lilly) and X14 insulin (Novo Nordisk).

Insulin lispro

Insulin lispro is made by exchanging the lysine and proline residues at positions 28 and 29, respectively, in the B chain of the insulin molecule (see Fig. 2). This substitution changes the conformational properties of the molecule so that it dissociates more rapidly into its monomeric form. It thus has a much more rapid onset of action than conventional soluble insulin, and indeed can be injected immediately before or shortly after meals [1].

Several large clinical trials have now compared insulin lispro with conventional soluble insulin, in patients using basal-bolus insulin regimens [4]. These have consistently found significantly reduced rates of hypoglycaemia (by up to 30%) without any deterioration in HbA_{1c}. Many patients prefer the ultra short-acting insulins which allow more flexible planning of meals, snacks and exercise; their use should be considered in diabetic patients treated with basal-bolus regimens, particularly if hypoglycaemia is a problem. Insulin lispro has recently been licensed for use in children, but there is currently insufficient evidence of safety and freedom from teratogenicity for these analogues to be recommended during pregnancy.

Long-acting insulin analogues

Long-acting insulin analogues, designed to provide better replacement of basal insulin secretion, are in the late stages of development and are currently undergoing clinical trials. These agents have a prolonged duration of action as they bind to serum albumin, and can achieve adequate background levels for a full 24-hour period when injected subcutaneously once daily.

Other routes of insulin administration

Some alternative routes of insulin administration are being explored, notably a nasal spray including bile-salt derivatives that act as surfactants and promote transmucosal absorption and, more recently, an insulin inhalation device that has been shown to result in significant insulin absorption from the lungs. These approaches remain experimental.

Amylin: an orphan β-cell hormone?

It has recently been discovered that the β-cells in the pancreatic islets produce another peptide, amylin, in addition to insulin. Amylin, also known as islet amyloid polypeptide, was first characterised as the main component of the amyloid deposits that

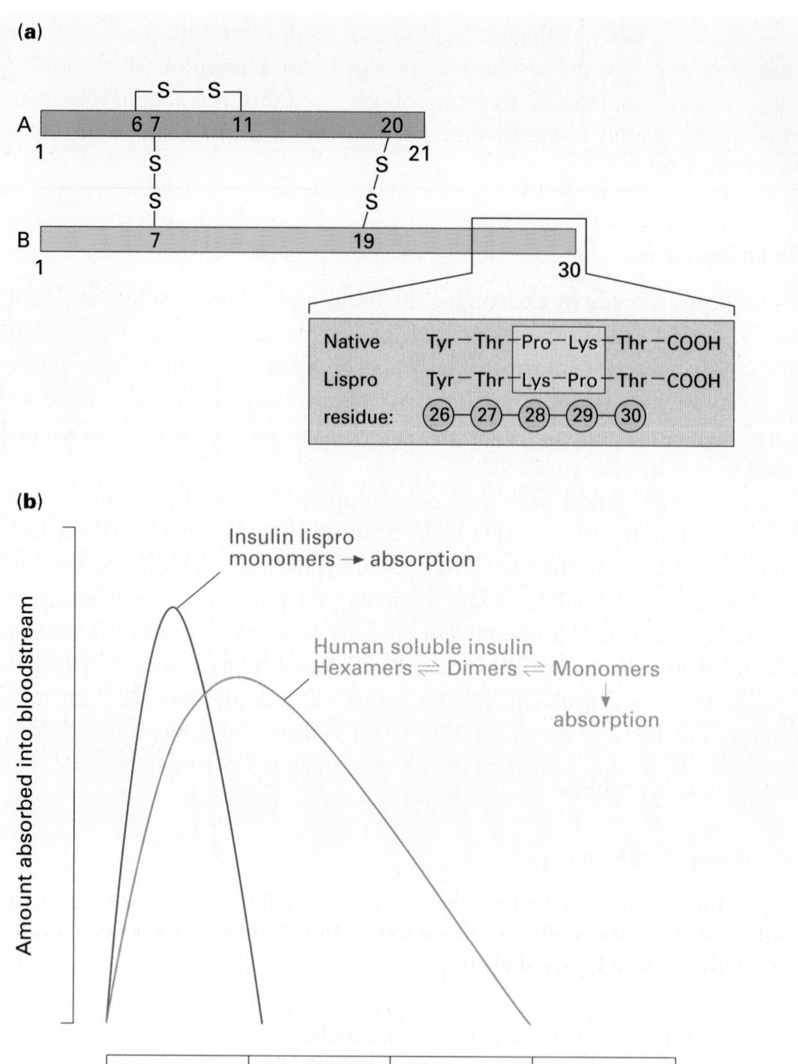

Fig. 2 (a) Structures of native human insulin and the fast-acting analogue, insulin lispro; **(b)** conventional soluble insulin forms hexamers when injected into subcutaneous tissue. It must dissociate into dimers and then monomers before it can be absorbed. Insulin lispro resists self-association, and so has a faster absorption profile.

commonly develop in the islets of patients with type 2 diabetes. There has been intensive research into the normal role and therapeutic potential of this peptide. Initial studies showed that amylin was generally secreted in parallel with insulin and suggested that it could induce insulin resistance in skeletal muscle. It now seems unlikely that this latter effect is significant at physiologically relevant concentrations in humans, and attention has shifted to other actions of amylin both within the islet and elsewhere.

In the islet, amylin apparently acts as a paracrine regulator of insulin secretion, inhibiting release of the hormone, an action clearly of limited relevance in type 1 diabetes. It may also function as a true hormone, as amylin-binding sites are found within the central nervous system (where a role in inhibiting feeding and regulating energy balance has been suggested), in the kidney and stomach. The synthetic amylin analogue, pramlintide, has been shown to delay gastric emptying.

The physiological importance of amylin is still uncertain, as is the significance of amylin deficiency in type 1 diabetes in which amylin levels fall in parallel with insulin. It has, however, been suggested that amylin deficiency might explain the unusually rapid gastric emptying seen in some type 1 diabetic patients, and which is postulated to worsen glycaemic control in these cases. Native amylin rapidly polymerises in solution to form fibrils, and thus has a short half-life, but various analogues have been developed that lack this property yet retain biological activity. An example is pramlintide, whose possible antihyperglycaemic effects in type 1 diabetes are currently being evaluated in clinical trials of up to six months' duration. When injected subcutaneously four times daily before meals, pramlintide has relatively modest effects, with a 0.3–0.4% fall in HbA_{1c} [5], unfortunately commonly associated with nausea and weight loss.

Amylin replacement therefore has some theoretical attractions, but its pharmacological rationale remains controversial, and the current lack of convincing benefit, together with the inconvenience of multiple daily injections, does not support its routine use in the treatment of type 1 diabetes. It might ultimately be useful for some patients, perhaps those in whom accelerated gastric emptying is thought to be a problem.

☐ NEW DRUGS FOR TYPE 2 DIABETES

Despite intensive research, only three classes of drugs other than insulin have been successfully used in type 2 diabetes:

- sulphonylureas, which stimulate insulin secretion;
- biguanides, which improve insulin action through still undefined mechanisms; and
- α-glucosidase inhibitors, which block the breakdown of complex carbohydrates in the gut, and so blunt the post-prandial rises in blood glucose.

Although the aetiology of type 2 diabetes remains unclear, recent advances in our understanding of the pathophysiology of this heterogeneous condition may ultimately lead to the development of new and more specific forms of treatment. The currently available drugs fall far short of the treatment targets proposed for type 2 diabetes (see Table 1); overall, treatment with a sulphonylurea or metformin generally lowers blood glucose levels by only 3–4 mmol/l and HbA_{1c} by 1%. Insulin can almost normalise blood glucose in type 2 diabetes, but very high dosages (>200 U/day) may be required in particularly insulin-resistant patients, and insulin treatment has important hazards including weight gain and hypoglycaemia.

Table 1 Treatment targets for the management of type 2 (non-insulin dependent) diabetes (from Ref 6).

	Good	Acceptable	Poor
Blood glucose (mmol/l)			
• Fasting	4.4–6.7	<7.8	>7.8
• Post-prandial peak	4.4–8.9	<10.0	>10.0
HbA_{1c} (standard deviations above non-diabetic mean for the laboratory)	<2.0	<4.0	>4.0
Serum cholesterol (mmol/l)			
• Total	<5.2	<6.5	>6.5
• High-density lipoproteins	>1.1	>0.9	<0.9
Fasting serum triglycerides (mmol/l)	<1.7	<2.2	>2.2
Body mass index (kg/m^2)			
• Men	<25	<27	>27
• Women	<24	<26	>26
Blood pressure (mm Hg)	<140/90	<160/95	>160/95

It is clear that both peripheral insulin resistance and β-cell dysfunction are present in type 2 diabetes, and that their relative importance may change during the clinical course of the disease. Thus, it is rational to target new therapies at both insulin resistance and insulin deficiency (see Fig. 3). The role of obesity as a powerful predisposing factor for type 2 diabetes should not be forgotten. The possible use of anti-obesity measures to treat or prevent diabetes is discussed briefly below (see also Chapter 9).

Thiazolidinediones

At present, the most promising new class of drugs for type 2 diabetes are the thiazolidinediones (glitazones). At the time of writing, discussion of these agents was inevitably coloured by the recent withdrawal in the UK and Europe of troglitazone, the first to reach the market. The thiazolidinediones are agonists at the peroxisome proliferator activated receptor (PPAR)-γ, one of a family of nuclear receptors that also includes the glucocorticoid and thyroid hormone receptors; the related PPAR-α receptor is the target for the fibrate drugs used to treat dyslipidaemias. PPAR-γ is expressed in fat, skeletal muscle and liver, and its activation by thiazolidinediones causes several complex changes in intracellular metabolism [7,8] (see Fig. 4). These include an increase in glucose transport, mediated by altered sensitivity of various intracellular cascades of protein phosphorylation caused by the binding of insulin to its receptor. Changes in handling of fatty acids also occur, the main effects being a

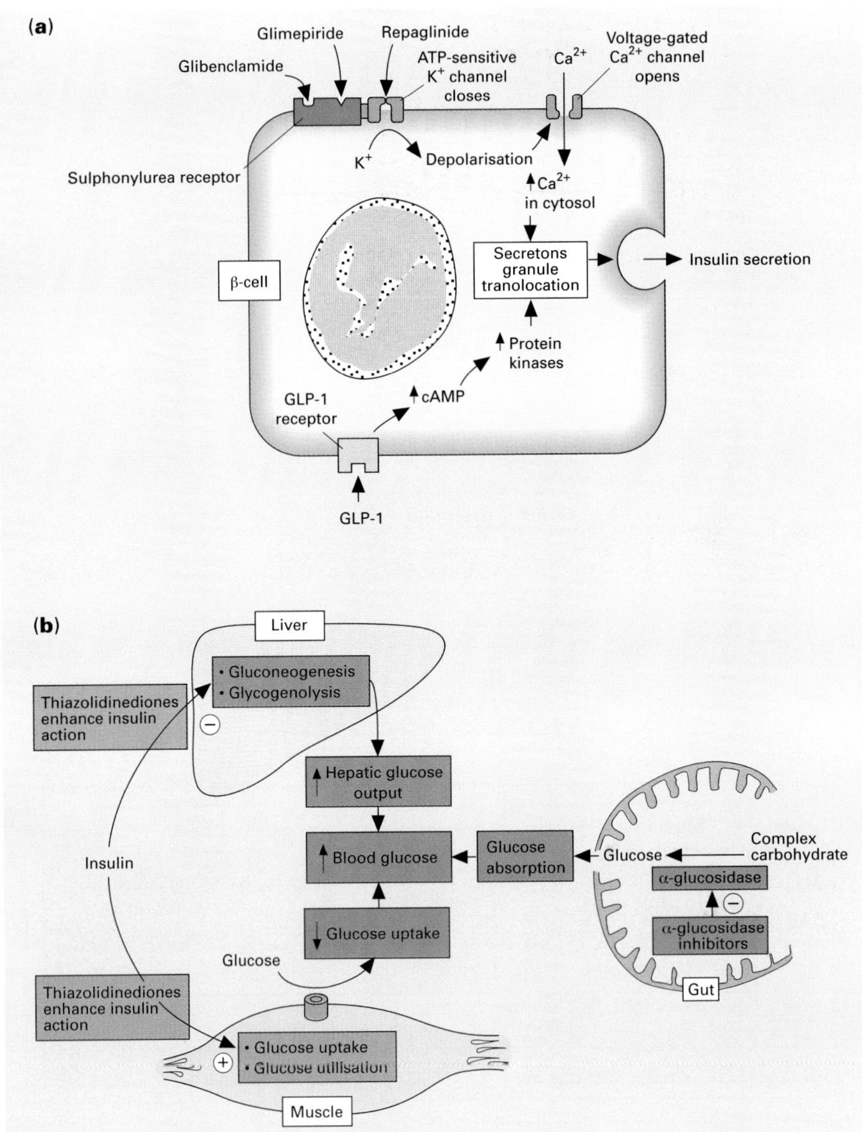

Fig. 3 Models of action of drugs to treat type 2 diabetes. These include **(a)** drugs that enhance insulin secretion or **(b)** act to reduce insulin resistance (thereby inhibiting hepatic glucose production and enhancing disposal of glucose into peripheral tissues) or decrease glucose absorption from the gut (GLP-1 = glucagon-like peptide).

reduction in lipolysis in adipose tissue and a net fall in circulating free fatty acid concentrations. Reduced free fatty acid levels may indirectly enhance certain biological actions of insulin via the Randle (glucose-fatty acid) cycle, in which free fatty acids are suggested to interfere with glucose metabolism at various levels in skeletal muscle (causing decreased glucose uptake) and liver (resulting in increased hepatic glucose production).

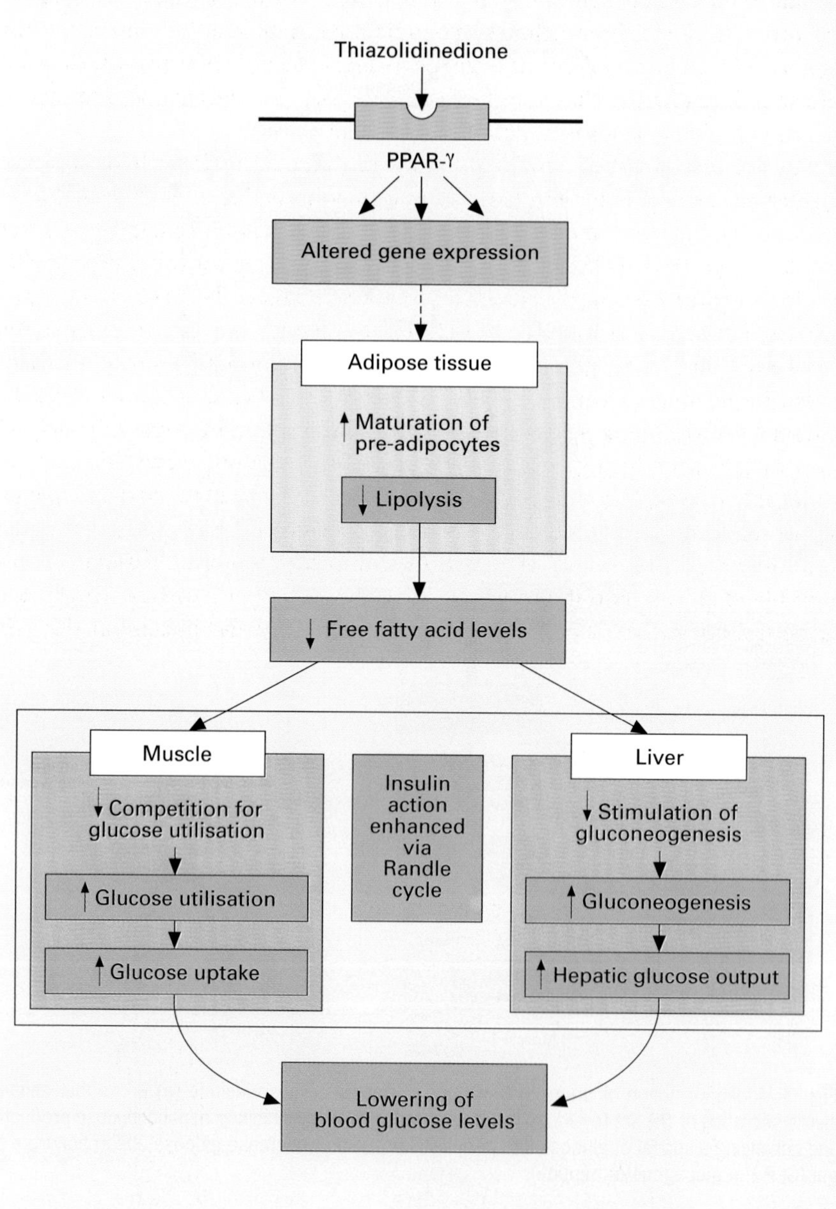

Fig. 4 Mode of action of thiazolidinediones. These agents (eg rosiglitazone) act on the peroxisome proliferator activated receptor (PPAR)-γ and affect the expression of several genes involved in metabolism in fat and other tissues. They are thought to improve insulin action in many ways, including direct effects on insulin receptor numbers and glucose transport in some tissues, and also effects on fatty acid metabolism which reduce circulating free fatty acids (FFA), thus indirectly improving insulin sensitivity via the glucose fatty acid (Randle) cycle.

Overall, the changes induced by thiazolidinediones result in improved insulin sensitivity. The actions of these drugs are most pronounced in states of insulin resistance and have little effect if insulin sensitivity is normal. The thiazolidinediones also promote the differentiation of pre-adipocytes into mature adipocytes; this, together with their inhibition of triglyceride breakdown, may explain their ability both to induce obesity when given at high dosages to animals and also to increase the ratio of subcutaneous to abdominal fat in man.

Most of the published clinical studies with thiazolidinediones have been with troglitazone. Several other agents (including rosiglitazone and pioglitazone) are in development, but it is too early to know whether these will differ significantly from troglitazone in their efficacy (ie maximal glucose-lowering capacity) or side effect profile. Troglitazone effectively reduces insulin resistance by 25–35% in type 2 diabetes, impaired glucose tolerance (IGT) and obesity (Fig. 5). In practice, this causes a fall in plasma glucose (generally with a 2–3 mmol/l decrease in fasting levels). In the longer term, HbA_{1c} falls by up to 2.7% when troglitazone is used in combination with other agents (metformin or insulin), and by approximately 1% when used as sole therapy. Insulin levels also fall in the long term; this may be a significant advantage, given the suspected atherogenic and other adverse effects of hyperinsulinaemia. For unexplained reasons, the glucose-lowering effect may take up to three weeks to become maximal. As with metformin, the thiazolidinediones lower blood glucose but, if given alone, do not cause hypoglycaemia. Troglitazone has been tested in type 2 diabetes both as a single agent and in combination with

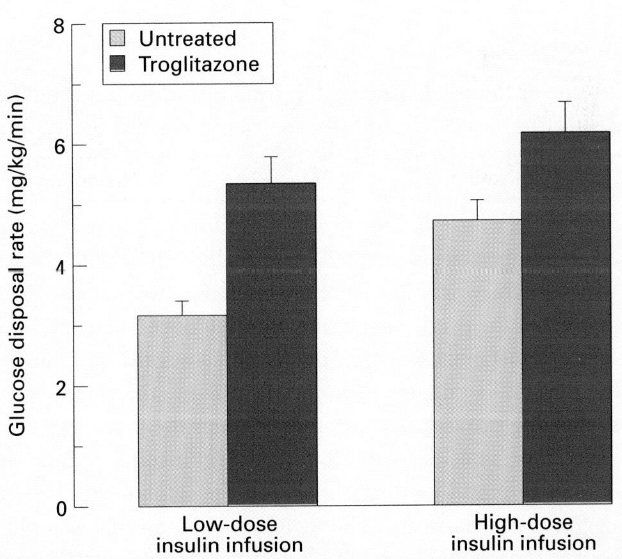

Fig. 5 Effects of troglitazone on insulin sensitivity in 11 subjects with type 2 diabetes, as measured by the euglycaemic clamp. During both high- and low-dose insulin infusions, troglitazone significantly stimulated peripheral glucose uptake as compared with the untreated state (NEFA = non-esterified fatty acids). (Data reproduced from Ref 9, with kind permission of the editor of *Diabetes Care*.)

sulphonylureas, insulin and metformin when it potentiates the action of the latter drugs and often leads to a reduction in their dose [10].

The main toxic effects of the thiazolidinediones appear to involve the liver. During clinical trials with troglitazone, up to 3% of patients experienced transient rises in serum transaminases, but significant hepatic dysfunction was much rarer. Nine cases of severe hepatic necrosis, either fatal or requiring liver transplantation, have been reported amongst over 300,000 patients exposed to the drug. This led to the withdrawal of troglitazone in Europe; paradoxically, its use continues in the USA where several fatal reactions have occurred. The potential links between troglitazone and these events are being carefully investigated. It is not clear at present whether this is an idiosyncratic reaction to troglitazone or a class effect, although it is encouraging to note that there is no evidence so far that the liver is a target for toxicity with any of the other thiazolidinediones currently under investigation.

Other adverse events of troglitazone observed in animal studies include a modest increase in circulating volume, accompanied by a fall in haematocrit, an increase in body fat, and an increase in left ventricular (LV) mass. In humans, a small fall in haemoglobin has been reported, together with modest weight gain and a redistribution of fat from abdominal to subcutaneous depots. However, clinical trials have demonstrated a potentially beneficial reduction in LV mass.

The place of the thiazolidinediones in treating diabetes and insulin resistance remains uncertain, but the continuing experience in the USA with troglitazone and ongoing clinical trials with other agents will undoubtedly provide further information in the near future.

Novel insulin secretagogues

β-cell failure is one of the fundamental abnormalities which lead to type 2 diabetes, and is apparently the crucial factor that determines whether an individual will progress from the prediabetic state of IGT to overt diabetes. Insulin secretagogues, notably the sulphonylureas, are therefore a rational therapeutic approach (see Fig. 3).

Several novel agents which increase insulin secretion in a similar way to the sulphonylureas have recently become available. These include the sulphonylurea derivative glimepiride, which interacts with the sulphonylurea receptor associated with the ATP-sensitive K^+ channel in the β-cell membrane. Binding of sulphonylureas, like the ATP produced by glucose metabolism within the β-cell, closes the K^+ channel, preventing the efflux of K^+ ions and so depolarising the membrane; this opens voltage-sensitive Ca^{2+} channels, allowing extracellular Ca^{2+} ions to enter the β-cell and drive the transport of the secretory vesicles that culminates in insulin release. Interestingly, glimepiride appears to bind to a different site on the sulphonylurea receptor protein from that recognised by 'classical' sulphonylureas such as glibenclamide. The non-sulphonylurea drug repaglinide does not bind to the sulphonylurea receptor, but also acts to close the ATP-sensitive K^+ channel. It is not yet clear whether either of these drugs has particular advantages over existing sulphonylureas.

A novel insulin secretagogue, which operates through a mechanism different from that of the sulphonylureas, is glucagon-like peptide 1 (7–36) amide (GLP-1).

GLP-1 is the principal 'incretin' hormone in humans and acts on specific receptors on the β-cell to stimulate insulin secretion and insulin synthesis. Incretins, which stimulate insulin release, are released by the gut in response to glucose, and also include gastric inhibitory peptide. Their existence was first suggested when it was observed that an oral glucose load was a more potent stimulus to insulin secretion than an equal glucose dose given intravenously. Other potentially glucose-lowering effects of GLP-1 include delayed gastric emptying, and possibly a modest improvement in non-insulin mediated glucose uptake in skeletal muscle.

GLP-1 secretion is normal in type 2 diabetes, but several studies have suggested that it may correct many of the metabolic abnormalities of type 2 diabetes and initial trials were promising. Overnight continuous intravenous infusion was shown to normalise blood glucose levels in type 2 diabetic patients; all the anti-diabetic mechanisms described above, together with suppression of glucagon production, were thought to be relevant contributors to this effect [11]. A longer-term, double-blind, placebo-controlled crossover study of GLP-1 therapy was carried out in type 2 diabetic patients poorly controlled by conventional oral hypoglycaemic agents. GLP-1 was injected subcutaneously three times daily before meals. Delayed and flattened post-prandial glucose responses were demonstrated [12], but there was little change in insulin or glucagon levels, suggesting that the main effect was via delayed gastric emptying (Fig. 6). A buccal GLP-1 preparation (to allow systemic absorption, while avoiding proteolytic destruction of GLP-1 in the stomach) has

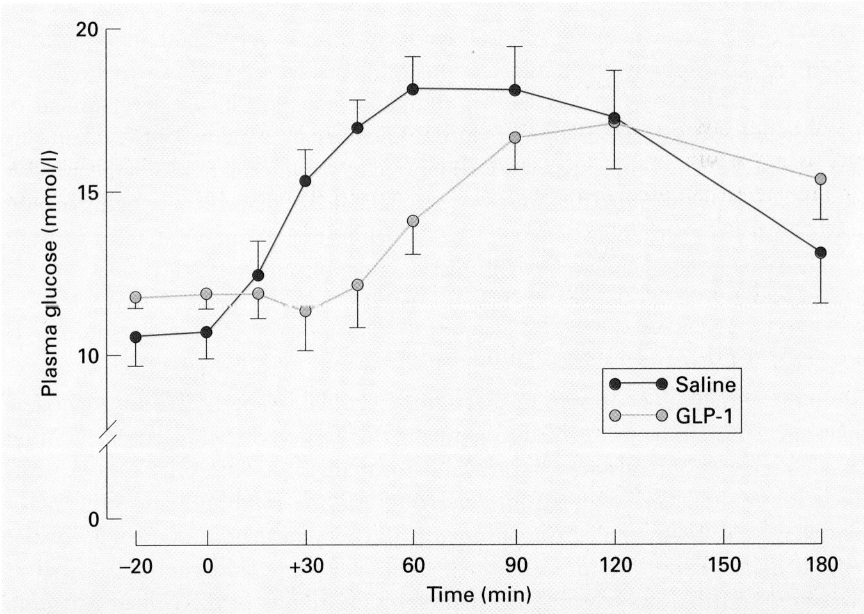

Fig. 6 Effects of subcutaneous glucagon-like peptide 1 (7–36) amide (GLP-1) on glucose levels in patients with type 2 (non-insulin dependent) diabetes. Compared with saline placebo, GLP-1 significantly delayed and reduced the post-prandial glycaemic peak ($p<0.02$). (Data redrawn from Ref 10, with kind permission of the editor of the *European Journal of Clinical Investigation.*)

recently been shown to lower fasting and post-prandial blood glucose concentrations by 1.4 and 4.2 mmol/l, respectively, in type 2 diabetes [13]. GLP-1 analogues and orally active GLP-1 agonists are also being actively investigated. However, the maximal glucose-lowering capacity of GLP-1 is no greater than with conventional oral hypoglycaemic drugs, and it remains to be seen whether it will prove useful in the therapy of type 2 diabetes.

Other approaches

Other agents include drugs which modify aspects of lipid metabolism (eg inhibitors of the mitochondrial carnitine 'shuttle' enzyme, CPT-1, that is crucial in fatty acid oxidation) and may lower glucose levels by interfering with the Randle cycle or other pathways. None of these has yet reached clinical stages of development. The use of amylin treatment is also being explored for type 2 diabetes, but the same caveats apply as with type 1 diabetes.

Anti-obesity drugs

It is important to remember that obesity is a major predisposing factor for diabetes, and that effective treatment of obesity in patients with type 2 diabetes can achieve substantial benefits in glycaemic control and the management of coexisting hypertension and dyslipidaemia.

The best evidence yet that treating obesity may ameliorate and even prevent diabetes comes from studies of surgical treatment (gastric bypass and fundoplication operations) in morbidly obese subjects. One retrospective US study, carried out over nine years in the USA, showed both a dramatic reduction in the development of diabetes and also a normalisation of glucose tolerance in many patients who already had the disease. This optimistic view is supported by the interim results of the Swedish Obesity Study, which show that the two-year incidence of diabetes developing in subjects with IGT or normoglycaemia at baseline fell from 6.5% in diet-treated controls to only 0.5% in those who underwent gastric reduction surgery [14].

□ TREATMENT OF CHRONIC DIABETIC COMPLICATIONS

Given the difficulties in optimising glycaemic control in diabetes, it is not surprising that much effort is being devoted to reducing the burden of complications in other ways. Specific treatments are now available for many problems, such as laser treatment for retinopathy, angiotensin-converting enzyme inhibitors and other antihypertensive drugs for diabetic nephropathy, and tricyclic drugs and other agents for painful neuropathy. The importance of tight blood pressure control, as well as glycaemic control, was recently highlighted by the results of the United Kingdom Prospective Diabetes Study. Advances in the understanding of the pathogenesis of diabetic complications, particularly the effects of hyperglycaemia at tissue and cellular levels, may soon lead to the development of new agents to reduce the organ damage caused by chronic hyperglycaemia.

Aldose reductase inhibitors

One theory relating to the cause of hyperglycaemia-induced tissue damage is the 'polyol' hypothesis (see Fig. 7). Polyols are sugar alcohols generated particularly in tissues in which glucose uptake is not regulated by insulin under the influence of the rate-limiting enzyme, aldose reductase (which, for example, converts glucose to sorbitol). In these tissues (notably nerve, retina and kidney), production of sorbitol and other polyols increases under hyperglycaemic conditions, and could potentially interfere with several crucial aspects of cellular metabolism.

Blockade of aldose reductase should theoretically lead to a reduction in the production of sorbitol, and thus reduce complications; this hypothesis is supported by various animal studies. Several aldose reductase inhibitors (eg sorbinil, tolrestat, ponalrestat) have undergone extensive clinical trials in humans, mainly focusing on neuropathy. Unfortunately, the results have been disappointing, with only marginal improvements in certain objective or symptomatic measures. It has been argued that larger, longer-term trials might show beneficial delays in the progression of neuropathy and other complications, but the effects seem likely to be modest; it seems improbable at present that these studies will ever be carried out [15].

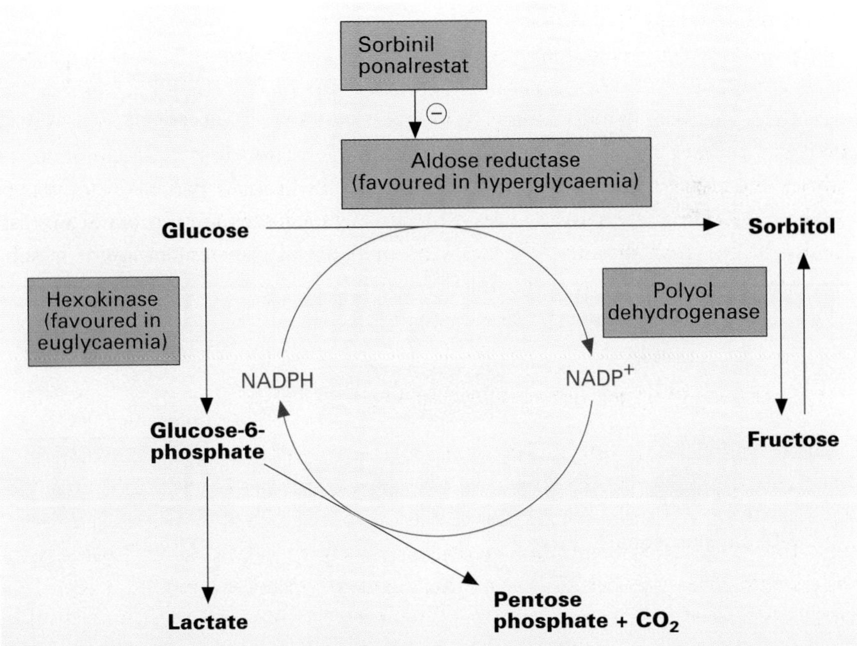

Fig. 7 The polyol pathway. Glucose is normally metabolised preferentially by hexokinase, which has a higher affinity for glucose than aldose reductase. Under conditions of hyperglycaemia, however, glucose flux through the polyol pathway is greatly increased. Aldose reductase inhibitors prevent the production from glucose of sorbitol, which has been implicated in the pathogenesis of some chronic diabetic complications.

Aminoguanidine and inhibitors of advanced glycation end-product formation

An alternative hypothesis that is gaining credibility is that diabetic tissue damage is related to the formation of cross-linked glycated proteins and other macromolecules, termed advanced glycation end-products (AGEs).

Excessive AGE formation may contribute to the stiffening of tissues frequently observed in diabetes, to basement membrane thickening, and ultimately to cellular and microvascular damage. AGE formation can be inhibited experimentally by aminoguanidine (Fig. 8), which has been shown to decrease both AGE accumulation and tissue damage in animal models of diabetes [16]. One short-term study in man has shown a reduction in the formation of cross-linked glycated haemoglobin, but effects on the all-important tissue proteins have not yet been reported. The results of further research with this and related compounds, particularly long-term clinical studies, are awaited with keen interest.

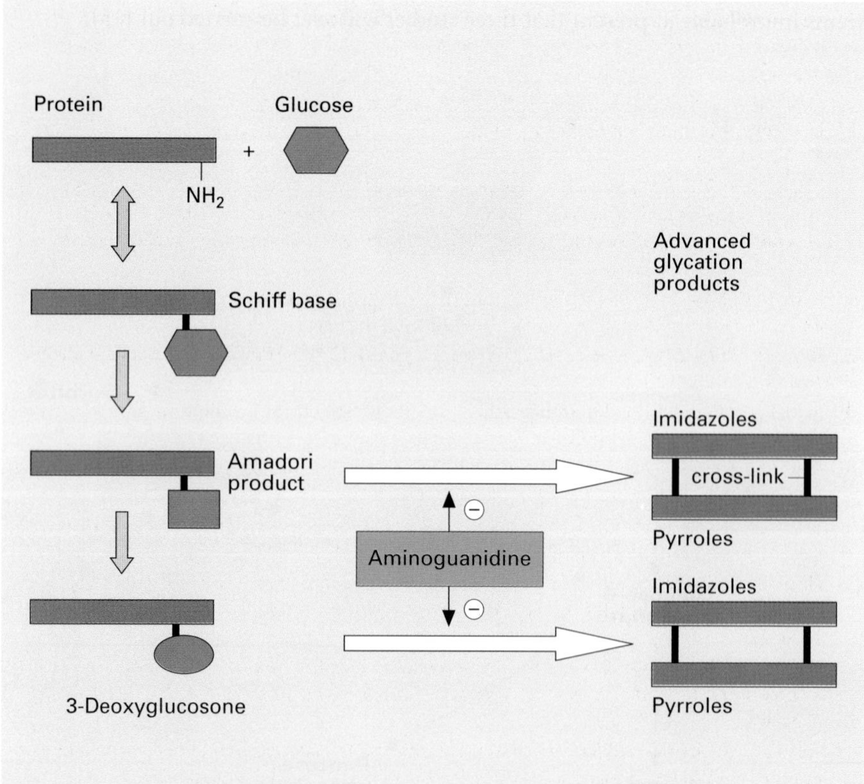

Fig. 8 Aminoguanidine prevents the formation of advanced glycation end-products (AGEs) by reacting with the Amadori products in such a way as to prevent further irreversible cross-linking between protein molecules. In the early stages of non-enzymatic glycation of proteins, glucose reacts with amino groups of protein molecules to form Schiff bases, which undergo molecular rearrangement to form the Amadori product and ultimately the highly reactive 3-deoxyglucosone derivative which cross-links proteins to form imidazole and pyrrole derivatives.

□ CONCLUSIONS

The pharmacological treatment of diabetes is now undergoing a quiet revolution, with a steady broadening of the range of therapeutic options available and a more critical appraisal of the long-term effectiveness of the established as well as the new anti-diabetic drugs. Hopefully, this will ultimately lead to a better quality of life for all people with diabetes but, as with many areas of rapid development, it is still unclear which of these new therapeutic avenues will lead to useful advances in the management of the disease.

REFERENCES

1 Bailey CJ, Williams G, Pickup JC. New drugs in the management of diabetes mellitus and its complications. In: Pickup JC, Williams G (eds). *Textbook of diabetes*, 2nd edn. Oxford: Blackwell Science, 1997: 84.1–84.30.

2 Petrie JR, Donnelly R. New pharmacological approaches to insulin and lipid metabolism. *Drugs* 1994; **47**: 701–10.

3 Diabetes Control and Complications Trial Research Group. The effect of intensive treatment of diabetes on the development and progression of long-term complications in insulin-dependent diabetes mellitus. *N Engl J Med* 1993; **329**: 977–86.

4 Garg SK, Carmain, JA, Braddy KC, *et al.* Pre-meal insulin analogue insulin lispro vs Humulin R insulin treatment in young subjects with type 1 diabetes. *Diabet Med* 1996; **13**: 47–52.

5 Thompson RG, Pearson L, Kolterman OG. Effects of 4 weeks administration of pramlintide, a human amylin analogue on glycaemic control in patients with IDDM: effects on plasma glucose profiles and serum fructosamine concentrations. *Diabetologia* 1997; **40**: 1278–85.

6 Alberti KGMM, Gries F. Management of non-insulin-dependent diabetes mellitus in Europe: a consensus view. *Diabet Med* 1988; **5**: 275–81.

7 Petrie J, Small M, Connell J. 'Glitazones': a prospect for non-insulin-dependent diabetes. *Lancet* 1997; **349**: 70–1.

8 Saltiel AR, Olefsky JM. Thiazolidinediones in the treatment of insulin resistance and type II diabetes. *Diabetes* 1996; **45**: 1661–9.

9 Suter SL, Nolan JJ, Wallace P, *et al.* Metabolic effects of new oral hypoglycemic agent CS-045 in NIDDM subjects. *Diabetes Care* 1992; **15**: 193–203.

10 Inzucchi SE, Maggs DG, Spollett GP, *et al.* Efficacy and metabolic effects of metformin and troglitazone in type II diabetes. *N Engl J Med* 1998; **338**: 867–72.

11 Gutniak M, Orskov C, Holst JJ, *et al.* Antidiabetogenic effect of glucagon-like peptide-1 (7–36) amide in normal subjects and patients with diabetes mellitus. *N Engl J Med* 1992; **326**: 1316–22.

12 Todd JF, Wilding JPH, Edwards CMB, *et al.* Glucagon-like peptide 1 7–36 amide (GLP-1): a three week trial in non-insulin dependent diabetes mellitus. *Eur J Clin Invest* 1997; **27**: 6533–6.

13 Gutniak MK, Larsson H, Sanders SW, *et al.* GLP-1 tablet in type 2 diabetes in fasting and post-prandial condition. *Diabetes Care* 1997; **20**: 1874–9.

14 Sjostrom L. The natural history of massive obesity. *Int J Obes Relat Metab Disord* 1995; **16**: 465–79.

15 Piefer MA, Schumer MP, Gelber DA. Aldose reductase inhibitors: the end of an era or the need for different trial designs? *Diabetes* 1997; **46** (Suppl 2): S82–9.

16 Vlassara H. Recent progress in advanced glycation end products and diabetic complications. *Diabetes* 1997; **46** (Suppl 2): S19–25.

☐ MULTIPLE CHOICE QUESTIONS

1 In the treatment of type 1 diabetes, lispro insulin:
   (a) Is absorbed more rapidly as it forms hexameric complexes when injected
   (b) Can be given immediately before meals
   (c) Improves glycaemic control
   (d) Reduces the risk of hypoglycaemia by 30%
   (e) Binds to serum albumin, thus slowing its action profile

2 Amylin:
   (a) Is produced by the pancreatic α-cells
   (b) May improve glycaemic control by delaying gastric emptying
   (c) Is deposited in the islets as islet amyloid in type 2 diabetes
   (d) Is the cause of insulin resistance in type 2 diabetes
   (e) Can be given as oral therapy for type 2 diabetes

3 Glucagon-like peptide-1:
   (a) Together with gastric inhibitory polypeptide, is the major incretin hormone in humans
   (b) Is produced by the pancreas
   (c) Lowers post-prandial blood glucose in diabetic patients
   (d) Secretion is abnormal in type 2 diabetes
   (e) Delays gastric emptying

4 Thiazolidinediones:
   (a) Have an immediate and long-lasting glucose-lowering effect
   (b) Act via a peroxisome proliferator activated nuclear receptor
   (c) Stimulate insulin secretion
   (d) May be used together with insulin in type 2 patients
   (e) Increase circulating volume and left ventricular mass in humans

5 Treatment of diabetic complications:
   (a) Aldose reductase inhibitors have proven benefit in diabetic neuropathy
   (b) Angiotensin-converting enzyme inhibitors slow the progression of diabetic nephropathy
   (c) Aminoguanidine prevents formation of advanced glycation end-products
   (d) The reaction linking glucose to proteins is irreversible
   (e) Cross-linked proteins are cleared only very slowly from the body

ANSWERS

1a False	2a False	3a True	4a False	5a False
b True	b True	b False	b True	b True
c False	c True	c True	c False	c True
d True	d False	d False	d True	d False
e False	e False	e True	e False	e True

Diabetic nephropathy: natural history and treatment

Jiten P Vora

□ INTRODUCTION

Diabetic nephropathy is defined as persistent albuminuria (>300 mg/24 h), on at least two occasions separated by 3–6 months, in the absence of other causes of proteinuria. This corresponds to total proteinuria of about 500 mg/24 h, when conventional urine analysis by dip-stick methods becomes positive. This simple definition belies the gravity of the condition. These patients, whether with type 1 (insulin-dependent – IDDM) or type 2 (non-insulin dependent – NIDDM) diabetes, invariably show a predictable and relentless decline in glomerular filtration rate (GFR) and a progressive increase in proteinuria; moreover, they invariably have hypertension and a dramatically higher mortality from cardiovascular disease. In addition, diabetic nephropathy remains the leading cause of end-stage renal disease (ESRD) in Western societies, with NIDDM patients forming the single largest group of patients enrolling on renal-support therapy programmes in Europe.

□ EPIDEMIOLOGY OF DIABETIC NEPHROPATHY

Historically, nephropathy has been said to occur in 30–40% of IDDM patients. Some recent studies, but not others, suggest that the cumulative incidence may have declined to approximately 25%; this may reflect success in lowering glycosylated haemoglobin (HbA_{1c}) levels over extended periods in some populations, thus reducing the incidence of all chronic microvascular complications including nephropathy [1].

In NIDDM, the risk of nephropathy was previously thought to be low, and this factor – perhaps compounded by the heterogeneity of NIDDM and the relatively frequent coexistence of other causes of renal impairment – has retarded the accumulation of information regarding the epidemiology and natural history of diabetic renal disease in this group of patients. Population-based studies demonstrate a 5–10% prevalence of nephropathy on diagnosis of NIDDM, perhaps reflecting the prolonged subclinical hyperglycaemia (probably averaging 5–7 years) before clinical presentation. Longitudinal studies show a cumulative incidence of nephropathy that reaches 25% after 20 years of NIDDM [1]; 10 years later, 20% of these patients progress to clinically significant renal impairment that requires renal support therapy [2].

Overall, the cumulative incidence of diabetic nephropathy (persistent proteinuria) appears to be similar in both IDDM and NIDDM (Fig. 1). However, the proportions of patients who enrol on renal support programmes with ESRD

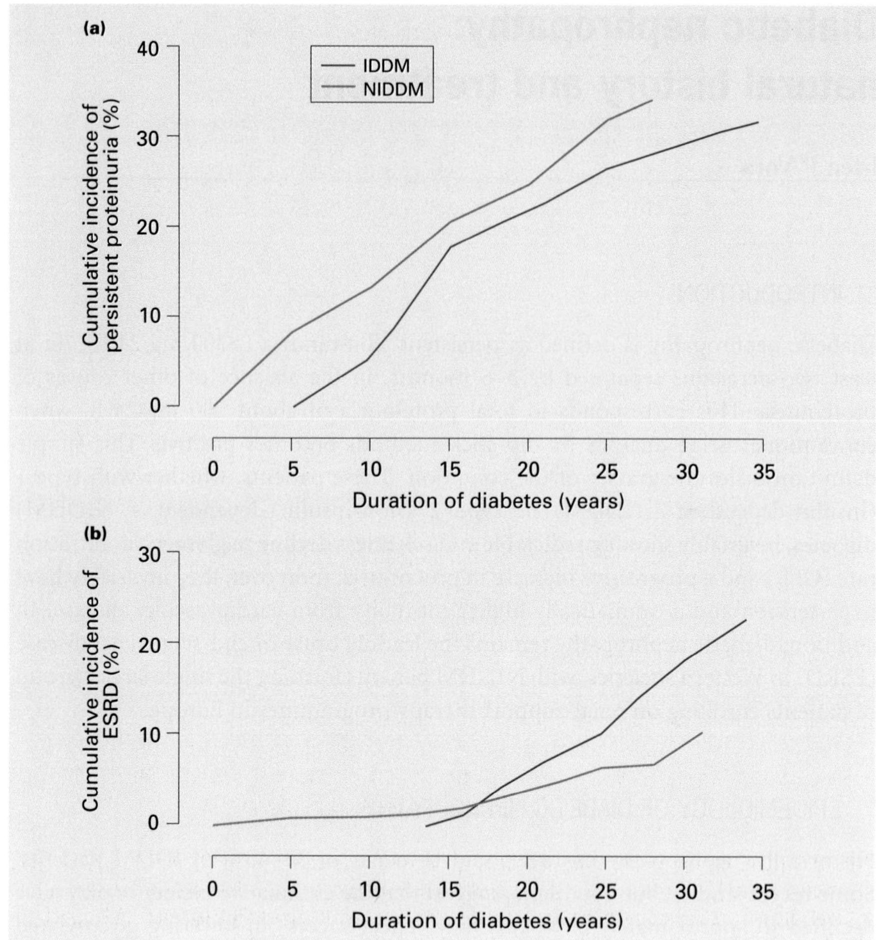

Fig. 1 Cumulative incidence of **(a)** persistent proteinuria (nephropathy) and **(b)** end-stage renal disease (ESRD) in insulin-dependent (IDDM) and non-insulin dependent (NIDDM) patients (Adapted from Ref 1.)

differ markedly between the two groups, being only 6–10% for patients with NIDDM but 20% for the IDDM patients.

□ NATURAL HISTORY OF DIABETIC NEPHROPATHY

Many aspects of the evolution of diabetic nephropathy are similar for the IDDM and NIDDM patients; those that differ will be described below.

Insulin-dependent diabetes

The natural history of renal dysfunction in IDDM has been well characterised, with the identification of five distinct stages [3] (Fig. 2).

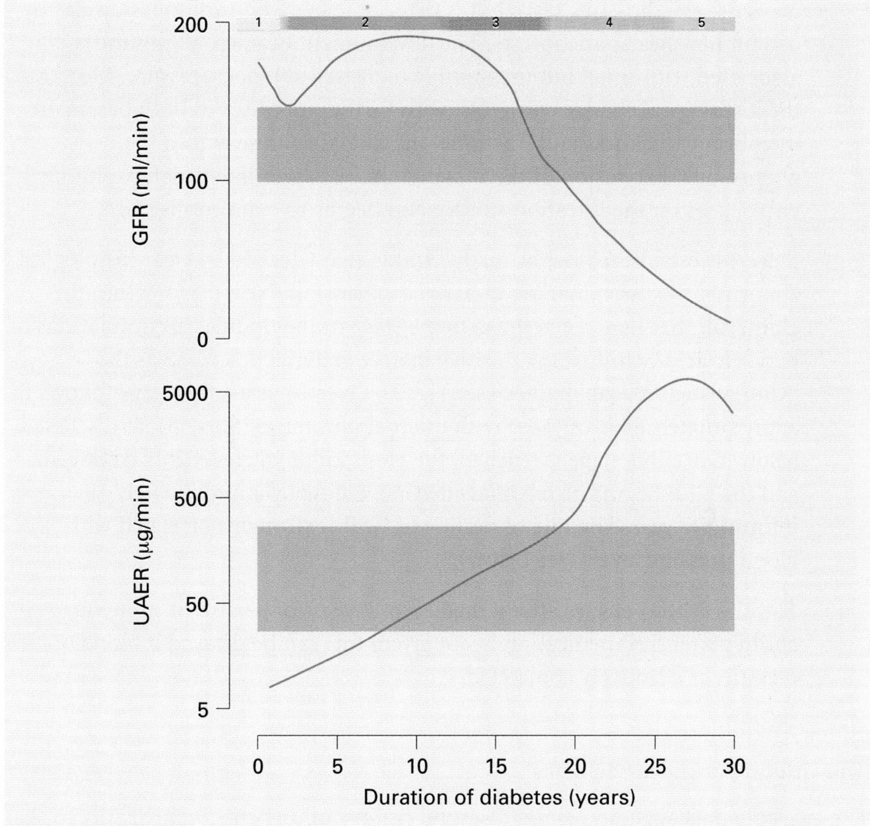

Fig. 2 Natural history of renal dysfunction: glomerular filtration rate (GFR) and urinary albumin excretion rate (UAER) in a cohort of patients with insulin-dependent diabetes mellitus; shaded areas: normal range for GFR and microalbuminuria (albumin excretion rate, 20–200 µg/min). (Adapted from Ref 3.) 1–5 represent the five different stages of renal dysfunction (see text).

- *Stage 1* relates to the renal hypertrophy and hyperfunction (elevated GFR) found in all IDDM patients at the time of diagnosis. Urinary albumin excretion rate (UAER) and blood pressure are both normal.

- *Stage 2* occurs when average glycaemic control is achieved with conventional insulin regimens and lasts for 10–15 years. During this 'silent phase', GFR remains elevated ('hyperfiltration'), with normal UAER and blood pressure levels. However, renal biopsy demonstrates early histological changes, with an increase in basement membrane thickness and expansion of the mesangium (characteristic features of diabetic nephropathy: see Fig. 3) after 2–4 years.

- *Stage 3*, described as 'incipient' nephropathy or microalbuminuria, occurs after 6–15 years of IDDM. UAER during this stage is 20–200 µg/min, (30–300 mg/24 h). This level of proteinuria is far below the sensitivity of the conventional dip-stick tests, but is detectable by radioimmunoassay and by certain new near-patient tests. The development of microalbuminuria is associated with small but measurable increases in blood pressure. Moreover, the histological changes progress, with further increases in both basement membrane thickness and fractional mesangial volume within the glomerulus. Expansion of the mesangium by extracellular matrix ultimately encroaches on the filtration surface and begins to compromise GFR.

- *Stage 4* is established nephropathy, and is characterised by clear histological abnormalities, with marked mesangial expansion ('sclerosis') within the glomeruli that may reach the extreme stage of the nodular accumulations of periodic acid-Schiff (PAS)-positive matrix material described as the 'Kimmelstiel-Wilson' kidney (see Fig. 3). Over 10 years, this stage follows in approximately 80% of those with microalbuminuria (Stage 3), as discussed below. Once this stage is reached, the glomerulus is irreversibly damaged, and the GFR begins its relentless decline, falling by approximately 10 ml/min per year. The rate of decline of GFR is strongly correlated with blood pressure levels (see below).
- *Stage 5* (ESRD) ensues after a median of 7 years of persistent proteinuria, if antihypertensive medication is not given; this can be delayed if blood pressure is effectively controlled.

Non-insulin dependent diabetes

The available data suggest a similar natural history of diabetic nephropathy to that in IDDM. At presentation of NIDDM, the kidneys are enlarged and GFR is 30–40% higher than in matched controls, but falls when initial therapy for diabetes is started [4]. Thereafter, persistent elevation ('hyperfiltration') is evident in 25% of cases, mainly young patients; in these cases, effective renal plasma flow (ERPF) is not increased in such patients, and the filtration fraction (GFR/ERPF), which reflects the glomerular capillary pressure, is therefore raised. As in IDDM, increased glomerular capillary pressure not only favours the filtration of albumin, but may itself be an aetiological factor in the initiation and progression of renal injury. As in IDDM, GFR remains stable up to and possibly during the phase of microalbuminuria, or until hypertension or proteinuria supervene [5] (Fig. 4).

The rate of decline of GFR in established nephropathy shows wider variability (5–10 ml/min/year) in NIDDM compared with IDDM patients (Fig. 2); however, it is still generally predictable in individual patients. The rate of decline accelerates with raised blood pressure, especially systolic [2]. As GFR falls, proteinuria progressively increases by 40% per annum until the development of ESRD. As in IDDM, the reported cases of decline of GFR would predict that ESRD would be reached a median of 7 years after the onset of persistent proteinuria.

The picture presented above indicates that the natural history of renal dysfunction is broadly similar in IDDM and NIDDM, but with some important differences in detail. The same is true of the histological features of renal damage. As

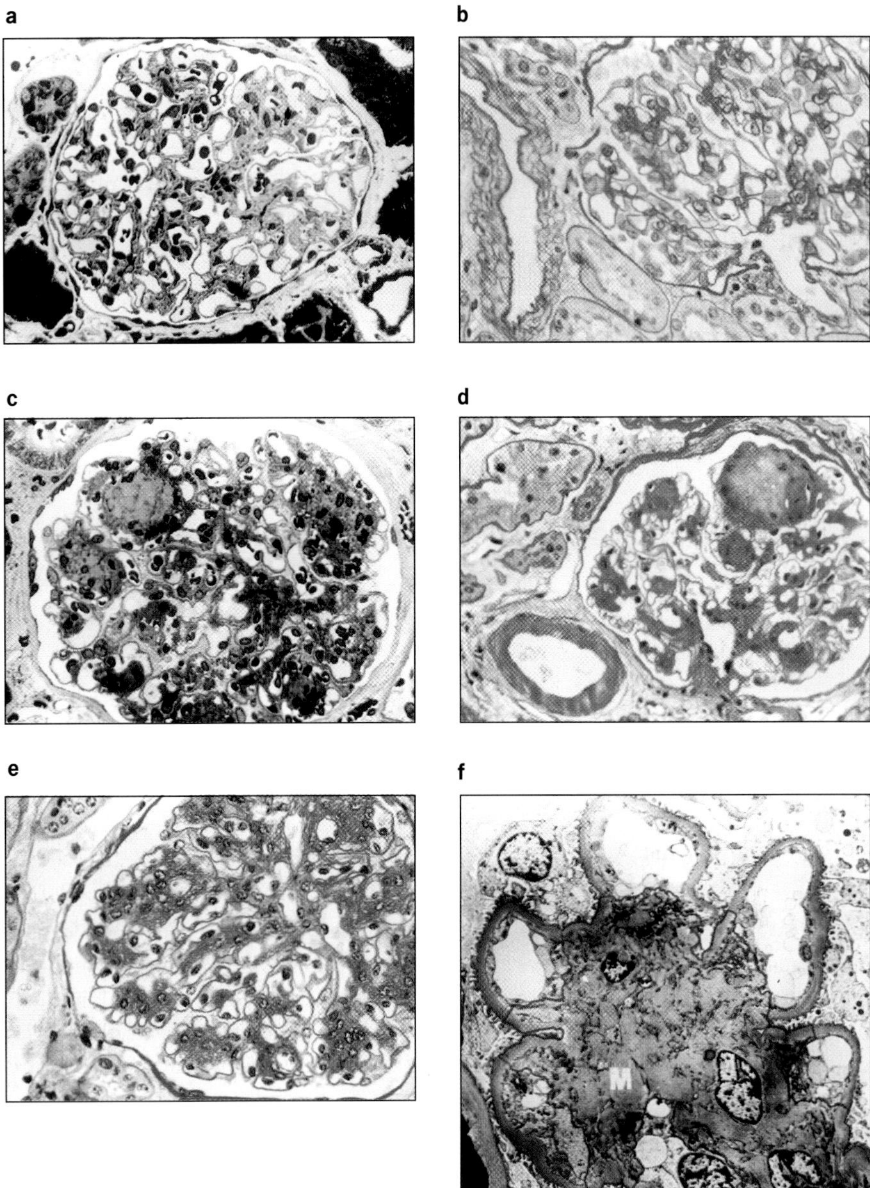

Fig. 3 Structural changes of diabetic nephropathy, on light microscopy **(a–e)** and electron microscopy **(f)**. **(a)** and **(b)** represent normal human glomerulus, with toludine blue staining and periodic acid-Schiff (PAS) staining after paraffin embedding, respectively; **(c)** demonstrates a human glomerulus from a patient with overt proteinuria (toludine blue stain). Note diminution of capillary number, nodule formation in top left-hand corner and widespread mesangial expansion; **(d)** represents a paraffin-embedded PAS-stained section from a kidney transplanted into a diabetic patient aged 14 years (note the typical nodule formation and widespread mesangial expansion); **(e)** is from a native kidney in a patient with microalbuminuria, demonstrating established mesangial expansion (paraffin-embedded PAS staining). The electron micrograph **(f)** illustrates dense increase in mesangial matrix (marked M), basement membrane thickening and encroachment of capillary space by the expanding mesangium.

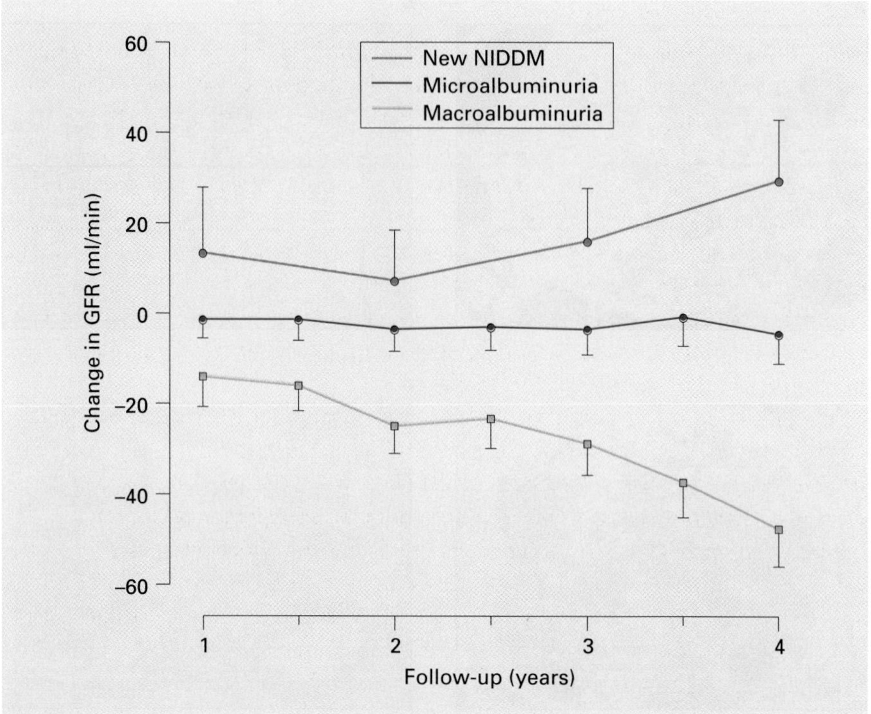

Fig. 4 Changes in glomerular filtration rate in newly diagnosed, microalbuminuric and macroalbuminuric non-insulin dependent diabetes mellitus (NIDDM) patients of Pima Indian origin. (Adapted from Ref 5.)

in IDDM, the kidneys of NIDDM patients show increased thickness of the glomerular basement membrane and expansion of the mesangium by matrix, ultimately encroaching on the capillary tuft that is responsible for glomerular filtration, and finally leading to glomerular sclerosis. These characteristic glomerular changes are seen in about one-third of NIDDM patients, while another one-third show predominantly tubulo-interstitial changes of tubular cell hyperplasia, incorporating the glycogen rich Armanni-Ebstein droplets (reversed with periods of improved glycaemic control), interstitial space cellular infiltrate and fibrosis, with superimposed signs of ischaemia (for example, arteriolar hyalinosis); the remainder have evidence of a non-diabetic cause for their renal impairment such as myeloma, immunoglobulin (Ig) A nephropathy.

□ MICROALBUMINURIA

This is a crucial stage, not only in the natural history of the condition, but also because it can now be readily identified and because various interventions have been shown to reduce the risks of progressing to clinically significant overt nephropathy. As above, IDDM and NIDDM will be discussed separately.

Insulin-dependent diabetes mellitus

Estimates of the prevalence of microalbuminuria in IDDM patients vary considerably, but recent methodologically sound studies have reported rates of 9–15% [6,7]. In IDDM, 2–3% of patients each year progress from normo- to micro-albuminuria, or 5 cases per 1,000 person years of IDDM. Normoalbuminuric patients who progress to microalbuminuria have higher HbA_{1c} and initial UAER levels while within the (broad) normal range.

Patients with IDDM and microalbuminuria are generally older, with longer durations of diabetes and worse glycaemic control (raised HbA_{1c} levels); they also tend to have marginal elevations of blood pressure (see below), and tend to be male smokers. Many also have left ventricular hypertrophy, and an increased incidence of silent myocardial ischaemia has been reported.

Overall, overt nephropathy will develop in approximately 40% and 80% of microalbuminuria IDDM patients after 5 and 10 years, respectively [8]. The pattern of albumin excretion – that is, its level, whether it lies persistently within the microalbuminuric range (30–300 mg/24 h) or whether it rises progressively or falls – appears to predict the outcome of this stage. In IDDM patients with persistent micro-albuminuria, UAER increases on average by 20–40% per annum (Fig. 5). By contrast, patients who do not demonstrate a progressive increase in UAER during the micro-albuminuric phase have only a small chance (approximately 10%) of progressing to nephropathy [8]. Indeed, it has been proposed that only patients with UAER in excess of 50 μg/min (75 mg/24 h) have a high risk (95%) of deteriorating to overt nephropathy. Intermittent microalbuminuria (ie varying between normo- and micro-albuminuria over time) is shown by 4–5% of IDDM patients. It is not necessarily a benign state, as 18% of these patients will develop persistent micro-albuminuria within 6 months. Conversely, some studies have reported that up to 20% of subjects with microalbuminuria return to within the normoalbuminuric range. These features, and the generally wide intra-individual variability in UAER, highlight the need for at least two samples separated by 3–6 months to show UAER in the range 20–200 μg/min (30–300 mg/24 h) before microalbuminuria can be confidently diagnosed.

Blood pressure plays an important role in determining the evolution of nephropathy once the microalbuminuric stage is reached, although it does not appear to distinguish patients who progress to microalbuminuria from those who remain persistently normoalbuminuric. Once microalbuminuria develops, blood pressure may remain initially in the conventional 'normal' range (<160/90 mmHg, as defined by the World Health Organization (WHO)). There are, however, minor increases in blood pressure (measured 'casually') within the normal range and 24 h ambulatory blood pressure monitoring shows clear abnormalities of diurnal rhythms. IDDM patients who remain persistently normoalbuminuric have daytime blood pressures comparable to healthy control subjects, although about 15% of these patients may lose the normal nocturnal dip. Blood pressure rises in parallel with development of microalbuminuria; on average, these patients have systolic and diastolic blood pressures that are respectively 8 and 5 mmHg higher than normo-albuminuric controls, and most show loss of the nocturnal fall (Fig. 6). The

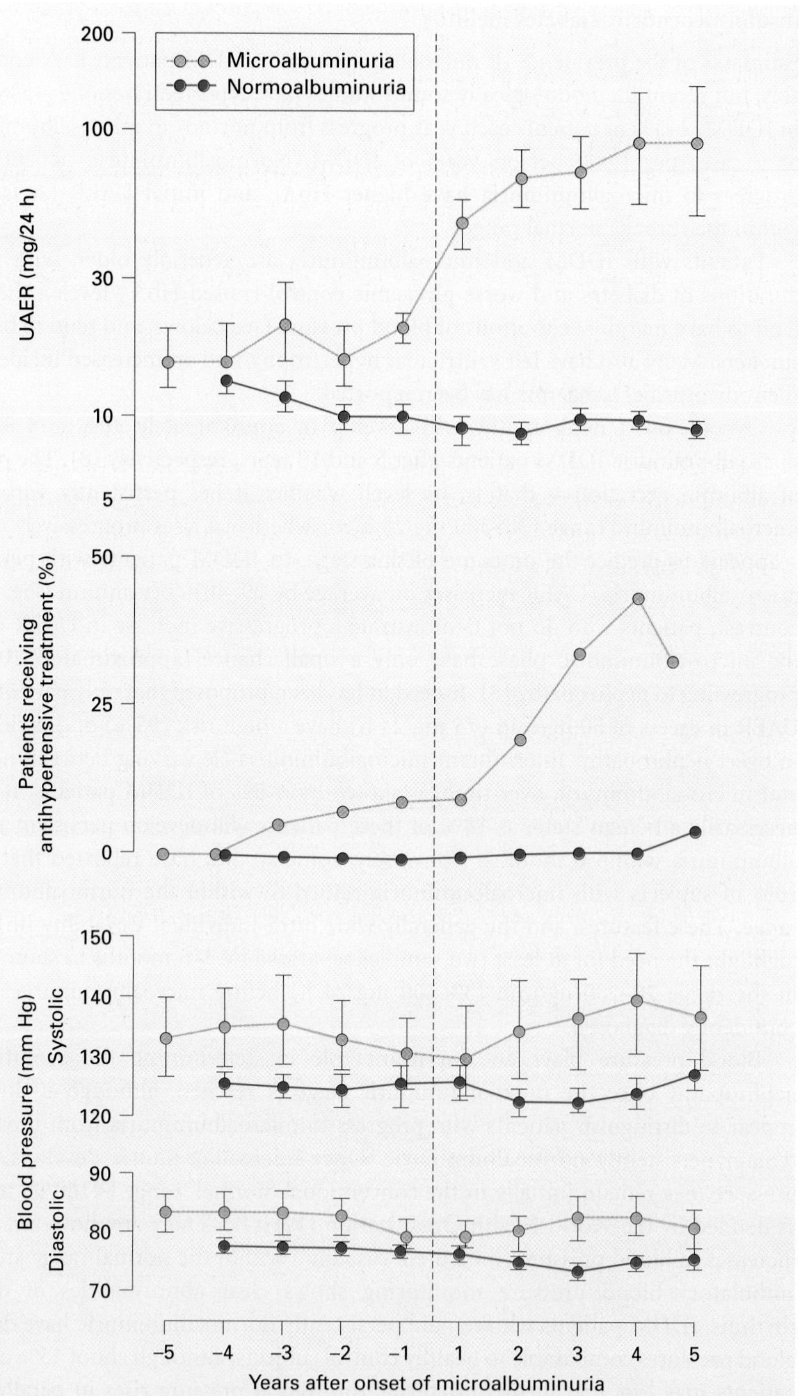

Fig. 5 Urinary albumin excretion rate (UAER), prevalence of antihypertensive therapy, systolic and diastolic blood pressure in a group of insulin-dependent diabetic patients who proceeded to develop microalbuminuria and those who remained normoalbuminuric. (Adapted from Ref 8.)

prevalence of antihypertensive therapy increases rapidly after the development of microalbuminuria and rises to 45–50% at 4–5 years (Fig. 5) [8], compared with only 8–10% of patients who remain normoalbuminuric.

There is now no doubt that the phase of microalbuminuria indicates early, but definite, renal dysfunction in IDDM. This conclusion is based not only on the clinical findings of increasing prevalence of hypertension with microalbuminuria and its value in predicting overt nephropathy, but also on the histological evidence of mesangial expansion (which will adversely affect glomerular filtration) in addition to the less specific increase in glomerular basement membrane thickness (see Fig. 3).

Non-insulin dependent diabetes

The prevalence of microalbuminuria in NIDDM patients is probably about 20–25% (substantially higher than the 10–15% in IDDM) although the prevalence reported in various cross-sectional studies ranges widely (10–50%). This variability may reflect the general heterogeneity of NIDDM, particularly in relation to duration of hyperglycaemia before diagnosis, the presence of hypertension and other diseases, and perhaps ethnic background.

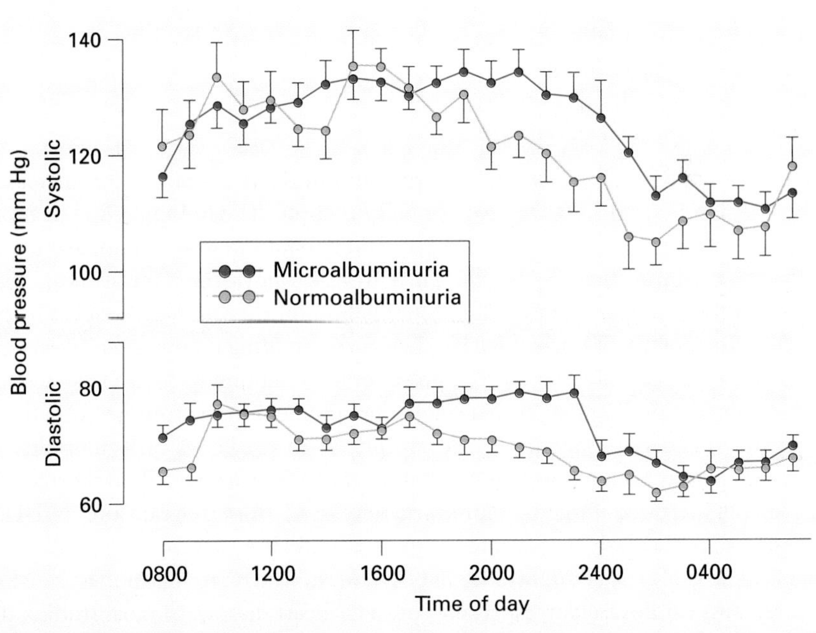

Fig. 6 Diurnal blood pressure profile in Type 1 insulin-dependent diabetic patients with microalbuminuria showing elevations of blood pressure, with loss of the normal nocturnal 'dip', compared with normoalbuminuric counterparts.

At diagnosis of NIDDM, the prevalence of microalbuminuria is in the range 20–40%; there is clearly a functional element to the increased UAER at this stage, as it often falls after routine anti-diabetic therapy is started.

About 20–40% of the NIDDM patients with microalbuminuria develop overt nephropathy over 10 years. These patients show a 15–40% increase in UAER in each year, the rate of rise being relatively steady for an individual, and often have higher baseline levels of UAER. Increasing UAER is associated with rising systolic and diastolic blood pressure as in IDDM. NIDDM patients with microalbuminuria also tend to differ from their normoalbuminuric counterparts, by their greater age and longer disease duration, and by further deterioration of conventional cardiovascular risk factors, including dyslipidaemia and smoking. They show some features of the metabolic 'syndrome X', with central obesity and relatively greater insulin resistance. There is also evidence of endothelial dysfunction (eg impaired vasodilatory and increased vasoconstrictive responses to locally infused vasoactive agents), consistent with the view that microalbuminuria is simply one manifestation of global vascular dysfunction throughout the body, and perhaps explaining the powerful association of microalbuminuria with premature cardiovascular death (see below).

The 20–40% of microalbuminuric NIDDM patients who deteriorate to overt nephropathy are characterised by increased HbA_{1c} levels, increased blood pressure (particularly systolic), higher initial UAER, hyperlipidaemia and smoking [9]. Recent reports have demonstrated familial clustering of renal disease in NIDDM, in conjunction with a parental history of hypertension and cardiovascular events. Familial, presumably genetic, influences have also been identified in IDDM; various candidate genes (eg angiotensin converting enzyme (ACE)) have been investigated but not yet conclusively implicated.

Implications for outcome in NIDDM

Recently, it has become clear that microalbuminuria is a marker for increased cardiovascular risk, not just worsening renal function. Its development appears to have particularly grave consequences in NIDDM patients, to whom it imparts a 2-to 5-fold increase in mortality, predominantly from cardiovascular causes [10]. Ten-year mortality is as high as 70–80% in microalbuminuric patients, compared with only 20% for those with normal UAER. The corresponding figures after 4 years are 25% and 4%, respectively (Fig. 7). The power of microalbuminuria as a risk factor is illustrated by the finding that even a single measurement in the routine outpatients setting showing a raised albumin to creatinine ratio predicts a 50% mortality at 8 years [10]. It has been reported that the impact of abnormal UAER on mortality is considerably increased if microalbuminuria develops 5 or more years after NIDDM is diagnosed, particularly if associated with increased HbA_{1c} levels.

This issue is of crucial importance in NIDDM, in which the commonest cause of death remains cardiovascular, especially coronary heart disease. In most studies, the contribution of the increased UAER to mortality is considerably greater than the traditional cardiovascular risk factors. On the other hand, patients with normal UAER are at low risk; not only are they unlikely to develop nephropathy, but they do not suffer increased mortality over 8–10 years.

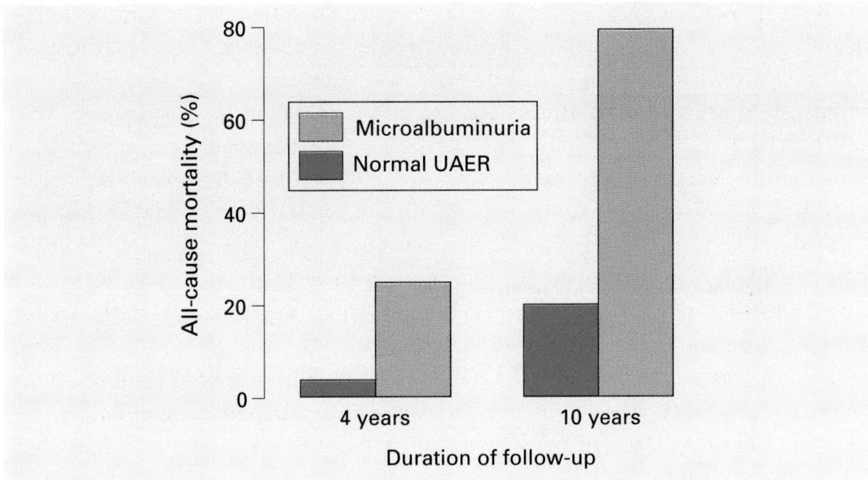

Fig. 7 Impact of microalbuminuria on mortality (from all causes) after 4 and 10 years in patients with non-insulin dependent diabetes mellitus (NIDDM). Patient deaths are predominantly due to cardiovascular disease (UAER = urinary albumin excretion rate).

☐ SCREENING AND DIAGNOSIS OF DIABETIC RENAL DISEASE

It will be obvious from the above that the early detection of diabetic renal dysfunction is important for several reasons: in particular, it will identify high-risk populations who may progress from microalbuminuria to overt nephropathy; those who will need careful attention to detect and treat hypertension and other risk factors, as well as long-term monitoring for possible renal support therapy in those with established nephropathy. Guidelines issued by specialist diabetes associations unanimously support regular screening for microalbuminuria. Cost-benefit analyses underline the financial savings made by early detection and intervention for microalbuminuria in IDDM patients [11], and there can be little doubt that the same arguments apply (perhaps even more convincingly) to NIDDM.

Thus, all patients with diabetes mellitus should be screened annually for microalbuminuria. Many strategies for screening microalbuminuria have been proposed, and one such is depicted in Fig. 8. However, most authors now favour the measurement of an albumin to creatinine ratio in an early morning spot urine sample, as it is sensitive and specific enough for screening purposes [11].

Once microalbuminuria has been identified, confirmation and close monitoring of albumin excretion is necessary, for example with serial measurements, at least once a year, of the albumin to creatinine ratio, or albumin concentrations in 24 h or timed overnight urine collections.

Demonstration of persistent proteinuria by routine dip-stick methods confirms the presence of established nephropathy. In such patients, serum creatinine concentrations must also be measured regularly, and any tendency to rise followed up. Declining glomerular filtration can be monitored by plotting inverse creatinine ratios (eg 1000 ÷ serum creatinine) or formal measurements of GFR, ideally with

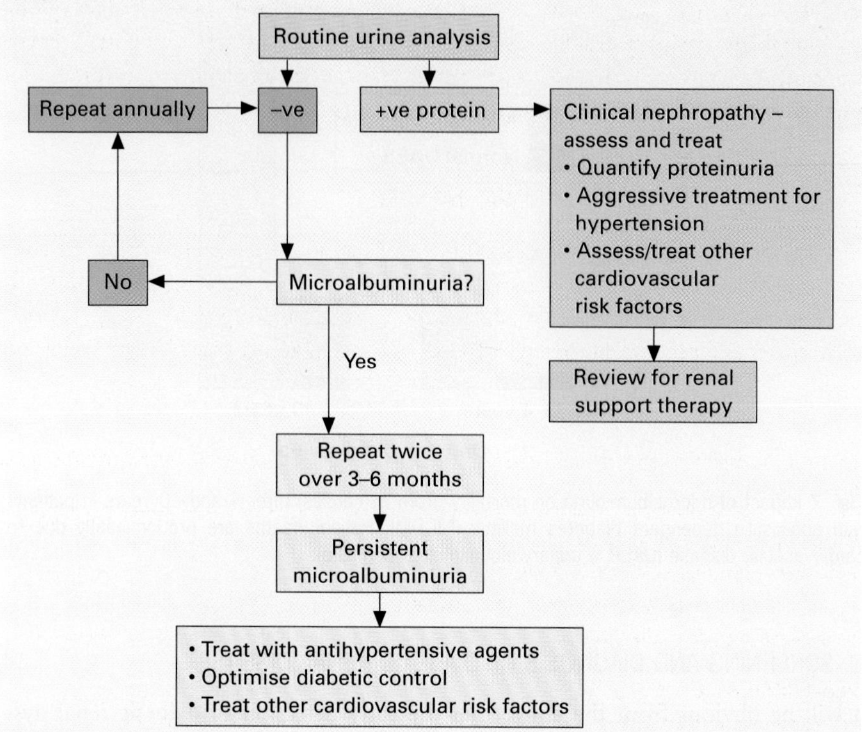

Fig. 8 Proposed scheme for the screening and management of microalbuminuria in diabetes mellitus. (Adapted from Ref 11.)

Cr-EDTA or equivalent methods, as creatinine clearance is unreliable in some diabetic patients. These measures characteristically show a linear decline at a rate that is constant for each subject and can be used to predict when renal support will become necessary (corresponding to a GFR of <10 ml/min, or serum creatinine of 400 μmol/l). Any deterioration in renal function that departs from the predicted linear decline should raise the suspicion of an additional, superimposed cause such as a urinary tract infection or obstruction.

The possibility should also be considered that renal impairment in a diabetic patient is not due to diabetic nephropathy. This applies particularly to NIDDM: in hospital based clinics, 25–30% of proteinuric NIDDM patients have non-diabetic renal disease as the cause. Atypical features that should raise this suspicion include:

- the absence of significant retinopathy;
- haematuria, possibly associated with an abnormal urinary sediment;
- the rapid onset of proteinuria;
- a normal blood pressure; and
- departure from the linear decline in glomerular filtration described above.

In these patients, other diseases must be actively excluded. These include glomerulonephritis, urinary tract infection (including tuberculosis), vasculitis, urinary tract outflow obstruction and renovascular disease. Detailed further investigation, including renal biopsy, may be necessary (see Table 1).

□ TREATMENT OF DIABETIC RENAL DISEASE

Management of diabetic renal disease has two distinct phases, with different aims: first, in the early stages of the condition, to delay its progression; and secondly, in patients who have already reached end-stage renal failure, to provide an appropriate form of renal replacement therapy. Also important, and discussed briefly below, are

Table 1 Diagnostic tests to be considered in diabetic patients with proteinuria and/or renal dysfunction.

Midstream urine sample
- Microscopy: sediment, red and white blood cells
- Phase-contrast microscopy: fragmented red cells
- Culture, including tuberculosis

Renal ultrasound

Intravenous pyelogram
Renal artery imaging (including digital subtraction/ spiral CT scanning)
} NB: potential risks of contrast medium; discontinuation of metformin

Glomerular filtration rate
- Isotopic clearance (eg Cr-EDTA)
- Creatinine clearance

Markers for vasculitis and other glomerulonephritis
- Erythrocyte sedimentation rate
- Autoantibody screen, including anti-glomerular basement membrane
- ANCA
- Complement levels
- Immunoglobulins

Renal biopsy

NB: Features suggesting non-diabetic causes of renal dysfunction
- Abnormal renal function without proteinuria
- Absence of diabetic retinopathy
- Normal blood pressure
- Haematuria
- Cellular urinary sediment
- Rapid onset (esp. proteinuria); departure from linear decline

ANCA = anti-neutrophil cytoplasmic antibody
CT = computed tomography

primary preventive measures that might reduce the risk of diabetic nephropathy developing in the first place.

Interventions to slow the progression of renal disease

The key approaches currently available are, first, improved glycaemic control and the effective use of antihypertensive agents and, second, reducing dietary protein intake and treatment with lipid-lowering drugs. The latter have both been shown in small, short-term studies to decrease urinary protein excretion rates, but these findings need to be confirmed in a broader setting before these interventions can become accepted in clinical practice.

Improved glycaemic control

The beneficial effects of good glycaemic control on the evolution of nephropathy in IDDM are now proven beyond doubt; the same principle applies to NIDDM.

Insulin-dependent diabetes. The Diabetes Control and Complications Trial (DCCT) conclusively demonstrated that improved glycaemic control achieved with intensive insulin treatment reduced the risks of microvascular complications, including microalbuminuria, over a 9-year period [12] (Fig. 9). Particular benefits were seen in the 'primary intervention cohort', that is, subjects with short-duration IDDM (<5 years) and no evidence of renal disease at entry to the study. Intensified insulin therapy (which reduced mean HbA_{1c} to about 1% above the non-diabetic range) decreased the 9-year risk of developing microalbuminuria to 16%, compared with the cumulative incidence in the conventionally treated group of 26% – a 34% reduction in risk over this period. In a secondary intervention cohort (with longer duration of diabetes and some early evidence of microvascular disease), the risk of developing microalbuminuria was reduced by 43% in the intensively treated group (cumulative incidence of 22%, compared with 42% in the conventionally treated group). These benefits of intensive treatment were at the expense of more frequent hypoglycaemia (up to threefold in subjects with the lowest HbA_{1c} values) and a significant weight gain that averaged 4.5 kg after 5 years; moreover, glycaemic control was improved (not normalised) only with extensive support from a multi-disciplinary diabetes team that is difficult to match outside a trial setting.

It has been suggested that there may be a 'threshold' value for glycaemic control (eg an HbA_{1c} concentration of 7.5–8%) below which the risk of microvascular complications, including nephropathy, is markedly reduced. The consensus view now argues against this, and suggests that the risk of developing nephropathy increases progressively as glycaemia rises.

The role of improved glycaemic control on the progression of nephropathy at or beyond the stage of microalbuminuria is more contentious. Recent studies have not been able to confirm previous findings suggesting a beneficial effect of improved glycaemic control on the progression of established microalbuminuria. In the DCCT study, the progression of microalbuminuria to overt nephropathy in a small sub-

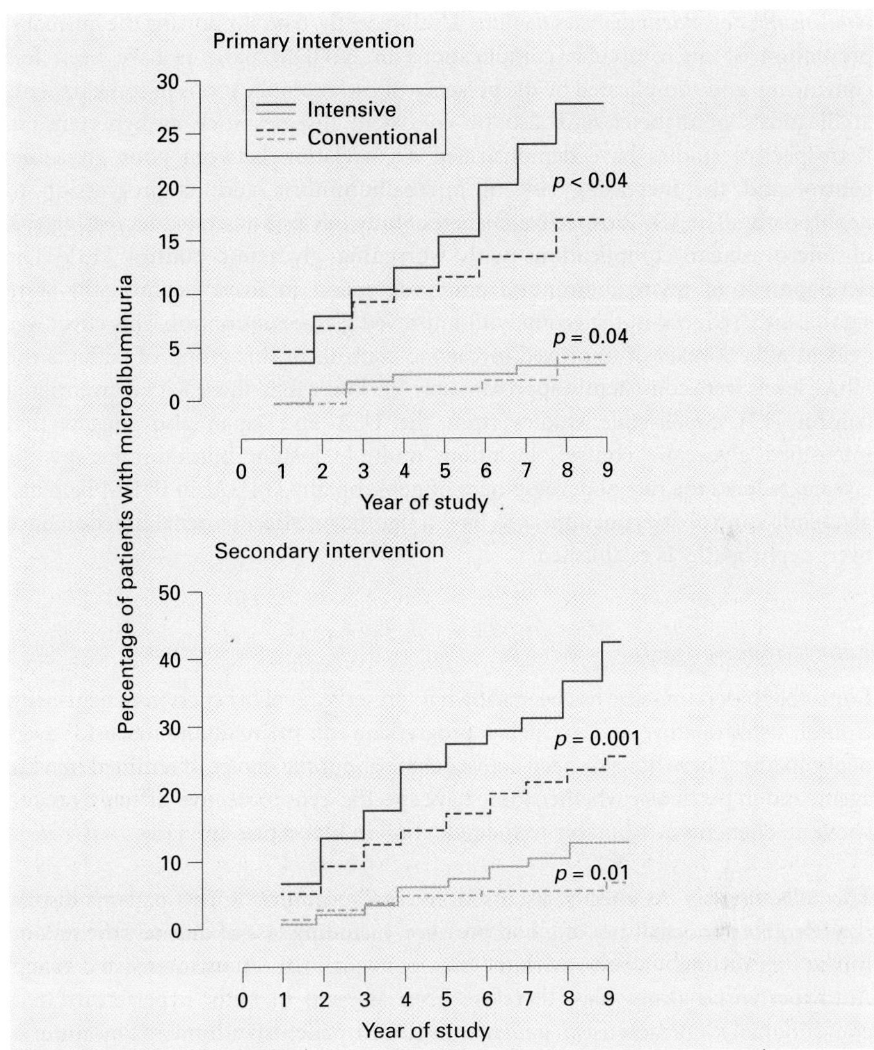

Fig. 9 The Diabetes Control and Complications Trial (DCCT). Beneficial effects on the development of microalbuminuria of intensive insulin treatment in patients with IDDM. Results are presented separately for primary and secondary intervention cohorts. (Adapted from Ref 11.)

group of 73 patients was similar for the intensively and the conventionally treated groups over a mean follow-up period of 6.5 years. Similar results were reported for the Microalbuminuria Collaborative Study group in the UK, although this study sustained significant glycaemic separation between the intensively and the conventionally treated groups for only 3 years.

Once clinical nephropathy is established, there is no evidence that glycaemic control influences renal function. Its impact on other microvascular complications may well continue, and thus it would be appropriate to achieve the best glycaemic control feasible.

Non-insulin dependent diabetes mellitus. Until recently, data supporting the 'primary' prevention of microvascular complications in NIDDM patients have been less convincing, and complicated by the presence of such complications in some patients at diagnosis of diabetes and also by coexistent diseases such as hypertension. Retrospective studies have demonstrated a correlation between poor glycaemic control and the increasing risk of microalbuminuria and its progression to nephropathy. The UK Prospective Diabetes Study has demonstrated increasing risk of microvascular complications with worsening glycaemic control [13]. The development of microalbuminuria and progression to overt nephropathy were significantly reduced in the group with improved glycaemic control. This effect was evident after 9 years of improved glycaemic control. In this group of patients the HbA_{1c} levels were consistently approximately 1% lower than those with conventional control [13]. Small-scale studies from the USA and Japan also suggest that intensified glycaemic control, including multiple insulin injection therapy for 6 years, reduces the rate of development of nephropathy [14]. As in IDDM patients, glycaemic control does not appear to have a significant effect on renal function once overt nephropathy is established.

Antihypertensive agents

Control of blood pressure has been shown to preserve renal function in patients with clinical nephropathy, and to delay progression of microalbuminuria to overt nephropathy. There has also been active debate about the choice of antihypertensive agent, and in particular whether some have specific 'renoprotective' effects over and above any benefits attributable to the reduction in blood pressure [15].

Microalbuminuria. As already discussed, microalbuminuric IDDM patients display considerable abnormalities of blood pressure, including loss of diurnal rhythm and minor elevations albeit within the conventional 'normotensive' range. Antihypertensive drugs have therefore been assessed in both 'hypertensive' and conventionally 'normotensive' patients. In IDDM patients with microalbuminuria, short-term studies using various antihypertensive agents have demonstrated a reduction in UAER, as have longer-term studies particularly of ACE inhibitors and calcium-channel blockers. For example, captopril (50 mg twice daily) given to 'normotensive' patients with microalbuminuria demonstrated a 63% reduction in the risk of progression to overt nephropathy, as compared with placebo [16] (Fig. 10]. In the actively treated group, blood pressure was reduced by a few mmHg, which was not surprising given the blood pressure abnormalities in microalbuminuric patients. A similar reduction in the risk of progression of microalbuminuria has recently been reported by the EUCLID Study Group, with the ACE inhibitor lisinopril [6]. It has been suggested that ACE inhibitors might have specific renoprotective effects. However, the Italian Microalbuminuria Study Group also reported identical reductions in the progression of microalbuminuria with the dihydropyridine calcium-channel blocker nifedipine (in its slow-release formulation) and lisinopril [7] (Fig. 11). However, regression of microalbuminuria

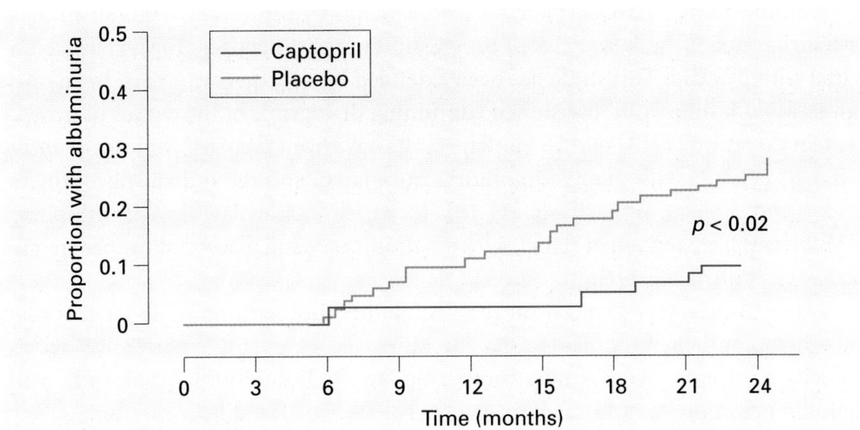

Fig. 10 Progression to nephropathy in normotensive insulin-dependent diabetic patients with microalbuminuria, receiving either captopril or placebo. Blood pressure was below 140/90 mmHg for subjects under 35 years of age, and below 160/95 mmHg for those over 35 years. (Data from the Microalbuminuria Captopril Study Group [16].)

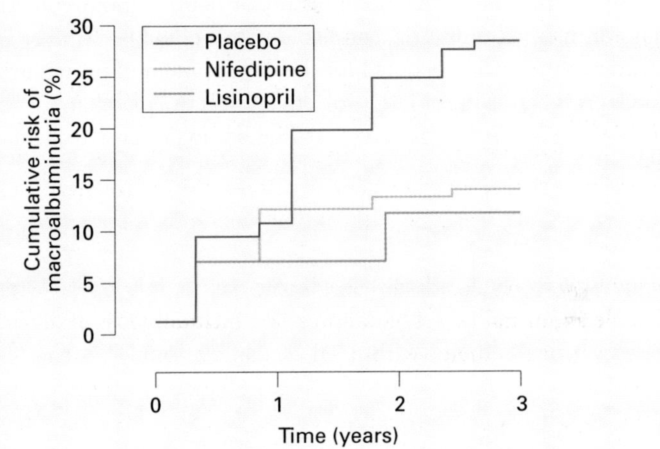

Fig. 11 Cumulative risk of developing nephropathy in normotensive microalbuminuric insulin-dependent diabetes mellitus (IDDM) patients, receiving placebo, lisinopril or nifedipine. (Adapted from Ref 7.)

into normoalbuminuria was observed more frequently with lisinopril than nifedipine.

It remains to be established whether this reduction in the otherwise progressive increase in UAER translates into structural protection, but the favourable comparisons with the placebo-treated group suggest that antihypertensive agents (consistently the ACE inhibitors) delay the onset of nephropathy in this 'normotensive' group.

Similar results have been reported for normotensive NIDDM patients with microalbuminuria, over periods of up to 7 years [17–19]. In relatively young microalbuminuric NIDDM patients whose blood pressure was <140/90 mmHg, enalapril reduced the 5-year risk of progression to overt nephropathy by 60%, compared with placebo. This study has been extended by a further two years, in an open randomised fashion, and has shown continuing divergence of the curves of urinary protein excretion [19] (Fig. 12). Similar results have been reported for normotensive NIDDM patients with microalbuminuria from Japan and the Indian subcontinent, over 4 and 5 years, respectively [17,18]. In patients treated with ACE inhibitors, UAER levels have remained stable, whereas those receiving placebo show progressive increases in protein excretion.

These studies have centred on ACE inhibitors, but various short-term studies have now confirmed similar results for other classes of antihypertensive agents. Indeed, a recent 7-year study comparing an ACE inhibitor (cilazapril) with amlodipine, a long-acting calcium-channel blocker of the dihydropyridine group, reported a greater reduction in UAER with the former but comparable preservation of GFR by the two agents [20].

The Hypertension in Diabetes Study, embedded within the UK prospective diabetes study, has demonstrated a reduction in the development of microalbuminuria in a group of hypertensive NIDDM patients, after 4.5 years of tight blood pressure control [21]. A blood pressure of 144/82 mmHg conferred a 30% risk reduction for microalbuminuria, compared with a blood pressure of 154/87 mmHg. No significant difference was noted for the development of proteinuria between the two blood pressure groups. The protective effect was similar for either an ACE inhibitor or a beta-blocker used as first-line antihypertensive agents. However, in

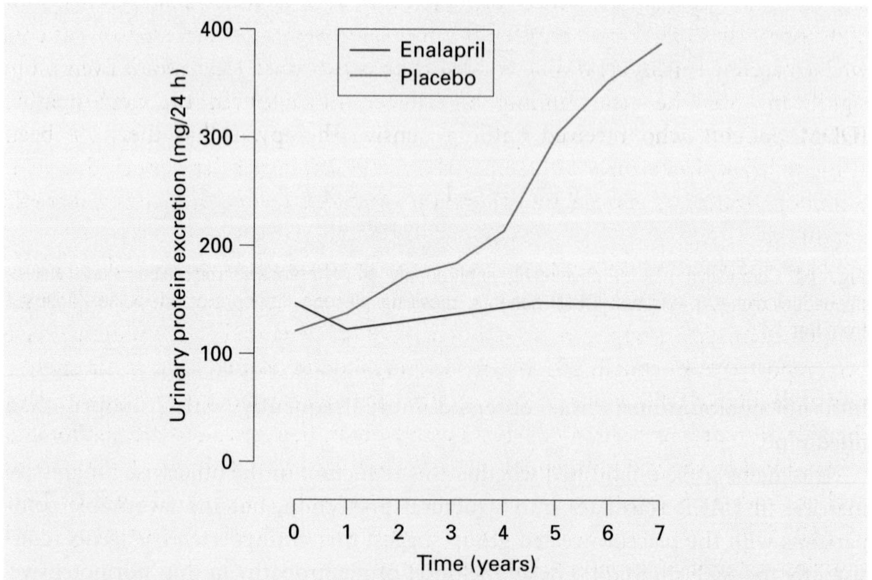

Fig. 12 Progression of proteinuria in normotensive microalbuminuric non-insulin dependent diabetes mellitus (NIDDM) patients, who were normotensive by World Health Organization criteria, receiving either enalapril or placebo. (Adapted from Ref 19.)

order to achieve the 'tight' blood pressure control, multiple antihypertensive agents were required (up to three agents).

Established nephropathy. It is well recognised that aggressive antihypertensive therapy in diabetic patients, both IDDM and NIDDM, who have established nephropathy and hypertension will reduce the rate of decline in GFR from 5–10 ml/min per year to approximately 1 ml/min per year, with a parallel reduction in proteinuria. Protection of renal function is evident in those patients who show a decline in urinary protein excretion. This property provides a surrogate marker enabling the evaluation of the renoprotective effect of the antihypertensive agents used and blood pressure levels attained.

These studies have also established target blood pressure levels for diabetic patients with nephropathy that will most effectively prevent the fall in GFR. Routine measurement blood pressure levels should be below 130/80 mmHg [15]. Retrospective studies in IDDM patients suggest that the cumulative death rate has fallen progressively over the past 20 years with increasing use of antihypertensive treatment, from 80% to less than 10% [15]. The benefits of aggressive blood pressure control are therefore incontrovertible.

Recent studies have attempted to address the issue of specific renoprotective effects of particular antihypertensive agents, as with microalbuminuria. In a group of 409 IDDM patients with established nephropathy who were given conventional antihypertensive therapy to control blood pressure (<140/90 mmHg), the addition of an ACE inhibitor for up to 4 years halved the risk of serum creatinine levels increasing twofold, and also decreased progression to renal support therapy (dialysis or transplantation) [22]. The beneficial effects of additional captopril therapy (25 mg thrice daily) were concentrated in patients whose baseline serum creatinine concentrations exceeded 133 μmol/l. Even more significant was the clear finding of reduced mortality in the nephropathic IDDM patients who received antihypertensive therapy. It has therefore been suggested that, in keeping with most other chronic glomerular nephritides, ACE inhibitors appear to have a specific renoprotective effect in established diabetic nephropathy.

Most information on antihypertensive therapy in established diabetic nephropathy derives from IDDM, but similar data are now emerging for NIDDM patients. In them, non-dihydropyridine calcium-channel blockers and ACE inhibitors have been reported to be equally effective in lowering blood pressure, proteinuria and the rate of decline of GFR, while both were better than a beta-blocker combined with a thiazide diuretic. However, more recent comparisons between an ACE inhibitor and a beta-blocker showed comparable maintenance of GFR (halving of the rate of decline) with both agents. At least three other studies have suggested similar effects of ACE inhibitors and conventional antihypertensive drugs in protecting renal function in NIDDM patients with nephropathy.

Overall, as with IDDM, antihypertensive therapy is of paramount importance in protecting renal function in NIDDM patients with hypertension and nephropathy. Specific roles of various classes of antihypertensive agents have not been clearly established for the NIDDM patients; in particular the effects of different drugs on mortality are unknown.

Other measures

As already mentioned, the main causes of death in patients with diabetic nephropathy are renal failure and arterial disease, particularly myocardial infarction. The high cardiovascular risks of microalbuminuria and proteinuria in NIDDM have been described above, and it has also been shown that the development of persistent proteinuria confers a 50-fold increase in cardiovascular mortality on IDDM patients.

Conventional cardiovascular risk factors other than blood pressure (smoking, dyslipidaemia, obesity) should therefore be actively tackled, although the effects of these interventions on mortality in patients with renal disease are as yet uncertain.

Cardiovascular disease is a common cause of death in patients who have received a renal transplant or are receiving haemodialysis, and cardiovascular risk (including coronary angiography, if indicated) should be carefully assessed in patients being considered for renal replacement therapy. The potential of silent myocardial ischaemia should also be considered in such patients.

Renal support therapy

The options for the diabetic patient approaching end-stage renal failure are the same as for non-diabetic people (Table 2). There was previous widespread reluctance to consider diabetic patients for renal transplantation or haemodialysis, but this prejudice is now diminishing. A detailed discussion of this topic is beyond the scope of this chapter, but can be found in the recent review [23].

Table 2 Treatment modalities available for renal support for diabetic patients.

Peritoneal dialysis

- Intermittent peritoneal dialysis (IPD)
- Continuous ambulatory peritoneal dialysis (CAPD)
- Continuous cyclic peritoneal dialysis (CCPD)

Haemodialysis

- Home haemodialysis
- Institutional haemodialysis

Renal transplantation

- Cadaver donor kidney
- Living donor kidney

Combined pancreas/kidney transplantation

- Type 1 insulin-dependent patients

□ CONCLUSIONS

Diabetic nephropathy is a common and important complication which has undoubtedly been neglected and inadequately treated in the past. Nowadays, simple and effective screening and specific forms of therapy that can help to slow the natural history of the condition can bring substantial benefits to these patients.

REFERENCES

1 Krowlewski AS, Warram JH. Natural history of diabetic nephropathy. How much can it be changed? *Diabetes Rev* 1995; **3**: 446–59.

2 Gall M-A, Nielsen FS, Smidt UN, Parving H-H. The course of kidney function in Type 2 (non-insulin dependent) diabetic patients with diabetic nephropathy. *Diabetologia* 1993; **36**: 1071–8.

3 Mogensen CE, Christensen CK, Vittinghus E. The stages in diabetic renal disease. With emphasis on the stage of incipient diabetic nephropathy. *Diabetes* 1983; **32**(suppl): 64–78.

4 Vora JP, Dolben J, Williams JD, *et al.* Impact of initial treatment on renal function in newly diagnosed non-insulin dependent (Type 2) diabetic patients. *Diabetologia* 1993; **36**: 734–40.

5 Nelson RG, Bennett PH, Beck GJ, *et al.* Development and progression of renal disease in Pima Indians with non-insulin dependent diabetes mellitus. *N Engl J Med* 1996; **335**: 1636–42.

6 The EUCLID study group. Randomised placebo-controlled trial of Lisinopril in normotensive patients with insulin-dependent diabetes and normoalbuminuria or microalbuminuria. *Lancet* 1997; **349**: 1787–92.

7 The Italian Microalbuminuria Study Group in IDDM. Effects of Lisinopril and Nifedipine on the progression of overt albuminuria in IDDM patients with incipient nephropathy and normal blood pressure. *Diabetes Care* 1998; **21**: 104–10.

8 Mathiesen ER, Ronn B, Storm B, *et al.* The natural course of microalbuminuria in insulin dependent diabetes: a 10 year prospective study. *Diabetic Med* 1995; **12**: 482–7.

9 Klein R, Klein BEK, Moss SE, Cruickshank J. Ten-year incidence of gross proteinuria in people with diabetes. *Diabetes* 1995; **44**: 916–23.

10 Alzaid AA. Microalbuminuria in non-insulin dependent diabetes. *Diabetes Care* 1996; **19**: 79–89.

11 Bennett PH, Haffner S, Kasiske BL, *et al.* Screening and management of microalbuminuria in patients with diabetes mellitus. *Am J Kidney Dis* 1995; **25**: 107–12.

12 The Diabetes Control and Complications Trial Research Group. The effect of intensive treatment of diabetes on the development and progression of long-term complications in insulin dependent diabetes mellitus. *N Engl J Med* 1993; **329**: 977–86.

13 UK Prospective Diabetes Study (UKPDS) Group. Intensive blood-glucose control with sulphonylureas or insulin compared with conventional treatment and risk of complications in patients with type 2 diabetes (UKPDS 33). *Lancet* 1998; **352**: 837–53.

14 Ohkubo Y, Kishikawa H, Araki E, *et al.* Intensive insulin therapy prevents the progression of diabetic microvascular complications in Japanese patients with non insulin dependent diabetes mellitus – a randomised prospective 6 year study. *Diabetes Res Clin Pract* 1995; **28**: 103–17.

15 Parving H-H, Possing P. The use of antihypertensive agents in prevention and treatment of diabetic nephropathy. *Curr Opin Nephrol Hypertens* 1994; **3**: 292–300.

16 The Microalbuminuria Captopril Study Group. Captopril reduces the risk of nephropathy in IDDM patients with microalbuminuria. *Diabetologia* 1996; **39**: 587–93.

17 Sano T, Hotta N, Kawamura T, *et al.* Effects of long-term Enalapril treatment on persistent microalbuminuria in normotensive Type 2 diabetic patients: results of a 4 year prospective randomised study. *Diabetic Med* 1996; **13**: 120–4.

18 Ahmad J, Siddiqui MA, Ahmad H. Effective postponement of diabetic nephropathy with Enalapril in normotensive Type 2 diabetic patients with microalbuminuria. *Diabetes Care* 1997; **20**: 1567–81.

19 Ravid M, Lang R, Rachmani R, Lishner M. Long-term renoprotective effect of angiotensin-converting enzyme inhibition in non-insulin dependent diabetes mellitus. A 7 year follow-up study. *Arch Intern Med* 1996; **156**: 286–9.

20 Velussi M, Brocco E, Frigato F, *et al.* Effects of Cilazapril and Amlodipine on kidney function in hypertensive NIDDM patients. *Diabetes* 1996; **45**: 216–22.

21 UK Prospective Diabetes Study (UKPDS) Group. Tight blood pressure control and risk of macrovascular and microvascular complications in type 2 diabetes: UKPDS 38. *Br Med J* 1998; **317**: 703–13.

22 Lewis EJ, Hunsicker LG, Bain RP, Rhode RD. The effect of angiotensin converting enzyme inhibition on diabetic nephropathy. *N Engl J Med* 1993; **329**: 1456–62.

23 Freidman EA. Management choices in diabetic end-stage renal disease. *Nephrol Dial Transplant* 1995; **10** (Suppl 7): 61–9.

Epilepsy: new understanding from new genes

Mark Gardiner

□ INTRODUCTION

The epilepsies are one of the most common serious neurological disorders, with up to 60 million people affected worldwide. Genetic factors may contribute to the aetiology in up to 40% of patients, and there has recently been significant progress in elucidating the genetic basis of specific epilepsies at a molecular level [1].

Epilepsy may be the end result of many different pathological processes, and it is not surprising that epilepsy genes have been found to fall into several distinct categories. These include genes in which mutations cause maldevelopment of the brain or progressive neurodegeneration, usually associated with gross structural changes in the brain and severe neurological deficits in addition to recurrent seizures. However, the most exciting development is the accumulating evidence that certain variants of idiopathic or primary epilepsy – the commonest form of the disease – arise from mutations in genes for ion channels.

A brief review will be provided of the genetics of human epilepsies, together with an overview of the current status of gene mapping and isolation in this field. This is followed by an account of the available evidence for the involvement of two classes of ion channel in human epilepsy, namely neuronal nicotinic acetylcholine receptors and voltage-gated calcium channels. The acetylcholine receptor is a ligand-gated ion channel which is most permeable to chloride ions; it is likely, but difficult to prove, that Ca^{2+} ions flow through it *in vivo*.

□ GENETICS OF HUMAN EPILEPSIES

There are over 120 single-gene Mendelian disorders that include epilepsy as part of the phenotype. Most of these diseases are rare and, in most cases, epilepsy is just one component of a more complex neurological disorder. Autosomal dominant, autosomal recessive and X-linked patterns of inheritance are found.

Progress has been particularly rapid in the genetic analysis of these Mendelian epilepsies, as illustrated in Table 1. Genes have been isolated for a number of progressive myoclonic epilepsies including Unverricht-Lundborg disease and the neuronal ceroid lipofuscinoses, while others are currently being targeted by the positional cloning approach. The genes have also been isolated for several major genetic neurological diseases that cause epilepsy, notably fragile X syndrome and tuberous sclerosis.

Most important, the genes responsible for specific variants of idiopathic epilepsy with Mendelian inheritance have been identified. Mutations in the neuronal

Table 1. Map location and identity of genes for Mendelian inherited epilepsies.

Disease	Mode of inheritance	Gene location	Gene symbol (gene product)	MIM number
Primary epilepsies				
Benign familial neonatal convulsions	AD	20q13	EBN1 (potassium channel)	121200
		8q24	EBN2	121201
Benign familial infantile convulsions	AD	19q		
Autosomal dominant nocturnal frontal lobe epilepsy	AD	20q13	CHRNA4 (nAChR α4 subunit)	600513
Partial epilepsy with auditory symptoms	AD	10q		600512
Progressive myoclonic epilepsies				
Unverricht-Lundborg disease (Baltic myoclonus, Mediterranean myoclonus)	AR	21q22	EPM1 (cystatin B)	254800
Neuronal ceroid lipofuscinosis				
Infantile	AR	1p32	CLN1 (palmitoyl protein thioesterase)	256730
Late infantile	AR	11p15	CLN2 (lysosomal protease)	204500
Variant late infantile	AR	15q21–23	CLN6	
Juvenile	AR	16p12	CLN3	204200
Finnish variant	AR	13q22	CLN5	256731
Lafora disease	AR	6q23–25		254780
Progressive epilepsy with mental retardation (Northern epilepsy)	AR	8p	EPMR	600143
Disorders including epilepsy as part of the phenotype				
Tuberous sclerosis	AD	9q34	TSC1 (hamartin)	191100
		16p13	TSC2 (tuberin)	191092
Angelman syndrome	AD	15q13	ANCR E6-AP (ubiquitin-protein ligase)	105830
Neurofibromatosis type 1	AD	17q11	NF1 (neurofibromin)	162200
Fragile X	X-linked	Xq27	FMR-1 (fragile X mental retardation protein)	309550

AD = autosomal dominant
AR = autosomal recessive
MIM = Mendelian Inheritance in Man

nicotinic acetylcholine receptor α4 subunit gene, *CHRNA4*, cause autosomal dominant nocturnal frontal lobe epilepsy (ADNFLE). Mutations in a novel potassium channel gene cause benign familial neonatal convulsions (BFNC), which also shows autosomal dominant transmission. These genes are likely to provide clues to the genes underlying the more common familial epilepsies.

Most familial epilepsies display a 'complex' pattern of inheritance, suggesting the interplay of several genetic loci and environmental factors. These include such well defined phenotypes as juvenile myoclonic epilepsy (JME) and childhood absence epilepsy, as well as other less distinct forms of idiopathic or primary generalised epilepsies which tend to show familial clustering. Progress in the analysis of these inherited epilepsies has been less rapid, reflecting the difficulties encountered in applying molecular genetic techniques to non-Mendelian diseases.

□ EPILEPSIES AS ION CHANNEL DISEASES

Ion channels play a key role in the function of excitable tissues; from first principles, mutations in genes encoding ion channels might therefore be predicted to cause disorders characterised by paroxysmal disturbances of function in these tissues. Several Mendelian diseases affecting skeletal and cardiac muscle, spinal cord and peripheral nerve have now been shown to be ion-channelopathies, and preliminary evidence in man (and mouse) suggests that a proportion of the inherited epilepsies are also ion channel diseases.

In skeletal muscle, sodium channel mutations cause hyperkalaemic periodic paralysis, while chloride channel mutations cause Thomsen and Becker disease and a calcium channel mutation leads to hypokalaemic periodic paralysis [2]. In cardiac muscle, the long QT syndrome can result from mutations in either a sodium channel or two types of potassium channel gene (*HERG* and *KVLQT1*). Episodic ataxia-myokymia syndrome is due to mutations in a potassium channel gene, *KCNA1*. Hereditary hyperekplexia or familial startle syndrome has been shown to arise from mutations in the gene encoding the α1 subunit of the glycine receptor (*GLRA1*) [3]; the *spasmodic* mouse, which displays a similar phenotype to startle syndrome, has mutations in the homologous murine gene, *glra1*.

At present, two forms of Mendelian inheritance human epilepsy have been shown to arise from ion channel gene mutations in at least some of the affected families. ADNFLE is caused by mutations in the gene encoding the α4 subunit of the neuronal nicotinic acetylcholine receptor (*CHRNA4*). Benign familial neonatal convulsions is caused by mutations in novel potassium channel genes (*KCNQ2* and *KCNQ3*), closely related to one of the potassium channels involved in the long QT syndrome [4,5]. In addition, preliminary evidence suggests that the gene encoding the α7 subunit of the neuronal nicotinic acetylcholine receptor may be involved in some families with juvenile myoclonic epilepsy.

Evidence for involvement of voltage-gated calcium channels in epilepsy has come from studies of two murine models of spike-wave epilepsy, *tottering* (tg) and *lethargic* (le), which have been shown to arise from mutations in *Cacna1a* and *Cacnb4* respectively.

The role of neuronal nicotinic acetylcholine receptors and voltage-gated calcium channels in inherited epilepsies of man and mouse will now be considered in more depth.

Neuronal nicotinic acetylcholine receptors and epilepsy

It has been known for a decade that nicotinic receptors are abundant in many parts of the brain, but their function remains uncertain [6]. Neuronal nicotinic acetylcholine receptors (nAChRs) are heteromultimeric complexes, each composed of 5 subunits (Fig. 1). At least 11 different subunits (α2–α9, β2–β4) are found in nAChRs. The predominant form consists of two α4 and three β2 subunits, but it is known that α7, α8 and α9 subunits can each self-associate to form homomultimers *in vitro*. Available evidence indicates that nAChRs serve as presynaptic 'modulators' of neuronal activity, rather than postsynaptic 'mediators' of transmission. Homomeric α7 channels have an unusually high calcium permeability.

Role in autosomal dominant nocturnal frontal lobe epilepsy

Initial evidence that nAChRs may be implicated in epilepsy has come from investigation of an uncommon idiopathic partial epilepsy, ADNFLE. This was first

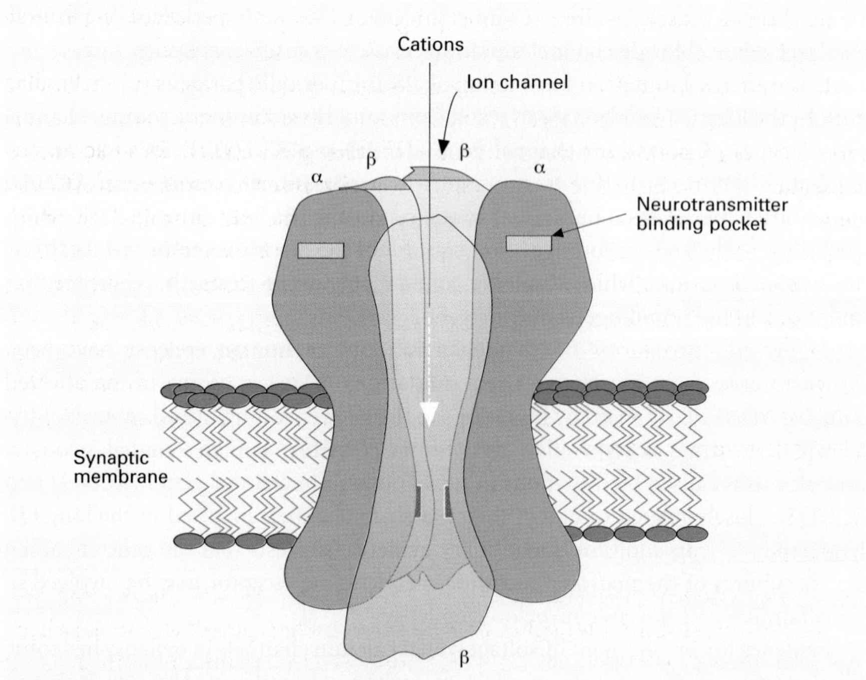

Fig. 1 Structures of neuronal nicotinic acetylcholine receptors (nAChRs). (Reprinted from Ref 12, with the permission of Oxford University Press).

described as a distinct syndrome by Scheffer *et al* [7] in a report of six families and was the first partial epilepsy shown to follow a Mendelian (autosomal dominant) pattern of inheritance. Frequent, violent brief seizures occur at night, usually beginning in childhood. Study of a very large Australian kindred [8] showed that a gene for ADNFLE mapped to chromosome 20q13.2–q13.3. This region of chromosome 20q was investigated as a candidate region; interestingly, another autosomal dominant idiopathic epilepsy, BFNC, had previously been shown to map to this site in a proportion of families. The neuronal nicotinic acetylcholine receptor α4 subunit (*CHRNA4*), already located to the same region of chromosome 20q, represented a 'positional candidate' and was therefore analysed for mutations. A missense mutation was found in all 21 available affected family members [9]. This C→T substitution causes replacement of a serine with phenylalanine at codon 248, a highly conserved amino acid residue in the second transmembrane domain (see Fig. 1). This represented a very important advance, as it was the first gene to be identified for an inherited idiopathic epilepsy in humans. But how does this mutation explain the electrophysiological and clinical features of ADNFLE? The properties of wild-type receptors composed of native α4 and β2 subunits have been compared to those of mutant receptors in which the α4 subunits carried the mutation at serine 248. When the wild-type and mutated receptors were expressed in *Xenopus* oocytes [10], the mutation apeared to cause loss of function: the receptor converts faster to an unresponsive state and remains longer in this inactive conformation. This defect may disturb the balance between inhibitory and excitatory synaptic transmission, but why this epileptogenic effect predominates in the frontal lobe and shows such a striking dependence on sleep remains a mystery.

It is now apparent that there is both allelic and locus heterogeneity underlying ADNFLE (ie the same phenotype may be produced by mutations of various types in more than one gene). A distinct mutation in another part of the *CHRNA4* gene has subsequently been identified in a Norwegian family: insertion of three nucleotides causes a leucine insertion at the C-terminal end of the M2 domain [11] which indirectly decreases function by reducing channel permeability to calcium. Moreover, some families with typical ADNFLE are not linked to chromosome 20q13.2–13.3. It has recently emerged that the BFNC phenotype, which maps to this region of chromosome 20q and thereby renders it a candidate region for linkage analysis of ADNFLE, is not caused by mutations in *CHRNA4*. In some families, 20q-linked BFNC is caused by mutations in the novel potassium channel gene *KCNQ2* located very close to *CHRNA4*.

Role in juvenile myoclonic epilepsy

The above results highlighted the genes encoding nAChR subunits as important candidates for familial idiopathic epilepsies, and their potential role has been explored in the aetiology of JME, a distinctive and common familial form of idiopathic generalised epilepsy (IGE). JME, characterised by myoclonic jerks on awakening, has a prevalence of 0.5–1.0 per 1,000 and a ratio of sibling risk to population prevalence (λs) of 42. Its mode of inheritance is uncertain;

autosomal dominant or recessive, two-locus and polygenic models have all been suggested.

Chromosomal regions harbouring genes for nAChR subunits were tested for linkage to the JME trait in 19 pedigrees. Negative pairwise LOD scores were obtained for all loci except *D15S118* and *D15S128* in the region of *CHRNA7* on chromosome 15q14. A further seven marker loci spanning a 20 cM region around *D15S118* were analysed in a total of 34 pedigrees. Significant evidence for linkage with heterogeneity was found using multipoint parametric and non-parametric analysis: HLOD = 4.4 at $\alpha = 0.65$; $Z_{all} = 2.94$; $p = 0.0005$ [12]. These data provide strong evidence in favour of a susceptibility locus for JME in this region – which encompasses *CHRNA7* – in most but not all families (Fig. 2(a) and (b)). Mutational analysis of *CHRNA7* is in progress but has been complicated by the existence of an adjacent expressed pseudogene.

In summary, there is unequivocal evidence for involvement of the *CHRNA4* gene in a Mendelian inheritance idiopathic partial epilepsy and suggestive evidence for the involvement of *CHRNA7* in an IGE. The putative modulatory role of these receptors in the brain provides a plausible functional basis for phenotypes characterised by episodic disturbance of neuronal excitability with intact cognitive and other functions.

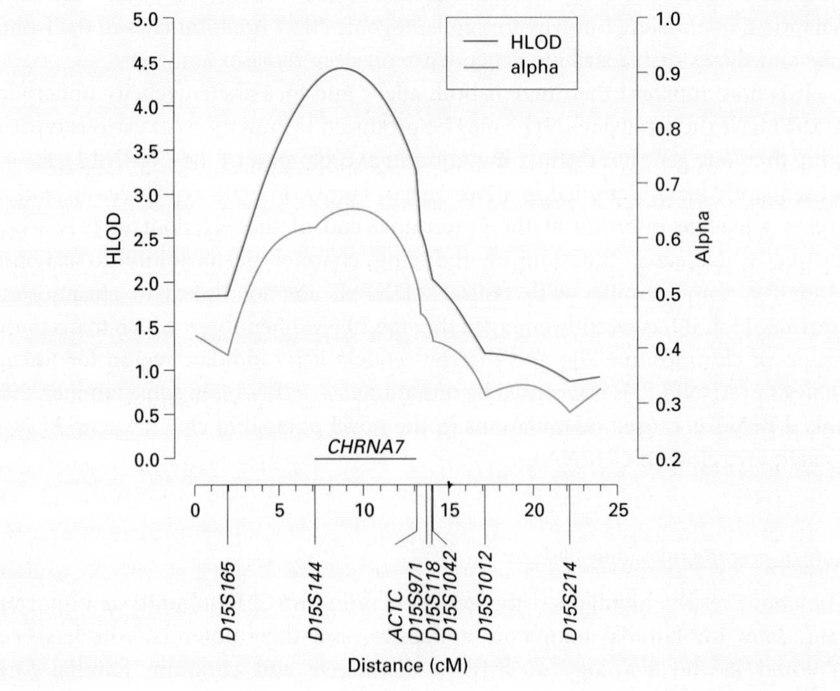

Fig. 2a Graphs of multipoint LOD score (HLOD) and corresponding values of alpha (proportion of linked families) against genetic location on chromosome 15q. Genetic distance between loci in centimorgans (cM). For clarity the vertical axis denoting values of α has a baseline set at 0.2.

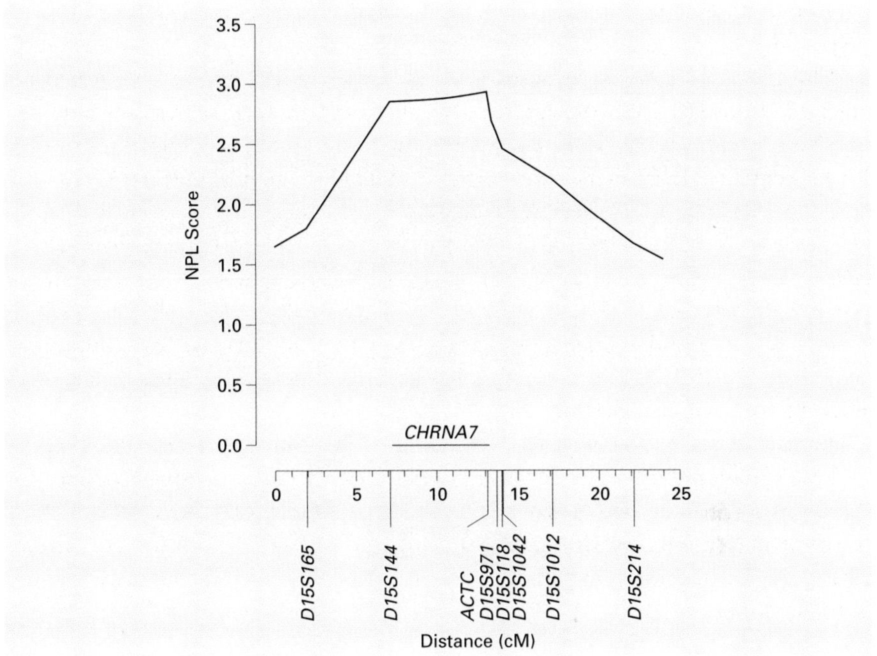

Fig. 2b Non-parametric linkage (NPL) score against genetic location on chromosome 15q.

Voltage-gated calcium channels and epilepsy

Another class of neuronal ion channels, the voltage-gated calcium channels, has been implicated in spike-wave epilepsy on the basis of molecular genetic analysis of single-gene models of epilepsy in the mouse. Mutations of these channels also cause various neurological and muscular diseases in man, but a role in any of the human inherited epilepsies has yet to be demonstrated.

Voltage-sensitive Ca^{2+} channels in excitable tissues regulate a number of cellular functions including neurotransmitter release and rhythmic firing. They are classified, according to their kinetics, voltage dependence and sensitivity to various agonists and antagonists, into T, L, N, P, Q and R types. They are hetero-oligomers of up to five subunits including the α1 subunit – a transmembrane protein which acts as the pore and voltage sensor (see Fig. 3) – and the smaller cytoplasmic β subunit which modulates channel activity; G-protein coupled receptors also influence channel activity. The α1 subunits (α1A–E and 5) are encoded by six genes (symbols *CACN1A 1–6*) and the β subunits (β1–4) by four genes (*CACN1B–4B*). Each gene displays alternative splicing, and the tissue distribution and time course of their expression vary (see Table 2).

There are six well documented single-locus models of idiopathic generalised spike-wave epilepsy in the mouse, which not only indicates that single-gene defects may cause epilepsy but emphasises the fact that locus heterogeneity may underlie a

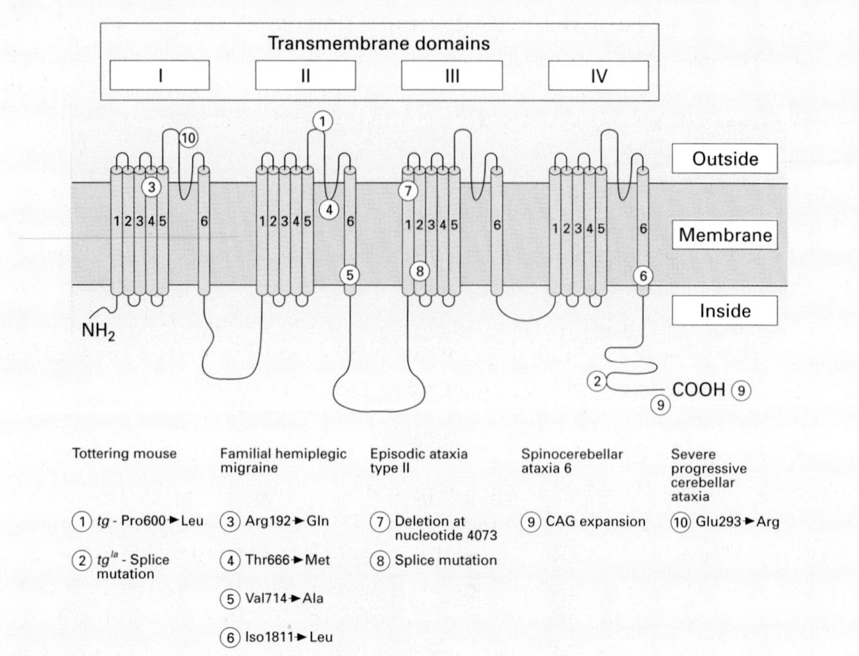

Fig. 3 Structure of the α1A subunit of the voltage-gated calcium channel, showing the positions of key mutations in the mouse gene (*Cacna1a*) and its human homologue (*CACN1A1*).

homogeneous phenotype. Five of the genes for these mouse models of epilepsy have recently been cloned (see Table 2), of which two encode voltage-gated channels: the *tottering* mouse is caused by mutations in the gene encoding the α1A subunit, *Cacna1a* [13], and the *lethargic* mouse by mutations in the gene encoding the β subunit, *Cchb4* [14]. It is noteworthy that both these mice display ataxia in addition to spike-wave seizures, and that these subunits are expressed at high levels in the cerebellum.

It remains uncertain exactly how these mutations disturb neuronal excitability and generate spike-wave seizures, but pre-existing human and animal data have

Table 2. Single-gene mutations causing spike-wave epilepsies in mice.

Mouse mutant		Chromosome	Gene
Tottering	*tg*	8	Ca channel, α1A subunit
Lethargic	*le*	2	Ca channel, β4 subunit
Mocha	*mh*	10	AP-3, δ subunit
Slow-wave	*Swe*	4	Na^+/H^+ exchanger
Stargazer	*Stg*	15	Novel gene
Ducky	*du*	9	Unknown

implicated voltage-gated calcium channels in the generation of the aberrant thalamocortical rhythms which are thought to underlie spike-wave and absence seizures. Voltage-dependent calcium channels are involved in control of the burst and tonic firing of thalamocortical rhythms. During burst mode, low- and high-voltage activated channels are switched on, whereas during the tonic mode only the latter are triggered. Moreover, ethosuximide – which appears to block T-type calcium channels – has a selective and specific action in suppressing this variety of seizure. In addition to any functional effect, Purkinje cell degeneration is seen, indicating that progressive neuronal loss also contributes to the final phenotype. In the *lethargic* mouse, the mutation generates a β4 subunit which is truncated and lacks the site of interaction with α1 subunits. The functional consequences of this are rather unpredictable, but the mutated β4 subunit may interact preferentially with other β subunits in particular neuronal populations.

At present, there is no direct evidence that mutations of calcium channels cause epilepsy in humans as well as mice. The human homologue of the *tottering* gene, *CACNA1A*, is known to underlie three diseases other than epilepsy: familial hemiplegic migraine, episodic ataxia type II (EA II) and autosomal dominant spinocerebellar ataxia (SCA6). Different mutant alleles underlie the three phenotypes (Fig. 3). The underlying mechanisms remain mysterious. In the ataxias (EA II and SCA6), it is clear that dysfunction is most obvious in the cerebellum. The α1A subunit forms P-type channels which have been shown to mediate serotonin release, providing a plausible link with the pathophysiology of migraine. The role of voltage-gated calcium channels in human absence epilepsies is currently being examined.

□ CONCLUSIONS

Evidence is emerging that certain inherited epilepsies in humans are due to abnormal function of neurotransmitter receptors and voltage-gated ion channels. Elucidation of the role of ion channels in human epilepsy should give rise to a more exact molecular classification and the development of specific therapy based on the underlying molecular pathophysiology.

REFERENCES

1 Elmslie FV, Gardiner RM. The epilepsies. In: Rimoin DL, Connor JM, Pyeritz RE (Eds). *Emery and Rimoin's Principles and Practice of Medical Genetics.* New York: Churchill Livingstone, 1997: 2177–96.

2 Barchi RL. Ion channel mutations and diseases of skeletal muscle. *Neurobiol Dis* 1997; **4**: 254–64.

3 Shiang R, Ryan S, Zhu Y-Z, *et al.* Mutations in the α_1 subunit of the inhibitory glycine receptor cause the dominant neurologic disorder, hyperekplexia. *Nat Genet* 1993; **5**: 351–7.

4 Singh NA, Charlier C, Stauffer D, *et al.* A novel potassium channel gene, *KCNQ2*, is mutated in an inherited epilepsy of newborns. *Nat Genet* 1998; **18**: 25–9.

5 Charlier C, Singh NA, Ryan SG, *et al.* A pore mutation in a novel *KQT*-like potassium channel gene in an idiopathic epilepsy family. *Nat Genet* 1998; **18**: 53–5.

6 Sivilotti L, Colquhoun D. Acetylcholine receptors: too many channels, too few functions. *Science* 1995; **269**: 1681–2.

7 Scheffer IE, Bhatia KP, Lopes-Cendes I, *et al.* Autosomal dominant nocturnal frontal lobe epilepsy: a distinctive clinical disorder. *Brain* 1995; **118**: 61–73.

8 Phillips HA, Scheffer IE, Berkovic SF, *et al.* Localization of a gene for autosomal dominant nocturnal frontal lobe epilepsy to chromosome 20q13.2. *Nat Genet* 1995; **10**: 117–8.

9 Steinlein OK, Mulley JC, Propping P, *et al.* A missense mutation in the neuronal nicotinic receptor $\alpha 4$ subunit is associated with autosomal dominant nocturnal frontal lobe epilepsy. *Nat Genet* 1995; **11**: 201–3.

10 Weiland S, Witzemann V, Villarroel A, *et al.* An amino acid exchange in the second transmembrane segment of a neuronal nicotinic receptor causes partial epilepsy by altering its desensitization kinetics. *FEBS Lett* 1996; **398**: 91–6.

11 Steinlein O, Magnusson A, Stoodt J, *et al.* An insertion mutation of the *CHRNA4* gene in a family with autosomal dominant nocturnal frontal lobe epilepsy. *Hum Mol Genet* 1997; **6**: 943–7.

12 Elmslie FV, Rees M, Williamson MP, *et al.* Genetic mapping of a major susceptibility locus for juvenile myoclonic epilepsy on chromosome 15q. *Hum Mol Genet* 1997; **6**: 1329–34.

13 Fletcher CF, Lutz CM, O'Sullivan TN, *et al.* Absence epilepsy in *tottering* mutant mice is associated with calcium channel defects. *Cell* 1996; **87**: 607–17.

14 Burgess DL, Jones JM, Meisler MH, Noebels JL. Mutation of the Ca^{2+} channel β subunit gene *Cchb4* is associated with ataxia and seizures in the lethargic (*lh*) mouse. *Cell* 1997; **88**: 385–92.

☐ MULTIPLE CHOICE QUESTIONS

1 Human genetic epilepsies:
- (a) Account for 20% of patients with epilepsy
- (b) Always display Mendelian inheritance
- (c) Are all idiopathic generalised epilepsies
- (d) Often have onset in childhood
- (e) May display a maternal pattern of inheritance

2 Mutations in genes encoding ion channels:
- (a) Cause inherited myotonias
- (b) Cause inherited periodic paralysis
- (c) Are always autosomal recessive
- (d) Have only been described in voltage-gated ion channels
- (e) Are always 'gain of function' mutations

3 Familial hyperekplexia (startle disease) is caused by mutations in:
- (a) *CHRNA2*
- (b) *GLRA1*
- (c) *KCNQ2*
- (d) *CACNA1A*
- (e) *HERG*

4 Neuronal nicotinic acetylcholine receptors:
- (a) Are located predominantly in the frontal lobe
- (b) Comprise six identical subunits
- (c) Mediate fast transmission in the brain
- (d) Are mutated in a form of mouse epilepsy
- (e) Are mostly composed of $\alpha 4$ and $\beta 2$ subunits

5 Genes mutated in the diseases stated:
   (a) *CHRNA7* in autosomal dominant nocturnal frontal lobe epilepsy
   (b) *Cchb4* in the *lethargic* mouse
   (c) *CACNA1A* in familial hemiplegic migraine
   (d) *CACNA1A* in episodic ataxia type II
   (e) *KCNQ2* in benign familial neonatal convulsions

ANSWERS

1a False	2a True	3a False	4a False	5a False
b False	b True	b True	b False	b True
c False	c False	c False	c False	c True
d True	d False	d False	d False	d True
e True	e False	e False	e True	e True

Use of new anti-epileptic drugs

David Chadwick

□ INTRODUCTION

Epilepsy is the commonest of neurological disorders and the one with the longest established therapeutic potential. It is heterogeneous in nature, and its management should therefore benefit from the widest possible range of drugs with diverse mechanisms of action. This chapter will discuss some of the newer anti-epilepsy drugs, and compare and contrast them with the established agents. Their modes of action will be briefly described, but the main aim is to focus on the key aspects of efficacy, value for money, safety and tolerability; these are the main preoccupation of prescribers and will ultimately determine their survival in both the formulary and the pharmaceutical market-place.

The field of anti-epileptic drug therapy has been unusual, being long dominated by old drugs such as phenobarbitone and phenytoin (introduced in 1912 and 1938, respectively). Until recently, carbamazepine and valproate were regarded as 'new' drugs, even though they entered clinical practice over a quarter of a century ago. All these drugs were developed from empirical screening programmes without any clear understanding of their mechanisms of action, although these have now been clarified. Phenytoin and carbamazepine influence fast voltage-sensitive sodium channels to block repetitive firing of neurones, an action shared by the new drug, lamotrigine (see Fig. 1). Phenobarbitone and benzodiazepines allosterically enhance the affinity of γ-aminobutyric acid (GABA), an inhibitory neurotransmitter for its binding site (Fig. 2). Valproate probably has multiple mechanisms of action including effects at both sodium and calcium channels [1].

Within the last few years, several new and potentially exciting anti-epileptic drugs with novel mechanisms of action have become widely available. The molecular structures of some of them, together with some older ones, is shown in Fig. 3. Their mechanisms of action have mostly been characterised. These are summarised in Table 1, from which it will be apparent that many share targets (eg neurotransmitter receptors, voltage-sensitive ion channels) with some of the longer established drugs, and that some act at more than one site. The interactions of various drugs with the $GABA_A$ receptor are illustrated in Fig. 2, and the types of epilepsy in which the various old and new drugs are effective are shown in Fig. 4.

After an initial predictable burst of enthusiasm for the new drugs, the stage is now being reached where a more realistic assessment of their effectiveness should be made. Increasingly, purchasers of health care are demanding systematic proof that new drugs have clear benefits that justify their inevitably greater cost. Epilepsy is so common that indiscriminate switching from old to new anti-epileptic drugs would have considerable economic implications. This is reflected by a survey

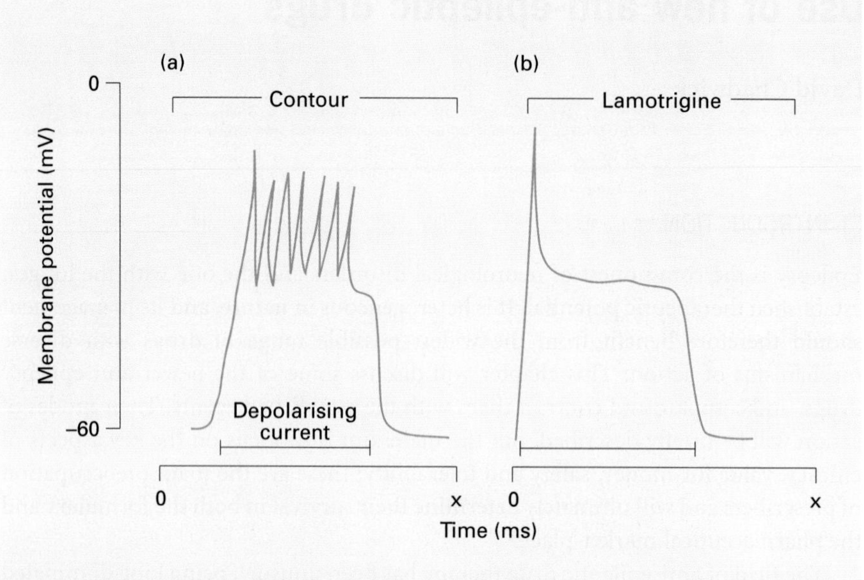

Fig. 1 Intracellular recording from **(a)** a single neurone in response to a depolarising current and **(b)** the suppression of its burst firing by lamotrigine.

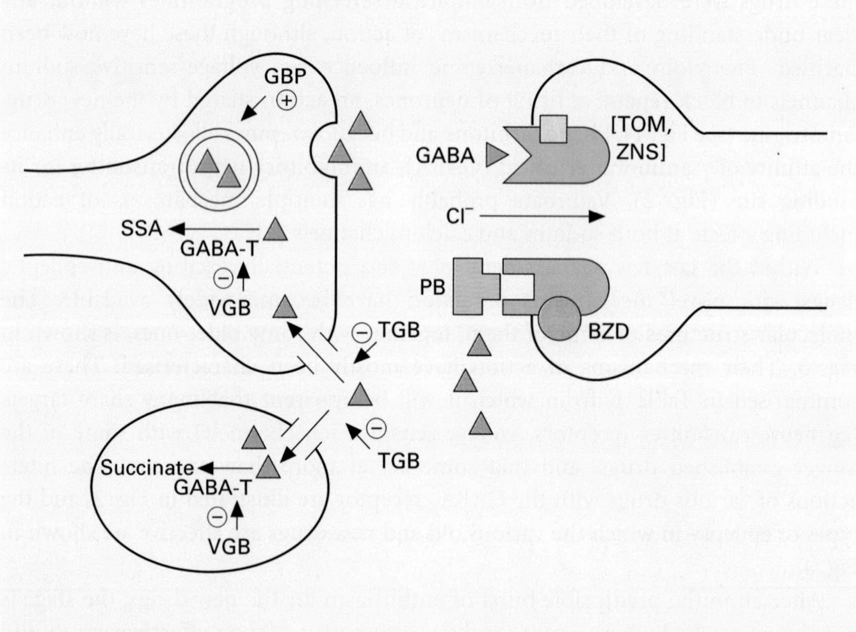

Fig. 2 Some anti-epileptic drugs that interact with γ-aminobutyric acid (GABA), an inhibitory neurotransmitter that hyperpolarises and stabilises the post-synaptic membrane by increasing Cl^- ion entry. Tiagabin and vigabatrin respectively block reuptake and degradation of GABA, while phenobarbitone and benzodiazepines enhance the action of GABA by enhancing its binding to the $GABA_A$ receptor.

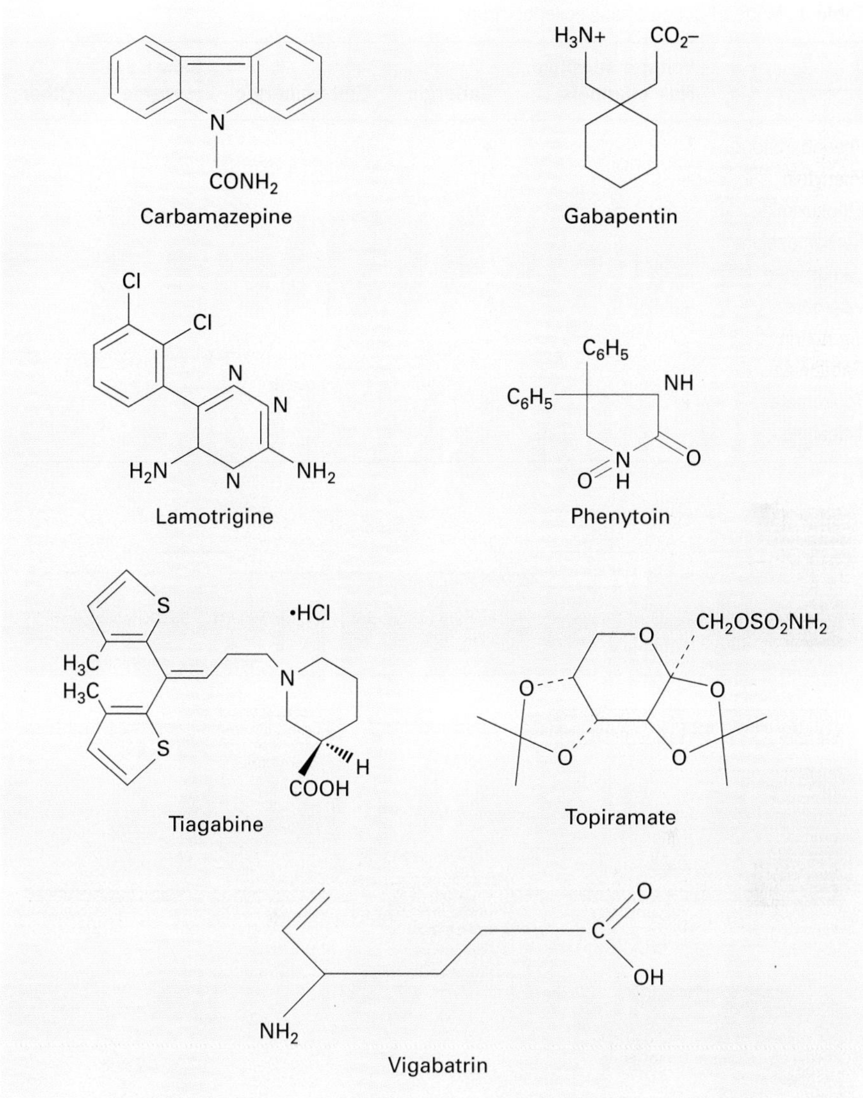

Fig. 3 Molecular structure of some old and new anti-epileptic drugs.

undertaken in the UK in 1992 which showed that the new drugs represented only 7% of prescriptions to people with epilepsy, but absorbed 39% of these patients' total drug costs, which in turn accounted for one-third of the direct medical costs of the disease [2].

To justify their extra cost, new anti-epileptic drugs will need to demonstrate greater efficacy against particular seizure types or epilepsy syndromes, or better tolerability or safety than existing agents. Other, less tangible aspects of their value may also need to be taken into account in justifying their expense (see below).

Table 1. Mode of action of anti-epileptic drugs.

	Voltage-sensitive Na+ channels	Gabergic	Glutaminergic	Slow Ca++ currents	Other
Phenobarbitone	?	+			
Phenytoin	+				
Ethosuximide				+	
Carbamazepine	+				
Lamotrigine	+		+		
Valproate	+	?	?	?+	
Vigabatrin		+			
Gabapentin					+
Topiramate	+	+	?+		
Tiagabine		+ .			

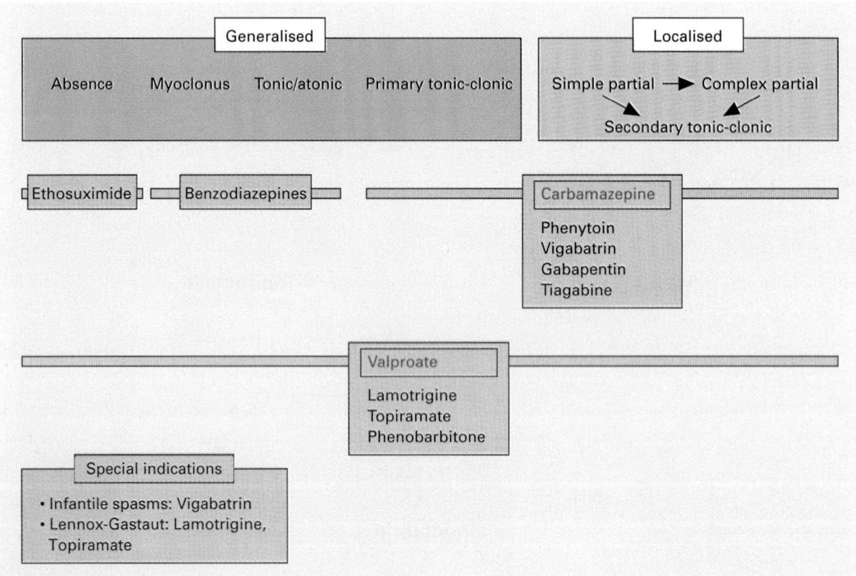

Fig. 4 Spectrum of efficacy of anti-epileptic drugs against various types of seizure. (Drugs in red are current drugs of choice.)

☐ EFFICACY OF NEW DRUGS

In the modern era, new anti-epileptic drugs receive regulatory approval as a result of placebo-controlled, add-on, double-blind studies, almost always conducted in populations of patients with refractory partial epilepsies. This study design is open to considerable criticism [2,3], but in essence aims to show that an individual drug, when used in combination with a number of other anti-epileptic drugs, is better than nothing (placebo) and is reasonably well tolerated and apparently safe. These studies do not allow efficacy and tolerability to be compared between different drugs, nor do they define the range of effectiveness of a drug against different seizure types and syndromes. In an age when meta-analysis is becoming fashionable, some estimates can be made about the various treatment effects of new anti-epileptic drugs from placebo-controlled studies [4,5].

Nearly 4,000 patients have been included in studies of new anti-epileptic drugs in placebo-controlled, add-on trials in refractory partial epilepsy. Efficacy can be defined as the proportion of patients in parallel-group studies showing a 50% reduction from baseline in seizure frequency; this can be compared with the rate in placebo-treated patients to give an odds ratio. On this basis, there is a trend for differences in efficacy and tolerability, with drugs such as topiramate and vigabatrin (odds ratio, 3.5–4.0) appearing more effective but less well tolerated than others such as gabapentin and lamotrigine (odds ratio, 2.0–2.5). Any differences may, however, be simply because the former drugs have been tested at near-maximal tolerated dosages, while the latter drugs have been studied in clinical trials at doses much closer to the minimal effective level. Unfortunately, standard anti-epileptic drugs have rarely been studied in similar placebo-controlled, add-on studies in comparable populations of patients. The exception is valproate, whose estimated efficacy seems broadly equivalent to those of newer drugs [4].

More clinically informative studies have become available after new drugs have received licences. Comparative studies of monotherapy against carbamazepine have been published for lamotrigine [6,7], vigabatrin [8,9], and gabapentin [10] in patients presenting with epilepsy for the first time. The results show that, overall, none of the new drugs can claim greater efficacy than carbamazepine – and indeed vigabatrin appears significantly less effective. All these drugs are, however, better tolerated than carbamazepine, with fewer withdrawals because of adverse events.

Equivalence of efficacy with better tolerability may be sufficient to promote a new drug to the ranks of first-line therapy. This will, however, depend both on tight and rigorous definitions of equivalence of efficacy [11] and on better understanding of the psychosocial and economic costs of drug failure due to poor tolerability. Lamotrigine currently has the strongest case for becoming a first-line drug, as it has a longer 'retention time' than carbamazepine in a population of newly-diagnosed patients [6]. This outcome reflects both efficacy and tolerability, and is therefore of considerable clinical relevance. The difference in favour of lamotrigine was comparable to that of carbamazepine versus phenobarbitone [12].

Some anti-epileptic drugs can have value outside the area of the treatment of partial epilepsies (see Table 1), and newer anti-epileptic drugs may increasingly move to occupy niches in particular epilepsy syndromes. Thus, vigabatrin may be highly effective in the treatment of infantile spasms, a malignant childhood epilepsy [13–15] previously treated with steroids, often with severe adverse effects. Similarly, randomised clinical trials suggest that felbamate [16], lamotrigine [17] and topiramate [18] are effective in Lennox-Gastaut syndrome, a generalised childhood epilepsy which is often refractory to established drugs. This use for specific syndromes will particularly apply where there are no well-designed randomised clinical trials (RCTs) of standard agents in these disorders.

SAFETY OF NEW DRUGS

Safety issues are rarely thoroughly explored within the context of RCTs, because risks of rare – but potentially serious – idiosyncratic adverse effects, chronic toxicity, and teratogenicity may only be identified during the course of post-marketing surveillance. Chronic toxic effects of new anti-epileptic drugs have so far been poorly studied, and recent experience confirms the need for continued vigilance in this area.

Felbamate, not yet registered in the UK, has been associated with risk of aplastic anaemia in between 1 in 3,000 and 1 and 5,000 patient exposures [19]. The identification of such a risk clearly influences the value and use of a new drug.

Lamotrigine is associated with acute idiosyncratic skin reactions, although possibly less frequently than seen with carbamazepine [6,7]. These reactions are occasionally severe and include Stevens-Johnson and toxic epidermal necrolysis syndromes (the risk is about 1 in 1,000 exposures). Comedication with valproate undoubtedly increases the risk of all adverse reactions, apparently through a pharmacokinetic interaction that raises lamotrigine levels. Introducing the drug slowly and titrating its dosage carefully appear to reduce but not abolish the risk.

Vigabatrin has been associated with occasional psychotic reactions and depression, and should probably be avoided in patients with a previous psychiatric history [20]. More recently, concern has arisen because of reports that vigabatrin may result in severe and irreversible visual field constriction, possibly due to retinal damage associated with prolonged high dose-treatment [21].

Topiramate may be associated with a risk of renal calculus because of its carbonic anhydrase activity, and may also lead to weight loss.

Standard anti-epileptic drugs are all associated with increased risk of fetal anomalies and major abnormalities. Some new drugs such as gabapentin, lamotrigine and vigabatrin may, in the long term, prove more satisfactory for women in the child-bearing years; animal screening has shown a lower incidence of these problems than with the standard drugs under similar conditions. How much reassurance may be taken from this remains to be seen, and it will clearly be many years before we can be confident about the relative risks to pregnancy from new and standard anti-epileptic drugs.

EASE OF USE

Standard anti-epileptic drugs have not always proved easy to use. Some have complex pharmacokinetic properties, with associated potential for interaction with other anti-epileptic agents, drugs and unrelated therapeutic substances. This contributes to the need for monitoring of drug levels in the blood [22]. Many anti-epileptic drugs (phenytoin is the most obvious example) are enzyme-inducers, and therefore interact with oral contraceptives. Drugs such as gabapentin and vigabatrin, which possess simple pharmacokinetics, may not need drug monitoring, and lend themselves particularly to add-on treatment because of the lack of risk of drug interaction. On the other hand, some new anti-epileptic drugs, including gabapentin and tiagabine, have relatively short pharmacokinetic half-lives, which may make them unsuitable for once- or twice-daily dosing.

Not all new anti-epileptic drugs are simple to use, and interactions with other agents can be troublesome (Fig. 5). The metabolism of lamotrigine, tiagabine and topiramate is accelerated by enzyme-inducers such as carbamazepine and phenytoin, necessitating higher dosages when given together with those drugs. More problematic is the potential for lamotrigine metabolism to be inhibited by valproate; this is of major clinical importance because it enhances the risk of acute idiosyncratic skin reactions (see above).

None of the new anti-epileptic drugs has potent enzyme-inducing or -inhibiting properties of their own, although topiramate may have a mild effect in inducing oestrogen metabolism.

☐ ADDITIONAL BENEFITS OF NEW DRUGS

We now have a much more comprehensive understanding of the mechanism of action of both new and standard anti-epileptic drugs [1] (see Table 1). This has led directly to the concept of rational polytherapy, which suggests that combining drugs with different mechanisms of action may be particularly beneficial. There is already some clinical evidence to support this approach. Thus, vigabatrin, a gabergic drug which was tested in add-on trials largely in combination with sodium-channel drugs (carbamazepine and phenytoin), appears to be one of the more effective add-on agents [4], but as monotherapy it may be less effective than a sodium-channel drug (carbamazepine) [8,9]. On the other hand, lamotrigine, another sodium-channel drug, is less effective when added to other sodium-channel drugs but may compare favourably with carbamazepine as monotherapy. The combination of valproate and lamotrigine may also be particularly effective in treating refractory idiopathic generalised epilepsies, an effect unlikely to be explained purely by their pharmacokinetic interaction. Thus, new drugs with new mechanisms of action may not simply

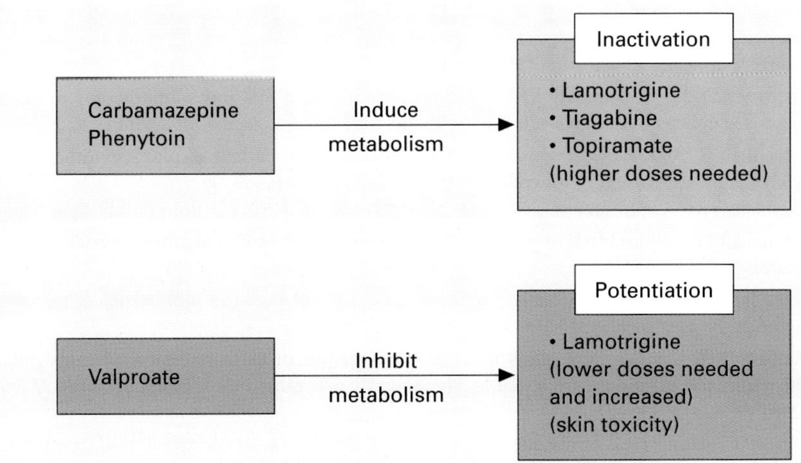

Fig. 5 Some interactions of new anti-epileptic drugs with established agents.

have value in their own right as monotherapy, but may allow additional health gains because of their potential for rational use as add-on therapy.

□ CONCLUSIONS

New anti-epileptic drugs have significantly increased the choice of agents to treat patients with epilepsy. Currently, they are largely used for patients with refractory epilepsy requiring polytherapy, where their better tolerability than longer-established drugs is particularly beneficial; increasingly, they may be used as monotherapy. There is no evidence that they are superior in efficacy to existing first-line agents such as carbamazepine or valproate, but they may be more acceptable to the patient – a key consideration in those presenting with seizures for the first time. Further comparative controlled trials with clinically important long-term outcomes are needed before any of the new drugs can replace carbamazepine or valproate. The exception to this is infantile spasm syndrome, where vigabatrin may be seen as the best available treatment.

REFERENCES

1 White HS. Mechanisms of antiepileptic drugs. In: Porter RJ, Chadwick D (eds). *The Epilepsies 2.* New York: Butterworth-Heinemann ,1997: l–30.

2 Jacoby A, Buck D, Baker G, *et al.* Uptake and costs of care for epilepsy: findings from a UK regional study. *Epilepsia* 1998; **39**: 776–86.

3 Mignot G. Drug trials in epilepsy. *Br Med J* 1996; **313**: 1158.

4 Marson AG, Kadir ZA, Hutton JL, Chadwick DW. The new antiepileptic drugs: a systematic review of their efficacy and tolerability. *Epilepsia* 1997; **38**: 859–80.

5 Elferink JA, Van Zwieten-Boot BJ. New 'AEDs'. Analysis based on number needed to treat, shows differences between drugs studied. *Br Med J* 1997; **314**: 603.

6 Brodie MJ, Richens A, Yuen AW. Double-blind comparison of lamotrigine and carbamazepine in newly diagnosed epilepsy. UK Lamotrigine/Carbamazepine Trial Group. *Lancet* 1995: **345**: 476.

7 Reunanen M, Dam M, Yuen AW. A randomised open multicentre comparative trial of lamotrigine and carbamazepine as monotherapy in patients with newly diagnosed or recurrent epilepsy. *Epilepsy Res* 1996; **23**: 149–55.

8 Chadwick D, Roi L, Kennedy KM. Vigabatrin (Sabril) as a first-line monotherapy in newly diagnosed epilepsy: A double-blind comparison with carbamazepine. *Epilepsia* 1996; **37**: 6.

9 Kalviainen R, Aikia M, Mervaala E, *et al.* Vigabatrin versus carbamazepine monotherapy in newly diagnosed patients with epilepsy. *Arch Neurol* 1995; **52**: 989–96.

10 Chadwick DW, Anhut H, Greiner MPH, *et al.* International Gabapentin Monotherapy Study Group. A double-blind trial of gabapentin monotherapy for newly diagnosed partial seizures. *Neurology* 1998; **51**: 1282–8.

11 Jones B, Jarvis P, Lewis JA, *et al.* Trials to assess equivalence: the importance of rigorous methods. *Br Med J* 1996; **313**: 36–9.

12 Mattson RH, Cramer JA, Collins JF, *et al.* Comparison of carbamazepine, phenobarbital, phenytoin and primidone in partial and secondarily generalised tonic clonic seizures. *N Engl J Med* 1985; **313**: 145–51.

13 Chiron C, Dumas C, Jambaque I, Mumford J, Dulac O. Randomized trial comparing vigabatrin and hydrocortisone in infantile spasms due to tuberose sclerosis. *Epilepsy Research* 1997; **26**: 39–95.

14 Vigevano F, Cilio MR. Vigabatrin versus ACTH as first-line treatment for infantile spasms: a randomized, prospective study. *Epilepsia* 1997; **38**: 1270–4.

15 Appleton RE (for The Infantile Spasm Study Group), Thornton L. Double blind comparison of vigabatrin versus placebo in newly diagnosed and previously untreated infantile spasms. *Epilepsia* 1996; **37**: 125.

16 Felbamate Study Group. Efficacy of felbamate in childhood epileptic encephalopathy (Lennox-Gastaut syndrome). *N Engl J Med* 1993; **328**: 29–33.

17 Motte J, Trevathan E, Arvidsson JFV, *et al*, and the Lamictal Lennox-Gastaut Study Group. Lamotrigine for generalised seizures associated with the Lennox-Gastaut syndrome. *N Engl J Med* 1997; **337**: 1807–12. [Published erratum appears in *N Engl J Med* 1998; **339**: 851–2.].

18 Glauser TA. Preliminary observations on topiramate in pediatric epilepsies. *Epilepsia* 1997; **38**: S37–41.

19 Stables JP, Bailer M, Johannessen SI, *et al.* Progress report on new antiepileptic drugs: a summary of the Second Eilat Conference. *Epilepsy Res* 1995; **22**: 235.

20 Riehens A. Vigabatrin and lamotrigine. In: Porter RJ, Chadwick D (eds). *The Epilepsies 2.* New York: Butterworth Heinemann, 1997: 201–22.

21 Eke T, Talbot JF, Lawden MC. Severe persistent visual field constriction associated with vigabatrin. *Br Med J* 1997; **314**: 180–1.

22 Richens A, Perueca E. Clinical pharmacology and medical treatment. In: Laidlaw J, Richens A, Chadwick D (eds). *A Textbook of Epilepsy.* Edinburgh: Churchill Livingstone, 1993: 495–560.

Imaging the brain at work

Richard S J Frackowiak

□ INTRODUCTION

Until recently, our knowledge of the functional organisation of the human brain was pieced together from observing the effects of neurological lesions, limited studies of brain stimulation pioneered by Penfield and others, and extrapolation from experiments in sub-human primates. These approaches identified brain areas involved in particular functions and showed that early sensory input and final motor output are arranged in topographically organised maps (Figs 1 and 2). However, they give little insight into how specific functions are embodied in the physical structure of the brain, and particularly how higher cognitive activities such as memory, language and emotion are organised.

Functional neuro-imaging – 'brain mapping' – exploits a range of complementary non-invasive techniques to visualise and characterise local physiological changes in the brain that are associated with the activity of selected sensory, motor or cognitive circuits. These techniques are beginning to clarify the functional architecture of the brain and its many levels of both spatial and temporal organisation [1]. At present, functional neuro-imaging is being applied to map relatively large neuronal systems and pathways, such as the visual cortex and its connections with regions that serve associated functions such as the perception and recognition of colour, shape and movement [2]. Important areas of enquiry include: how sensory input is mapped on to the human brain and how complex sensory representations are built up; interactions between sensory and motor representations during sense-guided motor output; the ways in which cognitive functions such as memory, language and emotion are organised; and the role of consciousness in forming human behaviour.

So far, brain mapping has been little used in clinical practice, but its potential is great; it is already causing a revolution in the fields of psychology and neuropsychology that is no less dramatic than that caused in neuroanatomy and neuropathology by the introduction of CT and MR scanning. Ultimately, it should become possible to examine the function of smaller structures (eg individual brain nuclei) as the resolution and acquisition speed of mapping methods improve through technological advances.

This chapter will first review some of the methods used to image brain structure and function (see Table 1), and will then illustrate how they have been applied to study particular sensory, motor and cognitive functions.

□ VISUALISING THE ANATOMY OF THE LIVING BRAIN

High-resolution images of the brain, generated by computed tomographic (CT)

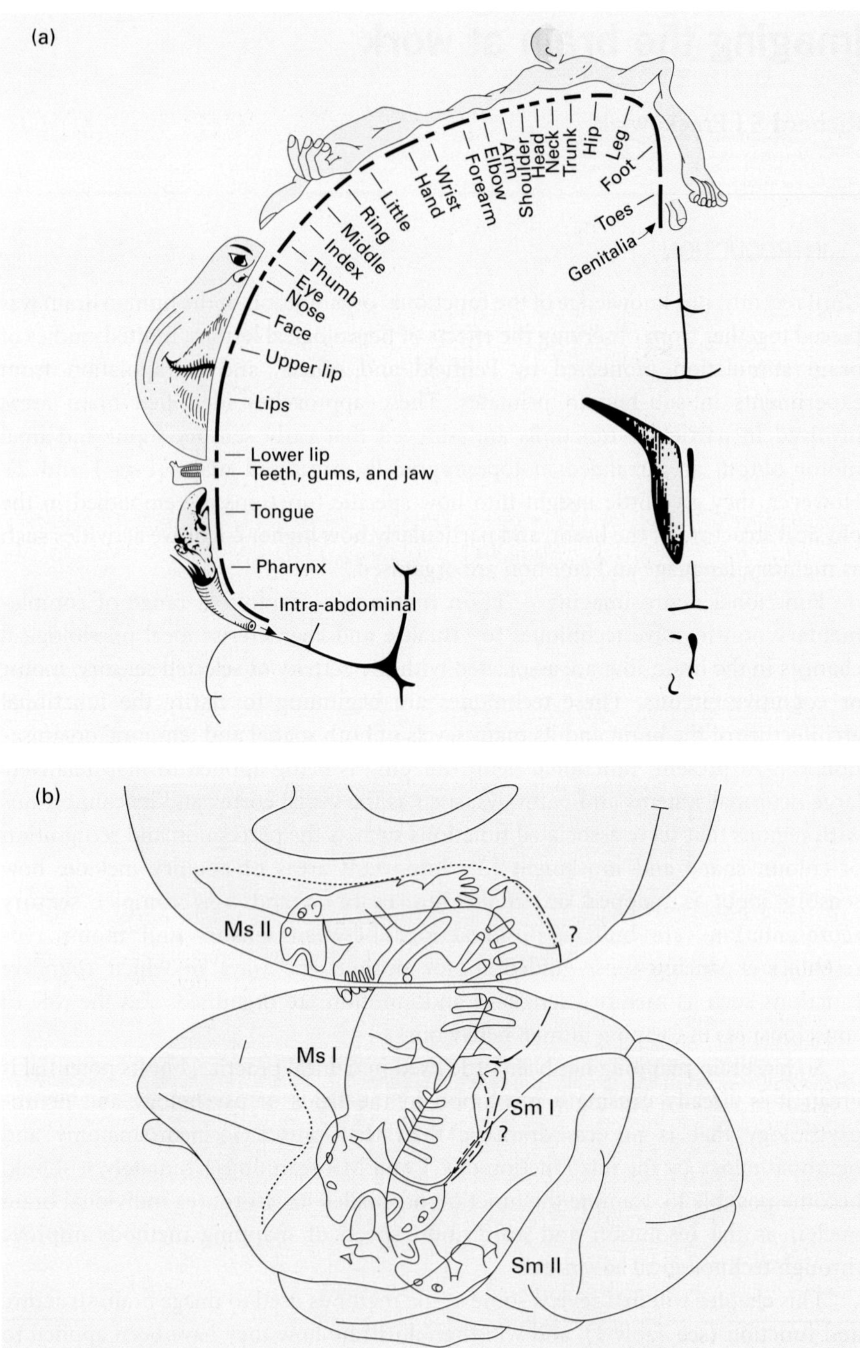

Fig. 1 (a) Classical views of cortical areas involved in sensation in humans. **(b)** The sensorimotor areas (SmI and SmII) and primary and secondary motor areas (MsI and MsII) in the monkey. Both species show somatotopic organisation. The human data were obtained by stimulating the exposed cortex in conscious patients undergoing brain surgery [3]. The monkey data were obtained from evoked potentials and from cortical stimulation [4].

(a)

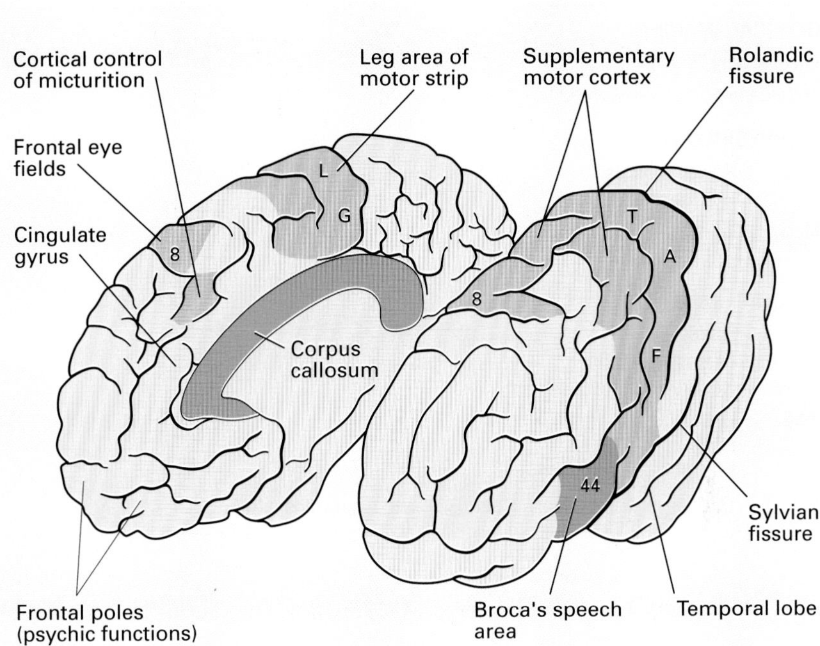

(b)

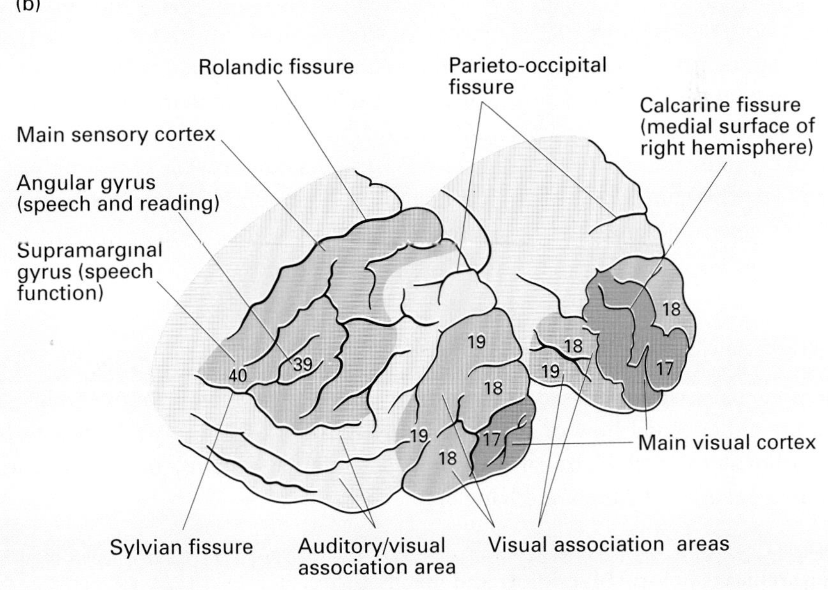

Fig. 2 The classical view of the functional subdivisions of the human cerebral cortex [5]. **(a)** Frontal lobes (shown pulled apart); **(b)** parietal and occipital lobes (from behind and above).

Table 1. Methods used to investigate structure and function in the living human brain.

ANATOMICAL IMAGING

- CT Scanning
- MRI Scanning eg T_1–weighted

NEUROPHYSIOLOGY

- EEG – Power analysis
  – ER Potentials
- MEG – Dipole analysis
  – ER Responses

FUNCTIONAL IMAGING

- PET – Perfusion
  – Glucose utilisation
  – Neurotransmitter function
- fMRI – EPI and BOLD contrast
  – FLASH etc
  – EPISTAR perfusion imaging
- SPECT – Qualitative distributions of perfusion and neurotransmitters

scanning or magnetic resonance imaging (MRI) are now familiar in clinical practice. CT scanning distinguishes anatomical structures by capitalising on the differential ability of tissues to attenuate X-rays directed through them; a three-dimensional image is then reconstructed using complex back-projection algorithms devised by Hounsfield and Cormack.

Magnetic resonance imaging uses a different principle to distinguish different tissues, but employs tomographic reconstruction methods to generate a variety of structural images of the brain. MRI is the method of choice for describing normal brain anatomy, because of a much wider range of information that can be obtained, the greater contrast between grey and white matter and cerebrospinal fluid, and the lack of exposure to ionising radiation (see Fig. 3). It is now possible to register functional maps obtained with other techniques on to structural images provided by MRI, to determine precisely the neuroanatomical sites of particular activities (see Figs 6 and 7).

□ VISUALISING FUNCTIONAL ACTIVITY IN THE LIVING BRAIN

The principal techniques used are shown in Table 1. They comprise methods that measure either blood flow or metabolic activity (both of which are known to be proportional to local neuronal activation) in selected regions, or the electrical impulses generated by the underlying brain.

Measurements of local blood flow and metabolism

Positron emission tomography

Positron emission tomography (PET) is a very sensitive functional imaging method,

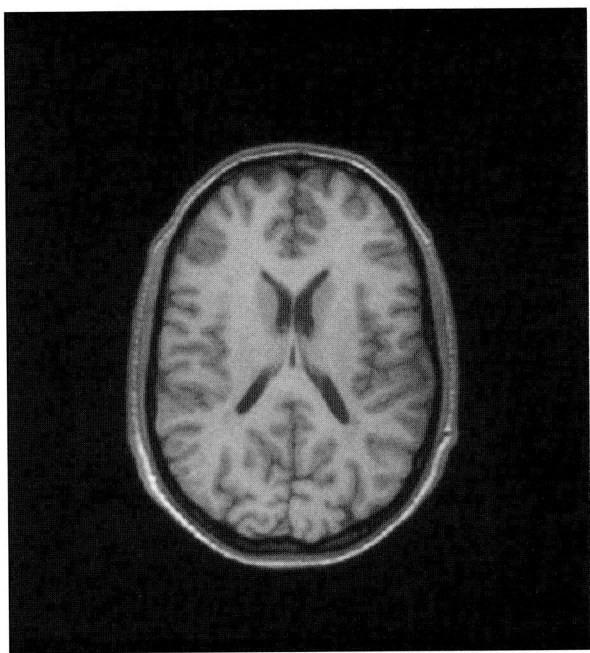

Fig. 3 High-resolution MRI scan, showing anatomy of the human brain through the level of the basal ganglia. This is a T_1-weighted image with high contrast between cerebrospinal fluid, cortex, grey and white matter.

based on the detection of very low levels of ionising radiation from positron-emitting isotopes (eg oxygen-15, ^{15}O; fluorine-18, ^{18}F) that are used to label tracer molecules of biological interest.

The labelled tracer is introduced into the brain via the bloodstream, and the regional distribution of radioactivity recorded by high-resolution scanning (see Fig. 4). Functional mapping (also known as activation studies) can study different aspects of brain activity, depending on the tracer used. The commonest variable examined is regional perfusion, which is conveniently measured using water tagged with ^{15}O. The short half-life of 2.1 minutes allows the entire brain to be scanned a dozen or more times in one session, with safe and acceptable radiation exposure. Regional metabolic activity of the brain can be measured using the glucose analogue 2-deoxyglucose labelled with ^{18}F (which is only partly metabolised and remains trapped in cells that have taken up glucose).

PET is quantitative, unlike the related technique of single photon emission computed tomography (SPECT). However, the temporal and spatial resolution of the functional images obtained with PET are limited. Generally, signals must be integrated over tens of seconds to generate images; methods now exist for mapping the distribution of random, short-lived (1 second or less) brain events but, even in ideal circumstances, events lasting milliseconds cannot be demonstrated with PET. Theoretically, PET images could achieve a spatial resolution of approximately 3 × 3 × 3 mm, but in practice this usually approximates to a sphere of diameter 8–16 mm.

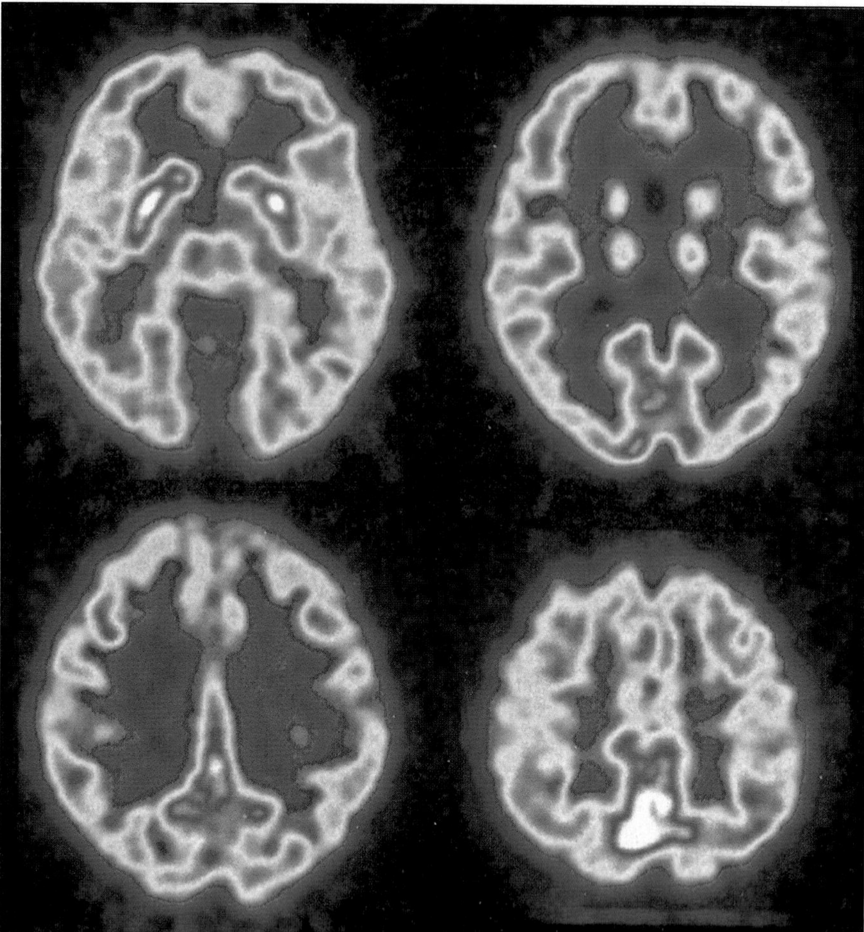

Fig. 4 Distribution of brain metabolism, measured by PET using the tracer deoxyglucose (an analogue of glucose) labelled with ^{18}F, in four transverse slices. The top of each image is anterior; left corresponds to the left side of the brain. Cortical metabolism is 3- to 4-fold greater than in the white matter. The resolution of these images is approximately 15 mm. Disturbances of this normal pattern are seen in a variety of brain disorders, including degenerative diseases.

Techniques have been developed to distinguish much closer foci of functional activation in the brain, by recording multiple images under different conditions of scanning.

Functional magnetic resonance imaging

Functional MRI (fMRI) is an adaptation of MRI which records changes in successive images that are related to specific tissue activities, especially local blood flow and brain oxygen level. fMRI requires a specialised scanner and magnet, and highly sophisticated software for data acquisition and reconstruction. There are a number of methods of fMRI scanning (see below and Table 1).

fMRI can be performed with intravascular injections of non-diffusible contrast material; at any time, the signal is determined by local blood volume, and changes in relative blood volume which reflect cerebral activation can be readily monitored. The method is at present limited by the load of intravenous contrast material that can be safely administered, and the speed with which it is cleared from the bloodstream.

EPISTAR is a new method which labels inflowing blood magnetically; this ingenious approach does not need contrast material and is totally non-invasive. A disadvantage of EPISTAR in its present form is that very few brain slices can be imaged at a time, which necessitates careful *a priori* selection of the areas to be studied.

BOLD is another totally non-invasive fMRI method which depends on brain oxygen level and produces images that reflect changes in a number of activity-dependent variables. These variables alter the local magnetic properties of brain tissue and hence produce recordable signals; they include local changes in blood volume and perfusion, and the blood levels of oxyhaemoglobin and haemoglobin. Alterations in brain activity generally produce smaller changes in image intensity with BOLD fMRI than with PET, but with higher spatial resolution (typically 1 × 1 mm transaxially and 3–10 mm axially) and better signal-to-noise discrimination.

BOLD fMRI images can be acquired very rapidly using 'echo-planar' imaging (EPI): an entire brain slice can be scanned in only 50 ms, with a recovery time of about 700 ms before another image can be recorded from it [6]. The impact of behavioural or physiological changes induced during scanning can therefore be monitored by repeated, fast imaging of the whole brain in sequentially acquired slices. Unfortunately, the BOLD signal has a long half-life of several seconds, and this limits the temporal resolution of the method; however, improved techniques for recording event-related images are rapidly being developed.

Outstanding issues limiting the usefulness of fMRI include artefacts due to bone-air interfaces (eg below the frontal cortex) and movement, which is difficult to avoid in ill patients. It is probable that many of these limitations will be overcome soon.

Electrical mapping of rapid events

The brain's activities are organised in a temporal hierarchy, in the same way that it has several structural levels. The temporal hierarchy includes electrical activities with periodicities ranging from milliseconds (eg the action potential) and hundreds of milliseconds (evoked potentials) to seconds (the EEG delta wave).

Mapping and analysis of such rapid brain events require techniques such as magnetoencephalography (MEG) and electroencephalography (EEG). Both these methods record and can be used to map spontaneous brain activity. Their ability to sample brain activity is limited physically by the number of electrodes that can be attached to the scalp, which means that it is mathematically impossible to pinpoint precisely the active brain areas responsible for a given pattern of electrical activity. This so-called 'inverse problem' is compounded in MEG by the fact that it only detects signals generated by the cortex lying perpendicular to the scalp surface. On the other hand, EEG signals are dispersed and attenuated by the scalp and skull, so the outermost cortex contributes most to the recordings. It is difficult to record brain activity from deep structures with either method [7].

Evoked potential (ERP) mapping is one way of enhancing the significance of electrical activity detected at the scalp by EEG. A cognitive or physiological task of interest is repeated, and the evoked activity is recorded during a defined interval after each stimulus or response. After a series of stimuli (typically 50), the records are digitised and averaged (which cancels out underlying measurement noise and maximises the signal of interest) and mapped. Recently, the prospect of localising sources of electrical or magnetic activity by using functional imaging techniques in addition has become more realisable.

Non-invasive measurement of local brain activity

Sokoloff and colleagues [8] have shown in the rat sensory system and hypothalamus that local synaptic activity is reflected by local glucose consumption, as measured using the labelled glucose analogues mentioned above (see Fig. 4).

Several caveats must, however, be observed. Activity-dependent glucose uptake is localised at the synapses and therefore at the projection sites of activated neurones rather than around their cell bodies. The mathematical relationship between metabolism and the number of impulses crossing a synapse is also unknown, as is the contribution, if any, of local glial metabolism to the changes in glucose uptake. As energy is consumed by activity at both excitatory and inhibitory synapses, electrophysiological excitation and inhibition do not equate with cerebral activation and de-activation as defined by changes in cerebral energy metabolism. Activation of an inhibitory synapse will cause a local increase in energy consumption but, by inhibiting the target neurones, will reduce synaptic activity and therefore glucose consumption at their projection sites. Furthermore, a local neuronal population may contain afferent excitatory and inhibitory synapses from distant sites, as well as excitatory and inhibitory interneurones.

Local changes in energy metabolism therefore reflect net activity in all contained synaptic populations. Local changes in cerebral perfusion, which are much easier and quicker to measure in practice, mirror changes in glucose metabolism and are therefore used for mapping the human brain.

□ MAPPING THE VISUAL CORTEX IN MAN

Our sensory world is dependent on sensory signals that are mapped on to the primary sensory areas of the brain. Maps of the early stages of sensory processing in the human brain are now being constructed for all the sensory modalities. Human visual maps have already extended 'classical' knowledge obtained from experiments in monkeys and by observations of brain-damaged humans. The visual system has been extensively studied by functional neuro-imaging and will be used here to illustrate principles underlying investigation of early sensory processing in other systems.

The simplest visual maps are constructed by measuring the distribution of brain activity during passive exposure to a visual stimulus and subtracting from it the image recorded in the resting state [9]. In the case of early visual sensory processing, this simple subtractive approach is relatively free of assumptions, but it becomes harder to interpret with more complex functions that recognise colour, shape or movement of objects.

The main cortical areas involved in the perception of vision are shown in Fig. 5. It is now possible to co-register accurately the functional images obtained by measuring perfusion with anatomical MRI scans, and this has largely confirmed the organisation of the visual areas deduced from the 'classical' approaches [10]. These studies have established that the visual cortex is subdivided into functionally specialised regions (see Figs 6 and 7).

The primary visual cortex

The well known retinoptic organisation of the primary visual (striate) cortex (V1) has been confirmed with functional imaging by presenting a visual stimulus (eg an

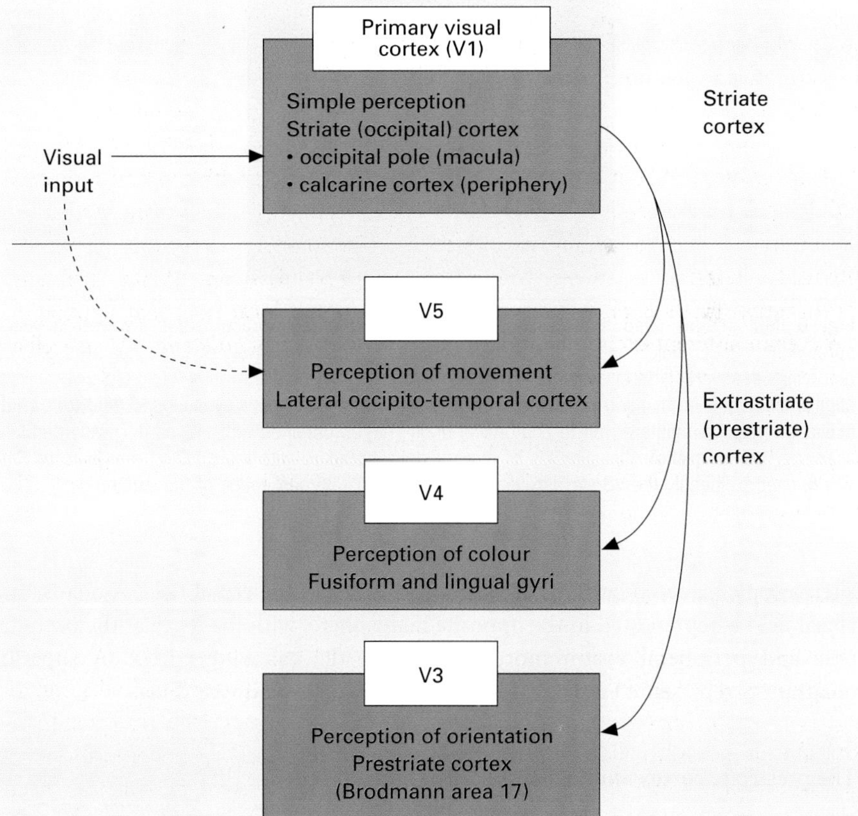

Fig. 5 Scheme of the organisation and connections between the cortical areas involved in visual perception in humans.

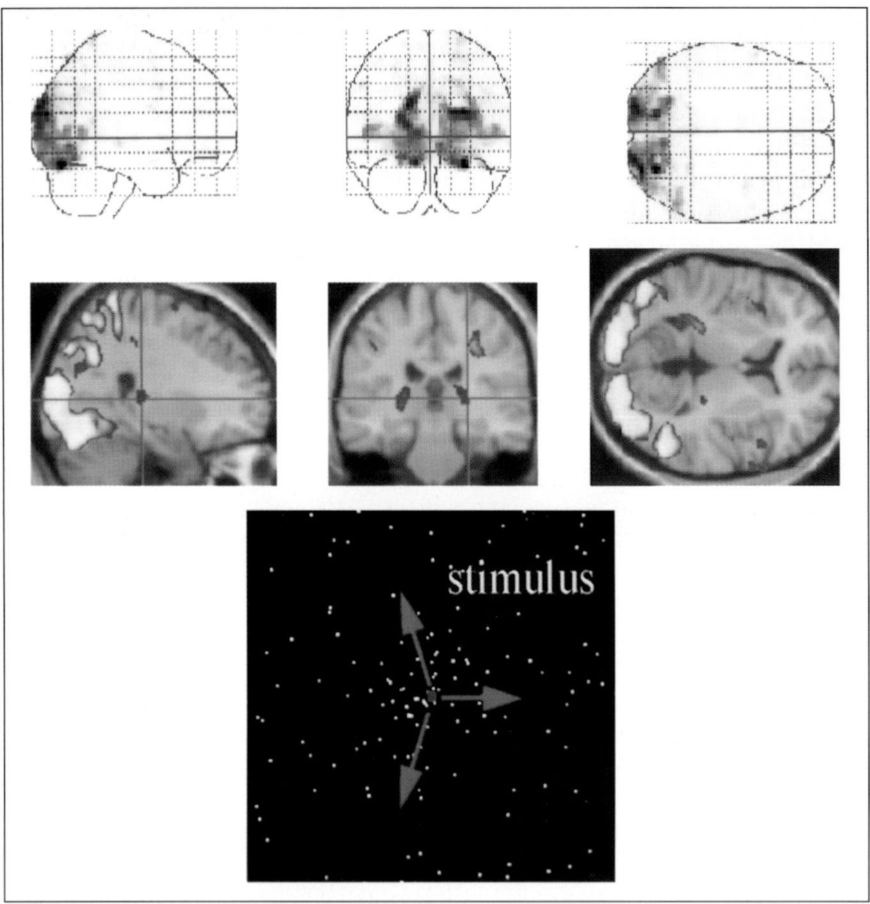

Fig. 6 fMRI images used to map the striate and extrastriate cortical areas involved in visual perception. These images were obtained by complex statistical analysis of large numbers of fMRI recordings in several different subjects. **Top panel**: areas of cortical activation (black) following visual stimulation, identified by subtracting the 'control' image with the subject's eyes closed. **Middle panel**: activation map co-registered on to anatomical brain images obtained with standard T_1-weighted MRI scanning. **Lower panel**: the stimulus of moving dots (compare with the opening moments of *Star Wars*), used to identify the V5 extrastriate area associated with perception of movement.

alternating chequered pattern) at various positions in the visual field. A quadrantic visual field is represented in the opposite hemisphere, with the fovea at the occipital pole and peripheral vision more rostrally in the calcarine cortex. A superior quadrant is represented in the inferior calcarine cortex and vice versa.

The prestriate cortex and visual specialisation

The prestriate (extrastriate) occipital cortex has also been mapped in man. Area V5, associated with the perception of movement, has been characterised by comparing scans with a visual target first in motion and then stationary. V5 lies on the lateral

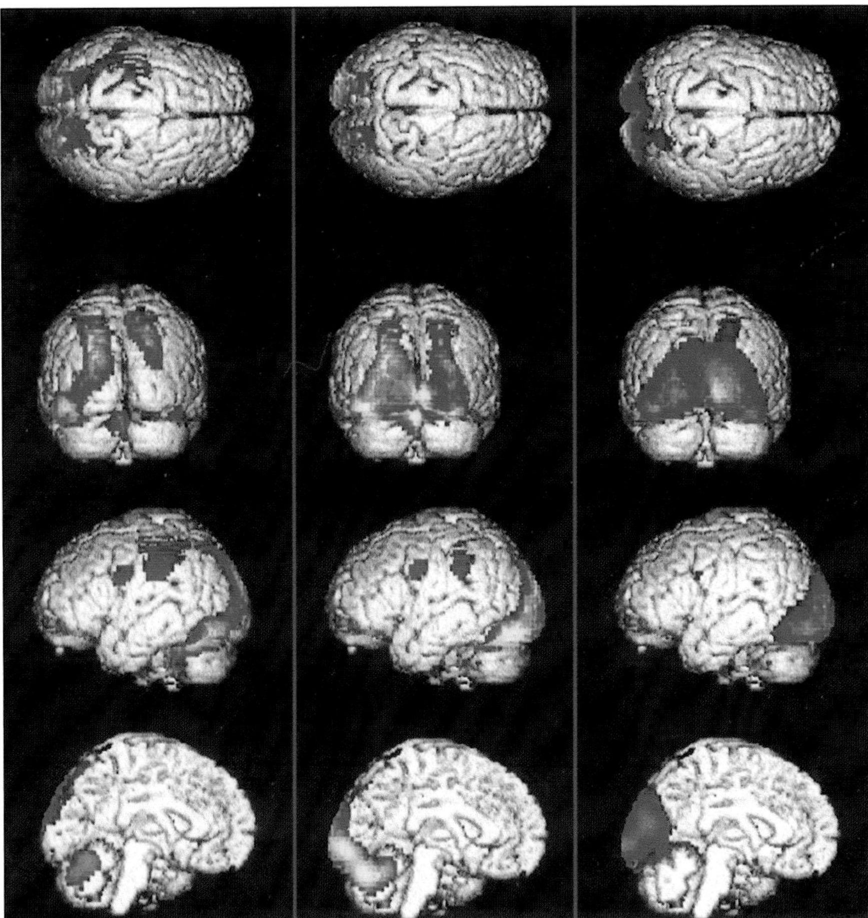

Fig. 7 Plasticity in the visual system. These functional neuro-imaging scans show results from (left to right) congenitally blind people, people with acquired blindness and normally sighted people. They have all performed reading tasks and the activations are compared with those during 'reading' of nonsense words. The blind read Braille using touch; the normally sighted read using vision. The activations in the normally sighted are centred on the primary and association visual cortices, as are those of people with acquired blindness. This raises the possibility that visual cortex that no longer receives retinal signals has undergone a change of function, now processing touch rather than visual stimuli relevant to reading. However, the visual cortex is not activated in the congenitally blind, who are the most proficient Braille readers. This finding suggests that visual cortex activation in people with acquired blindness is not due to processing of touch signals as such, but instead reflects compensatory strategies such as the use of visual imagery in interpreting the Braille symbols. A visual cortex that has never been exposed to patterns of firing mediated by a light-stimulated retina does not seem to be taken over by a completely different sensory modality. (Image courtesy of Dr C Buchel.)

surface of the brain; its position is quite variable in normal individuals, though it bears a constant relationship to the ascending limb of the inferior temporal sulcus and the inferior occipital sulcus [11]. A case has been described of a patient with bilateral lesions in the V5 areas who had grossly disturbed perception of movement but could still recognise other visual attributes of objects (dyskinetopsia) [12].

Colour perception, ie the ability to perceive the same colour of an object whatever the ambient light conditions, is associated with activation of the fusiform and adjacent parts of the lingual gyri at the back of the brain, so-called area V4. This area correlates closely with the position of lesions that cause achromatopsia (inability to perceive colours) [13].

The position of area V3, which is involved in recognising shapes and orientation, has been defined by experiments in which visual stimuli with different orientations and form are used.

Although significant advances have been made, much remains to be done in mapping other parts of the human visual extrastriate cortex, to determine their functional attribution and evolutionary developments compared with the monkey's visual cortex, the organisation of which is relatively well understood.

Mapping visual pathways

The activation of functionally specialised areas in the extrastriate cortex with appropriate stimuli also confirms that there is parallel organisation of efferent pathways from the primary visual cortex. The ways in which the brain reconstitutes a spatially and temporally congruent visual percept has now become a central issue for vision research. Initial evidence obtained from patients with occipital lesions indicates that minor visual pathways (compared with the optic radiation) reach extrastriate areas directly from the retina, bypassing the primary visual cortex. Activity in V5 without activation of V1 has been shown in a patient who had total destruction of the primary visual cortex (documented on anatomical MRI) and a dense hemianopia. The patient remained sufficiently aware of motion in his otherwise blind hemifield to be able to describe accurately its presence and direction. This observation leads to the interesting conclusion that functionally relevant visual signals can reach specialised parts of the extrastriate cortex directly and may therefore modulate activity that reaches V5 by the classical route through V1 [14]. Additionally, the perception of visual motion (albeit a degraded form of perception) is, at least in part, a property of activity in a specialised area alone and divorced from other earlier components of the visual processing pathways. Moreover, it appears that, in these abnormal circumstances, signals from V5 can reach and 'inform' function in extravisual areas of the brain, such as those associated with language.

Pathways beyond the prestriate cortex

Processing of visual signals beyond the extrastriate cortex has been explored non-invasively in man, in an attempt to relate this to separate pathways, anatomically defined in monkeys, that are postulated to deal with recognising the position of an object or with knowledge of its identity [15]. Two of these pathways may be affected in the syndromes of simultanagnosia (ie the inability to integrate parts of a visual scene into a coherent whole; part of Balint's syndrome) or visual object agnosia, in stroke patients with lesions to the posterior parietal and temporal regions respectively. A third pathway has been demonstrated in humans, and is associated with tasks that involve reaching for and drawing of objects in different positions of space; these activities cause activation of the ventral posterior parietal lobes.

Further functional specialisations will undoubtedly be identified in the human brain, representing the integration of visual signals with various aspects of behaviour which occurs at multiple anatomical levels. Each specialised area has reciprocal connections with other multiply dispersed areas, and draws on signals from these areas as behavioural contingencies demand (see Fig. 7).

□ MAPPING THE MOTOR CORTICAL AREAS

Studies of simple limb movements have confirmed a degree of somatotopy along the motor cortex, with sites of maximal activation corresponding to Penfield's homunculus (Fig. 1). The activated areas overlap but their centres are clearly separated along the central sulcus. The supplementary motor areas on the mesial surface of the cortex also display somatotopy, with the arm represented in a dorsoventral axis and the shoulder lying ventralmost [16].

Multiple motor representations in the human brain can be demonstrated by selection of appropriate behavioural conditions during scanning [17]. Activations have been found at sites in the insula, the ventral and dorsal premotor cortex, the primary motor and sensory cortices, the rostralmost parts of the dorsolateral parietal cortex and at least three sites on the mesial cortex, in anterior and posterior supplementary motor area (SMA) and in dorsal and ventral cingulate cortex. There is preliminary evidence that some, if not all of these areas are somatotopically organised into maps, with separate peaks in each activation cluster that correspond to movements of different body parts. This finding has obvious implications for the potential to reorganise and restore function following brain injury.

Extensive activation of motor-related areas is found when self-selected actions are made, without external instruction or spatial constraint [18]. In addition to the motor areas already described, there is activation of both dorsolateral prefrontal cortices, areas of mesial frontal cortex extending down to the level of the genu of the corpus callosum and into the frontal pole, and parts of the lateral and mesial parietal cortex including the inferior as well as the superior parietal lobules. Activations of the basal structures, especially the putamen and thalamus, are most evident when movements are self-paced or when a constant rather than phasic force is exerted [19]. There are also major activations of the cerebellar hemisphere ipsilateral to a moving limb and of the cerebellar vermis.

□ MOTOR AREAS ASSOCIATED WITH DIFFERENT ASPECTS OF ACTION

Imaging a movement can help to improve performance, a fact well known to musicians and athletes and sometimes exploited by physiotherapists. The brain activity associated with imagined actions surrounds areas that are associated solely with motor execution and execution of an imagined movement activates both the motor imagery areas and those associated with the movement itself [20]. There is functional specialisation in certain areas of this widespread motor system. The posterior supplementary motor area (pSMA) can be subdivided functionally into distinct rostral and caudal parts. The rostral pSMA is activated with imagined movement, while the more caudoventral pSMA is additionally activated by executing the movement. The cingulate shows a similar rostrocaudal distribution of function. These facts suggest a possible anatomical and functional basis for disorders of the conceptualisation of action (apraxias).

Preparing to make a movement produces prominent activations in the dorsolateral prefrontal cortex (DLPFC), anterior SMA and anterior cingulate cortex. The role of the prefrontal cortex in the initiation and selection of movements is substantial. Controversy exists about the nature of this contribution, as a role has been suggested for the same area in working memory; loading short-term memory beyond the span of working memory activates the DLPFC. Self-selected rather than externally instructed movements specifically activate the DLPFC and anterior cingulate cortex; conversely, there are failures of activation of these same areas in diseases characterised by poverty of spontaneous action, such as Parkinson's disease and retarded depression. These abnormalities can be reversed, in parallel with amelioration of symptoms, by dopaminergic drugs [21].

☐ INVESTIGATION OF FUNCTIONAL INTERACTIONS BETWEEN DIFFERENT BRAIN REGIONS

Functional neuro-imaging is being applied to characterise the connections between the brain regions serving motor, sensory and cognitive functions. These studies are complicated and technically demanding: in general, multiple scans recorded under different but related task conditions are required to study spatiotemporal correlations of cognitive aspects of brain activity.

Some intriguing links between motor and cognitive functions have already been identified. Externally instructed movements cause significantly greater activation of motor cortex than those that are self-selected. The same applies to extrinsically specified and internally generated word lists. The DLPFC is activated in the left, language-dominant hemisphere by internally generated language tasks, and this activation is accompanied by significant de-activation of the superior temporal gyrus, including the primary auditory and auditory association cortex. In the extrinsically specified task, there is prominent activation of the same temporal regions. These observations suggest an interaction between the DLPFC, which apparently initiates a movement or a verbal response, and the relevant modality-specific area of cortex that executes it. It also indicates a difference in cortical activity between actions that are internally generated and those that are a response to external stimuli. Such distinctions may be relevant to diseases with symptoms that include the misattribution of actions or thoughts, eg feelings of alien control in schizophrenia, the 'alien hand' syndrome that accompanies corticobasal degeneration, and delusions in states of impaired awareness.

☐ DOES THE BRAIN WORK HARDER WITH MORE DIFFICULT TASKS?

Improved quantitation of scan data has made it possible to examine the impact of graded cognitive tasks, and it has been shown that these are often associated with graded responses or physiological changes. Parametric scanning depends on recording task performances and correlating them with scan data, thus identifying regions in which activation is altered as a function of a task. The difficulty of a set task may itself be varied, for example, by presenting the subject with flashes of light at increasing frequencies; in this case, activity in the visual cortex reaches a maximum and falls off at frequencies where it is difficult to discriminate between individual flashes.

Similarly, activity in the primary auditory cortex increases linearly with the number of words spoken per unit time [22]. However, the posterior temporal (Wernicke's) cortex, to which the auditory cortex projects, shows a different response with such stimuli. Activation is apparent as soon as words are heard, but local brain activity does not increase further across a range of word frequencies. The conversion of a time-dependent response in the primary auditory cortex to one in which activity is time-independent suggests a possible mechanism for integration of frequency-determined neural activity into a form that could signal the fundamental properties of language, namely phonological or semantic identity. Breakdown of this system may be a basis for the aphasia encountered with damage to Wernicke's area.

□ LOCALISATION OF MEMORY AND LEARNING PROCESSES TO BRAIN AREAS

The final part of this chapter will deal with the functional neuro-anatomy of human memory, a topic made complicated by the great variety of memory processes now identified and the interactions between them.

Working memory

Like many cognitive processes, memory is apparently composed of a number of sub-processes. A theoretical model of verbal working memory developed by Baddeley and colleagues proposes at least two sub-processes: a 'rehearsal' system, which refreshes a 'phonological store' that acts as a memory buffer of limited size and with a half-life of approximately 2 seconds [23].

This conceptual framework has been verified by imaging experiments that have shown a critical role for Broca's area in the rehearsal function, and for the inferior parietal lobe in the phonological store [24]. People with developmental dyslexia appear to have a functional disconnection between Broca's area and the inferior parietal cortex, so these regions do not activate together as is the case in normal readers. In addition, dyslexic subjects show impaired working memory, which is entirely consistent with the pattern of dysfunction observed. Thus, cognitive processes (in this case, those involved in working memory) may be components of larger cognitive abilities (see Fig. 8).

Impact of learning new skills

The repetitive performing of tasks that results in learning is shown by functional neuro-imaging to result in progressive habituation of activations and even

(a)

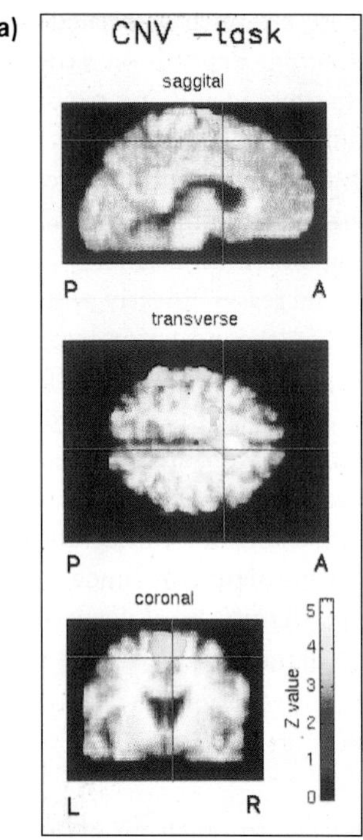

Fig. 8 Activation of common brain areas by **(a)** attention-demanding tasks and **(b)** memory retrieval. The demonstration of common areas of activation suggests that there may be shared cognitive processes in the systems underlying these two distinct and complex brain functions. The top figure (CNV-task) demonstrates a sagittal, transaxial and coronal brain slice activation of the midline prefrontal cortex. The CNV task demands considerable attentional resources. The lower figure shows in three transaxial slices that in the same midline prefrontal region (seen in the right-hand column) there is activation with retrieval of both facts from autobiographical memory (episodic memory) and from knowledge (semantic memory).

(b)

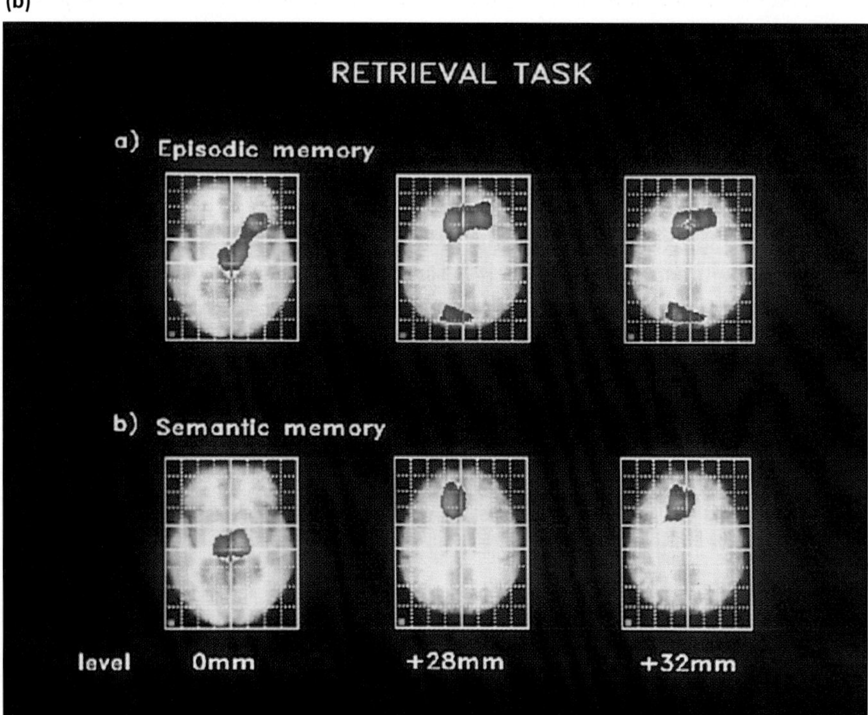

redistribution of activity between different brain areas. This is well shown by subjects asked to generate verbs in response to some target object. For example, the noun 'car' can be associated with the verbs 'drive', 'buy', 'wash' and 'crash'. Responses to novel categories produce activation in a distributed network that includes the DLPFC and various language-related areas. By contrast, responses to already overlearned words are associated with an attenuated pattern of activation resembling that obtained with the simple repetition of words, indicating that response selection has become automatic [25].

Learning specific motor skills results in improved performance that correlates with increased activity in primary and supplementary motor cortices. However, if the performance is kept constant during learning, progressive attenuation of cerebellar and premotor activation is observed, with an increase in SMA activity suggesting that this latter area is associated with the laying down of new motor programmes [26]. When a motor task is learned with feedback of errors (eg by an auditory signal), there is greater activation in the right premotor area than when the task has been overlearned, suggesting a role for this region in self-monitoring or attention.

When a task is novel and requires considerable attentional resources, there appear to be mechanisms for large-scale de-activation of whole systems that are not required for the task. When a task becomes overlearned, attentional needs decline, and activity in these other areas tends to normalise.

□ CONCLUSIONS

The field of functional brain mapping is in a state of rapid technical development. The data derived from the different mapping modalities are often complementary, and there is much evidence to suggest that further refinements will provide even better tools to explore the functional architecture of the human brain. In particular, advances in fMRI and in electrophysiological methods promise much-needed improvements in spatial and temporal resolution.

These techniques will undoubtedly help to unravel the complexities of brain functions that are unique to humans. At a more practical level, they may help in the understanding and treatment of disorders of cognitive function and other mental disease.

For example, grave neurological disorders such as schizophrenia that have few if any associated structural abnormalities detectable in life may well turn out to be 'functional' disorders due to abnormalities of cortical connectivity. Indeed, an abnormality of functional connectivity between the anterior cingulate cortex in the frontal lobe and the superior temporal cortex has been identified in schizophrenics; this defect is reversed by the administration of drugs acting on the dopaminergic systems and this reversal is accompanied by amelioration of symptoms [27].

REFERENCES

1 Frackowiak RSJ, Friston KJ, Frith CD, Dolan RJ, Mazziotta JC. *Human Brain Function.* San Diego: Academic Press, 1997: 1–521.

2 Zeki S. *A Vision of the Brain.* Oxford: Blackwells, 1993: 1–366.

3 Penfield W, Rasmussen T. *The Cerebral Cortex of Man.* New York: Macmillan, 1950.
4 Woolsey CN. In: Schaltenbrand G, Woolsey CN, eds. *Cerebral Localization and Organization.* Madison: University of Wisconsin Press, 1964.
5 Patten J. *Neurological Differential Diagnosis.* London: Harold Starke, 1977.
6 Schmitt F, Stehling MK, Turner R. *Echo-Planar Imaging: theory, technique and application.* Heidelberg: Springer Verlag, 1998: 1–662.
7 Toga AW, Mazziotta JC. *Brain Mapping: the methods.* San Diego: Academic Press, 1996: 1–471.
8 Schwartz WJ, Smith CB, Davidsen L, *et al.* Metabolic mapping of functional activity in the hypothalamo-neurohypophyseal system of the rat. *Science* 1979; **205**: 723–5.
9 Zeki S, Watson JDG, Lueck CJ, *et al.* A direct demonstration of functional specialization in human visual cortex. *J Neurosci* 1991; **11**: 641–9.
10 Tootell RB, Dale AM, Sereno MI, Malach R. New images from human visual cortex. *Trends Neurosci* 1996; **19**: 481–9.
11 Watson JDH, Myers R, Frackowiak RSJ, *et al.* Area V5 of the human brain: a combined study using positron emission tomography and magnetic resonance imaging. *Cerebral Cortex* 1993; **3**: 79–94.
12 Shipp S, de Jong BM, Zihl J, Frackowiak RSJ, Zeki S. The brain activity related to residual motion vision in a patient with bilateral lesions of V5. *Brain* 1994; **117**: 1023–38.
13 Lueck CJ, Zeki S, Friston KJ, *et al.* The colour centre in the cerebral cortex of man. *Nature* 1989; **340**: 386–9.
14 Barbur JL, Watson JDG, Frackowiak RSJ, Zeki S. Conscious visual perception without V1. *Brain* 1993; **116**: 1293–302.
15 Ungerleider LG, Mishkin M. Two cortical visual systems. In: Ingle DJ, Mansfield RJW, Goodale MD (eds). *The Analysis of Visual Behaviour.* Cambridge, MA: MIT Press, 1982.
16 Colebatch JG, Deiber MP, Passingham RE, Friston KJ, Frackowiak RSJ. Regional cerebral blood flow during voluntary arm and hand movements in human subjects. *J Neurophysiol* 1991; **65**: 1392–401.
17 Fink GR, Frackowiak RSJ, Pietrzyk U, Passingham RE. Multiple non-primary motor areas in the human cortex. *J Neurophysiol* 1997; **77**: 2164–74.
18 Frith CD, Friston KJ, Liddle PF, Frackowiak RSJ. Willed action and the prefrontal cortex in man. *Proc R Soc Lond (B)* 1991; **244**: 241–6.
19 Dettmers C, Lemon RN, Stephan KM, Fink GR, Frackowiak RSJ. Cerebral activation during the exertion of sustained static force in man. *NeuroReport* 1996; **7**: 2103–10.
20 Stephan K-M, Fink G, Passingham RE, *et al.* Functional anatomy of mental representation of upper extremity movements. *J Neurophysiol* 1995; **73**: 373–86.
21 Jenkins IH, Fernandez W, Playford ED, *et al.* Impaired activation of the supplementary motor area in Parkinson's disease is reversed when akinesia is treated with apomorphine. *Ann Neurol* 1992; **32**: 749–57.
22 Price C, Wise RJS, Ramsay S, *et al.* Regional response differences within the human auditory cortex when listening to words. *Neurosci Lett* 1992; **146**: 179–82.
23 Baddeley AD. *Working Memory. Oxford Psychology Series no. 11.* Oxford: Clarendon Press, 1986.
24 Paulesu E, Frith CD, Frackowiak RSJ. The neural correlates of the verbal component of working memory. *Nature* 1993; **362**: 342–5.
25 Petersen SE, van Mier H, Fiez JA, Raichle ME. The effects of practice on the functional anatomy of task performance. *Proc Natl Acad Sci USA* 1988; **95**: 853–60.
26 Friston KJ, Frith CD, Passingham RD, Liddle PF, Frackowiak RSJ. Motor practice and neurophysiological adaptation in the cerebellum: a PET study. *Proc R Soc Lond Biol* 1992; **243**: 223–8.
27 Dolan RJ, Fletcher P, Frith CD, *et al.* Dopaminergic modulation of impaired cognitive activation in the anterior cingulate cortex in schizophrenia. *Nature* 1995; **378**: 180–2.

Management of acute stroke

Peter Sandercock

☐ INTRODUCTION

Stroke is an enormous problem, affecting about 8 million people worldwide each year. Six months after a stroke, about two-thirds of patients are either dead or sufficiently disabled to need help with the activities of daily living. Common complications after stroke include painful shoulder, aspiration pneumonia and mood disorder, while others such as pulmonary embolism are rare but none the less important. The acute management of stroke aims to limit the volume of brain damaged by the primary stroke, to prevent complications and early stroke recurrence, and to start long-term secondary prevention measures. Combined with early, well coordinated rehabilitation, these measures should reduce long-term impairment, disability and handicap.

☐ CAUSES AND CONSEQUENCES OF STROKE

In the UK, about 85% of strokes are ischaemic [1]. Most are due to the thrombotic and embolic complications of atheromatous disease in the great arteries in the neck. About 20% are associated with a potential source of embolism within the heart, such as atrial fibrillation, although the presence of such a source does not necessarily mean that it caused the stroke [1]. About one-quarter of all ischaemic strokes are due to occlusion of a small deep penetrating artery within the brain (lacunar infarction). In the first 2 weeks after an ischaemic stroke, the risks are moderate: about 12% of patients suffer major complications, 9% die and 3% suffer a non-fatal recurrent stroke [1,2].

Cerebral haemorrhage accounts for most of the remaining strokes. A common cause of haemorrhagic stroke in the elderly is amyloid angiopathy of the cerebral vessels, which tends to cause recurrent haemorrhages. Other predisposing factors include hypertension and long-term therapy with aspirin or warfarin [1]. The risk of early death is higher in patients with haemorrhagic stroke than with ischaemic stroke, although the poorer prognosis is related more to the greater volume of tissue destruction, and the location of the bleed, than to the fact that the stroke is haemorrhagic; a small intracerebral bleed may have a similar, relatively benign, long-term prognosis to a comparably sized infarct [1].

☐ DIAGNOSIS AND ASSESSMENT

Obtain a clear history and ensure accurate clinical diagnosis

The clinical diagnosis of acute stroke may not be straightforward, especially within the first hour or two after onset [1]. It is crucial to obtain a clear history that the neurological deficit was *focal* and that it definitely came on *suddenly* or was first noted on waking from sleep; if the patient or family can give a clear time of onset, this is useful supporting evidence that onset really was sudden. Time spent in finding out precisely what happened, and when, is not wasted, as it will make diagnosis more accurate and management more appropriate. It is also important to consider stroke in patients who present with deficits other than hemiparesis: common stroke syndromes include isolated dysphasia or hemianopia, weakness of just a hand or arm, and sudden ataxia.

Perform computed tomography early to exclude intracranial haemorrhage

Current-generation computed tomography (CT) scanners can reliably identify even small intracerebral haemorrhages. These are initially hyperdense (ie they appear white on CT scan; Fig. 1), but their density declines progressively as the haemoglobin alters chemically: within a few days, the haematoma may become isodense with surrounding brain and therefore invisible, but after a week or two will be hypodense and may be indistinguishable from an infarct. Cerebral infarcts appear darker than normal brain (Fig. 2); a sudden increase in density indicates haemorrhage into the infarcted region (Fig. 1). To differentiate infarction from haemorrhage, CT scans must therefore be done as soon as practicable, and no more than 2 weeks after onset [1]. Some doctors and radiologists favour delaying the CT scan in order to image the cerebral infarct, because the cerebral lesion following an acute ischaemic stroke may not be readily visible on a CT performed within the first hours (Fig. 2). This makes no sense; the aim of treating stroke patients acutely is to prevent (or at least limit) the extent of cerebral infarction, which of course becomes impossible if diagnostic scanning is first performed after irreversible cerebral infarction has occurred.

Patients with transient ischaemic attacks (TIAs) and minor ischaemic strokes need to be clinically assessed with urgency, but do not need to be admitted to have their CT; this can be performed as an outpatient but, as the aim in both types of patient is to exclude haemorrhage, it must be done within 2 weeks. Patients with a severe carotid stenosis and whose stroke symptoms arise from parts of the brain (or eye) fed by the carotid artery are likely to benefit from carotid endarterectomy; current guidelines from the European Carotid Surgery Trial (ECST) suggest that operation should be considered for arteries showing 80% or more stenosis. Patients with atrial fibrillation should be given long-term oral anticoagulants, unless these are contraindicated (see chapter 25).

□ MANAGEMENT OF ACUTE STROKE

Admit to a stroke unit for coordinated multidisciplinary care

Organised stroke care saves lives and reduces the risk of death or institutionalisation by about one-third [3]. For every 1,000 patients admitted to a stroke rehabilitation unit, 71 avoid a poor long-term outcome [3]. The duration of hospital stay is no longer in rehabilitation units than in routine wards. The benefits of admission to an *acute* stroke unit are less clear. Such units may serve as a useful focus for research and education, but there is no clear evidence that they improve outcome.

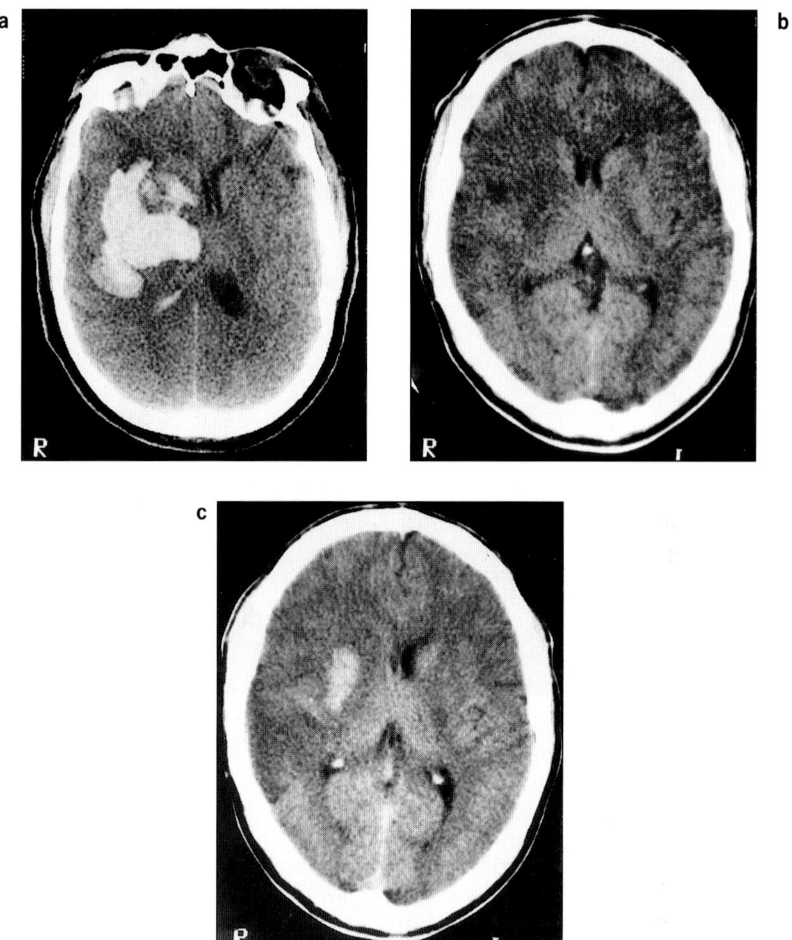

Fig. 1 Computed tomography scan appearances of stroke: **(a)** acute intracerebral haemorrhage in the right hemisphere, showing typical high-density (white) lesion; **(b)** typical low-attenuation (dark) infarct in the right hemisphere of another patient; **(c)** the same lesion a few days later, showing an increase in density due to subsequent haemorrhagic transformation.

Organised stroke care should be delivered by a multidisciplinary team that really functions as a team. There should be regular meetings for all members and a designated leader, and the team should preferably operate within a clearly defined space, ideally a dedicated stroke unit [3].

Assess swallowing, hydration and nutrition immediately

Swallowing difficulties lead to aspiration pneumonia and hypoxia as well as poor nutrition and dehydration, so careful assessment of swallowing within the first few hours of stroke is important. All stroke units have a protocol for the bedside

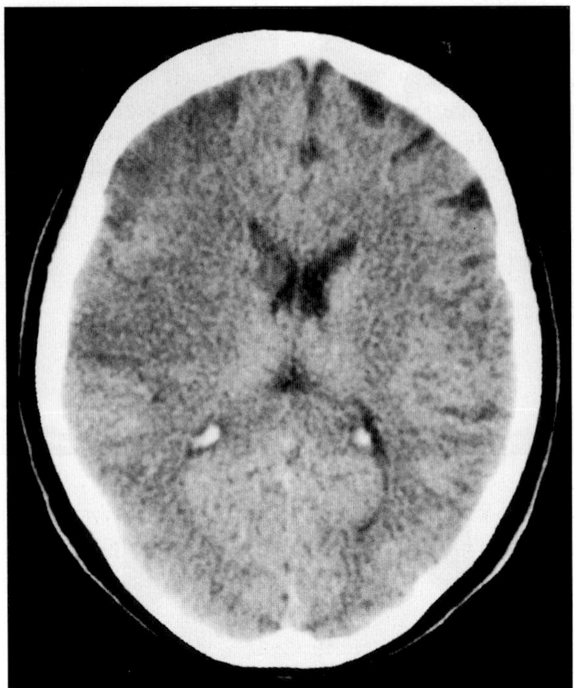

Fig. 2 Computed tomography scan showing subtle changes of early infarction in the right hemisphere (ie left side of picture).

assessment of swallowing function which can be done by doctors or nurses (nurses are preferable, as they tend to be more thorough and systematic).

The initial assessment usually consists of the supervised swallowing of small volumes of water. Coughing, choking or a 'wet voice' indicate swallowing problems and the need to avoid oral intake, at least until assessed in detail by a speech therapist. A modified barium swallow can be useful; a small volume of contrast medium should be given in the presence of a speech therapist, and the screening fluoroscopy recorded on videotape. Contrary to common belief, the gag reflex is useless in evaluating the safety of swallowing and has no value in the assessment of acute stroke.

The optimal fluid and feeding policy for stroke patients remains uncertain, and it has not yet been reliably determined whether food should be administered by percutaneous gastrostomy or by nasogastric tube. These issues are currently being examined in a large, international randomised trial, the Food Or Ordinary Diet trial (FOOD), which aims to recruit over 4,000 patients.

Rehabilitation should start immediately after admission

Stroke patients should no longer have to wait for rehabilitation; this process and planning for discharge must begin immediately on admission. Multidisciplinary rehabilitation obviously focuses on the patient, but must not neglect those who will look after the patient following discharge. Carers of stroke patients need to be educated about practical issues such as how to move and handle disabled stroke patients, and must also be informed about the services available to support them in the community after discharge. They must also know that behavioural complications – notably anger, irritation, depression and non-specific worries – occur frequently after stroke. These problems must be dealt with either by appropriate psychological management or, if low mood is persistent and severe, antidepressant therapy. Low mood in the patient can cause serious problems for the carer, who must not feel neglected in the process of rehabilitation.

Start antiplatelet therapy with oral or rectal aspirin as soon as practicable

The benefits of antiplatelet therapy with aspirin for long-term secondary prevention of stroke and other serious vascular events are clear; when started a few weeks after an ischaemic stroke, this is likely to avoid about 36 serious vascular events per 1,000 patients treated over the next 3 years [4]. Until recently, there has been uncertainty about when to start aspirin in patients presenting to hospital with an acute ischaemic stroke, in whom haemorrhage has been excluded by CT scanning. Two recent large randomised trials, the International Stroke Trial (IST) [2] and the Chinese Acute Stroke Trial (CAST) [5], each including 20,000 patients, have both provided reliable evidence that beginning aspirin within the first 48 hours is more beneficial than waiting for a few weeks. For every 1,000 patients starting aspirin early, an additional nine will avoid early death or recurrent stroke within the first few weeks, 13 will avoid death or dependency a few months after the stroke, and an additional 10 will recover completely from their stroke (see Fig. 3).

The dose of aspirin in the acute phase of stroke is probably not critical provided that it is at least 160 mg daily. This dose rapidly inhibits thromboxane biosynthesis, which is massively activated early in the acute phase of stroke. About one-third of patients with acute stroke cannot swallow safely, and they should receive aspirin as a 300 mg suppository daily. These suppositories are now available in most UK hospitals. Once started in hospital, aspirin should be continued indefinitely for secondary prevention. Effective doses of aspirin for long-term secondary prevention probably lie between 30 and 300 mg daily; side effects are likely to be less with the lower dose [4].

Avoid routine heparin therapy in acute ischaemic stroke

Subcutaneous heparin therapy has been advocated by some after acute stroke, particularly to prevent deep venous thrombosis and pulmonary embolism, two well recognised complications of reduced mobility. In the IST, patients were randomly allocated to 12,500 or 5,000 units of unfractionated heparin subcutaneously twice daily, or had no heparin for the first 14 days. Heparin treatment at either dosage was not associated with any net short- or long-term benefit, but conferred a significant risk of bleeding: for every 1,000 patients treated, heparin caused about eight extra

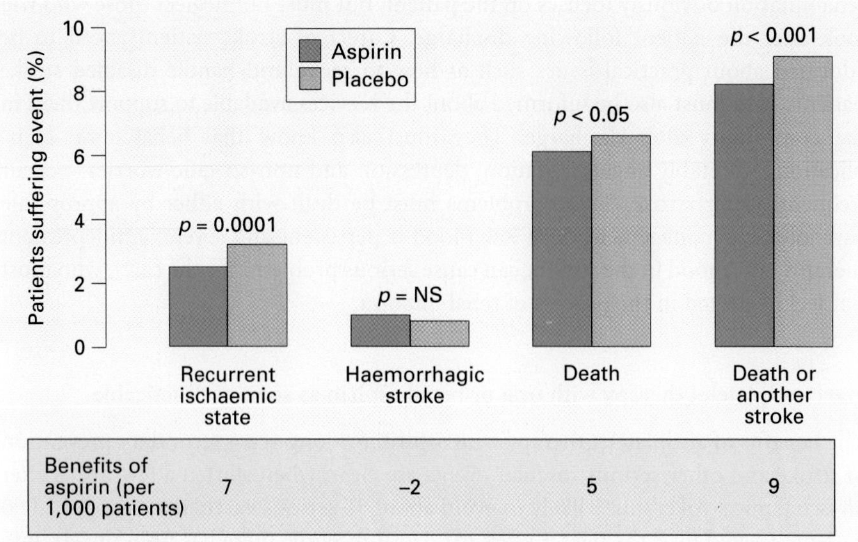

Fig. 3 Systematic review of the absolute effects of early aspirin treatment in acute ischaemic stroke on clinical events (indicated below histograms) occurring in the first 14 days. Data from CAST, IST and MAST. Redrawn from [5].

symptomatic intracranial haemorrhages and about nine extracranial haemorrhages. The risk of bleeds was much higher with the higher dose (Fig. 4). Data combined from several trials, including the IST, indicate that heparin reduced the risk of recurrent ischaemic stroke by about one-quarter, but more than doubled the risk of an intracranial bleed (Fig. 5). Overall, therefore, heparin does not produce clear net benefits and should not be used in acute ischaemic stroke.

In most stroke units nowadays, patients are given daily aspirin, mobilised early and provided with compression stockings to prevent deep vein thrombosis, and only rarely become dehydrated. All of these manoeuvres are likely to reduce the risk of deep venous thrombosis and pulmonary embolism, further questioning the need for routine use of subcutaneous heparin. Indeed, the risk of pulmonary embolism within 2 weeks reported in the IST was only 1%, though the true rate was probably higher because of underascertainment. Nonetheless, the data did not provide strong evidence to support a policy of routine heparin therapy to prevent pulmonary embolism, or even its selective use in patients at higher risk of thromboembolism because of leg paralysis [2,6]. On the other hand, there is good evidence that heparin reduces the risk of deep venous thrombosis in stroke [6]. Overall, it is reasonable to consider heparin in selected individuals at particularly high risk, such as those with previous thromboembolic episodes or thrombophilia, or perhaps evidence of asymptomatic calf vein thrombosis on ultrasound compression venography.

The newer low molecular weight heparin and heparinoids have not been adequately evaluated in acute stroke, and the limited data available do not provide clear evidence of net short- or long-term benefit [2,6].

Another contentious issue has been the use of early heparin in ischaemic stroke

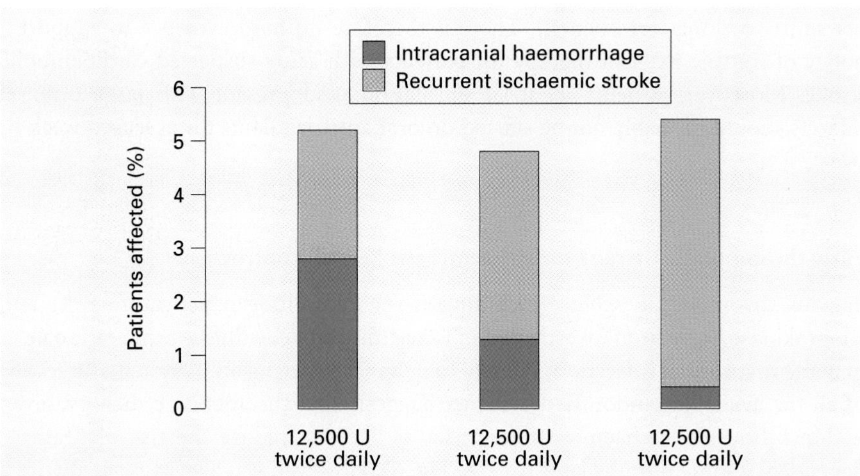

Fig. 4 Absolute effect of different heparin regimens on recurrent ischaemic stroke and on symptomatic intracranial haemorrhage within 14 days in 3,163 patients with atrial fibrillation in the IST. Data from IST [2].

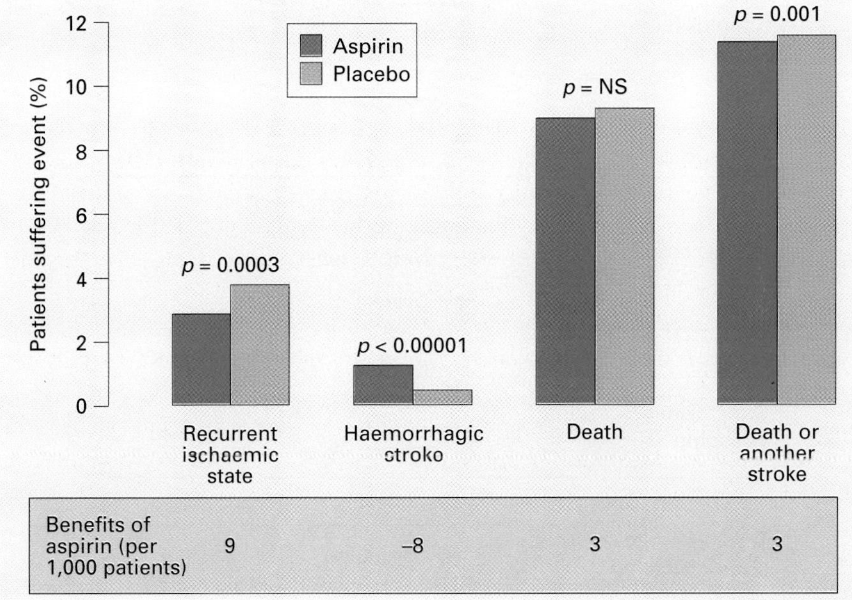

Fig. 5 Systematic review of the absolute effects of early heparin therapy in acute ischaemic stroke on clinical events during the first 14 days. Data from IST [2] and [6], totalling 21, 600 patients.

attributed to an embolus originating in the heart, particularly in patients who have atrial fibrillation. The IST included over 3,000 patients with atrial fibrillation and acute ischaemic stroke [1] in whom immediate heparin therapy significantly reduced the risk of early recurrent ischaemic stroke; however, this benefit was offset by a comparable increase in the risk of haemorrhagic stroke and there was no overall net short- or long-term benefit. There is therefore no hard evidence to support a policy of routine heparin therapy for patients with acute suspected cardioembolic stroke. Moreover, patients in atrial fibrillation who present with large cerebral infarcts should probably not be started on oral anticoagulants for at least a week or two.

Early thrombolytic therapy for ischaemic stroke: still controversial

Various thrombolytic agents, including tissue plasminogen activator (tPA) and streptokinase, have been investigated in ischaemic stroke, with the same rationale as in acute myocardial infarction, namely to enhance reperfusion. A systematic review of all the available randomised evidence suggests that thrombolytic therapy, given within 6 hours of ischaemic stroke onset, is likely to reduce the risk of death or dependency some months later [7] (see Fig. 6). However, it is also associated with a

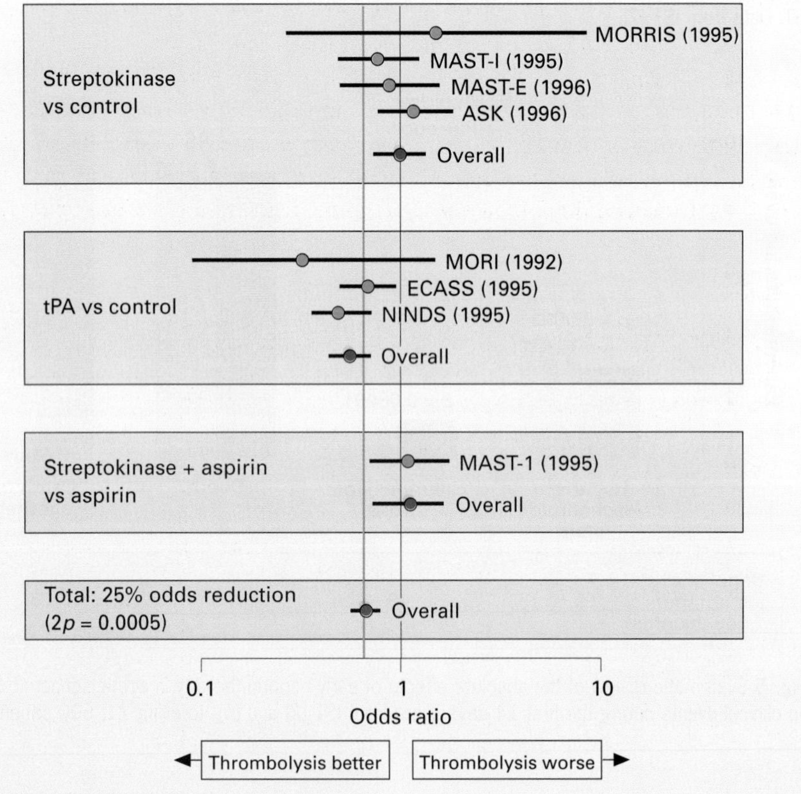

Fig. 6 Systematic review of trials of thrombolysis within 6 hours of onset: effects on death or dependency at the end of scheduled trial follow-up. Results expressed as odds ratio with 95% confidence interval (CI). Each study is shown as a blue circle, with the overall result for each treatment a red circle. Symbols to the left of the vertical line indicate benefit from therapy; those to the right, harm from therapy. If the 95% CI overlaps the vertical line, the result is not significant at the 5% level (tPA = tissue plasminogen activator). Redrawn from [7].

significant immediate risk of intracranial haemorrhage (see Fig. 7) and, at 3–6 months, with an excess of about 40 deaths per 1000 patients treated (95% confidence intervals, 20–83 per 1,000). The balance of risk and benefit is much more favourable if it is given within 3 hours (see Fig 8), but it still carries significant early hazards.

In my opinion, the balance of risk and benefit of thrombolytic therapy is unclear for most patients; I think that it is premature to recommend it routinely even for patients presenting within 3 hours, and that its use should be confined to randomised controlled trials until decisive evidence has been gathered. However, this is a controversial area, and many physicians in Europe and the US regard tPA as standard therapy for appropriately selected patients.

Thrombolytic therapy used outside a randomised trial should only be given in the context of a very well organised acute stroke service, with meticulous attention to diagnosis, selection of patients and minimising the delay between onset and treatment. As delaying thrombolytic drugs reduces the scope for benefit, early and accurate diagnosis is critical. In the first few hours after a cerebral infarct, the CT scan is likely to be normal or show only subtle changes of infarction; if the CT does not clearly show an infarct – which can be a very subjective judgement – the decision to give or withhold thrombolytic therapy depends almost entirely on the *clinical* diagnosis of 'acute stroke'. This places considerable responsibility on the clinician who makes the assessment: for example, an intracranial haemorrhage due to inappropriate use of thrombolytic therapy in a case whose hemiparesis was not due to an ischaemic stroke but to a Todd's paresis from an unrecognised epileptic seizure would be catastrophic for the patient (and could have serious medicolegal

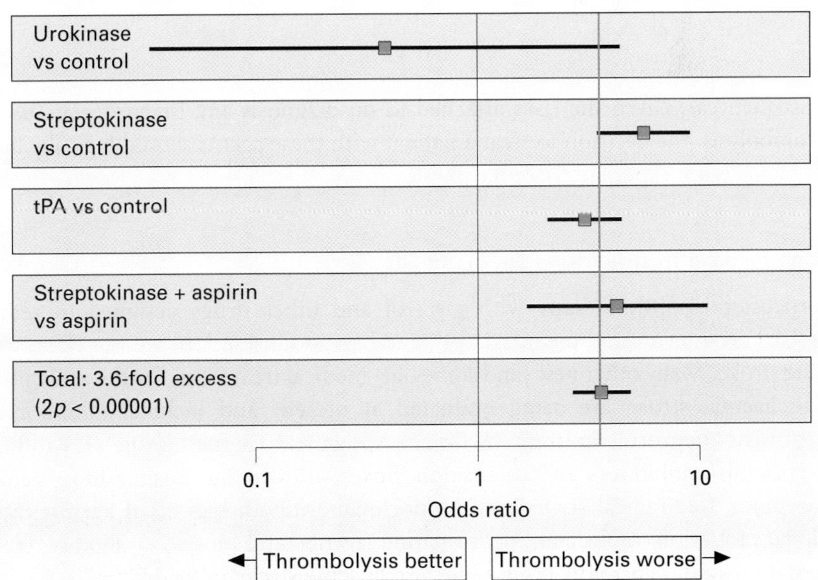

Fig. 7 Systematic reviews of trials of thrombolysis within 6 hours of onset: effects on symptomatic intracranial haemorrhage (tPA = tissue plasminogen activator).

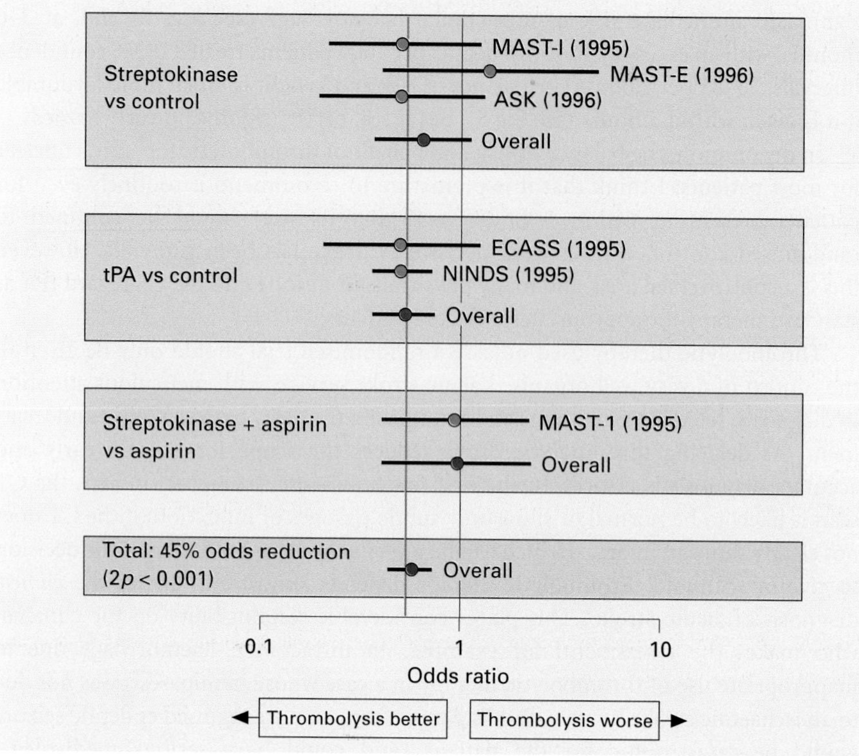

Fig. 8 Systematic review of trials of thrombolysis within 3 hours of onset: effects on death or dependency at the end of scheduled trial follow-up (CI = confidence interval; tPA = tissue plasminogen activator).

consequences). Given the risks attached to misdiagnosis and inappropriate use of thrombolysis, the decision to treat a patient with these agents should logically be in the hands of an experienced stroke physician.

Other medical treatments for the acute phase

Corticosteroids [8], therapy with glycerol and other drugs designed to reduce cerebral oedema around the infarct [9], and haemodilution [10] are not effective in acute stroke. Many other new (and some old) medical treatments for the acute phase of ischaemic stroke are being evaluated at present and include: inhibitors of excitotoxic neurotransmitters (Selfotel, Aptiganel, Clomethiazole, GV150526, magnesium), inhibitors of various ion fluxes, intravenous magnesium, benzodiazepines, free-radical scavengers, monoclonal antibodies directed against intercellular adhesion molecules, defibrinating agents and drugs to modify blood pressure. None is currently licensed for use in acute stroke in the UK.

The optimum management of blood pressure in acute stroke is the subject of an ongoing collaborative systematic review of all the randomised evidence (Blood

Pressure in Acute Stroke collaboration) [11]. At present no definite conclusions can be drawn about how to manage acute stroke patients with 'high', 'normal' or 'low' blood pressure [11].

Plan long-term secondary prevention before discharge

Several important steps in the secondary prevention of further events in patients with ischaemic stroke have been mentioned above. They include: long-term aspirin; performing carotid ultrasound in patients with carotid territory stroke to identify severe symptomatic carotid stenosis and evaluate the patient's suitability for endarterectomy; and treating patients in atrial fibrillation with long-term oral anticoagulants.

Attention to vascular risk factors is probably even more important, particularly hypertension [12] and smoking. Patients with symptomatic coronary artery disease should be considered for cholesterol lowering treatment with a statin; whether all survivors of ischaemic stroke should have statins is controversial [13].

☐ ACKNOWLEDGEMENT

Thanks go to Dr C Sudlow for help in creating the diagrams of the thrombolysis systematic review.

REFERENCES

1 Warlow CP, Dennis MS, van Gijn J, *et al. Stroke: A Practical Guide to Management.* Oxford: Blackwell Scientific, 1996.

2 International Stroke Trial Collaborative Group. The International Stroke Trial (IST): a randomised trial of aspirin, subcutaneous heparin, both, or neither among 19,435 patients with acute ischaemic stroke. *Lancet* 1997; **349**: 1569–81.

3 Stroke Unit Trialists' Collaboration. Collaborative systematic review of the randomised trials of organised inpatient (stroke unit) care after stroke. *Br Med J* 1997; **314**: 1151–9.

4 Antiplatelet Trialists' Collaboration. Collaborative overview of randomised trials of antiplatelet therapy. I. Prevention of death, myocardial infarction and stroke by prolonged antiplatelet therapy in various categories of patients. *Br Med J* 1994; **308**: 81-106.

5 CAST (Chinese Acute Stroke Trial) Collaborative Group. Randomised placebo-controlled trial of early aspirin use in 20,000 patients with acute ischaemic stroke. *Lancet* 1997; **349**: 1641–9.

6 Counsell C, Sandercock P. Anticoagulant therapy compared to control in patients with acute presumed ischaemic stroke. In: Warlow C, van Gijn J, Sandercock P, Candelise L, Langhorne P (Eds.) *Stroke Module of the Cochrane Database of Systematic Reviews,* (updated 03 June 1997). Available in the Cochrane Library; database on disk and CD ROM. The Cochrane Collaboration; Issue 3. Oxford: Update Software, 1997. Updated quarterly.

7 Wardlaw JM, Warlow C, Counsell C. Systematic review of evidence on thrombolytic therapy for acute ischaemic stroke. *Lancet* 1997; **350**: 607–14.

8 Qizilbash N, Lewington SL, Lopez-Arrieta JM. Corticosteroids following acute presumed ischaemic stroke. *The Cochrane Database (see reference 6).*

9 a'Rogvi-Hansen B, Boysen G. Glycerol treatment in acute ischaemic stroke. *Cochrane Database (see reference 6).*

10 Asplund K, Israelsson K, Schampi I. Haemodilution in acute ischaemic stroke. *Cochrane Database (see reference 6).*

11 Blood Pressure in Acute Stroke Collaboration (BASC). Blood pressure management in acute stroke. Part I. Assessment of trials designed to alter blood pressure. *Cochrane Database (see reference 6).*

12 Neal B, MacMahon S, PROGRESS Management Committee. PROGRESS (perindopril protection against recurrent stroke study): rationale and design. *J Hypertens* 1995; **13**: 1869–73.

13 Blauw GJ, Lagaay AM, Smelt AH, Westendorp RG. Stroke, statins and cholesterol: a meta-analysis of randomized, placebo-controlled, double-blind trials with HMG-CoA reductase inhibitors. *Stroke* 1997; **28**: 946–50.

☐ MULTIPLE CHOICE QUESTIONS

1 A CT scan of a patient with an acute focal neurological deficit:
(a) Showing a hyperdense (white) lesion in the relevant area indicates the stroke was due to intracerebral haemorrhage
(b) If normal, rules out stroke as the diagnosis
(c) Is better able to diagnose cerebral haemorrhage if the first scan is delayed for a few days
(d) Can be performed as an outpatient

2 Stroke rehabilitation units:
(a) The key element to the management of the stroke unit is that the senior physician adopts a ‘strong leadership’ role model
(b) Have been evaluated by randomised trials involving about 1,000 patients
(c) For every 1,000 patients treated, about 70 avoid death or institutionalisation
(d) Are effective, but generally need longer than average hospital stays to achieve their benefits

3 Swallowing assessment:
(a) The gag reflex is the simplest and most reliable way of assessing whether a stroke patient should be ‘nil by mouth’ or not
(b) For patients with prolonged swallowing problems after stroke, randomised trials have clearly shown percutaneous gastrostomy to be superior to nasogastric tube feeding
(c) The FOOD trial is evaluating multivitamin therapy and parenteral nutrition for stroke survivors
(d) A ‘wet voice’ after being given 5–10 ml of water is a reliable sign of swallowing problems

4 Aspirin, started within 48 hours of onset of acute ischaemic stroke:
(a) Should be given per rectum as a suppository in patients who are drowsy or cannot swallow safely
(b) Increases the chances of making a complete recovery from the stroke by 6 months
(c) Reduces the risk of pulmonary embolism
(d) Is effective at a dose of 160–300 mg daily

5 Heparin and thrombolysis in patients with acute ischaemic stroke:
(a) In IST, heparin was associated with an excess of 8 intracranial haemorrhages per 1,000 patients treated
(b) Thrombolytic therapy with tPA, given in appropriately selected patients, is not associated with any significant excess of intracranial bleeds
(c) In all patients with atrial fibrillation, heparin should be started immediately
(d) The risk of intracranial bleeding with heparin is dose-related

ANSWERS

1a True	2a False	3a False	4a True	5a True
b False	b False	b False	b True	b False
c False	c True	c False	c True	c False
d True	d False	d True	d True	d True

Emerging concepts in the management of acute myocardial infarction

Anthony H Gershlick

□ BACKGROUND

Thrombotic occlusion of the coronary arteries is usually caused by plaque disruption with release of the plaque's contents, resulting in activation of the coagulation systems (Fig. 1). This introduction will briefly review the background against which recent advances in the understanding and management of acute myocardial infarction will be set.

During the 1980s, thrombolytic drugs (particularly streptokinase and tissue plasminogen activator (tPA)) were tested for their benefits in large clinical trials and, when given sufficiently early were shown to reduce death rates by about 30%, to 10–12% or less [1]; 'real life' death rates are higher than those in trials because of patient selection and other factors. Thrombolytics should be given as soon as possible after infarction, though there may be benefit for up to 12 hours after the onset of symptoms. Audit standards suggest that an ECG should be performed within 15 minutes of arrival at hospital and thrombolytic therapy given within 30 minutes to patients with clinical and ECG evidence of acute infarction (Fig. 2). Educating the general public to seek help early after the onset of chest pain and

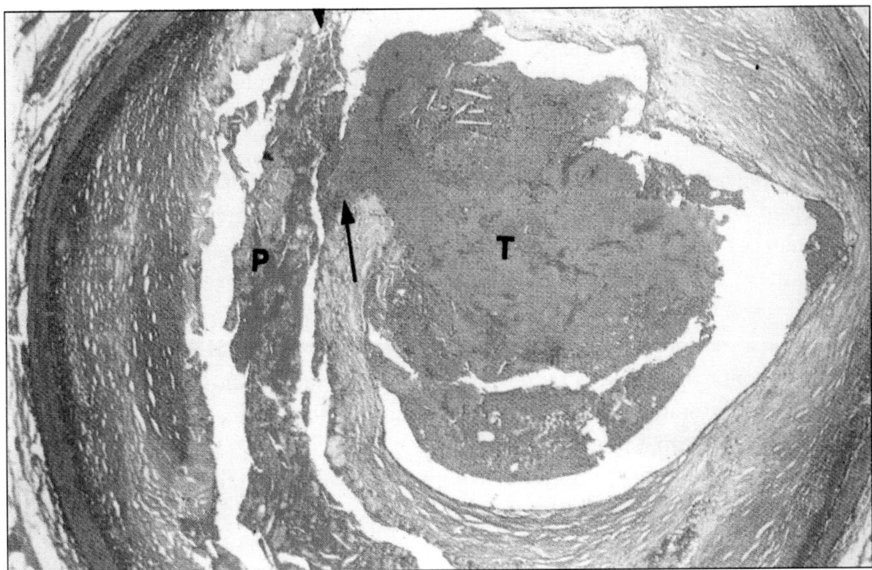

Fig. 1 Plaque events resulting in disruption and exposure to flowing blood procoagulant plaque contents are the most likely cause of coronary artery occlusions.

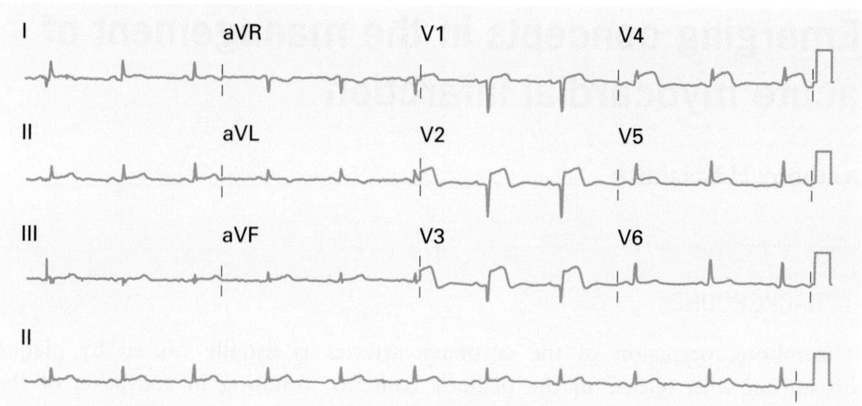

Fig. 2 Electrocardiographic evidence of acute coronary occlusion.

improving the speed of thrombolytic delivery remain important aims. tPA may have some advantages over streptokinase in certain patients, notably those who are younger, present early, have an anterior infarction or have received streptokinase for a previous infarct.

Aspirin appears to confer benefits equivalent to those of thrombolytics, and the case for lifelong aspirin therapy after a myocardial infarct now appears to be generally accepted. Its mode of action is unclear and may not be entirely related to its anticoagulant actions; acetylation of fibrinogen or effects on the red blood cell membrane may play a role.

Early angiotensin-converting enzyme (ACE) inhibitor administration in patients with impaired left ventricular function [2] or beta-blockers in those whose ventricular function is not severely impaired both improve long-term outcome.

Nitrates and prophylactic antiarrhythmics do not confer any benefit. The ISIS group have led a consensus against giving intravenous magnesium, as it has not been shown to improve outcome; however, some would argue for its use, especially in patients not receiving a thrombolytic.

The 'open artery' concept (ie the adoption of measures that restore and maintain patency of the occluded artery and allow reperfusion of the infarct territory) is important, as this has been shown to predict a good prognosis. The angiographic arm of the GUSTO trial [3] clearly demonstrated that improved flow through the infarct artery after intervention was associated with a lower mortality at 30 days. Reperfusion was quantitated in this and other trials by the TIMI grading, defined in Fig. 3. Patients with TIMI grade 0 flow (ie complete occlusion) at 90 min had a 30-day mortality rate of 8.4%, compared with only 4% in those with TIMI grade 3 (restoration of normal flow) (see Fig. 4).

TIMI grade 3 patency associated with the lowest mortality can currently be achieved in only 50% of patients with the best current thrombolytic strategy (accelerated tPA), and in only 30% of those treated with streptokinase; there clearly remains much room for improvement. In most trials, the greater vessel patency achieved with tPA compared with streptokinase has failed to translate into a

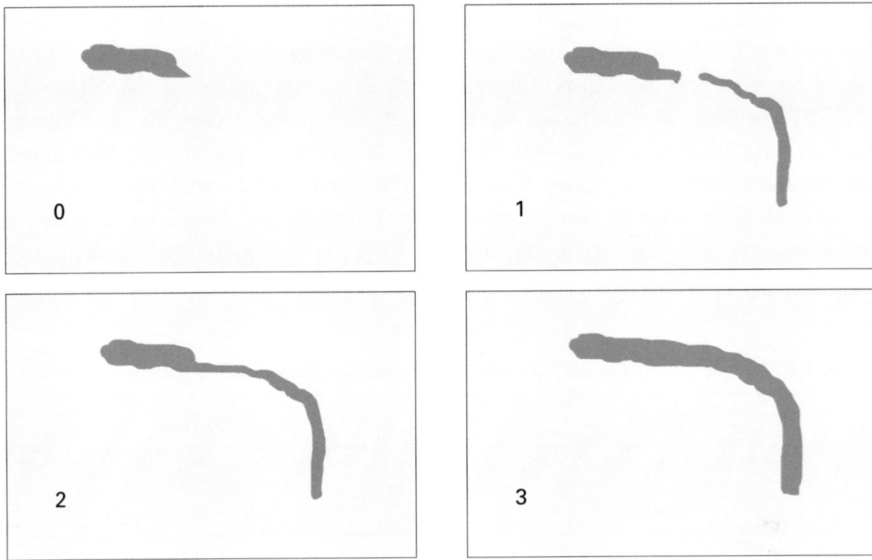

TIMI Grade

0 No flow of contrast beyond point of occlusion
1 Penetration with minimal perfusion (contrast fails to opacify entire coronary bed distal to the stenosis for duration of cine run)
2 Partial perfusions (contrast opacifies entire distal coronary but rate of entry and/or clearance is slower in the territory of the infarct artery than in nearby normally perfused vessels)
3 Complete perfusion (contrast filling and clearance are as rapid in the infarct-territory vessel as in normally perfused vessels)

Fig. 3 TIMI (thrombolysis in myocardial infarction) study grading system to measure restoration of patency in treated coronary arteries. Diagrammatic representation of angiographic images of coronary arteries. In clinical trials of thrombolytic drugs or angioplasty the TIMI grading is normally determined 90 minutes after intervention.

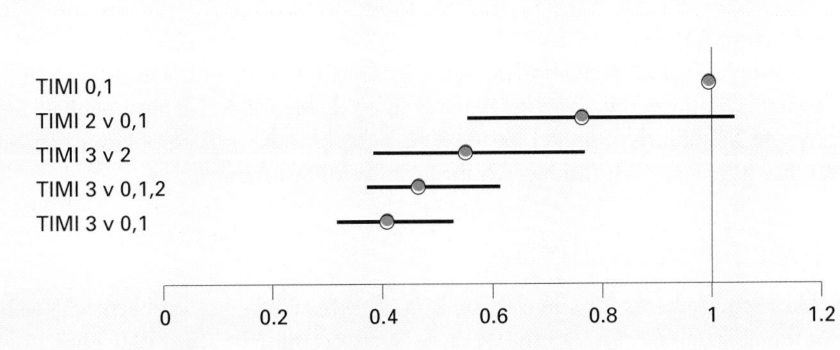

Fig. 4 Relationship between TIMI grade and 1 month mortality from the angiographic arm of the GUSTO trial; the higher the TIMI grade the better the outcome.

significant difference in mortality rates; the apparent benefit in the GUSTO-1 trial was partly offset by an excess of strokes in tPA treated patients (Table 1). The failure of tPA to produce a clear clinical benefit may relate in part to vessel reocclusion in the first few hours after initial opening, which is a particular problem with agents such as tPA that have a short half-life. In the longer term, reocclusion after acute myocardial infarction increases with time after intervention, with up to 30% of previously open arteries being occluded at 3 months [4]. Such reocclusion is important, since 3-year event-free survival (ie without reinfarction or stroke) is significantly lower in patients with an occluded artery at this time (68% v 92%).

Table 1 Comparison of 30-day mortality between tPA and streptokinase (SK) in three major trials.

	GISSI-2	ISIS-3	GUSTO-1
tPA	8.9%	10.3%	6.3% (0.7%*)
SK	8.5%	10.6%	7.3% (0.5%*)

*Incidence of intracranial bleeding.

☐ IMPROVING THE OUTCOME AFTER MYOCARDIAL INFARCTION

Currently available thrombolytics include streptokinase, tPA and more recently reteplase. In the UK, cost issues have meant that the less expensive streptokinase tends to be used as first-line agent in most patients, although the use of tPA has increased slightly following the GUSTO trial results [3]. tPA is used in patients previously given streptokinase, because of the risk of allergic reactions and reduced efficacy due to anti-streptokinase antibodies. Reteplase has yet to find its place.

So-called 'front loading' tPA, as in the GUSTO trial (ie giving the standard 100 mg dose over 90 min rather than over 3 h) appears to increase vessel patency, with the proportion of cases achieving TIMI grades 2 or 3 rising from 70% to 81%. Preliminary data suggest that a double-bolus regimen of 50 mg of tPA given 30 min apart may achieve TIMI grade 2/3 flow rates of 91%, but this needs to be confirmed in larger clinical trials.

Currently available thrombolytic regimens thus fall short of the ideal, by failing to re-establish and maintain vessel patency in a reliable fashion. The short half-life of tPA and the failure of higher early patency to translate into an obvious clinical advantage have stimulated the search for 'improved' thrombolytics.

☐ NEWER THROMBOLYTIC DRUGS

The ideal requirements for a new thrombolytic (which have not yet been achieved) are outlined in Table 2. Safety issues mean it is important to be aware of the potential narrow therapeutic window when more potent agents are being considered. Fibrin specificity (ie localisation of agent to clot) may only be a relative advantage since this may reduce half-life. Various new thrombolytics are currently in development or

Table 2 Ideal properties of a new thrombolytic drug.

- Non-antigenic
- Safe and well tolerated
- Resistant to plasminogen activator inhibitor (PAI-1)
- Fibrin specificity
- Long half-life to allow single-bolus administration
- High and maintained rates of coronary artery reperfusion
- Low cost

undergoing clinical trials. These include structurally modified variants of tPA, improved properties of which include resistance to inhibitors of thrombolysis such as plasminogen activator inhibitor-1 (PAI-1), or the need to bind to fibrin in order to become active, which would restrict their action to existing or forming thrombi; such modifications can enhance efficacy. Other approaches have involved molecular 're-design' of thrombolytic agents (eg alteration of the kringle 2 region of tPA) to reduce their plasma clearance and prolong half-life, although such modifications may lessen their thrombolytic capacity. Most of these modifications have increased clinical effectiveness, with increased rates of early patency (Figs 5 and 6).

Reteplase (rPA) is a non-glycosylated mutant of native tPA, which differs from it in the deletion of two molecular domains; this change contributes to the longer half-life of this agent [5]. Initial studies (RAPID-1 and RAPID-2) were open, randomised dose-finding studies. Data for rPA are encouraging, demonstrating vessel patency rates similar to those with accelerated tPA [6]. rPA has been assessed against streptokinase in the INJECT trial (6000 patients), which showed it to be as effective as streptokinase in reducing mortality with a trend towards improved mortality. rPA-treated patients had significantly fewer side-effects such as atrial fibrillation and cardiogenic shock, and showed complete resolution of ST segment elevation (an indirect measure of patency and a predictor of mortality) in a significantly higher proportion of cases.

Other agents such as lanoteplase (currently being assessed in the InTIME study) and TNK-tPA also have longer half-lives as a consequence of molecular manipulation. Lanoteplase achieves a particularly high 90-minute patency rate of 75% (Fig. 6), though this may turn out to be a disadvantage if higher efficacy also increases the risk of bleeding. The therapeutic choice in the next two or three years is likely to lie between these agents, though it is unlikely that either will be dramatically better than tPA and the problems of obtaining and maintaining very high patency safely will probably remain unresolved; in this case, the price of these drugs will become an important issue.

Naturally occurring thrombolytics such as the vampire bat plasminogen activator (bat-PA) have also attracted attention. This agent is similar to human tPA but does not have a plasmin-sensitive processing site; it thus appears to be resistant to PAI-1 and has greater fibrin selectivity than tPA. Experimental data have shown that bat-PA is effective without activating systemic plasminogen, and may therefore

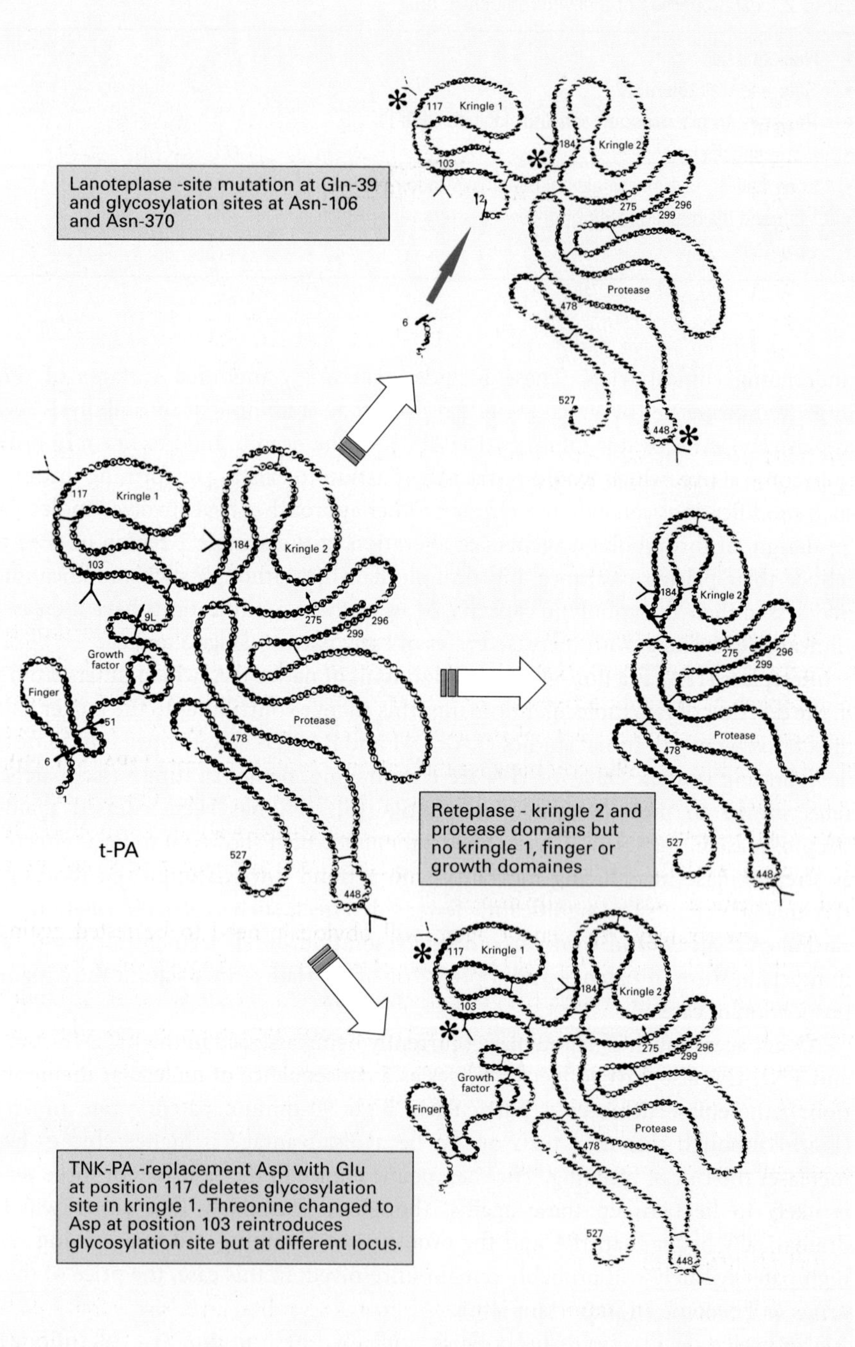

Fig. 5 Variations on the tPA molecule. The aim is to extend the half-life and to improve efficacy by promoting specific binding to fibrin in existing or forming clots (unfortunately these two aims may be mutually exclusive).

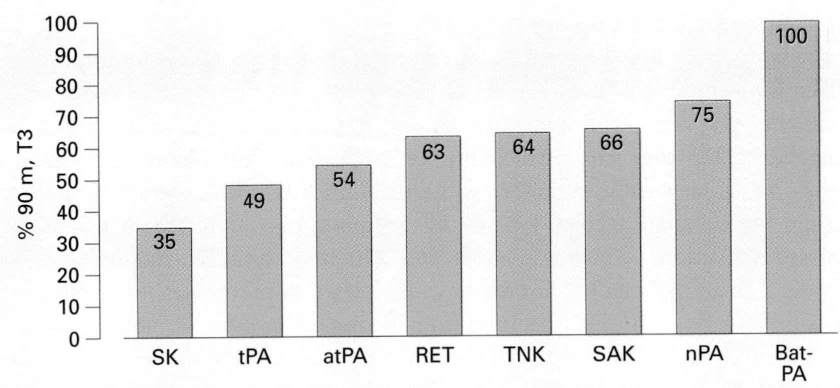

Fig. 6 TIMI grade 3 patency rates for some of the newer thrombolytics compared with established agents. (With kind permission of Professor B Wilcox)

have a lower bleeding complication rate. Early data suggest that it can achieve very high rates (90%) of TIMI grade 3 patency.

Staphylokinase, a protein produced by *Staphylococcus aureus*, has pro-fibrinolytic properties. A recombinant form (STAR), shown in experimental studies to be less immunogenic and more active against platelet-rich arterial clots than streptokinase, has now been evaluated in small-scale clinical trials. STAR (10–20 mg given over 30 min) produced similar coronary recanalisation rates to accelerated tPA, but without causing fibrinogen breakdown (indicating significantly greater fibrin specificity than tPA). Unfortunately, all patients developed STAR-neutralising antibodies after the second week following treatment, suggesting that this agent may not be as hypoallergenic as was originally hoped.

Any new strategy, regimen or agent will obviously need to be tested against currently used therapies; this field has now entered the era of equivalency trials [7]. These require substantial numbers of patients to show a mortality difference, but it seems likely that future clinical practice will incorporate some of the ideas and concepts outlined above. The current new competitor to accelerated tPA appears to be reteplase which, even though no more efficacious, is easier to give.

The 90-minute TIMI grade 3 patency rates for newer and the established thrombolytics are compared in Fig. 6.

☐ ANTITHROMBINS

Reocclusion after successful thrombolysis remains a problem. Heparin (followed by warfarin) and aspirin have been assessed in this context but did not significantly decrease the reocclusion rate at 3 months (25% v 32% with placebo) in the APRICOT study. Heparin, while relatively safe, has a number of disadvantages. It requires endogenous cofactors for activity (principally antithrombin III and heparin cofactor II). It is inactive against fibrin-bound thrombin and unable to displace thrombin bound to platelets, and its action can be neutralised by products released by activated platelets (eg platelet factor 4).

These disadvantages have led to interest in novel directly acting antithrombins. Currently preclinical and clinical research programmes are investigating a number of agents, in particular hirudin, argatroban and efegatran. All are antithrombin III independent, but they vary in their precise mechanisms for inhibiting thrombin. The last two are reversible inhibitors, while hirudin binds to both the active catalytic site and the substrate-recognition site of thrombin and inhibits both thrombin-catalysed activation of factors V, VIII and XIII and thrombin-induced platelet activation. In animal models, hirudin has been shown to prevent rethrombosis after tPA administration. Originally isolated from the leech *Hirudo medicinalis*, hirudin is now produced by recombinant DNA technology, and its desulphatohirudin form has been evaluated in clinical trials. Early results from the Thrombolysis in Myocardial Infarction (TIMI) 5 trial suggested that, following accelerated tPA administration, hirudin produced superior vessel patency at 18–36 hours compared with heparin (98% v 89%) and also reduced rates of mortality and reinfarction. Encouraging results were also obtained with hirudin versus heparin plus streptokinase in the TIMI-6 trial. Recently, three large clinical trials including hirudin (GUSTO-2, TIMI-9 and HIT-3) had to be discontinued and restarted at lower dosages because of an excess of intracerebral bleeding; unfortunately, preliminary results from the GUSTO 2b study have suggested that this lower dose confers no extra clinical benefit [8].

The narrow therapeutic window for these new antithrombins makes it difficult at present to define their exact role in clinical practice.

□ NEW ANTIPLATELET TREATMENTS

Platelets are central to thrombus generation after arterial injury. It has been known for some time that aspirin fundamentally affects only one route to platelet activation (the arachidonic acid pathway) and cannot, for example, block the stimulatory effects of high doses of collagen and thrombin on platelets. Work by Collen during the early 1980s revolutionised our understanding of effective antiplatelet therapy, by showing that the fibrinogen (glycoprotein IIb/III) receptor on platelets was central to platelet-platelet aggregation as well as to the development of the fibrin-platelet mesh that progresses to a mature thrombus.

A more effective antiplatelet approach would involve inhibition of the final common pathway which normally leads to GP IIb/IIIa activation (Fig. 7). A humanised monoclonal antibody against the receptor (7E3) has been shown in animal and preliminary human studies to improve vessel patency when given alone after coronary occlusion [9]. There have been reports of profound platelet inhibition and low rates of bleeding and recurrent ischaemia when 7E3 was used after tPA in small clinical studies. GUSTO-4 will test 7E3 (ReoPro) as adjunctive therapy to thrombolytic (either tPA or reteplase). Such studies will not be designed to replace aspirin – the benefits of which are proven – but rather to determine whether additional antiplatelet therapy acting through alternative pathways confers further advantages.

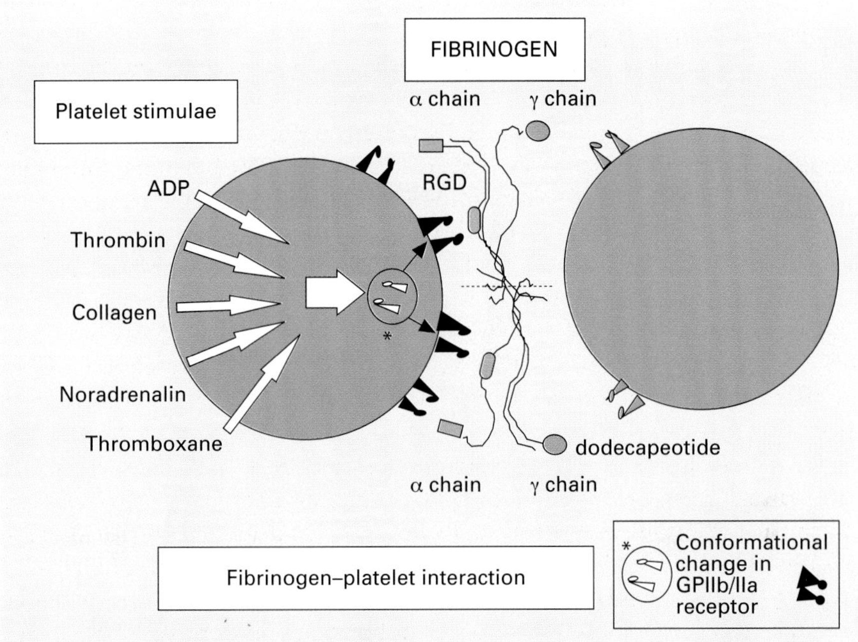

Fig. 7 Platelet activation pathways. The final common pathway involves the expression of the glycoprotein IIb/IIIa receptor which through fibrinogen binds platelets to each other. Inhibitors of this pathway are powerful inhibitors of platelet aggregation and more effective than aspirin which inhibits only one intraplatelet pathway.

Synthetic GP IIb/IIIa antagonists such as the peptide integrelin and the non-peptide compounds tirofiban and lamifiban hold promise as agents to supplement or possibly ultimately replace aspirin in treating myocardial infarction. The early pilot results using 7E3 and integrelin in acute myocardial infarction patients are encouraging and point to improvements in coronary artery patency and reductions in recurrent ischaemic events; bleeding complications will need to be carefully assessed.

Of the various therapeutic options that might be considered adjunctive to thrombolysis, these powerful platelet receptor blockers appear to have true potential.

☐ PRIMARY ANGIOPLASTY

An alternative therapy to thrombolysis in acute myocardial infarction (AMI) is angioplasty, whereby a wire and balloon mechanically removes the thrombus and dilates the underlying stenosis [8] (Fig. 8). This intervention requires taking the patient to a cardiac catheter laboratory, and needs to be performed as rapidly as possible.

Angioplasty can produce patency rates of 99% (with 97% being TIMI grade 3) [10], compared with the best current patency rates achieved with thrombolytic drugs of 81% (54% TIMI grade 3) (Fig. 9). Two trials have shown that these higher

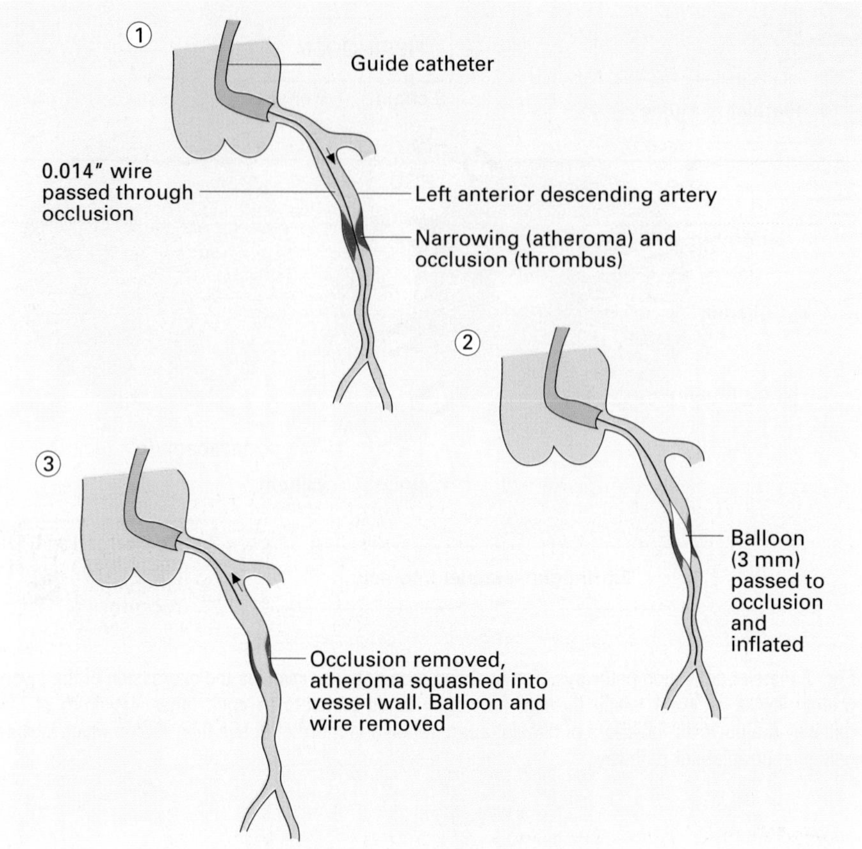
1
Guide catheter
0.014" wire passed through occlusion
Left anterior descending artery
Narrowing (atheroma) and occlusion (thrombus)
2
Balloon (3 mm) passed to occlusion and inflated
3
Occlusion removed, atheroma squashed into vessel wall. Balloon and wire removed

Fig. 8. Diagram showing the principle of coronary balloon angioplasty.

patency rates reduce 30-day mortality to 2.6% (cf 6.5% for tPA [11]), and decrease the relative risk from cardiac death by a factor of 6.1 (CI 2.9–12.7) compared with streptokinase. In the Zwolle study, angioplasty achieved TIMI grade 3 flow in 90% of patients (cf 55% in the streptokinase treated group), and was also associated with lower cardiac enzyme rises, better left ventricular function, less reinfarction (7% v 30%) and significantly lower 31-month mortality (5% v 13%; *p* 0.03). Whereas coronary artery reocclusion is common after thrombolytic therapy (30–40% by 3–6 months), it is less frequent (9–13%) after direct angioplasty [12]. In the longer term, event-free survival (ie absence of myocardial infarction, cardiac death or need for reintervention) has been shown by some authors to favour angioplasty, though other meta-analyses are less convincing, possibly because some small trials lacking statistical power were included. Pooling of the data suggests that high-risk patients (older, with larger and/or anterior infarcts) benefit particularly, both in terms of lower mortality and reinfarction rates. There is evidence that the outcome of angioplasty at a given centre depends on the volume of these interventions performed.

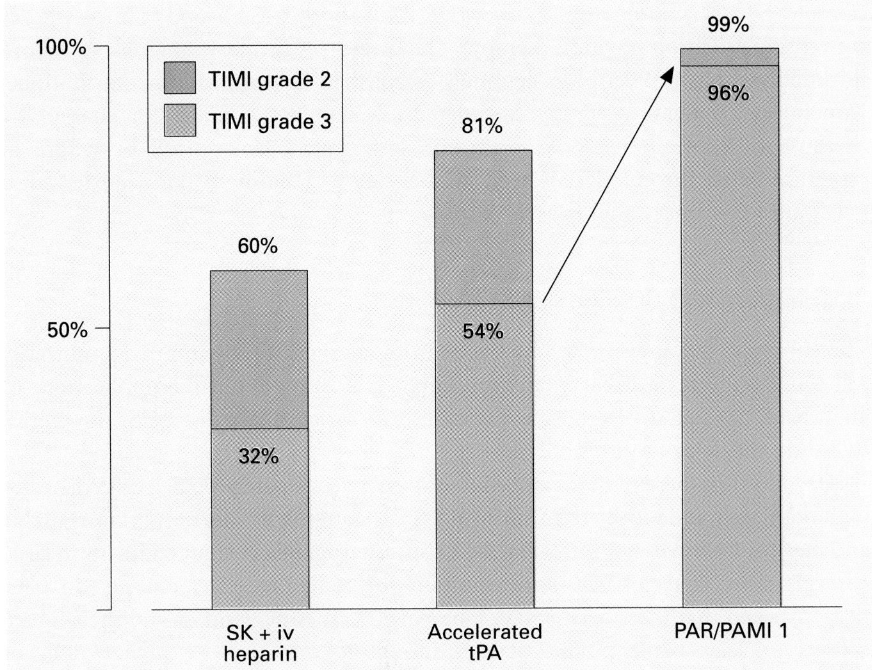

Fig. 9 How much better is balloon angioplasty than the current best available thrombolytic? Other trials indicate TIMI 3 patency in the setting of balloon angioplasty may be nearer 70%.

More recently, the GUSTO-2 trial failed to show significant benefits of angioplasty over tPA in total rate of death, reinfarction, and disabling strokes (10% v 13%; *p* 0.06). This may be related to the lower TIMI grade 3 patency rate achieved in this study (74%), compared with previous ones (>90%) [13]. Angioplasty for AMI has to be performed well and may need to involve deployment of stents; if it is to be undertaken, it must be performed by experienced operators who are more likely to achieve the TIMI grade 3 needed for acute and longer-term advantage.

□ HEALTH CARE RESOURCE IMPLICATIONS

Although the case for direct angioplasty for acute myocardial infarction appears compelling, particularly for selected high-risk cases, there are considerable problems related to limited resources, both in terms of personnel and finance.

A cost-benefit analysis undertaken in Europe and in the USA suggests that primary angioplasty appears no more expensive than thrombolysis in the longer term. However, the vast majority of acute infarct patients in the UK are admitted to units without invasive interventional facilities. Furthermore, current resources allow for only about 17,000 angioplasties per year in this country, concentrated in approximately 54 units.

Before we can rigorously evaluate primary angioplasty in the UK, we need to know its true financial cost and whether transferring patients from centres that cannot perform angioplasties to ones that can is both feasible and as successful as conventional (thrombolytic) therapy. The value of primary angioplasty above thrombolysis has not yet been definitely established, and the arguments continue. Nonetheless, patients currently considered as definite candidates for angioplasty (because of contraindications to thrombolysis, cardiogenic shock or failure to reperfuse after thrombolysis) need to be clearly identified and transferred if necessary for primary angioplasty.

□ SUMMARY AND CONCLUSIONS

Thrombolytic therapy with adjunctive aspirin has significantly improved mortality following acute myocardial infarction. Public education about the implications of chest pain, particularly in those with risk factors for coronary disease, is imperative to reduce the delay to thrombolysis.

Beyond this, there remains a need to optimise vessel patency since this correlates with both early and longer-term survival. New thrombolytics are becoming available and may improve patency but will need to be tested against current regimens in large clinical trails. Trials of new antithrombins for reducing vessel reocclusion have demonstrated that these agents have a narrow therapeutic window and their future role is unclear, while potent platelet inhibitors may achieve higher rates of immediate and sustained vessel patency; oral formulations of platelet inhibitors may soon be commercially available.

Primary angioplasty may prove the definitive treatment in selected cases provided that the procedure can be undertaken early enough to be of benefit; patients who fail to reperfuse after thrombolytic drugs may benefit particularly. Limited resources may be the inhibiting factor in widespread use of this treatment modality.

We have reached a watershed in the management of AMI, and further major breakthroughs will be unlikely within the next year or two. Thereafter, the need to reopen the occluded artery quickly, reliably and in a sustained manner will undoubtedly stimulate the further development of some of the novel strategies outlined above.

REFERENCES

1 ISIS-2 Collaborative Group. Randomised trial of intravenous streptokinase, oral aspirin, both or neither among 17,187 cases of suspected acute myocardial infarction. *Lancet* 1988; **2**; 349–60.

2 ISIS-4. A randomised trial comparing oral captopril versus placebo, oral mononitrate versus placebo, and intravenous magnesium sulphate versus control among 58,043 patients with suspected acute myocardial infarction. *Lancet* 1995; **345**: 669–85.

3 The GUSTO Angiographic Investigators. The effects of tissue plasminogen activator, streptokinase, or both on coronary patency, ventricular function, and survival after acute myocardial infarction. *N Engl J Med* 1993; **329**: 1615–22.

4 Meijer A, Verheugt FW, Werter CJ, *et al.* Aspirin versus coumadin in the prevention of reocclusion and recurrent ischemia after successful thrombolysis: a prospective placebo-controlled angiographic study. Results of the APRICOT study. *Circulation* 1993; **87**: 1524–30.

5 Martin U, Kohler J, Sponer G, *et al.* Pharmacokinetics of the novel recombinant plasminogen activator BM 06.022 in rats, dogs, and non-human primates. *Fibrinolysis* 1992; **6**: 39–43.

6 The Global Use of Strategies to Open Occluded Coronary Arteries (GUSTO-II) investigators. A comparison of reteplase with alteplase for acute myocardial infarction. *N Engl J Med* 1987; **337**: 1118–23.

7 Hampton JR. Thrombolytic therapy in acute myocardial infarction. *Cardiovasc Drugs Ther* 1997; **11**: 241–6.

8 Antman EM, Braunwald E. Trials and tribulations of thrombin inhibition. *Eur Heart J* 1996; **17**: 971–3.

9 Gold H, Cigarroa JE, Ferrell MA, *et al.* Enhanced endogenous coronary thrombolysis during acute myocardial infarction following selective platelet receptor blockade with ReoPro. Presented at the 69th scientific session at the American Heart Association meeting, November 1996.

10 O'Neill WW, Brodie BR, Ivanhoe R. Primary coronary angioplasty for acute myocardial infarction (the Primary Angioplasty Registry). *Am J Cardiol* 1994; **73**: 627–34.

11 Grines CL, Browne KF, Marco J. A comparison of immediate angioplasty with thrombolytic therapy for acute myocardial infarction. The Primary Angioplasty in Myocardial Infarction Study Group. *N Engl J Med* 1993; **328**: 673–9.

12 Brodie BR, Grines CL, Ivanhoe R. Six-month clinical and angiographic follow-up after direct angioplasty for acute myocardial infarction. Final results from the Primary Angioplasty Registry. *Circulation* 1994; **90**: 156–62.

13 Grines C. Primary angioplasty: the strategy of choice. Clinical debate. *N Engl J Med* 1996; **335**: 1313–6.

☐ MULTIPLE CHOICE QUESTIONS

1 Drugs shown conclusively to benefit prognosis after myocardial infarction:
(a) Magnesium
(b) Nitrates
(c) ACE inhibitors
(d) Staphylokinase
(e) Thrombolytic given within 18 hours

2 TIMI grade:
(a) Is a clinical measure of effective thrombolysis
(b) Has no bearing on prognosis
(c) Tells us something about how thrombolytic agents work
(d) Is measured at 90 minutes in trials
(e) Demonstrates the limitations of current thrombolytic agents

3 Of the new thrombolytics:
(a) Only reteplase has been evaluated in clinical trials against tPA
(b) Efficacy may be improved through increasing the half-life
(c) All have been shown to produce higher TIMI grades than tPA
(d) bat-PA is currently commercially available
(e) All are likely to produce better clinical outcome than streptokinase

4 Antiplatelet therapy:
(a) Is best based on inhibiting the glycoprotein IIb/IIIa receptor
(b) Has been shown with aspirin to improve outcome after AMI

(c) Will be tested as sole therapy in GUSTO-4
(d) Is likely to cause excess bleeding when used in combination with thrombolytic
(e) Can currently be given as oral glycoprotein IIb/IIIa receptor blockers

5 Primary angioplasty:
(a) Involves balloon treatment <u>after</u> thrombolysis
(b) Produces lower patency rates than thrombolytic
(c) Deals with the thrombus and the underlying plaque
(d) Is currently available to all patients
(e) Needs to be considered when patients fail to reperfuse

ANSWERS

1a False	2a False	3a True	4a True	5a False
b False	b False	b True	b True	b False
c True	c False	c False	c False	c True
d False	d True	d False	d True	d False
e False	e True	e True	e False	e True

Atrial fibrillation and its management

Gregory Y H Lip and Foo Leong Li-Saw-Hee

☐ INTRODUCTION

Atrial fibrillation (AF) is a common arrhythmia which has been recognised since ancient times as chaotic irregularity of the pulse that carries a poor prognosis. Perhaps its earliest description is found in the Yellow Emperor's Classic of Internal Medicine *(Huang Ti Nei Ching Su Wen)*, written by the legendary emperor physician who is believed to have ruled China around 1696 BC: 'When the pulse is irregular and tremulous and the beats occur at intervals, then the impulse of life fades; when the pulse is slender (smaller than feeble, but still perceptible, thin like a silk thread), then the impulse of life is small'. William Harvey was apparently the first to describe 'fibrillation of the auricles' in animals, in 1628. About 200 years ago, William Withering reported a patient whose irregular palpitation was successfully controlled by an extract of *Digitalis purpurea* (purple foxglove) leaf; this was probably the first account of drug treatment of AF. During the 1920s, the clinical and electrocardiographic features of AF and its management were well documented by Sir Thomas Lewis and Sir James Mackenzie. Subsequently, however, it received relatively little attention, perhaps because many physicians considered the condition benign.

Recently, there has been a resurgence of interest in AF, with the recognition that it confers a fivefold increase in premature mortality as well as substantial morbidity from stroke, thromboembolism, heart failure and exercise intolerance. Moreover, the increasing number of elderly people in the general population means that AF is becoming commoner, as its prevalence increases progressively with age.

Greater understanding of the epidemiology, pathophysiology, electrophysiology and complications of AF has led in the past decade to significant advances (and some controversies) in its management. Technological advances include radiofrequency atrioventricular (AV) nodal ablation in selected patients with AF, and the atrial defibrillator in some with paroxysmal AF. Perhaps, and more important, prevention strategies have been devised to reduce the risk of stroke and other complications.

☐ EPIDEMIOLOGY

There remains a need for rigorous surveys of the epidemiology of AF and its complications. Estimates of the prevalence of AF vary widely around the world, though all agree that it increases with age. The prevalence reported in the Framingham study increased from 0.5% at age 50–59 years to 8.8% at 80–89 years [1], while that in the Busselton community in Western Australia rose from 1.7% at age 60–64 years to 11.6% in those aged over 75 years. In the United Kingdom, there have been few large, representative epidemiological studies of atrial fibrillation. In the West Birmingham Atrial Fibrillation Project, we found a prevalence of AF of 2.4% in two general practices; the commonest causes were hypertension (37%) and ischaemic heart disease (29%) (another study is represented in Fig. 1). Interestingly, only one-third of these patients had ever presented to hospital, suggesting that hospital-based series may underestimate true frequency of the condition [2]. In this survey, cardiac failure was associated with AF in one-third of cases, while 18% had suffered at least one cerebrovascular event. Sudlow *et al* [3] suggest that atrial fibrillation may be commoner in the UK than in the United States or Australia, and may affect between 160,000 and 644,000 British subjects aged over 65 years.

The high prevalence of AF is particularly important, as it is present in about 15–20% of acute stroke victims, and is associated with a 1.5- to 3-fold higher mortality than for those in sinus rhythm [4].

□ CAUSES AND PATHOPHYSIOLOGY OF ATRIAL FIBRILLATION

Atrial fibrillation occurs in three broad clinical circumstances:

- □ Primary arrhythmia with no other identifiable heart disease, commonly referred to as 'lone AF'

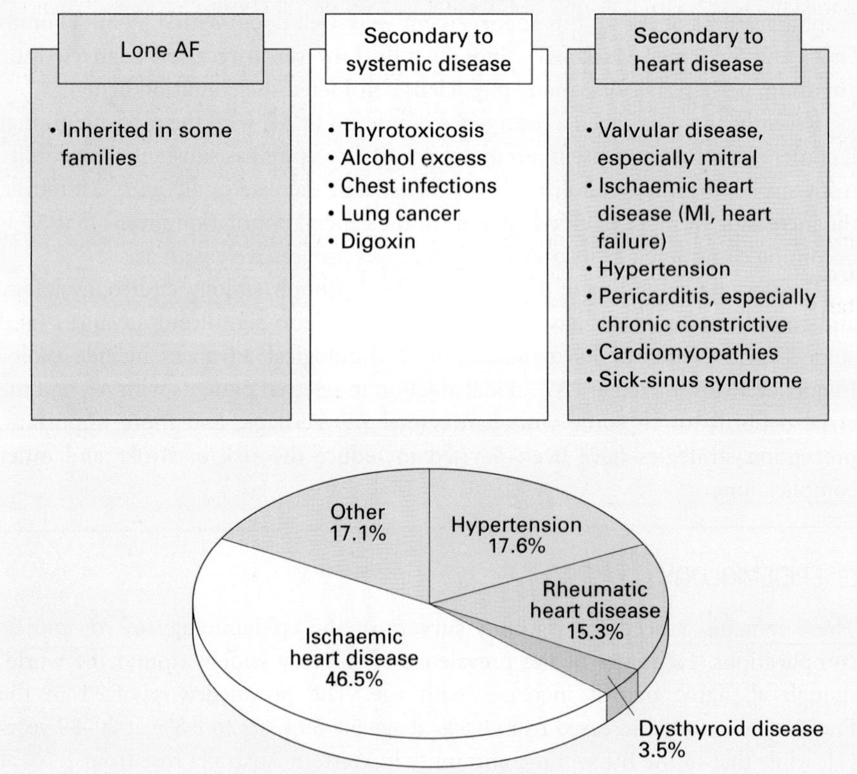

Fig. 1 Causes of atrial fibrillation among emergency admissions to a district general hospital in Glasgow, UK [5].

- Secondary arrhythmia, in the absence of structural heart disease but in the presence of a systemic abnormality that predisposes the individual to the AF
- Secondary arrhythmia with structural heart disease, including rheumatic valve disease and coronary artery disease. These conditions are usually associated with atrial dilatation and patchy fibrosis that ranges from scattered foci to diffuse involvement. This syndrome includes sino-atrial node dysfunction; in some patients, AF may be the first manifestation of the sick-sinus syndrome.

Electrophysiological basis of atrial fibrillation

The most widely accepted theory of the mechanism of AF is the 'multiple wavelet' hypothesis of Moe [6], which suggests that AF is perpetuated by multiple re-entrant impulses of various sizes wandering through the atria, creating continuous electrical activity (Fig. 2). The critical number of wavelets required to perpetuate AF is thought to be about six, and other crucial determinants include the wavelength of the wavelets, and the product of wavelet conduction velocity and refractory period. Factors that increase wavelet wavelength (eg antiarrhythmic agents) tend to prevent or terminate AF, whereas those that shorten the wavelength (eg increased parasympathetic tone, rapid atrial pacing or intra-atrial conduction abnormalities) tend to initiate and perpetuate AF.

Certain supraventricular arrhythmias, including atrial tachycardia and atrio-ventricular or AV nodal re-entry tachycardia, can degenerate into AF. Fast AF may be the presenting arrhythmia in patients with the Wolff-Parkinson-White syndrome (Fig. 3); ventricular rates in such cases are very fast and can degenerate into ventricular fibrillation if managed inappropriately (eg if digoxin is given). In a minority of patients, lone paroxysmal AF can be caused by an atrial focus firing irregularly but with a consistently centrifugal pattern of activation; in such cases, targeted radiofrequency ablation of the abnormal focus can be curative.

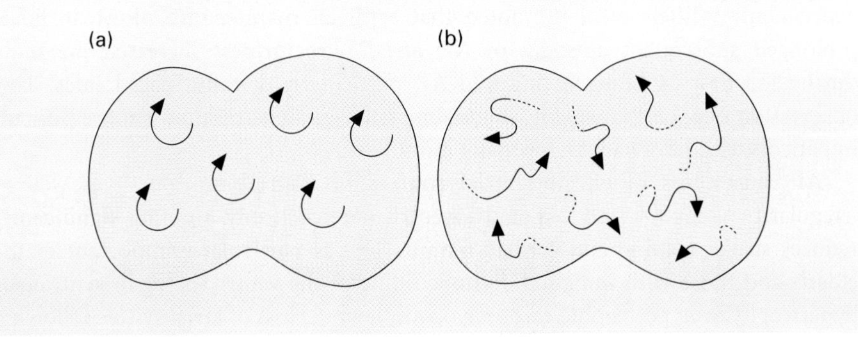

Fig. 2 Electrophysiology of atrial fibrillation. **(a)** Moe's model (1962): multiple coexisting re-entrant wavefronts of activation within atria. **(b)** Allessie's model (1985): multiple wavelets continually sweeping around atria in irregular, shifting patterns.

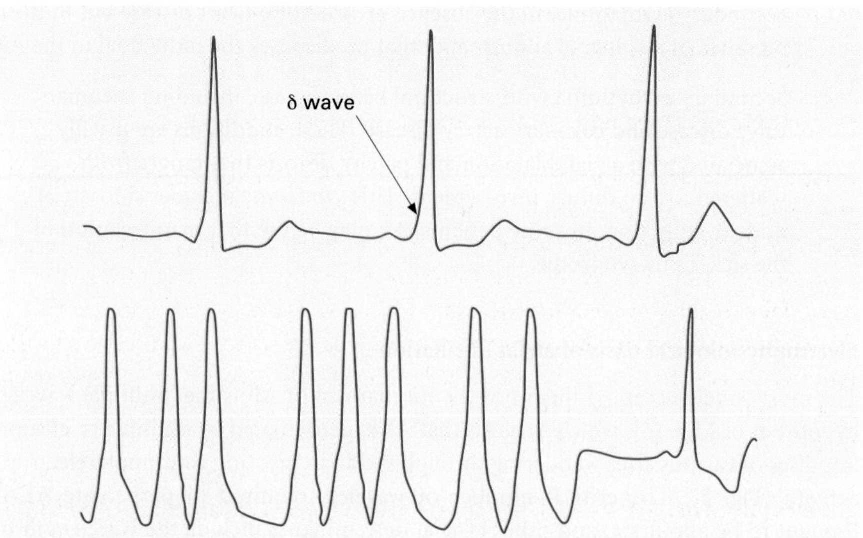

Fig. 3 Electrocardiogram showing fast AF in a patient with Wolff-Parkinson-White syndrome (with trace in sinus rhythm as well).

Genetic factors

Recently, genetic mapping by Brugada *et al* [7] has identified a locus for AF on chromosome 10 in a family of 26 members, of whom 10 were affected in an autosomal dominant pattern. Although the gene product remains unknown, this finding may help to elucidate the molecular basis of AF and provide some aetiological insight into the acquired forms.

Cardiac sequelae of atrial fibrillation

Prolonged AF may cause electrical and structural changes within the atria, which may perpetuate the arrhythmia; effectively, AF may beget AF. In an elegant experiment, Wijffels *et al* [8] noted that artificial maintenance of AF in goats prolonged subsequent episodes of AF; atrial refractoriness increased markedly during the first 24 hours of induced AF, particularly at rapid paced rates. This observation may partly explain why maintenance of sinus rhythm is more difficult in patients who have had AF for many months.

AF causes loss of effective atrial contraction ('atrial transport') as well as irregularity of rhythm and loss of atrioventricular synchrony, and thus significantly reduces stroke volume and cardiac output. This is particularly important in the elderly and those with impaired diastolic filling of the ventricles (eg in ventricular hypertrophy or hypertrophic cardiomyopathy), where loss of atrial systole following the onset of AF may reduce stroke volume by about 30%. Moreover, excessively fast heart rates in AF or any supraventricular tachycardia may cause ventricular dysfunction, characterised by global hypokinesia and cardiac dilatation; this tachycardia-induced cardiomyopathy or 'tachycardiopathy' is often reversible following effective control of ventricular rate [9].

□ CLINICAL PRESENTATIONS OF ATRIAL FIBRILLATION

Symptoms associated with AF can vary and depend on several factors, including the ventricular rate, cardiac function, concomitant medical problems and the individual patient's perception. Most subjects with AF experience palpitations, while pre-syncope, dizziness, fatigue, exercise intolerance and dyspnoea are not uncommon; heart failure is associated in one-third of cases. Some present with stroke or thromboembolic events; for example, the Oxfordshire Community Stroke Project reported pre-existing AF in approximately 15% of patients with thrombotic stroke and in up to 11% of those with stroke due to intracerebral haemorrhage [4]. Finally, many patients are asymptomatic and AF is only found by chance.

AF has been subdivided into 'vagal' and 'adrenergic' forms, largely on clinical grounds [10]. The vagal form affects predominantly men, with an age of onset of 40–50 years. There is a higher prevalence of lone AF; it is usually preceded by bradycardia, and it tends to occur at night, during rest, or after eating or drinking alcohol. Importantly, both beta-blockers and digoxin may paradoxically increase heart rate in the vagal form of AF. By contrast, the adrenergic form of AF is less common and generally occurs during daytime, being preceded by adrenergic stimuli such as exercise and emotional stress. Beta-blockers are usually the treatment of choice in adrenergic AF.

□ INVESTIGATION OF ATRIAL FIBRILLATION

Appropriate initial investigations are shown in Table 1. The aims are to determine whether AF is chronic or paroxysmal; to identify any remediable causes; to assess coexistent heart disease and other risk factors for thromboembolic and other complications of AF; and to optimise treatment.

□ MANAGEMENT OF ATRIAL FIBRILLATION

The management of AF depends upon the goals of treatment, which differ between paroxysmal and chronic AF (see Fig. 4). In paroxysmal AF, the objective is to suppress paroxysms and maintain sinus rhythm. In chronic AF, the clinician has to choose between cardioversion to sinus rhythm (in cases with persistent but potentially reversible AF) or rate control (in permanent AF). Antithrombotic therapy should be considered in all patients, as overall evidence suggests that both paroxysmal and chronic AF carry similar risks of stroke.

Uncertainty remains as to whether long-term morbidity and mortality are improved by aggressive rhythm control using cardioversion and antiarrhythmic drugs, as compared with rate control and anticoagulation. Large controlled studies, such as the Atrial Fibrillation Follow-up Investigation of Rhythm Management (AFFIRM) trial, are under way to evaluate the best management strategies for AF. At present, it is reasonable to individualise the approach to the patient with AF, basing

Table 1 Investigation of atrial fibrillation.

Clinical history and examination

- Intermittent or sustained AF?
- Relationship to ischaemic heart disease
- Valve lesions
- Heart failure
- Hypertension
- Precipitating factors present? (eg thyrotoxicosis, alcohol excess, infections)

Electrocardiography

- 24-hour ECG recording
- Cardiomemo or transtelephonic event recorder

Echocardiography (transthoracic or transoesophageal)

- Mitral valve disease
- Left ventricular dysfunction
- Clot in left atrium and atrial appendage

Exercise testing

- Coronary artery disease

Electrophysiological studies

- Pre-excitation syndrome
- Focal AF

therapy on symptoms, stroke risk, underlying heart disease and the patient's preference.

Restoration of sinus rhythm

Treatment of AF should control symptoms attributable to the arrhythmia and reduce the risk of thromboembolic complications. Conversion of AF to sinus rhythm directly accomplishes the first goal in the short term, and can theoretically achieve the second if sinus rhythm can be maintained. Restoration of sinus rhythm is well recognised to improve cardiac output and exercise capacity; these haemodynamic improvements may take days or weeks to occur, and are generally correlated with the restoration of atrial mechanical function.

Three strategies are available to convert AF to sinus rhythm:

- □ Simple control of ventricular response rate while awaiting spontaneous conversion
- □ Pharmacological conversion
- □ Electrical conversion

AF of recent onset frequently reverts to sinus rhythm; several placebo-controlled

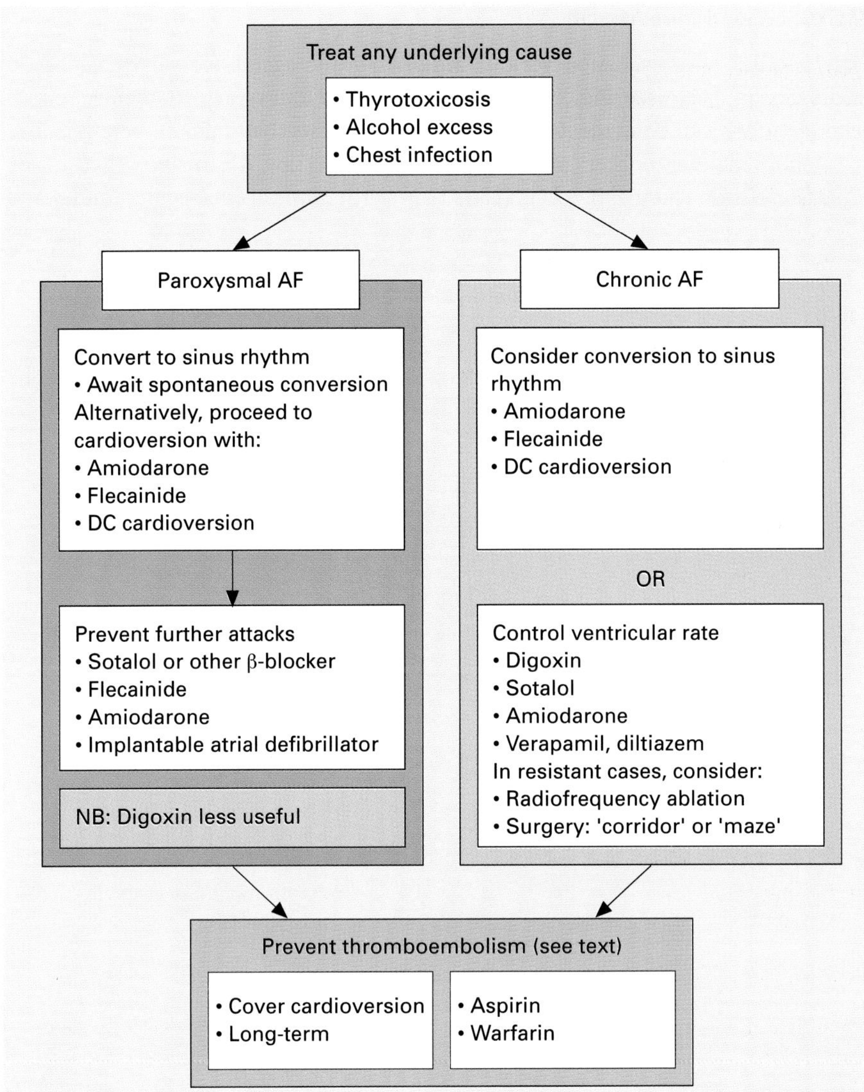

Fig. 4 Flow chart for the management of atrial fibrillation.

trials report spontaneous conversion rates of up to 48%, and this is about 40% for patients presenting less than 72 hours after onset of AF, especially if the ventricular rate is controlled. The most important factor determining successful cardioversion and maintenance of sinus rhythm appears to be a short duration of AF, whereas adverse predictors include increasing age, the presence of structural heart disease (including mitral valve disease, left atrial enlargement and dilation, poor left ventricular function), and the absence of an obvious precipitant such as fever or infection.

Pharmacological cardioversion

Many studies have evaluated various antiarrhythmic agents for pharmacological cardioversion [11] (see Fig. 5). Although response rates vary markedly, several generalisations can be made. Current evidence suggests that digoxin, beta-blockers or calcium channel blockers are not useful for converting AF to sinus rhythm. By contrast, sodium channel blockers (class I antiarrhythmic agents, eg flecainide) and

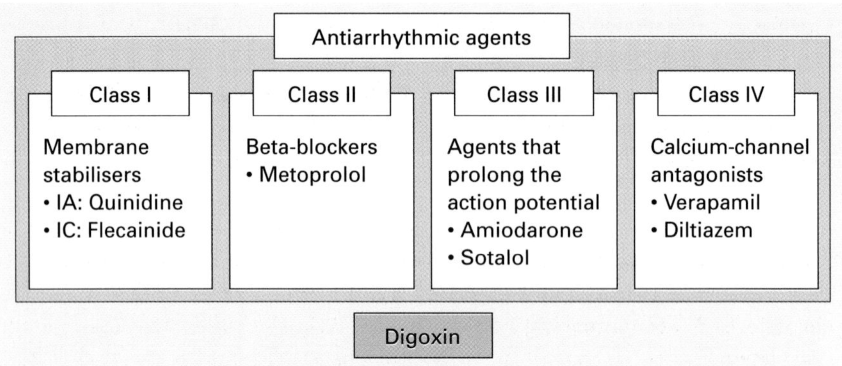

Drug	Advantages	Disadvantages and cautions
Digoxin	• Useful in heart failure	• Ineffective in exercise, fever, thyrotoxicosis • Less useful in paroxysmal AF, sick-sinus syndrome and Wolff-Parkinson-White syndrome (may worsen arrhythmias)
Beta-blockers	• Useful in angina, hypertension and hypertrophic cardio-myopathy • Secondary prevention of myocardial infarction (?)	• Reduces exercise tolerance • May occasionally worsen heart failure
Amiodarone	• Converts AF to sinus rhythm • Does not worsen heart failure	• Thyroid dysfunction (hyper- or hypo-thyroid) • Corneal microdeposits
Verapamil	• Useful in angina, hypertension • May improve exercise tolerance	• Contraindicated in patients receiving β-blockers (risk of asystole)
Flecainide and Propafenone	• Convert AF to sinus rhythm • Useful in paroxysmal AF	• Contraindicated in left ventricular dysfunction

Fig. 5 Antiarrhythmic drugs used for cardioversion.

amiodarone (class III) are effective in both acute and chronic AF; there is no convincing evidence that one agent is more successful than the others.

Electrical cardioversion

Direct current (DC) electrical cardioversion is the most reliable method to restore sinus rhythm in patients with AF. Initially introduced in 1962 by Lown [12], DC cardioversion terminates AF in 80–90% of patients. Energy requirements for successful dc cardioversion vary according to many factors, such as the duration of AF, transthoracic impedance (particularly related to the thickness of the chest wall), the appropriate placement of electrodes, and the prior use of antiarrhythmic agents. Energy requirements may also be predicted by the amplitude of the fibrillatory waves; the coarse (>2 mm) waves associated with recent onset AF generally indicate lower requirements for cardioversion.

To minimise the risk of thromboembolism, anticoagulation should be established for at least 3 weeks before and at least 4 weeks after elective cardioversion. Organisation and firm adhesion of atrial thrombus to the atrial wall is thought to occur over 2–3 weeks, making embolism less likely thereafter. More important, cardioversion leads to atrial 'stunning', which delays the return of atrial systolic function; this favours intra-atrial stasis immediately after cardioversion and therefore necessitates continued anticoagulation. Recently, transoesophageal echocardiography has been used in this setting to visualise the left atrium and left atrial appendage (see Fig. 6); if no thrombi are evident, 48 hours of anticoagulation with heparin before cardioversion may suffice, though full anticoagulation is still required for 4 weeks afterwards.

In cases of chronic AF resistant to external DC cardioversion, low-energy intracardiac cardioversion has been evaluated in specialist centres, and preliminary results show that this is effective and safe [13]. The concept of internal cardioversion has led to the development of the implantable atrial defibrillator for patients with paroxysmal AF; the device detects episodes of AF and performs low-energy conversion to sinus rhythm.

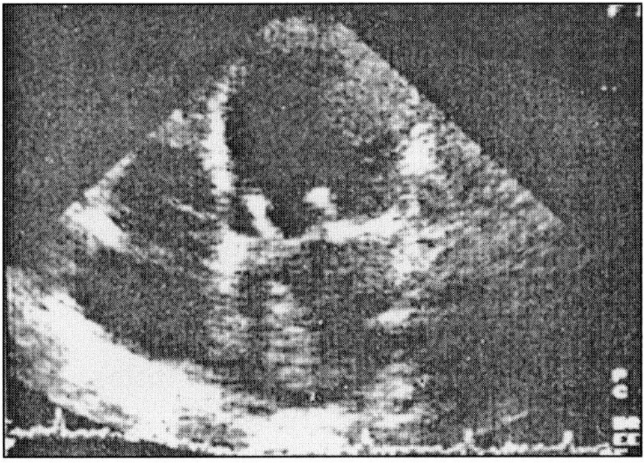

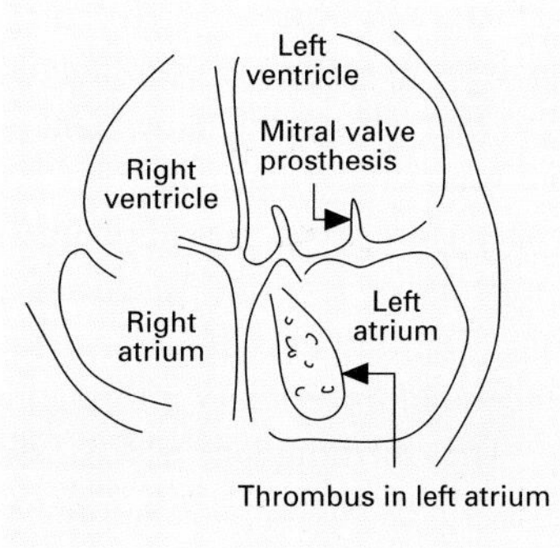

Fig. 6 Transthoracic echocardiogram, showing thrombus in left atrium, in a patient with a prosthetic mitral valve.

Control of ventricular rate in atrial fibrillation

Pharmacological control of heart rate with relief of symptoms is one strategy in the management of chronic AF. Drug options are generally limited to digoxin, beta-blockers or the calcium channel blockers diltiazem or verapamil (see Fig. 5). Anticoagulation is also required to prevent thromboembolism.

Traditionally, digoxin has been widely used to control heart rate in AF, though there is increasing evidence that it is ineffective in conditions of high sympathetic drive, including heart failure, exercise and fever. Digoxin is also ineffective in converting AF to sinus rhythm and may even be detrimental in paroxysmal AF, as it can induce paroxysms more frequently and at faster heart rates. It is also contraindicated in the Wolff-Parkinson-White syndrome, in which it may provoke ventricular fibrillation (see Fig. 3).

Beta-blockers control ventricular response rate but may exacerbate exercise intolerance, while calcium channel blockers control rate with some improvement in exercise capacity.

The presence of concomitant disease may influence the choice of drug. For example, patients with AF and coronary artery disease, hypertension or hypertrophic cardiomyopathy would also benefit from use of beta-blockers or calcium channel blockers. In patients with poor left ventricular function, digoxin (± amiodarone) is the drug of choice.

□ ANTITHROMBOTIC THERAPY IN ATRIAL FIBRILLATION

AF is associated with at least a fivefold increase in the risk of stroke compared with age-matched controls without AF. A meta-analysis of seven large, randomised trials of anticoagulation [14] for the prevention of stroke in AF has not only demonstrated the benefits of warfarin in preventing stroke prevention, but also introduced the concept of risk stratification for stroke. For example, warfarin is associated with a 64% reduction in stroke, while aspirin may reduce risk by 25% (although this latter decrease was not statistically significant on meta-analysis).

Various clinical and echocardiographic parameters have been associated with a higher risk of stroke in patients with AF, including pre-existing hypertension and diabetes and worsening left ventricular function [15] (Table 2). The most recent meta-analyses from the AF Investigators of 1066 patients from three clinical trials did not find that left atrial enlargement *per se* was an independent risk factor for stroke, but left ventricular impairment on 2D echocardiography did appear to be an independent risk factor. Most patients with AF can be classified on clinical criteria into high, moderate or low risk categories that can be used to guide antithrombotic treatment (Fig. 7). If not already performed, echocardiography should be considered, especially in cases of uncertainty, although it merely refines the clinical risk stratification.

The Birmingham risk-stratification criteria and guidelines for using antithrombotic therapy are summarised in Table 2. Using these criteria:

- □ High-risk patients with AF (annual risk of stroke 8–12%) should start warfarin with a target International Normalised Ratio (INR) of 2.0–3.0,

Table 2 Risk factors for stroke in patients with untreated atrial fibrillation.

	Stroke rate (per year) (%)	Relative Risk versus non-AF controls
Clinical parameters		
• Previous stroke or transient ischaemic attack	11.7	2.5
• Hypertension	5.6	1.6
• Diabetes	8.6	1.7
• Previous or current heart failure	6.8	1.4
• Increasing age	–	1.4*
Echocardiographic parameters		
• Global left ventricular dysfunction	12.6	2.0

*Relative risk based on decades of age.

which reduces risk to 1–4%. If there are contraindications to warfarin, such as bleeding, falls, poor compliance or serious concomitant disease, aspirin 75–300 mg/day should be prescribed instead.

- Moderate-risk patients (annual risk of stroke 4%) should be given either warfarin (target INR 2.0–3.0) or aspirin 75–300 mg/day, both of which reduce annual risk to 1–2%. In this group, there is less certainty that warfarin is better than aspirin, and individual circumstances must therefore be considered.

- Low-risk patients (annual risk 1%) are advised to take aspirin 75–300 mg/day if possible.

- If warfarin or aspirin are withheld because of contraindications (particularly gastrointestinal bleeding and allergy), this should be carefully documented in the patient's notes; specialist cardiology referral is suggested in cases of uncertainty.

The intensity of anticoagulation may be an important factor both in preventing stroke in non-valvular AF and in causing bleeding, which affects 2–3% of warfarin treated patients per year. In the multicentre trials, most strokes occurred in warfarin treated patients whose INR was <2.0, whereas bleeding was commoner in patients with INR values >3.0; the target INR range is therefore 2.0–3.0. Maintenance of desirable INR values is, however, difficult; for example, only 61% of values in the SPAF III study [16] were between 2.0 and 3.0, even though INR was monitored monthly and the warfarin dosage was carefully adjusted using a nomogram developed by the investigators.

The safety and tolerability of long-term anticoagulation titrated to conventional levels are less clear in subjects aged over 75 years, who comprise perhaps one-half of the AF-associated stroke patients. One trial reported a substantially greater risk of major haemorrhage during anticoagulation (with a mean INR of 2.7, range 2.0–4.5)

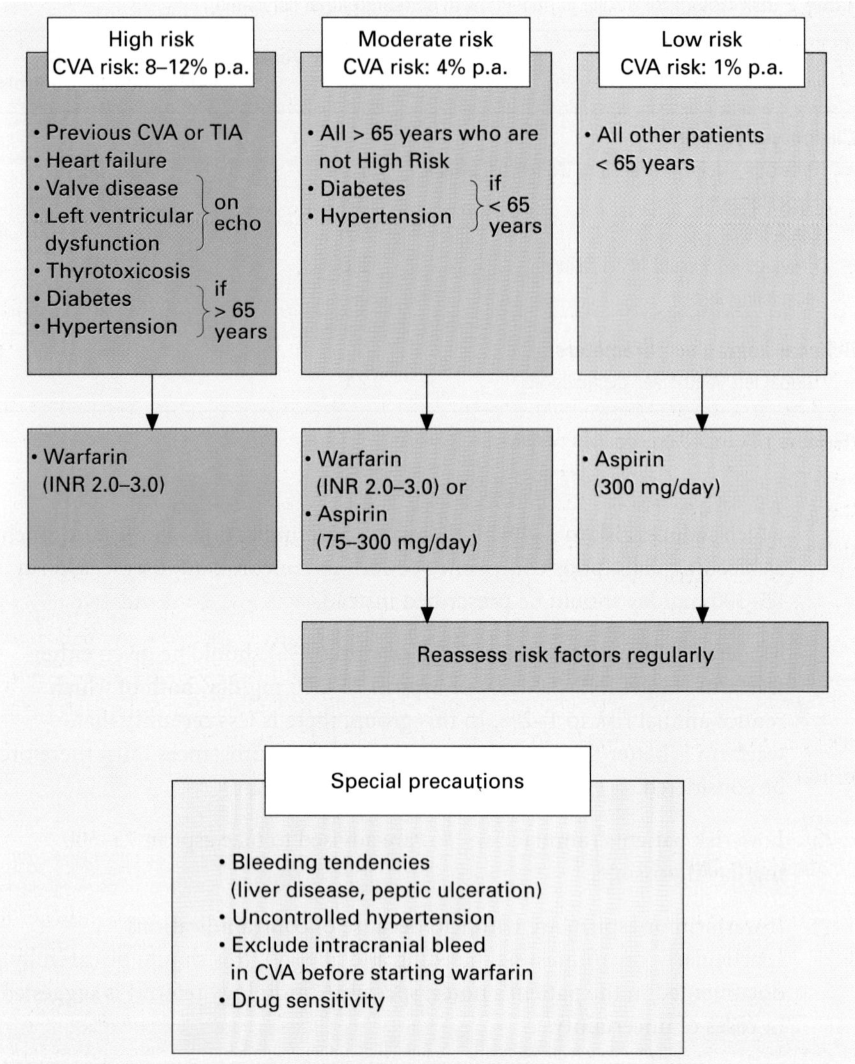

Fig. 7 Stratification of risk for stroke in patients with atrial fibrillation: the Birmingham guidelines.

in AF patients over 75 years of age, whereas pooled data from five other trials revealed only one intracranial haemorrhage in 223 warfarin treated patients in this age range [17]. Attempts to reduce the risk of bleeding by using low-intensity, fixed-dose warfarin that maintains the INR at 1.2–1.5, together with aspirin 325 mg/day, have been ineffective [16]. Thus, particular care must be taken and INR levels closely monitored when warfarin is used in the elderly. One strategy for AF patients aged >75 years, given the uncertainty about the safety of INRs >2.5, would be to use a target INR of 2.0 (range 1.6–2.5) which provides substantial efficacy (≥90%) for thromboprophylaxis.

Antithrombotic therapy continues to be underutilised in patients with AF, despite the compelling evidence that it prevents stroke. In a recent community-based survey from Newcastle [3], 44% of patients with AF aged 65–74 years, and only 11% of those over 75 years of age, were receiving warfarin; our survey of two general practices in West Birmingham [2] broadly agrees with these findings, as warfarin was prescribed to only 36% of 111 patients with AF. A survey of British consultant physicians suggested that more cardiologists than non-cardiologists considered anticoagulation (and cardioversion) in the management of AF.

Who should be responsible for monitoring anticoagulation therapy? There is clear evidence that many general practitioners can monitor coagulation more efficiently than hospital-based clinics, but few are prepared to undertake this role; possible solutions, including decision support for dosing and self-monitoring, need further evaluation.

The risk of stroke is ever present in patients with AF, and antithrombotic therapy is considered a lifelong commitment. It is not clear whether results from large clinical trials are readily applicable to everyday clinical practice, as the trials have involved only relatively small numbers of highly selective and highly motivated patients and a high standard of care which is not usually available. For example, the SPAF I study screened 17,046 patients with AF but only 1330 patients entered the study; many were excluded because of inadequate follow-up or anticipated compliance problems. Furthermore, despite the relatively short-term follow-up (averaging 2–3 years) of these trials, a high proportion (10–38%) of patients were withdrawn from warfarin. Very little information is available on patients who were withdrawn; they are likely to represent a sizeable number in routine clinical practice.

☐ NON-PHARMACOLOGICAL CONTROL OF VENTRICULAR RATE

Pharmacological approaches to control rate in AF do not always succeed, and non-pharmacological alternatives have been developed that employ pacemaker and other electrophysiological techniques.

In patients with sinus node dysfunction and paroxysmal AF, particular types of pacemaker may prevent the development of AF in some circumstances, and certain modes of pacing are better suited to patients who have episodic or chronic AF. For example, the randomised prospective study by Anderson *et al* [18] showed a lesser frequency of thromboembolic events and episodes of AF with atrial pacing than with ventricular pacing, though there were no significant differences in mortality or heart failure. After longer follow up, the same investigators recently reported a reduction in AF episodes, thromboembolism, heart failure and mortality. At present, the Canadian Trial of Physiological Pacing (CTOPP) is comparing VVIR (ventricular pacing that is inhibited by sensed ventricular impulses and is rate-responsive) pacing with physiological pacing (AAIR, atrial pacing that is inhibited by atrial impulses and is rate-responsive; or DDD, dual-chamber pacing where the unit paces and senses both chambers) in patients with either sinus-node or atrioventricular conduction disease, and their respective impacts on mortality, stroke and the development of AF. Pacing may suppress premature atrial contractions that can trigger some episodes of paroxysmal AF. Dual-site pacing is another approach, where pacing the right atrium and coronary sinus or nearer the ostium may reduce the frequency of AF, although many patients often require concomitant antiarrhythmic therapy [19]. As mentioned above, the atrial defibrillator has found a role in the management of paroxysmal AF.

Another method to control the ventricular rate in AF is by using radiofrequency electromagnetic radiation to destroy selected parts of the conduction pathways that propagate AF (see Fig. 8). Techniques employed include ablation of the atrioventricular

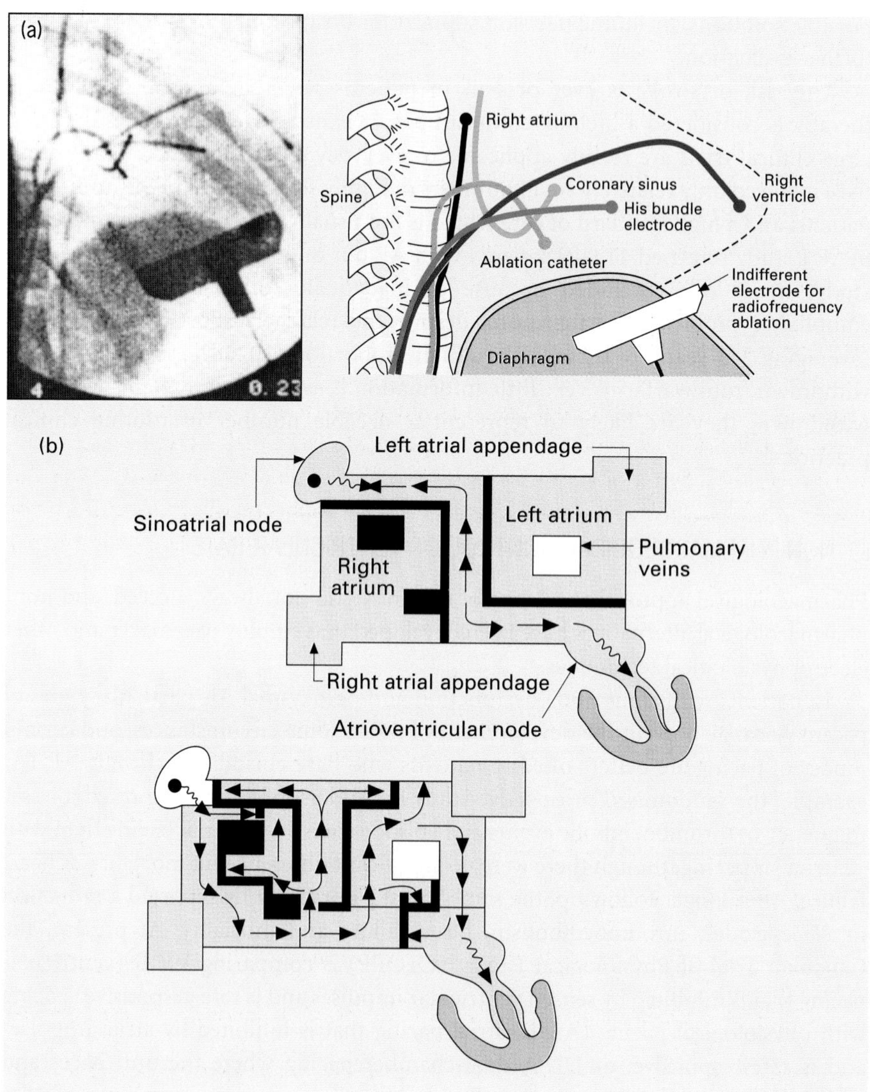

Fig. 8 (a) Radiofrequency ablation of accessory pathway. (b) Surgery for AF with the 'corridor' *(top)* and 'maze' *(bottom)* procedures.

(AV) node or of accessory pathways in pre-excitation syndromes with AF, modulation of the AV node, or ablation of AF foci.

Surgery of AF [20] is a major breakthrough, but remains the therapy of last resort in this condition. The two main techniques are the 'corridor' and 'maze' procedures (Fig. 8). The corridor approach isolates the fibrillating atria from a strip of tissue connecting the sinus and the AV nodes, whereas the maze procedure attempts to abolish AF by channelling the atrial activation impulses between a series of incisions.

□ FUTURE DIRECTIONS

Where do we go from here? The diverse clinical presentation of AF makes it difficult to develop generalised management strategies. At a practical level, investigation and management should be tailored to the patient's individual needs.

Warfarin remains an inconvenient drug, requiring frequent blood tests and carrying a modest risk of bleeding. The potential use of lower-dose warfarin, alone or with aspirin or other antiplatelet agents such as ticlopidine or clopidogrel, deserves further investigation. Interestingly, AF itself may confer a hypercoagulable state as it is associated with abnormalities of thrombogenesis, endothelial dysfunction and platelet activation [21]; measurements of these markers might complement existing clinical and echocardiography factors in the stratification of stroke risk for AF patients.

On the scientific front, basic research is needed to characterise the currents responsible for atrial depolarisation and repolarisation, in health and disease. The recent identification of a focal electrophysiological form of AF, as well as a familial type of AF, are major advances in this direction. The substantial advances over the past decade have made the management of this common cardiac arrhythmia one of the most interesting challenges of modern cardiology, and should lead to improved pharmacological and other strategies for treating the condition.

REFERENCES

1 Kannel WB, Abbott RD, Savage DD, McNamara PM. Epidemiology of chronic atrial fibrillation: the Framingham study. *N Engl J Med* 1982; **306**: 1018–22.

2 Lip GYH, Golding DJ, Nazir M, *et al.* A survey of atrial fibrillation in general practice: the West Birmingham Atrial Fibrillation Project. *Br J Gen Pract* 1997; **47**: 285–9.

3 Sudlow M, Rodgers H, Kenny RA, *et al.* Population based study of use of anticoagulants among patients with atrial fibrillation in the community. *Br Med J* 1997; **314**: 1529–30.

4 Sandercock P, Bamford J, Dennis M, *et al.* Atrial fibrillation and stroke: prevalence in different types of stroke and influence on early and long-term prognosis (Oxfordshire Community Stroke Project). *Br Med J* 1992; **305**: 1460–5.

5 Lip GYH, Tean KN, Dunn FG. Treatment of atrial fibrillation in a district general hospital. *Br Heart J* 1994; **71**: 92–5.

6 Moe GK. On the multiple wavelet hypothesis of atrial fibrillation. *Arch Int Pharmacodyn Ther* 1962; **140**: 183–8.

7 Brugada R, Tapscott T, Czernuszewicz GZ, *et al.* Identification of a genetic locus for familial atrial fibrillation. *N Engl J Med* 1997; **336**: 905–11.

8 Wijffels MCEF, Kirchhof CJHJ, Dorland R, Allessie MA. Atrial fibrillation begets atrial fibrillation: a study in awake chronically instrumented goats. *Circulation* 1995; **92**: 1954–68.

9 Packer DL, Bardy GH, Worsley SJ, *et al.* Tachycardia-induced cardiomyopathy: a reversible form of left ventricular dysfunction. *Am J Cardiol* 1986; **57**: 563–70.

10 Coumel P. Autonomic arrhythmogenic factors in paroxysmal atrial fibrillation. In: Olsson SB, Allessie MA, Campbell RWF (Eds). *Atrial Fibrillation: mechanisms and therapeutic strategies.* Armonk, New York: Futura Publishing Co, 1994: 171–85.

11 Suttorp MJ, Kingma JH, Jerrusen ER, *et al.* The value of class 1c antiarrhythmic drugs for acute conversion of paroxysmal atrial fibrillation or flutter to sinus rhythm. *J Am Coll Cardiol* 1990; **16**: 1722.

12 Lown B. Electrical reversion of cardiac arrhythmias. *Br Heart J* 1967; **29**: 469–89.

13 Alt E, Schmitt R, Ammer A, *et al.* Effect of electrode position on outcome of low-energy intracardiac conversion of atrial fibrillation. *Am J Cardiol* 1997; **79**: 621–5.

14 Barnett HJM, Eliasziw M, Meldrum HE. Drugs and surgery in the prevention of ischaemic stroke. *N Engl J Med* 1995; **332**: 238–48.

15 Atrial Fibrillation Investigators. Risk factors for stroke and efficacy of antithrombotic therapy in atrial fibrillation. *Arch Intern Med* 1994; **154**: 1449–57.

16 McBride R. Adjusted-dose warfarin versus low-intensity, fixed-dose warfarin plus aspirin for high risk patients with atrial fibrillation: Stroke Prevention in Atrial Fibrillation III Randomised Clinical Trial. *Lancet* 1996: **348**: 633–8.

17 Atrial Fibrillation Investigators. Risk factors for stroke and efficacy of antithrombotic therapy in atrial fibrillation: analysis of pooled data from five randomised controlled trials. *Arch Intern Med* 1994; **154**: 1449–57.

18 Anderson HR, Thuesen L, Bagger P, *et al.* Prospective randomised trial of atrial versus ventricular pacing in sick sinus syndrome. *Lancet* 1994; **344**: 1523–8.

19 Saksena S, Prakash A, Hill M, *et al.* Prevention of recurrent atrial fibrillation with chronic dual-site right atrial pacing. *J Am Coll Cardiol* 1996: **28**: 687–94.

20 Cox JL, Schuessler RB, D'Agostino HJ, *et al.* The surgical treatment of atrial fibrillation. III. Development of a definitive surgical procedure. *J Thorac Cardiovasc Surg* 1991; **101**: 569–83.

21 Lip GYH. Hypercoagulability and haemodynamic abnormalities in atrial fibrillation. *Heart* 1997; **77**: 395.

□ MULTIPLE CHOICE QUESTIONS

1 In the treatment of permanent atrial fibrillation (AF):
   (a) The target INR range for anticoagulation in patients with AF is between 2 and 3
   (b) The combination of aspirin and low-dose warfarin (ie 1 mg) is effective in reducing the risk of cerebrovascular embolic events
   (c) Aspirin has no role as an antithrombotic agent in patients intolerant to warfarin
   (d) Aspirin is adequate prophylaxis against stroke in a patient with AF and a previous cerebrovascular event
   (e) Dipyridamole is an acceptable alternative in patients unable to take warfarin

2 Clinical features that predict the possibility of reduced likelihood of maintenance of sinus rhythm after cardioversion:
   (a) Persistence of any illness or condition responsible for the onset of atrial fibrillation
   (b) Left atrial enlargement
   (c) Presence of left ventricular hypertrophy

(d) Increasing duration of atrial fibrillation (1 year or more)
(e) Presence of left ventricular impairment

3 Reversion of acute-onset fibrillation (AF) to sinus rhythm:
(a) Occurs spontaneously in more than 50% of patients
(b) AF of duration <48 hours can be safely cardioverted without any prior anti-coagulation
(c) Chemical cardioversion should always be attempted first before electrical cardioversion
(d) All patients must be given antiarrhythmic drug prophylaxis after successful reversion to sinus rhythm
(e) All patients should be anticoagulated for at least 4 weeks after successful reversion to sinus rhythm by either chemical or electrical means

4 Drugs effective in cardioversion of atrial fibrillation to sinus rhythm:
(a) Digoxin
(b) Amiodarone
(c) Diltiazem
(d) Flecainide
(e) Verapamil

5 Statements about atrial fibrillation:
(a) Uncontrolled atrial fibrillation with fast heart rate can lead to left ventricular dilatation and dysfunction
(b) AAI and dual-chamber pacemakers are thought to reduce the likelihood of the occurrence of atrial fibrillation
(c) There is a small subgroup of atrial fibrillation patients with a genetic aetiology
(d) Digoxin is a useful drug in controlling ventricular response rate both at rest and on exercise
(e) Verapamil should be avoided in patients with acute-onset atrial fibrillation where the ventricular response rate is high associated with broad ventricular complexes

ANSWERS

1a True	2a True	3a True	4a False	5a True
b False	b True	b True	b True	b True
c False	c False	c False	c False	c True
d False	d True	d False	d True	d False
e False	e True	e True	e False	e True

Primary pulmonary hypertension

Tim Higenbottam and Celia Emery

☐ INTRODUCTION

Primary pulmonary hypertension (PPH) has been widely neglected, undetected and inadequately treated. This is partly because of its rarity (annual incidence, two cases per million), its generally non-specific presentation and the tendency to overlook characteristic abnormalities on physical examination, chest X-ray and ECG. The lack of a useful non-invasive screening test has undoubtedly contributed, as has therapeutic nihilism engendered by the poor prognosis of untreated patients and the absence until recently of any effective treatment. Fortunately, this unhappy situation has been revolutionised, first, by the advent of transthoracic Doppler echocardiography (which can readily demonstrate raised pulmonary arterial pressure) and, secondly, by two treatments that greatly extend survival, namely, continuous intravenous (IV) infusion of prostacyclin (PGI_2) and heart-lung transplantation. Today, there is no excuse for missing the diagnosis or failing to treat the disease.

☐ PRIMARY PULMONARY HYPERTENSION: DEFINITIONS

Pulmonary hypertension commonly complicates chronic left ventricular failure, chronic hypoxic lung disease and chronic pulmonary thromboembolic disease, and in these settings is described as 'secondary' to these disorders (see Table 1). This nomenclature can be similarly applied to pulmonary hypertension which occurs as an isolated complication of systemic diseases such as systemic lupus erythematosus (SLE) and systemic sclerosis, particularly the CREST form. Secondary pulmonary hypertension is now also recognised to complicate HIV infection and advanced liver disease.

Conventionally, the term PPH has been reserved for patients in whom no cause can be discerned. It is still generally used to describe those forms of disease which are similar in natural history and pathology to 'idiopathic' PPH but in which specific environmental or genetic factors have now been identified. Examples include exposure to drugs, notably the fenfluramine appetite-suppressants and the chemically similar cocaine and amphetamine [1], and a form with familial inheritance now attributed to a locus on chromosome 2 [2]. Strictly speaking, these patients have secondary causes of pulmonary hypertension, but are still bracketed with PPH (see Table 1). The proportion of patients with 'primary' pulmonary hypertension will undoubtedly diminish as further advances in knowledge identify mechanisms and specific causes of the disorder.

☐ PATHOLOGY OF PULMONARY HYPERTENSION

Structural changes in the pulmonary vasculature

All forms of pulmonary hypertension, whether secondary or primary, show

Table 1 A classification of pulmonary hypertension.

'Primary'	'Secondary'
Idiopathic	***Lung disease***
(no cause identified)	• Chronic hypoxic state
Drug-induced	***Heart disease***
• Fenfluramines (±phentermine)	• Chronic left ventricular failure
• Cocaine	• Congenital cyanotic heart disease (eg Eisenmenger's complex)
• Amphetamine	
• Aminoplex	***Systemic diseases***
Genetic	• Systemic lupus erythematosus
• Linkage with 2q31–32	• Systemic sclerosis, especially CREST
	• Sarcoidosis
	• Obesity
	• HIV infection
	• Liver failure

characteristic endovascular eccentric or concentric thickening of the intima of pulmonary arteries, which narrows and can obliterate their lumen [3]. The intima, which is normally difficult to discern, lies between the muscular layer and the endothelium of the vessels; it is thickened in PPH by migrating and proliferating fibroblasts and smooth muscle cells (Fig. 1). The factors which initiate and sustain this process remain unknown, but the process is similar to the normal age-related changes seen in the pulmonary vasculature. Intravascular thrombosis (Fig. 1) is a common feature in pulmonary hypertension, especially in PPH and in forms secondary to chronic hypoxic lung disease or congenital heart disease. This explains the rationale for anticoagulation treatment in pulmonary hypertension, and perhaps also the improved survival with warfarin treatment [4].

'Plexiform lesions', commonly found in patients with longstanding severe pulmonary hypertension, consist of thin-walled vessels lying close to the resistance arteries and alveolar capillaries (Fig. 2). Their endothelial layer is structurally and functionally abnormal (see below). Plexiform lesions are characteristic of PPH, but are also found in secondary forms of the disorder. They may represent new vessel formation in an attempt to bypass the occluded arteries; alternatively, some have argued that they are the primary lesion in PPH and themselves induce further pathological abnormalities. Further work is needed to clarify the relationship between the plexiform lesions and arterial occlusion.

Haemodynamic consequences

The structural changes in the pulmonary arteries, notably thickening of the arterial wall (which reduces compliance) and occlusion, have important deleterious effects

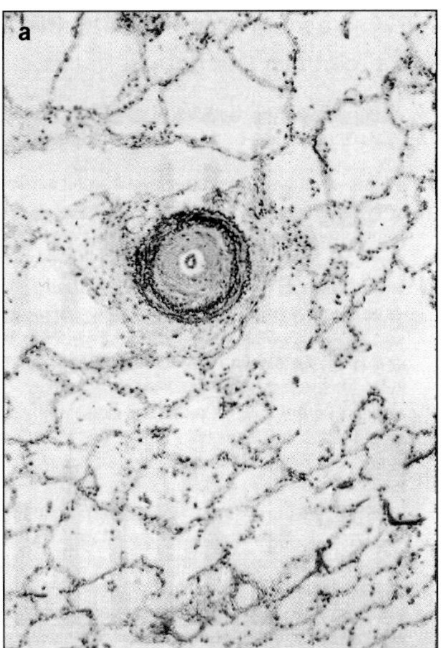

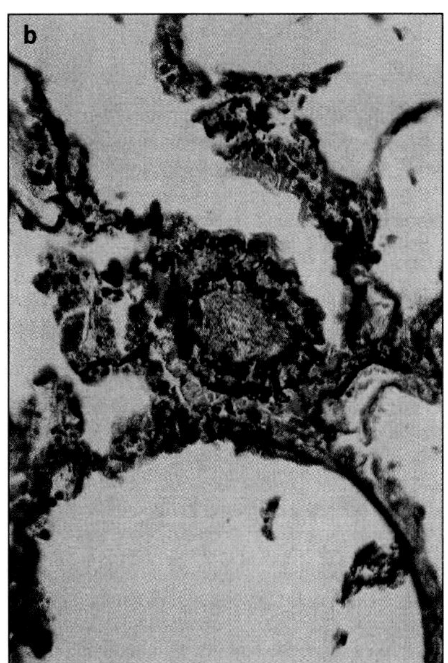

Fig. 1 Structural changes in the pulmonary arteries of a patient with primary pulmonary hypertension, showing **(a)** medial hypertrophy and concentric intimal thickening and **(b)** luminal obliteration (sections stained for elastin with Verhoeff's stain). (Reproduced from Ref 3, with kind permission of the editor of the *American Journal of Pathology.*)

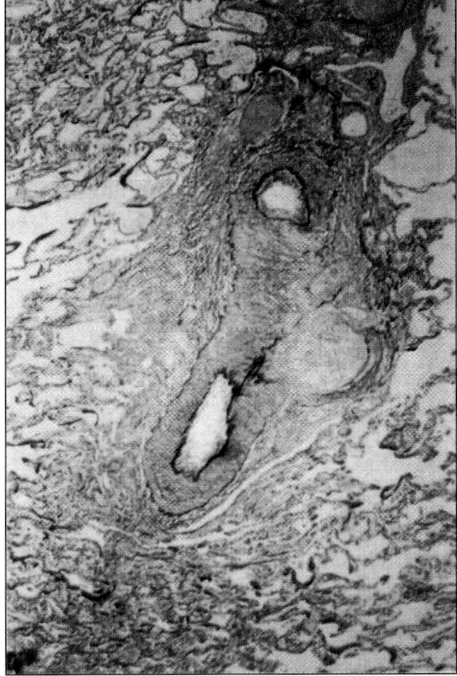

Fig. 2 Plexiform lesion associated with a muscular pulmonary artery (stained for elastin with Verhoeff's stain). The elastic laminae are absent from the arterial wall where the lesion arises. (Reproduced from Ref 3, with kind permission of the editor of the *American Journal of Pathology.*)

on blood flow through the lungs. In the typical patient presenting with PPH, vascular occlusion has obliterated up to 80% of precapillary pulmonary arteries. This loss of the vascular bed raises pulmonary vascular resistance, and reduces the capacity of the lungs to adapt to the rise in cardiac output during exercise. In healthy subjects, the pulmonary circulation has an enormous capacity to accept this increased blood flow, and the pressure gradient across the pulmonary vascular bed does not rise. In patients with PPH, however, pulmonary arterial pressure rises steeply with exercise and increases right ventricular work. Initially, this explains the symptoms of fatigue and breathlessness on exertion; later, exercise can precipitate acute right ventricular failure. As the disease progresses, right heart failure develops even at rest; this stage indicates an extremely poor prognosis.

Endothelial cell function

Distinct patterns of endothelial dysfunction have become evident in PPH and secondary forms of pulmonary hypertension, and they appear to play a crucial role in the pathogenesis of these disorders. The endothelial cell produces numerous vasoactive and anti-proliferative factors. It also acts as an important interface between blood cells and the arteries and veins, modulating platelet aggregation and the release of their stored vasoactive chemicals.

Endothelial production of nitric oxide

The endothelium is a major source of nitric oxide (NO), which is produced by many cell types from L-arginine and molecular oxygen under the influence of nitric oxide synthase (NOS). Three isoforms of NOS are recognised, the inducible (iNOS, or NOS II), the neural (nNOS, or NOS I) and the endothelial (eNOS, or NOS III) [5]. These isoforms are encoded by separate genes on different chromosomes; although their structure is highly conserved, there are important differences in specific regulatory regions of their respective genes and in their tissue distribution.

NO has many and varied physiological roles, including the regulation of vascular tone, neurotransmission and the cytotoxic activity of inflammatory cells. Many of these activities are mediated through activation of the enzyme-soluble guanylate cyclase, which raises intracellular levels of cyclic guanidine monophosphate (cGMP). Guanylate cyclase is activated by NO, which reacts with the haem moiety of the enzyme. NO has 6,000 times greater affinity for haemoglobin than oxygen, and the reaction of NO with red-cell haemoglobin is the principal method of removing and inactivating the molecule; this process largely confines the action of NO released by the endothelium to the abluminal side of the blood vessel, where it acts as a potent vasodilator on the vascular smooth muscle cells. Endothelial NO appears to modulate systemic vascular resistance and may play an important role in regulating the pulmonary circulation of man, pig and sheep [6].

The powerful vasodilator effects of NO, together with its anti-proliferative and anti-platelet properties, suggest that it could potentially impede and prevent the remodelling of the pulmonary vasculature in pulmonary hypertension, and that abnormalities of NO generation could contribute to its pathogenesis. Some evidence for dysfunction of NOS and NO has come from studies of diseased lungs removed from PPH patients receiving heart-lung transplants. Basal release of NO from pulmonary endothelium is apparently maintained in PPH (and in secondary forms of pulmonary hypertension), but there is blunting of the enhanced release normally evoked by pharmacological stimulation [7,8]. The severity of impairment of stimulated NO release is related to the degree of hypoxia experienced by the patient before surgery. Moreover, the expression of eNOS gene, as measured by both the protein and its mRNA, is reduced in the lungs of patients with pulmonary hypertension, including PPH [9]. Intriguingly, the distribution of eNOS expression is patchy, being decreased in the pulmonary arteries, but markedly increased in the plexiform lesions [9]. The significance of these observations remains to be determined. These marked phenotypic changes in the endothelial cells could contribute to the pulmonary vascular abnormalities of PPH, but it is not clear whether they are primary or secondary to the remodelling process.

Prostacyclin and thromboxane

Vasoactive prostanoids are also produced by the endothelium and have been implicated in the pathogenesis of PPH. Research in this field has been rewarded by the development of PGI_2 as effective therapy for the disease. Arachidonic acid (AA) is released from cell membrane phospholipids by phospholipases A_2 and C, enzymes that are activated by both humoral and physical stimuli. AA is a substrate of the two isoforms of cyclo-oxygenase (COX). The constitutive isoform (COX-1) converts AA to prostaglandin H_2 (PGH_2). In the endothelial cell, prostacyclin synthase converts PGH_2 to PGI_2, a potent vasodilator and inhibitor of platelet aggregation; by contrast, the platelet converts PGH_2 via thromboxane synthase to the vasoconstrictor and enhancer of platelet aggregation, thromboxane A_2 (TXA_2).

The opposing actions of PGI_2 and TXA_2 on vessel calibre and coagulation suggest that they may play a role in PPH. Unfortunately, these compounds are difficult to study: circulating PGI_2 levels are very low (picomolar), while instrumentation of blood vessels provokes release of both PGI_2 and TXA_2. An indirect approach, measuring their specific metabolites in the urine, suggests that exercise increases the production of both compounds, but that PGI_2 predominates. This process appears sensitive to alveolar oxygen tension, as less PGI_2 is produced than TXA_2 when the oxygen level falls. Patients with PPH have reduced rates of PGI_2 production relative to TXA_2 [10], and overall decreased expression of the prostacyclin synthase in the pulmonary vessels (although, as with eNOS, it is increased in the plexiform lesions). As discussed below, the therapeutic success of PGI_2 infusions in PPH provides gratifying proof of this concept.

Endothelin-1

Endothelial cells also produce endothelin-1 (ET-I), a 21 amino acid peptide, a powerful vasoconstrictor and mitogen. As with both NO and PGI_2, accurate measurement of the rate of release of ET-1 is hindered by its short plasma half-life, but immunoreactive ET-1 levels are elevated in patients with either PPH or secondary pulmonary hypertension [11]. ET-1 expression is markedly increased in the pulmonary circulation of lungs explanted from patients with pulmonary hypertension, including PPH [12]. However, this may be a non-specific response to hypoxia, as raised ET-1 levels are also found in patients with chronic obstructive lung disease, and following acute hypoxia in normal subjects. Expression of pre-proendothelin, the precursor of ET-1, is known to be enhanced by hypoxia, cytokines and circulating factors such as the biogenic amines noradrenaline and serotonin. Conversely, its expression is inhibited by NO and PGI_2.

The overexpression of ET-1 in primary and secondary forms of pulmonary hypertension raises the notion that this is the common pathway of disturbed endothelial function that leads to the characteristic vasoconstriction and arterial remodelling. This view is supported by the demonstration that ET-1 antagonists can reverse experimentally-induced pulmonary hypertension in the rat [13].

□ SPECIFIC FORMS OF 'PRIMARY' PULMONARY HYPERTENSION

Drug-induced primary pulmonary hypertension

There is now strong evidence that various phenylamine- and phenylethylamine-derived appetite-suppressant and psychotropic agents are associated with the development of PPH. These include the anti-obesity drugs, aminorex fumarate (long obsolete), fenfluramine and dexfenfluramine (recently withdrawn), and amphetamine and cocaine. All increase the release and/or inhibit the uptake of biogenic amines including catecholamines (eg noradrenaline) and serotonin (5-hydroxytryptamine, 5-HT), thus enhancing the actions of these amines. These transmitters increase vascular smooth muscle tone and can induce smooth muscle proliferation, suggesting a link with the pathological changes of PPH in the pulmonary vasculature (see Fig. 3).

Serotonin has been particularly implicated: PPH has been reported in the carcinoid syndrome, where plasma serotonin levels are dramatically raised (together with substance P and other vasoactive mediators), whereas the raised catecholamine levels of phaeochromocytoma cause only systemic hypertension. There is, however, growing evidence that a combined disturbance of both adrenergic and serotonergic activity may predispose to PPH, as exemplified by the very high risk of PPH associated with the combined use of dexfenfluramine and phentermine (see below).

Impaired clearance of biogenic amines may be a critical factor. Circulating biogenic amines mostly originate from the chromaffin cells of the gut (serotonin) and adrenal medulla (catecholamines). About 80% of them are cleared by the liver, but uptake by the platelets and the lung is important in regulating their blood concentrations. Cellular uptake is achieved through specific membrane-bound transporters, members of a family of Na^+, Cl^- and ATP-dependent biogenic amine transporters. They share a number of similarities, including inhibition by cocaine, tricyclic antidepressants and phenylethylamines. This parallel inhibition of catecholamine and serotonin uptake may explain why the phenylethylamine-derived

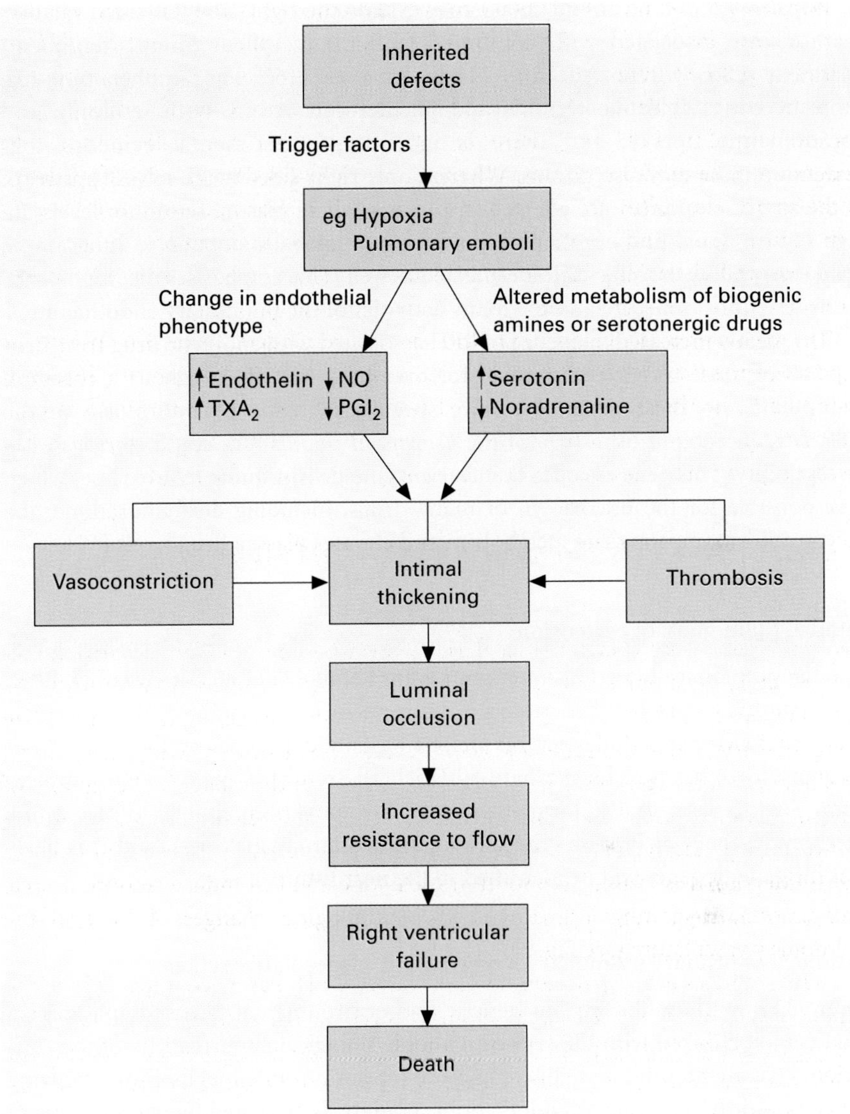

Fig. 3 Some factors that may contribute to the development of pulmonary hypertension (NO = nitric oxide; PGI_2 = prostacyclin; TXA_2 = thromboxane A_2).

fenfluramine, but not specific serotonin uptake inhibitors such as fluoxetine or paroxetine, is associated with PPH. Hypoxia, a common cause of pulmonary hypertension secondary to cardiopulmonary disease, also reduces lung and platelet biogenic amine uptake and elevates plasma catecholamines and possibly serotonin. A defect in platelet amine storage, which leads to raised plasma serotonin, has been associated with PPH [14]. Furthermore, patients with PPH have elevated levels of serotonin that persist after successful heart-lung transplantation [15].

Impairment of lung amine uptake may explain the right- and left-sided valvular heart disease associated with combined fenfluramine-phentermine ('fen/phen') treatment recently reported from North America [16]. The amphetamine-like anorectic drugs chlorphentermine and phentermine reduce both serotonin and noradrenaline uptake, and there is increasing experimental evidence that dexfenfluramine may also do this. Whereas only right-sided heart valves (upstream of the site of clearance) are affected in diseases where plasma serotonin levels are high (eg carcinoid and ergotamine poisoning), a global reduction in lung amine uptake may allow the left side to be affected as well. This emphasises the importance of the functional integrity and the many activities of the pulmonary endothelium.

The greatly increased incidence of PPH associated with anorectic drug treatment (1:8,000 of those using fenfluramine for over three months) suggests a common susceptibility to these drugs. We have speculated that a polymorphism of the *CYP2D6* gene, found in 5–10% of the Caucasian population, could confer such a susceptibility. This gene encodes the liver enzyme debrisoquine hydroxylase, which is responsible for the breakdown of many drugs, including dexfenfluramine; the polymorphism impairs drug metabolism and elevates plasma drug levels [17].

Familial pulmonary hypertension

Familial pulmonary hypertension accounts for about 6% of all patients with PPH. Initial studies in six families localised the gene to chromosome 2 [2]. A critical region of 5 cM that includes several interesting candidate genes on the long arm of chromosome 2 has now been identified (Richard Trembath: personal communication). The markers used to localise the gene have now been applied to predict the later development of PPH in clinically unaffected family members, and it is likely that the gene or genes will be identified in the near future.

Aetiology of primary pulmonary hypertension: a speculative scheme

Figure 3 shows how the various genetic and environmental factors implicated in PPH could be linked with the known pathophysiological abnormalities of the condition. Overall, an inherited abnormality of biogenic amine metabolism, involving platelets and the pulmonary endothelium, potentially triggered by anorectic drugs or hypoxia, could lead to the characteristic structural and biochemical features.

□ INVESTIGATION AND DIAGNOSIS OF PRIMARY PULMONARY HYPERTENSION

The investigation of suspected PPH serves four main purposes:

- to confirm the diagnosis;
- to exclude secondary causes of pulmonary hypertension;
- to indicate prognosis; and
- to optimise treatment.

A diagnostic pathway is suggested in Fig. 4. The main symptoms are dyspnoea, fatigue, chest pains and syncope. Their non-specific nature often causes the diagnosis to be overlooked, but their occurrence in patients in the third or fourth decade of life should raise the suspicion of pulmonary hypertension. Physical examination can be helpful, and usually reveals a small-volume peripheral pulse and a loud second heart sound in the pulmonary area. Causes of secondary pulmonary hypertension may also be apparent.

Routine investigations may be useful. The chest radiograph often shows enlarged central pulmonary arteries, sometimes with 'pruning' of peripheral vascular markings (Fig. 5), while the ECG demonstrates right ventricular hypertrophy or right bundle branch block in over 85% of patients [18] (see Fig. 6).

Non-invasive diagnosis has been greatly aided by transthoracic echocardiography, which can identify dilatation of the right atrium and right ventricle. More specifically, Doppler flow measurements can be used to estimate systolic pulmonary artery pressure, and show other features such as a regurgitant tricuspid valve (Fig. 7). The measurement of pulmonary artery pressure offers a simple screening test for patients in whom there is a high index of suspicion, although adequate echocardiographic views may be difficult to obtain in obese patients. A pulmonary arterial pressure greater than 25 mm Hg is abnormal.

Additional investigations are used to exclude secondary causes of pulmonary hypertension. Echocardiography will show septal defects in congenital heart disease, as well as left ventricular failure. High-resolution computed tomographic scanning of the thorax is undertaken to exclude mediastinal lymphadenopathy and other features of sarcoidosis which can be associated with pulmonary hypertension. Full pulmonary function tests and arterial blood gas tensions will identify coexistent lung disease and alveolar hypoventilation. An auto-antibody screen for sytemic sclerosis, systemic lupus erythematosus and the antiphospholipid syndrome should be carried out, together with tests for liver function and HIV.

A ventilation-perfusion (V/Q) lung scan is undertaken to determine if the pulmonary hypertension is a result of chronic pulmonary thromboembolic disease. This is suggested by one or more segmental or subsegmental perfusion defects with normal ventilation (Fig. 8), and these patients should proceed to pulmonary angiography (Fig. 9). Selective views are required to identify any obstructive lesions in the main branches of the pulmonary artery; even if these occur down to the subsegmental level, thrombo-endarterectomy is a possible treatment (see below).

Right heart catheterisation must be performed in all patients strongly suspected of having PPH. This will not only confirm the diagnosis, but also indicate prognosis and guide therapy. Pulmonary hypertension is defined as a mean pulmonary artery pressure about 25 mm Hg at rest, and in the presence of a normal pulmonary wedge pressure.

□ ASSESSING PROGNOSIS IN PRIMARY PULMONARY HYPERTENSION

Prognosis, an important determinant of treatment, can be assessed in several ways (see Table 2).

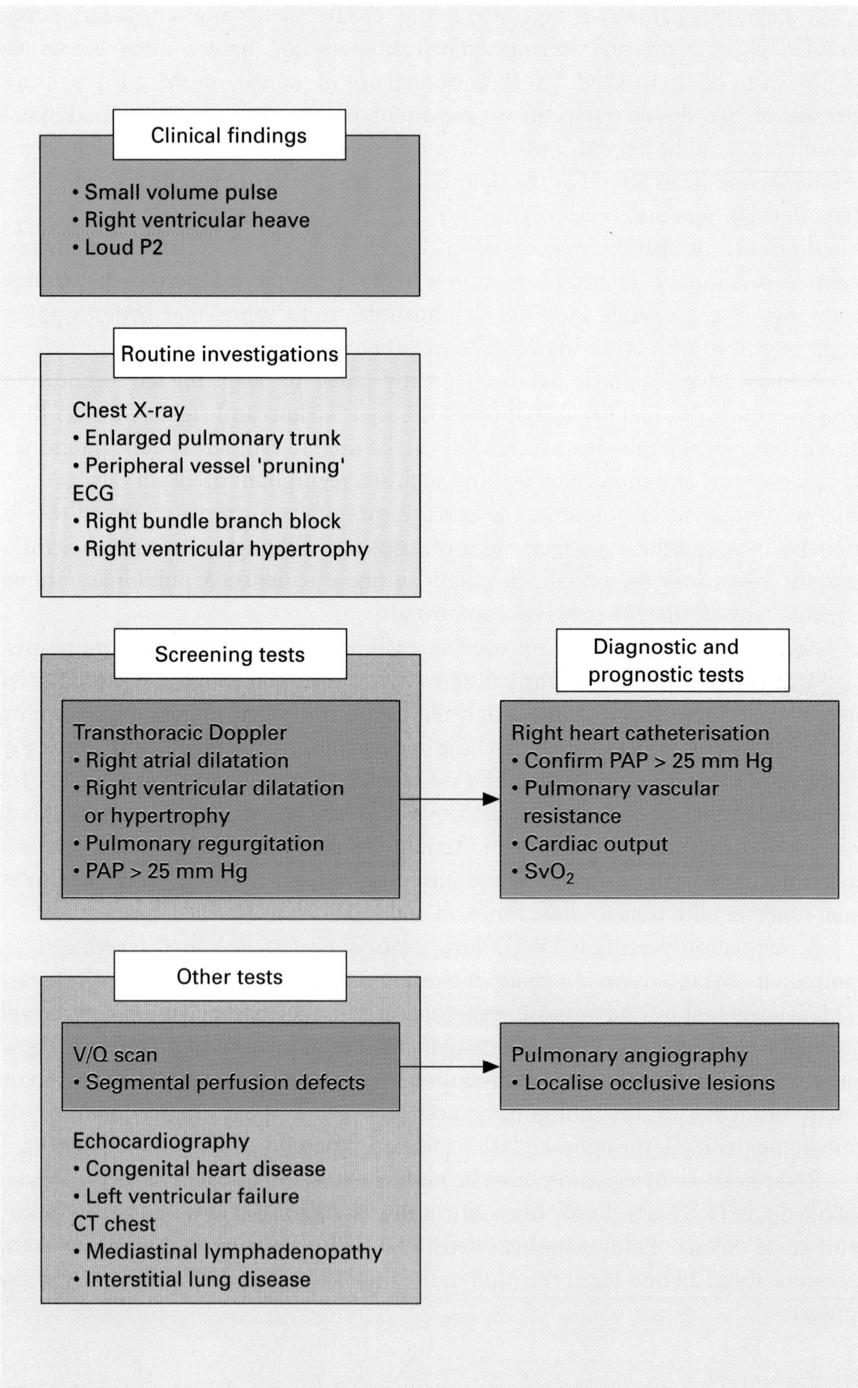

Fig. 4 Flow chart for the investigation and diagnosis of pulmonary hypertension (CT = computed tomography; PAP = pulmonary arterial pressure; SvO_2 = mixed pulmonary venous oxygen saturation).

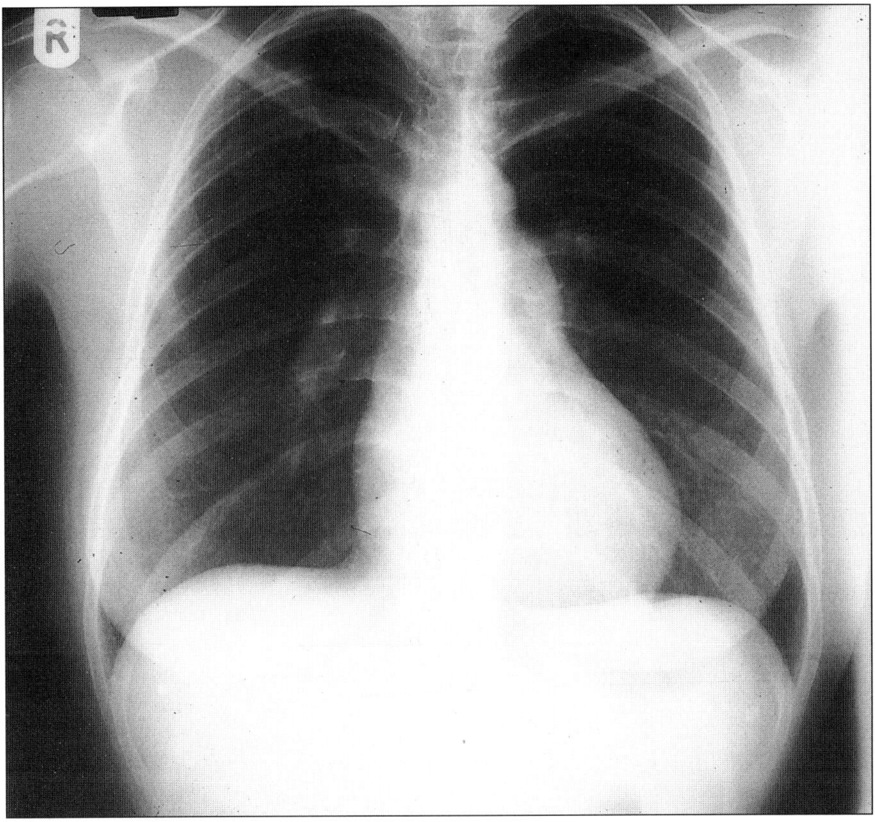

Fig. 5 Chest radiograph in a patient with primary pulmonary hypertension, showing enlargement of the central pulmonary vessels and attenuation ('pruning') of the peripheral vessels.

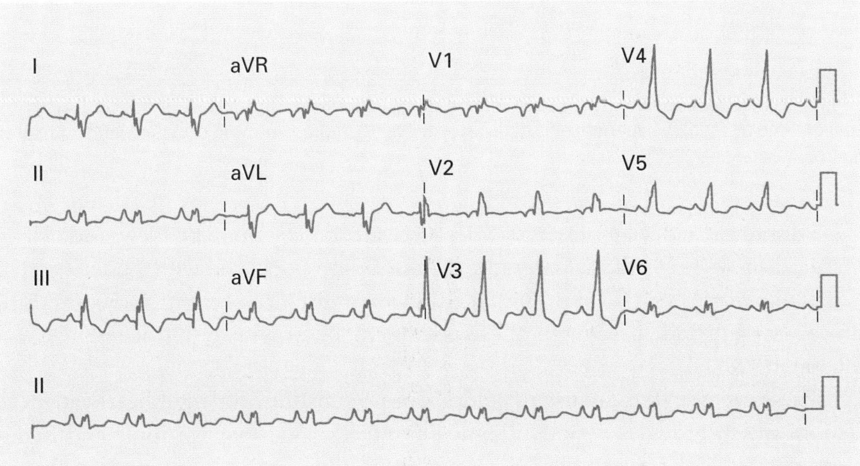

Fig. 6 Typical ECG in a patient with primary pulmonary hypertension, showing right bundle branch block and right ventricular hypertrophy.

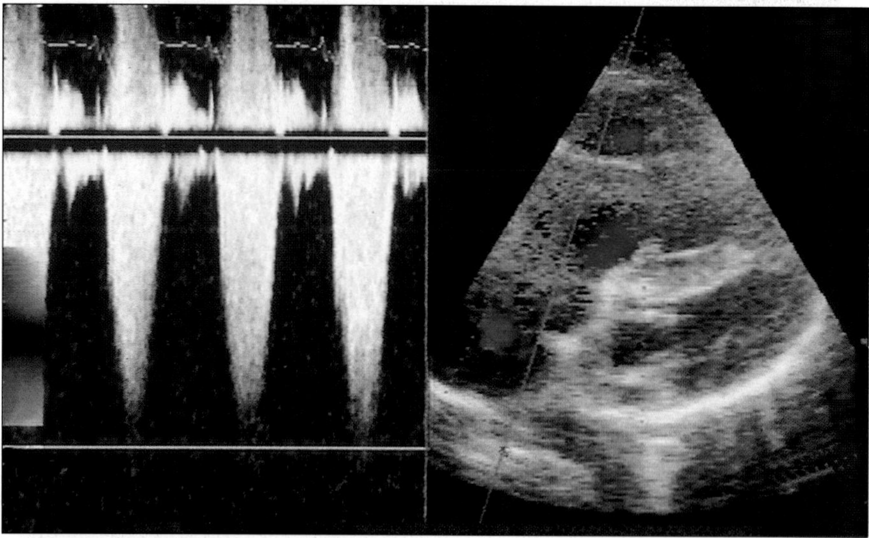

Fig. 7 Transthoracic Doppler scan showing severe pulmonary regurgitation in a patient with primary pulmonary hypertension whose mean pulmonary arterial pressure (PAP) was 60 mm Hg on right heart catheterisation.

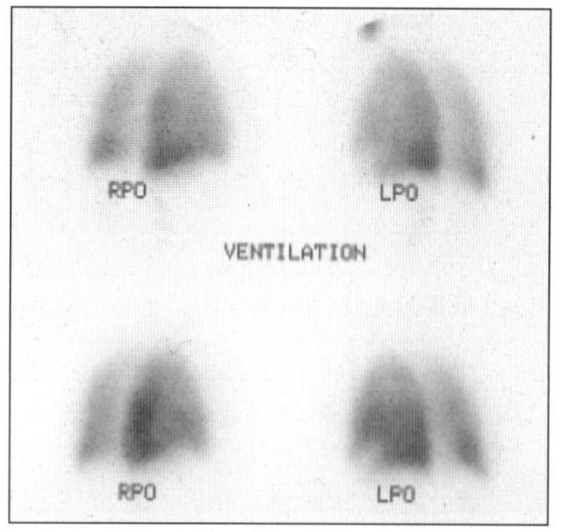

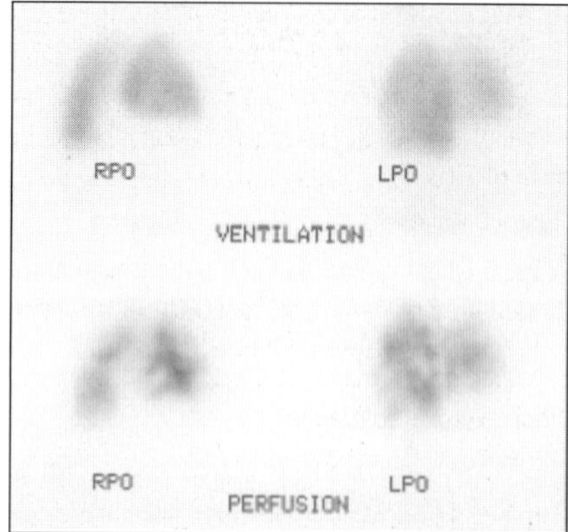

Fig. 8 Ventilation-perfusion (V/Q) scan showing segmental and lobar areas of non-perfusion in a patient with pulmonary hypertension secondary to chronic thromboembolic disease (right) compared with a normal scan (left).

Symptoms, especially exercise tolerance, are important. The New York Heart Association (NYHA) disability grades III and IV are associated with a poor survival (only one or two years) [19]. This equates with a distance of less than 500 m using the 12-minute walk assessment of exercise tolerance, or with a 'shuttle test' distance of 300 m [20].

These exercise tests are useful guides, but no substitute for right heart catheterisation, which provides various prognostic indices. One that is simple and highly reproducible is the mixed venous oxygen saturation (SvO_2) in pulmonary arterial blood: saturations below 60% indicate three-year survival of less than 33%. Other useful prognostic measures are:

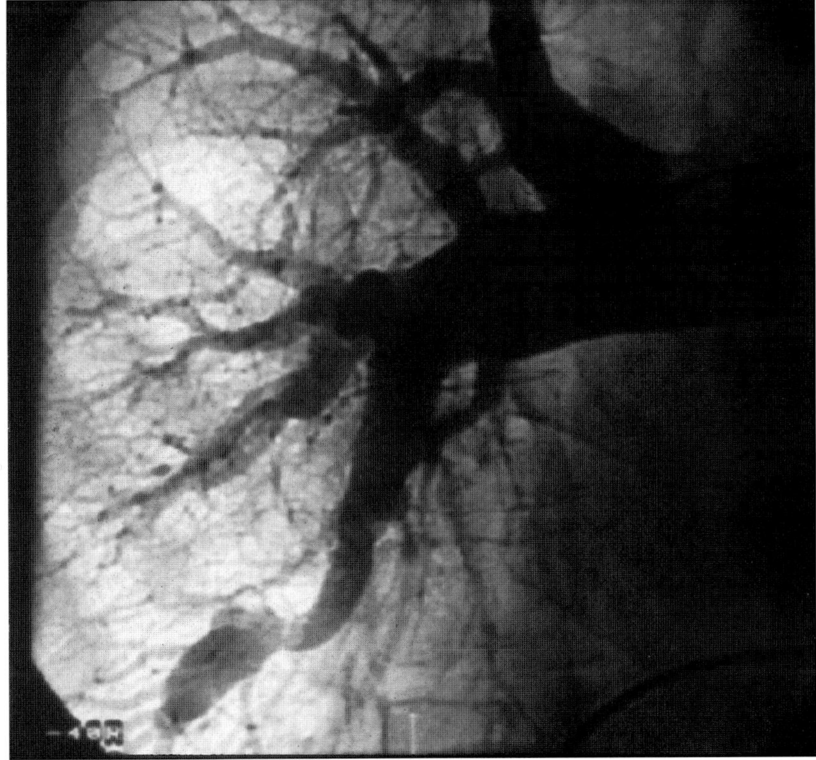

Fig. 9 Pulmonary angiogram showing occlusion of the right lower lobe artery by a web, with post-stenotic dilatation.

Table 2 Features indicating poor prognosis (median survival 1–2 years) in patients with primary pulmonary hypertension (see also Fig 10).

Poor exercise tolerance

- NYHA grade III/IV
- <500 m with 12-minute walk
- <300 m with 'shuttle' test

Right-heart catheterisation

- SvO_2 <60%
- cardiac index <2 l/min/m^2
- right atrial pressure >20 mm Hg
- PAP >85 mmHg

Poor response to vasodilators

- <20% rise in cardiac index after prostacyclin
- <30% fall in PAP after NO inhalation

NO = nitric oxide
NYHA = New York Heart Association
SvO_2 = mixed pulmonary venous oxygen saturation
PAP = pulmonary arterial pressure

- reduced cardiac index (CI);
- elevated right atrial pressure (RAP);
- raised pulmonary arterial pressure; and
- high pulmonary vascular resistance (PVR), calculated from the cardiac output and the difference between the mean pulmonary artery pressure and wedge pressure.

These measures effectively indicate the onset of right ventricular failure. Figure 10 and Table 2 show the effects of these measures, and the levels that indicate poor prognosis.

Trial of vasodilators

In patients with a normal RAP and a CI about 2 l/min/m^2, the effects of PGI_2 infusion [21] or inhaled NO are assessed. Cumulative dose-response curves are performed; dosages of PGI_2 may be limited if systolic systemic arterial pressure falls below 90 mm Hg. A positive vasodilator response (ie 20% rise in CI with PGI_2, or 30% fall in mean pulmonary artery pressure with NO) is associated with a better prognosis than when this response is absent. A positive result also indicates that long-term treatment with oral vasodilators such as nifedipine or diltiazem may enhance survival [4].

TREATMENT OF PULMONARY HYPERTENSION

Anticoagulants

Anticoagulation improves survival in PPH, irrespective of the severity of disease [4]. Its value is uncertain in secondary pulmonary hypertension, but its use is now being extended to patients with systemic sclerosis and Eisenmenger's syndrome.

Prostacyclin and its analogues

The rationale for vasodilators, notably PGI_2 and NO, has been discussed above [21]. A large randomised controlled trial has shown that continuous intravenous infusion of PGI_2 improves survival in patients with advanced PPH [22]. Poor-prognosis patients (ie NYHA grade III or IV; SvO_2 <60%; CI <2.0 l/min/m^2; and RAP >15 mm Hg) benefit with extended survival (>80% at 2 years) and improved quality of life (Table 3). PGI_2 is delivered with a portable pump into a central vein. It is expensive: together with the infusion system, annual costs are £35,000 ($55,000). The decision to treat should therefore be made in a specialised centre [23].

Progressive loss of efficacy over time, with increasing doses failing to control symptoms, is an indication for lung transplantation. The patient's status is conveniently monitored by testing exercise tolerance.

Other vasodilators

A small, non-randomised (but none the less convincing) study has shown that both nifidepine and diltiazem prolong survival in PPH [4]. These drugs are effective in

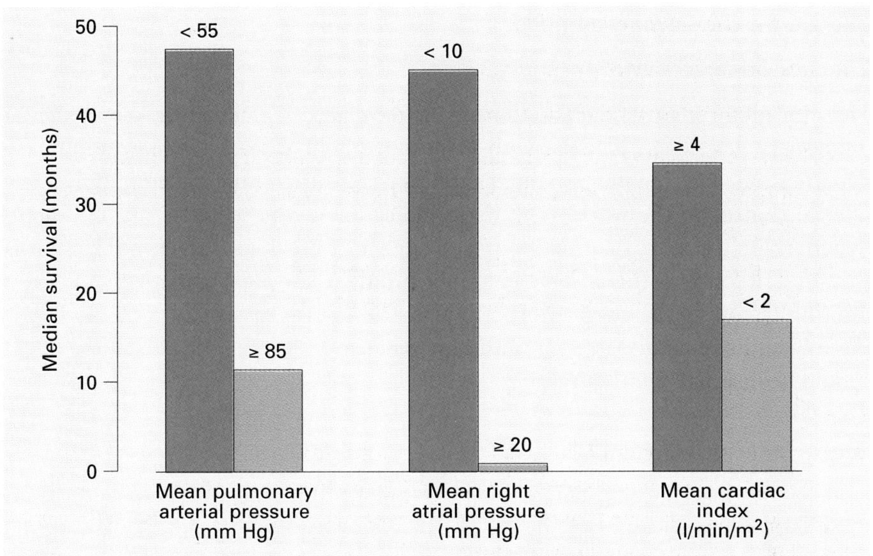

Fig. 10 Prognostic impact of raised pulmonary arterial pressure, raised right atrial pressure and decreased cardiac index in patients with primary pulmonary hypertension. (Adapted from Ref 19.)

Table 3 Quality of life indices derived from the Nottingham Health Profile scores in primary pulmonary hypertension patients treated with either prostacyclin or conventional therapy, analysed by three methods to achieve a single index [23].

	Prostacyclin group				**Conventional therapy**			
Quality of life	A	B	C	*Mean*	A	B	C	*Mean*
At day 1	0.67	0.67	0.65	*0.67*	0.72	0.71	0.69	*0.70*
At day 87	0.82	0.82	0.81	*0.82*	0.72	0.70	0.68	*0.70*

A, B and C are three statistical methodologies taken from Appendix C in O'Brien *et al, J Chron Dis* 1987; **40** (Suppl 1): 137S–153S, in which the authors cautiously attempt to aggregate the profile dimensions into a single score.

patients with no evidence of right ventricular failure and a positive vasodilator response.

Heart-lung and lung transplantation

The choice of technique depends on the centre. Overall data suggest that double-lung transplantation provides the best results, although both heart-lung and single-lung transplantation achieve survival figures of over 60% at two years [24]. Long-term survival is limited by the development of obliterative bronchiolitis, probably the result of chronic rejection. Transplantation surgery is also expensive, and is now reserved principally for patients whose symptoms no longer respond to PGI_2.

Therapy for coexistent conditions

Thrombo-endarterectomy

The aim of thrombo-endarterectomy is to recanalise segmental or subsegmental pulmonary arteries in patients with thromboembolic disease causing pulmonary hypertension. This highly specialised surgical procedure is undertaken in only a few referral centres in the world. The main indication is the presence of pulmonary hypertension for more than six months. Evidence of previous deep vein thrombosis is not a criterion, as this history is found in only a few affected patients. Age is a limiting factor, as the surgical procedure carries a risk of stroke from the hypothermia and circulatory arrest. An inferior vena cava filter (eg the Greenfield filter) should be inserted before surgery.

Long-term oxygen therapy

Evidence is emerging that patients with secondary pulmonary hypertension from Eisenmenger's syndrome and other forms of congenital heart disease are chronically hypoxaemic, particularly at night. This group can benefit from long-term oxygen therapy, where oxygen is given at home for at least 14 hours per day. Arterial oxygen saturation can be assessed at home, with levels of less than 90% indicating the need for treatment.

Novel treatments

Inhaled iloprost

Iloprost, an analogue of PGI_2, is more stable and has a longer half-life; it is also easier to use and slightly cheaper. It can be given either by intravenous infusion [25], or by inhalation from a nebuliser, when up to 15 doses per day are required to control PPH [26].

Oral prostacyclin analogues

Oral PGI_2 analogues are now available, and have been shown to be effective in controlling the symptoms of PPH [27].

Inhaled nitric oxide

NO has a very short duration of action and must be continuously inhaled. This is relatively straightforward for patients supported on a ventilator, but ambulatory subjects need to receive the gas safely and in a way that allows the dose to be increased with exercise. We have developed a portable system that delivers a brief 'spike' of gas at the beginning of each breath [28]. A similar apparatus has been successfully applied in PPH patients in a long-term pilot study [29].

Balloon atrial septostomy

This procedure, in which a left-right atrial connection is formed using a blade/balloon introduced via an intravascular catheter, appears to be successful in patients without right ventricular failure, although controlled data are not available [30]. It seems to be appropriate for patients in whom transplantation and PGI_2 are realistic options.

☐ CONCLUSIONS

Some of the mystique and much of the pessimism surrounding PPH have recently been swept away. Specialists in the field have developed a multi-staged plan of care for patients with PPH, which offers them a greater chance of survival and much improved quality of life (Fig. 11). Moreover, some of the treatments can now be extended to secondary forms of pulmonary hypertension. The impending identification of the genes involved in pulmonary hypertension may also bring the possibility of novel forms of treatment as well as greater understanding of the disease process itself. Overall, the future is looking much brighter for these unfortunate patients.

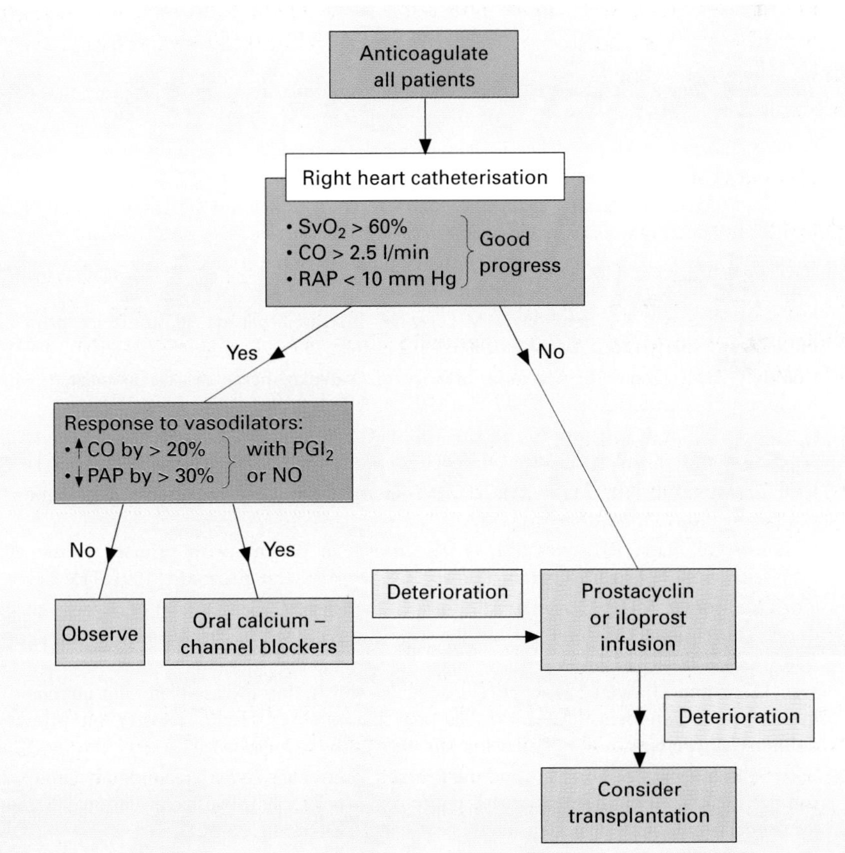

Fig. 11 Treatment decision tree for patients with primary pulmonary hypertension (CO = cardiac output; RAP = right atrial pressure; PAP = pulmonary arterial pressure; PGI_2 = prostacyclin; SvO_2 = mixed pulmonary venous oxygen saturation).

REFERENCES

1 Abenhaim L, Moride Y, Brenot F, *et al.* for the International Primary Pulmonary Hypertension Study Group. *N Engl J Med* 1996; **335**: 609–16.

2 Nichols WC, Koller DL, Slovis B, *et al.* Localization of the gene for familial primary pulmonary hypertension to chromosome 2q31-32. *Nature Genet* 1997; **15**: 277–80.

3 Chazova I, Loyd JE, Zhdanov VS, *et al.* Pulmonary artery adventitial changes and venous involvement in primary pulmonary hypertension. *Am J Pathol* 1992; **146**: 389–97.

4 Rich S, Kaufmann E, Levy P. The effect of high doses of calcium channel blockers on survival in pulmonary hypertension. *N Engl J Med* 1992; **327**: 76–81.

5 Moncada S, Higgs EA. The L-arginine/nitric oxide pathway. *N Engl J Med* 1993; **329**: 2002–12.

6 Cremona G, Wood AM, Hall LW, *et al.* Effect of inhibitors of nitric oxide release and action on vascular tone in isolated lungs of pig, sheep, dog and man. *J Physiol* 1994; **481**:185–95.

7 Cremona G, Higenbottam TW, Bower EA, *et al.* Basal and stimulated release of pulmonary endothelial nitric oxide from isolated human lungs. *Circulation* (in press).

8 Dinh-Xuan AT, Higenbottam TW, Clelland CA, *et al.* Impairment of endothelium dependent pulmonary artery relaxation in chronic obstructive lung disease. *N Engl J Med* 1991; **24**: 1539–47.

9 Springall DR, Mason NA, Burke M, *et al.* Endothelial (type iii) nitric oxide synthase is highly expressed in plexiform lesions in pulmonary hypertension. *J Pathol* 1996; **179**: A7.

10 Christman BW, McPherson CD, Newman JH, *et al.* An imbalance between the excretion of thromboxane and prostacyclin metabolites in pulmonary hypertension. *N Engl J Med* 1992; **327**: 70–5.

11 Stewart DJ, Levy R, Cernacek P, Langleben D. Increased plasma endothelin-1 in pulmonary hypertension – marker or mediator of disease? *Ann Intern Med* 1991; **114**: 464–9.

12 Giaid A, Yanagisawa M, Langleben D, *et al.* Expression of endothelin-1 in the lungs of patients with pulmonary hypertension. *N Engl J Med* 1993; **28**: 173–6.

13 Chen S, Chen Y, Meng QC, *et al.* Endothelin receptor antagonist bosentan prevents and reverses hypoxic pulmonary hypertension in rats. *J Appl Physiol* 1995; **79**: 2122–31.

14 Herve P, Drouet L, Dosquet C, *et al.* Primary pulmonary hypertension in a patient with a familial platelet storage pool disease: role of serotonin. *Am J Med* 1990; **89**: 117–20.

15 Herve P, Launay J-M, Scrobohaci M-L, *et al.* Increased plasma serotonin in primary pulmonary hypertension. *Am J Med* 1995; **99**: 249–54.

16 Connolly HM, Crary JL, McGoon MD, *et al.* Valvular heart disease associated with fenfluramine–phentermine. *N Engl J Med* 1997; **337**: 581–8.

17 Gross AS, Phillips AC, Rieutord A, Shenfield GM. The influence of the sparteine/debrisoquine genetic polymorphism on the disposition of dexfenfluramine *Br J Pharmacol* 1993; **41**: 311–17.

18 Rich E, Dantzker DR, Ayres SM, *et al.* Primary pulmonary hypertension: a national prospective study. *Ann Intern Med* 1987; **107**: 216–23.

19 D'Alonzo GE, Barst RJ, Ayres SM, *et al.* Survival in patients with primary pulmonary hypertension. Results from a national prospective registry. *Ann Intern Med* 1991; **115**: 343–9.

20 Singh SJ, Morgan MDL, Hardman AE, Rowe C, Bardsley PA. Comparison of oxygen uptake during conventional treadmill test and the shuttle walking test in chronic airflow limitation. *Eur Respir J* 1994; 7: 2016–20.

21 Weir EK, Rubin LJ, Ayers SM, *et al.* The acute administration of vasodilators in pulmonary hypertension. Experience from the National Institutes of Health registry on primary pulmonary hypertension. *Am Rev Respir Dis* 1989; **140**: 1623–30.

22 Barst R, Rubin LJ, McGoon MD, and the Primary Pulmonary Hypertension Study Group. A comparison of continuous intravenous epoprostenol (prostacyclin) with conventional therapy for primary pulmonary hypertension. *N Engl J Med* 1996; **334**: 296–301.

23 Higenbottam TW, Ward SE, Brennan A, *et al.* *Prostacyclin treatment of primary pulmonary hypertension; guidance to purchaser.* Trent Region (97/02), 1997.

24 Hosenpud JD, Novick RJ, Bren TJ, *et al.* The Registry of the International Society for Heart and Lung Transplantation. 12th Annual Report, 1995. *J Heart Lung Transplant* 1995; **14**: 805–15.

25 Higenbottam TW, Butt AY, Dinh-Xuan AT, *et al.* Treatment of pulmonary hypertension with the continuous infusion of a prostacyclin analogue, iloprost. *Heart* 1998; **79**: 175–9.
26 Olschewski H, Walmrath D, Schermuky R, *et al.* Aerosolised prostacyclin and iloprost in severe pulmonary hypertension. *Ann Intern Med* 1996; **53**: 820–4.
27 Okano Y, Yoshioka T, Shimouchi A, *et al.* Orally active prostacyclin analogue in primary pulmonary hypertension. *Lancet* 1997; **349**: 1365.
28 Katayama Y, Higenbottam TW, Cremona G, *et al.* Minimising the inhaled dose of inhaled nitric oxide, with a breath by breath delivery of spikes of concentrated gas. *Circulation* 1998; **98**(22): 2429–32.
29 Channick RN, Newhart JW, Johnson FW, *et al.* Pulsed delivery of inhaled nitric oxide to patients with pulmonary hypertension. *Chest* 1996; **109**: 1545–9.
30 Kerstein D, Levy PS, Hsu DT, *et al.* Blade balloon atrial septostomy in patients with severe primary pulmonary hypertension. *Circulation* 1995; **91**: 2028–35.

☐ MULTIPLE CHOICE QUESTIONS

1 Pulmonary hypertension is defined by:
(a) Presence of peripheral oedema
(b) Central cyanosis
(c) Mean pulmonary artery pressure over 25 mm Hg
(d) Enlarged right ventricle on echocardiogram
(e) Pulmonale on ECG

2 A recent epidemic of primary pulmonary hypertension has been described due to:
(a) Use of growth hormone
(b) Oral contraceptive pills
(c) Bush tea consumption
(d) Phenylethylamine anorectics
(e) Altitude skiing

3 A pulmonary angiogram is indicated in pulmonary hypertension when there is:
(a) Left ventricular failure
(b) Segmental perfusion defects on lung scans
(c) Peripheral oedema
(d) Enlargement of pulmonary arteries on chest X-ray
(e) ECG shows s_i t_{iii} q_{iii} pattern

4 Patients should be considered for lung transplantation when they have:
(a) Leg oedema
(b) A good vasodilator capacity at right heart catheter
(c) Left ventricular failure
(d) Failure to respond chronically to intravenous prostacyclin or iloprost
(e) Evidence of chronic thromboembolic disease

5 Inhaled nitric oxide has proved to be an effective treatment in:
(a) Infantile pulmonary hypertension
(b) Left ventricular failure
(c) Deep vein thrombosis

(d) Adult respiratory distress syndrome
(e) Chronic obstructive pulmonary disease

ANSWERS

1a False	2a False	3a False	4a False	5a True
b False	b False	b True	b False	b False
c True	c False	c False	c False	c False
d False	d True	d False	d True	d False
e False	e False	e False	e False	e False

Cystic fibrosis

Duncan Geddes

□ INTRODUCTION

The past ten years have seen an explosion in knowledge about cystic fibrosis (CF), notably in three main areas which will be the focus of this review. The first encompasses the basic genetic defect and the function of the affected protein, cystic fibrosis transmembrane regulator (CFTR). The second concerns the pathogenesis of the disease and the way in which defects in CFTR contribute to organ pathology. The third is the development of new treatments and the optimisation of conventional management. This chapter will concentrate on pulmonary disease, which is both the main source of morbidity and mortality and the area of greatest research progress.

□ MOLECULAR PATHOLOGY OF CYSTIC FIBROSIS

The CF gene lies on chromosome 7 and was identified in 1989. Its product, CFTR, is a 1480-residue protein and is now known to be a chloride channel that is inserted into the apical (luminal) membrane of epithelial cells in the bronchial and other mucosae. CFTR is regulated by cyclic AMP, and in turn influences the activity of other ion channels in the apical membrane, including a sodium channel which is sensitive to amiloride. Fully functional CFTR promotes the outward transport of Cl^- and inhibits the inward transport of Na^+ entry; defects due to mutations in the CFTR gene cause Cl^- retention within the epithelial cell and enhanced Na^+ entry (Fig. 1). These local electrolyte disturbances affect the physiochemical and bactericidal properties of airways mucus; possible mechanisms include inactivation of the peptides termed 'defensins' (*eg* β-defensin-1) which have antimicrobial actions.

To date, over 750 mutations in the CFTR gene have been identified, which can be classified into four groups (Fig. 1).

1. Defective protein production, eg nul and frame-shift mutations such as G542X (ie a glycine=stop mutation at codon 542) and 3905insT (a thymidine insertion at nucleotide position 3905), respectively.

2. Defective trafficking or processing. The mutant protein is trapped within the endoplasmic reticulum and is subsequently degraded, eg ΔF 508.

3. Defective regulation. The mutant protein reaches the cell membrane but cannot be phosphorylated to act as an ion channel, eg G551D.

4. Defective ion channel function. The protein reaches the cell membrane and is phosphorylated but, because of alterations in its structure, chloride transport is deranged, eg R117H.

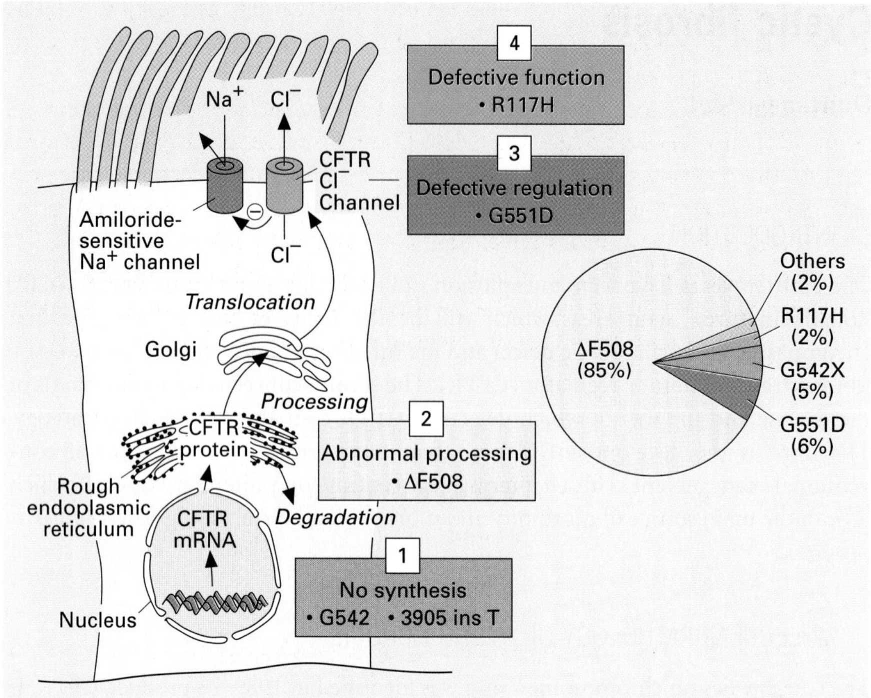

Fig. 1 Types of mutations causing defects in the synthesis, processing, regulation (phosphorylation) and Cl^- conductance function of the cystic fibrosis transmembrane regulator (CFTR). Frequencies of the commonest mutations in Caucasian populations are indicated at right.

The commonest is the ΔF 508 mutation, which accounts for about 85% of alleles in Northern European and 50% in Mediterranean populations. The next commonest are G551D (6%), G542X (5%) and R117H (2%). The resulting disease can be broadly classified into 'pancreatic insufficient' and characterised by relatively severe pulmonary involvement, typically caused by homozygosity for ΔF 508, and 'pancreatic sufficient' with milder lung disease. There are also 'dominant mild' mutations, where individuals who are compound heterozygotes may have equivocal sweat test results and mild disease irrespective of the other allele. This genetic heterogeneity implies that mutation analysis has only a limited role in diagnosis, and that clinical assessment together with sweat testing remain essential.

□ SCREENING

Neonatal screening

This has long been possible by measuring serum immunoreactive trypsin; levels are raised in CF neonates, presumably because pancreatic duct blockage leads to back-leakage of acinar enzymes. The test is simple and cheap, and can be performed using dried blood spots. Those testing positive can then proceed to genetic analysis and finally sweat testing. Several studies have shown the feasibility of this approach, the detection rate of which approaches 100%; the recall rate for further investigation is approximately one in a thousand (Fig. 2).

Nevertheless, neonatal screening is not yet in routine use. The arguments in favour of such screening are that early detection may influence parents' subsequent reproductive decisions (which would probably have very little impact) and that early diagnosis improves the delivery of care and therefore long-term prognosis. Various studies have shown benefits for screened as compared with unscreened groups, but these benefits are slight. Moreover, diagnosis by screening will detect all CF subjects, whether mild or severe, whereas clinical diagnosis inevitably identifies the more severely affected, thus introducing bias in favour of the screened group.

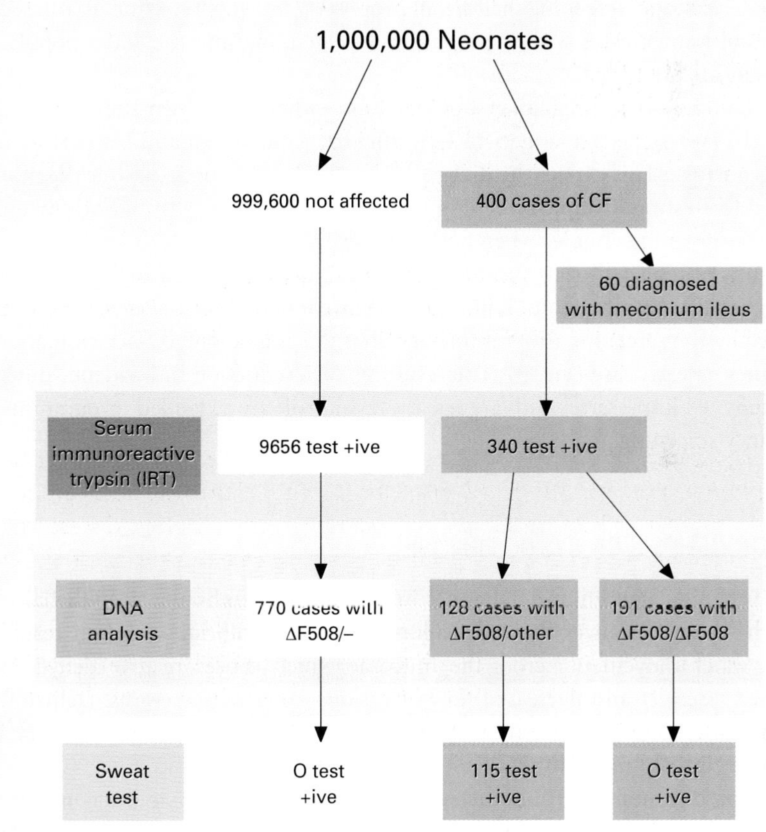

Fig. 2 Neonatal screening procedure, using immunoreactive trypsin initially, followed sequentially by DNA genotyping for the commonest CFTR mutations (see Fig. 1) and finally sweat-testing. The numbers shown are those anticipated for Caucasian populations. CFTR mutations: ΔF508/ΔF508 = homozygotes; Δ508/other = compound heterozygote with another mutation that impairs CFTR function (see Fig. 1), having milder disease and a negative sweat test; ΔF508/ — = simple heterozygote, clinically unaffected.

ANTENATAL AND POPULATION SCREENING STRATEGIES

These aim to identify couples where both partners are heterozygous, to warn them of the risk of having a CF child and to inform them of reproductive options ranging from *in vitro* fertilisation or artificial insemination using donated gametes to termination of affected pregnancies. There are, however, problems in both accuracy and uptake. There are too many mutations to allow comprehensive heterozygote screening, although the commonest three will encompass over 95% of heterozygotes. Some authorities have suggested population screening at school age to accompany biology lessons; in practice, however, screening is only likely to be accepted during pregnancy or when a family member has CF. Pilot trials of routine screening during pregnancy have shown that about 75% of couples want to be tested if they are approached personally, while fewer than 10% respond to letters or leaflets; people who know that they are carriers frequently ask for their partners to be screened. Cascade screening has been proposed, in which testing is offered to relatives of known cases with the intention of extending into the wider population as carriers are identified.

Screening during pregnancy can be done either by a 'two-step' or 'couple' approach. Two-step screening involves testing the woman first and her partner only if she is positive. This carries the disadvantage of delay and anxiety while the partner is called for testing. Couple screening involves taking samples from both members and only informing couples when both test positive.

Results of reported trials show take-up rates ranging from 60 to 99%. The most comprehensive results, from Edinburgh, showed that 70% of cases of CF were detected by the screening programme and that the couple opted for termination of pregnancy in each case (Fig. 3). The resulting 70% reduction in incidence of CF in this study is impressive and argues in favour of an extended programme of pregnancy screening.

PATHOGENESIS OF CYSTIC FIBROSIS

CFTR is a regulated chloride channel in the apical membrane of epithelial cells, through which Cl^- leaves the cell. Failure of normal chloride secretion results in altered water movement across the mucosae which causes relative dehydration, increased viscosity and decreased flow of various exocrine secretions. Dehydration of pancreatic secretion and intrahepatic bile lead to pancreatic insufficiency and periportal fibrosis, respectively.

The pathogenesis of pulmonary disease appears to be more complicated. Impaired chloride secretion in the airways is accompanied by enhanced sodium absorption, so compounding the relative dehydration of airway surface liquid. This may contribute to impaired clearance, although the pattern of CF lung disease is unlike that of the classic clearance defect, primary ciliary dyskinesia.

In CF, the airways are colonised early in life by potentially pathogenic bacteria, particularly *Staphylococcus aureus* and *Pseudomonas aeruginosa.* This suggests specific defects in antibacterial defences, for which various mechanisms have been

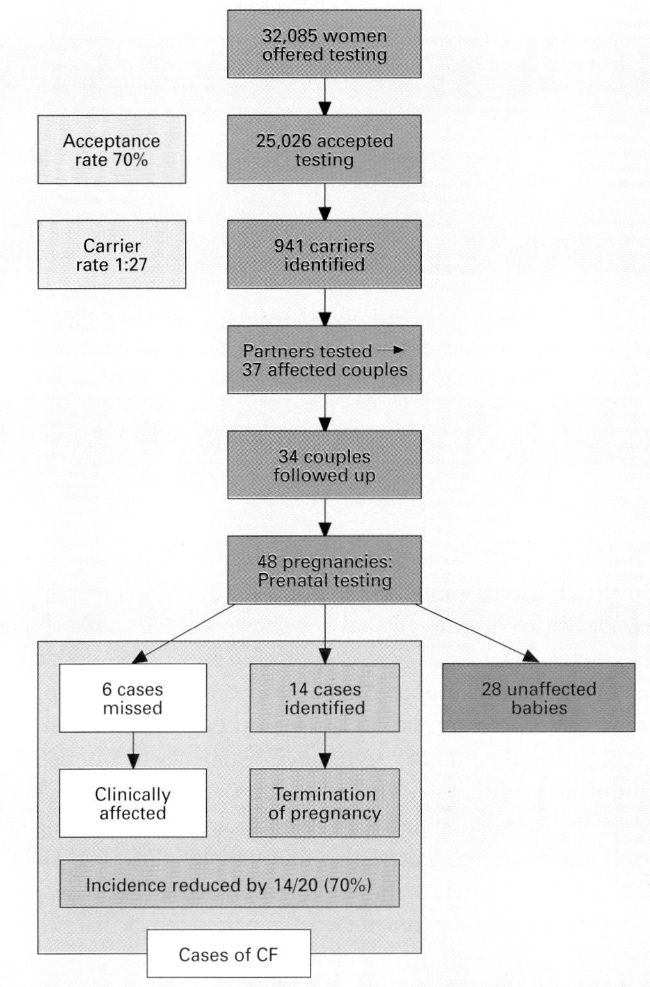

Fig. 3 Outcome of antenatal testing in Edinburgh [1]. Of the 20 affected cases, 14 were identified prenatally by DNA analysis and these pregnancies were terminated, thus reducing the incidence of CF by 70%. Six cases were missed; three were potentially detectable by prenatal testing, but one of these was missed while the other two were not tested.

proposed (Fig. 4). These include enhanced bacterial adherence, impaired antibacterial activity of airway surface liquid, and disordered bacterial ingestion by epithelial cells. *Pseudomonas* adheres to cells by their pili which are recognised by specific receptors on the cell surface. These receptors are increased in number in CF, resulting in enhanced binding of bacteria, as has been demonstrated in a number of models; the defect can be corrected by transfer of the normal CF gene. The ability of airway epithelial cells to kill bacteria is also impaired in CF, and this too can be corrected by transfer of the normal CF gene. One explanation is that altered local concentrations of sodium chloride interfere with the action of epithelium-derived

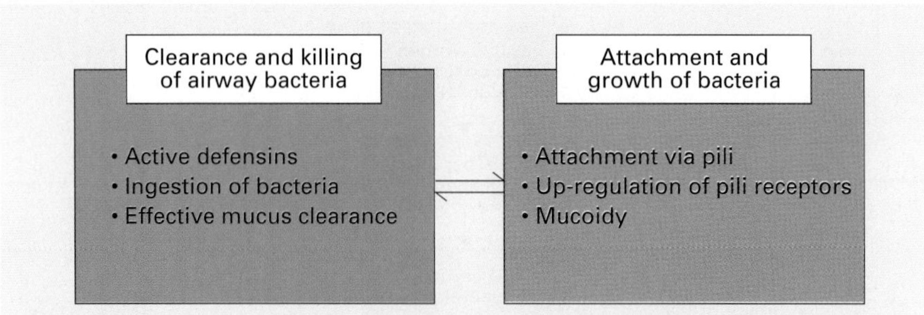

Fig. 4 The fine balance between host-bacterial interactions in patients with CF. Bacteria are removed by mechanisms including the antimicrobial 'defensin' peptides, ingestion of bacteria by airways epithelial cells and effective mucociliary clearance. Factors that favour bacterial survival and proliferation include the up-regulation on epithelial cells of the receptors that bind the pili of *Psdudomonas* species, the formation of a protective bacterial coating ('mucoidy') and impaired mucociliary clearance.

lysozymes and defensins. This hypothesis is attractive, as it links the ion transport defect to impaired bacterial killing, but it awaits confirmation; current methodology (which may not be precise enough) has not shown obvious ionic abnormalities of airway surface liquid in CF.

The local inflammatory response that follows early bacterial colonisation seems to make things worse. Bronchoalveolar lavage in young children with CF has shown high levels of pro-inflammatory cytokines, particularly interleukin-8 (IL-8), together with neutrophil elastase. The latter can partly abrogate the host's immune defences in various ways, eg by cleaving chemotactic factors, breaking down certain complement components and inactivating immunoglobulins (Fig. 5). Furthermore, neutrophil elastase is a potent stimulus for submucosal gland secretion; if such secretions are dehydrated, they contribute to impaired mucociliary clearance.

Ultimately, the combination of enhanced bacterial adherence and defective killing leads to bacterial colonisation with subsequent inflammation which further impairs clearance of bacteria and contributes to airway damage leading to small airway obliteration, bronchiectasis and persistent low-grade infection (Fig. 6).

□ TREATMENT OF CYSTIC FIBROSIS

Four factors have contributed to the continuing improvement in survival and quality of life of CF subjects over the past ten years:

- □ various new treatments for CF lung disease have been developed or are currently under investigation;
- □ the conventional treatment of lung colonisation and infection is continually being refined;
- □ lung transplantation has become established as an option for those with end-stage disease,

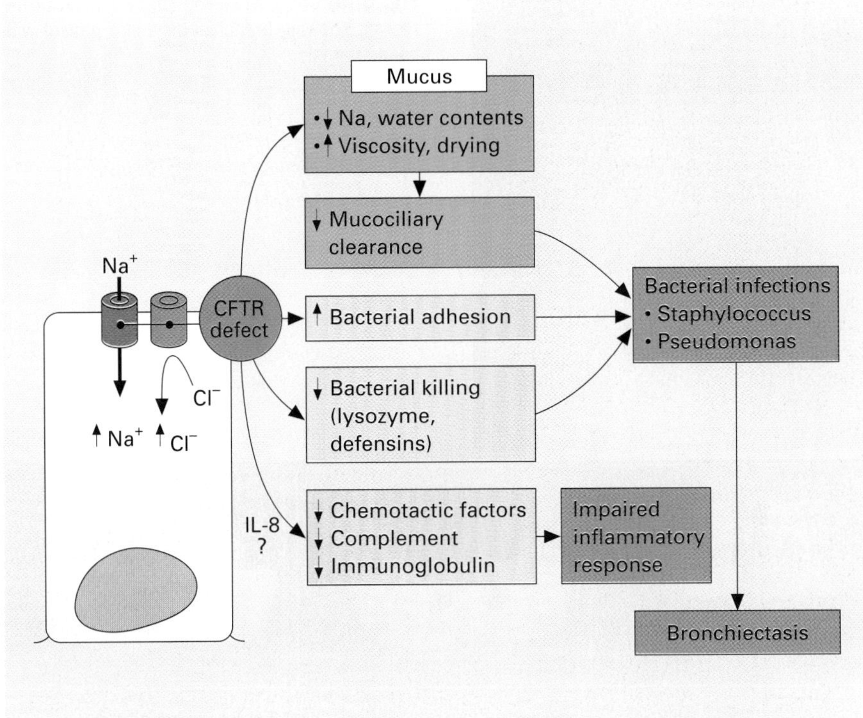

Fig. 5 Factors contributing to bacterial infections in cystic fibrosis, and that relationship with defects in the CFTR protein.

- CF care is increasingly being delivered by specialist units, resulting in greater uniformity of care and early application of new treatments.

New treatments

Gene therapy

The demonstration that transfer of the normal version of the CF gene into epithelial cells can correct the cellular phenotype of the disease has led to large-scale efforts to develop gene therapy. Results so far have established that the gene can be transferred *in vivo*, resulting in expression of the mRNA and protein together with some degree of functional correction. However, early optimism based on laboratory *in vitro* studies has been dampened by *in vivo* problems, including inefficient gene transfer, inflammation and immunity.

The two main methods for delivering CFTR cDNA to the interior of epithelial cells are illustrated in Fig. 7. 'Viral gene transfer' involves inserting the cDNA into the genome of an adenovirus or other non-pathogenic viruses. 'Non-viral transfer' employs carriers such as liposomes, lipid envelopes that can fuse with the cell membrane. Both methods are developing fast. With virologists deleting proteins in

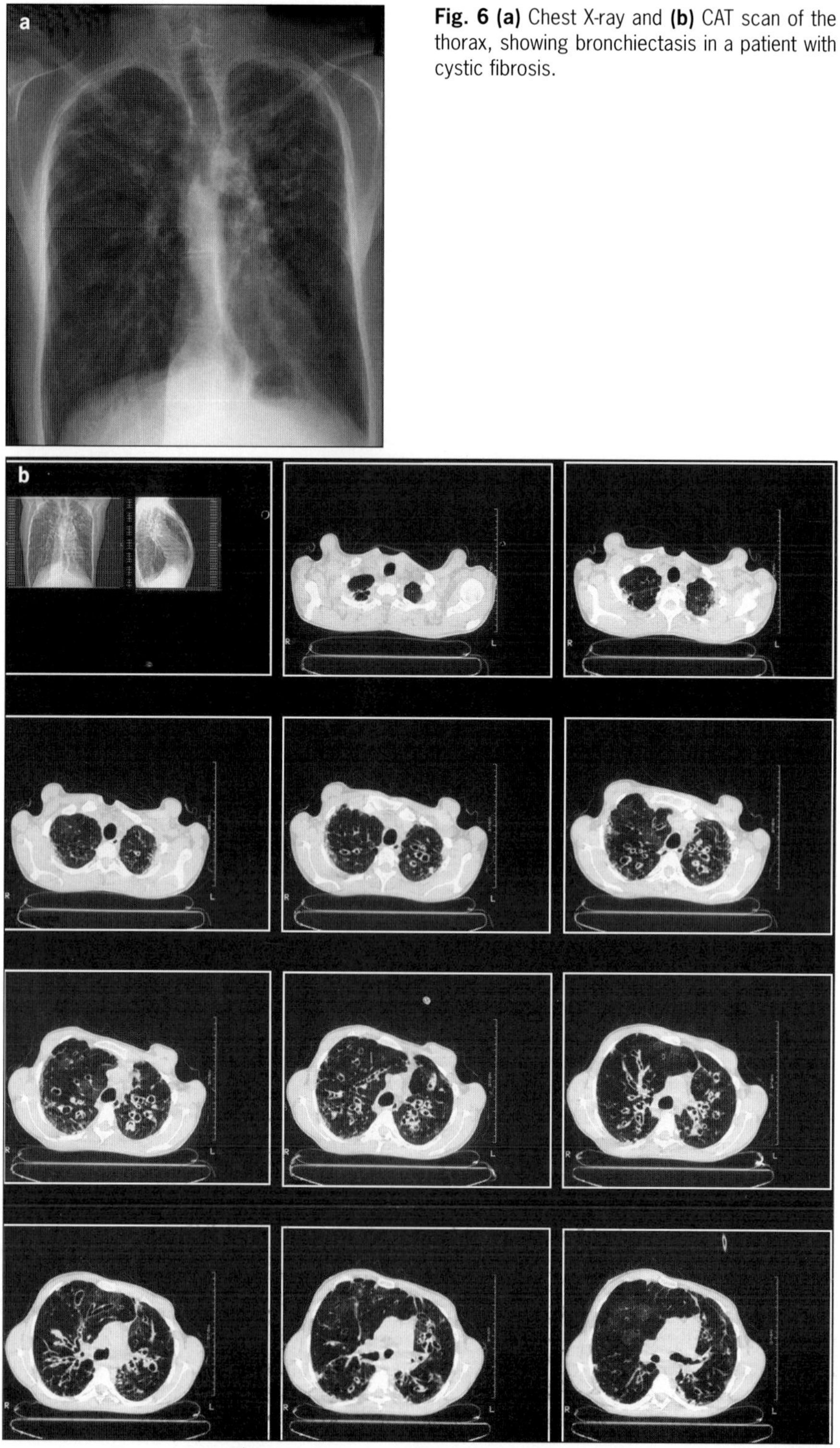

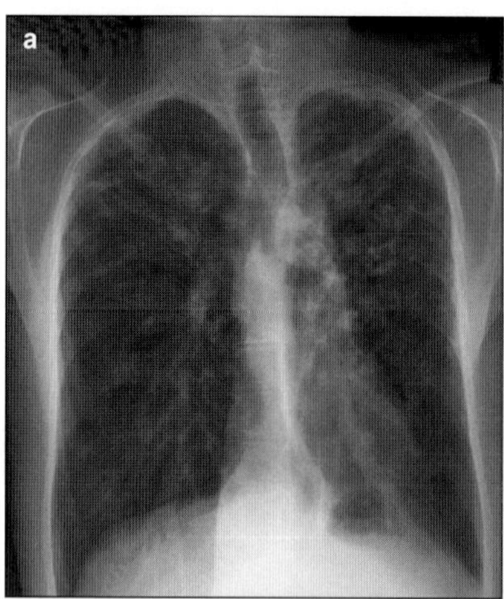

Fig. 6 (a) Chest X-ray and **(b)** CAT scan of the thorax, showing bronchiectasis in a patient with cystic fibrosis.

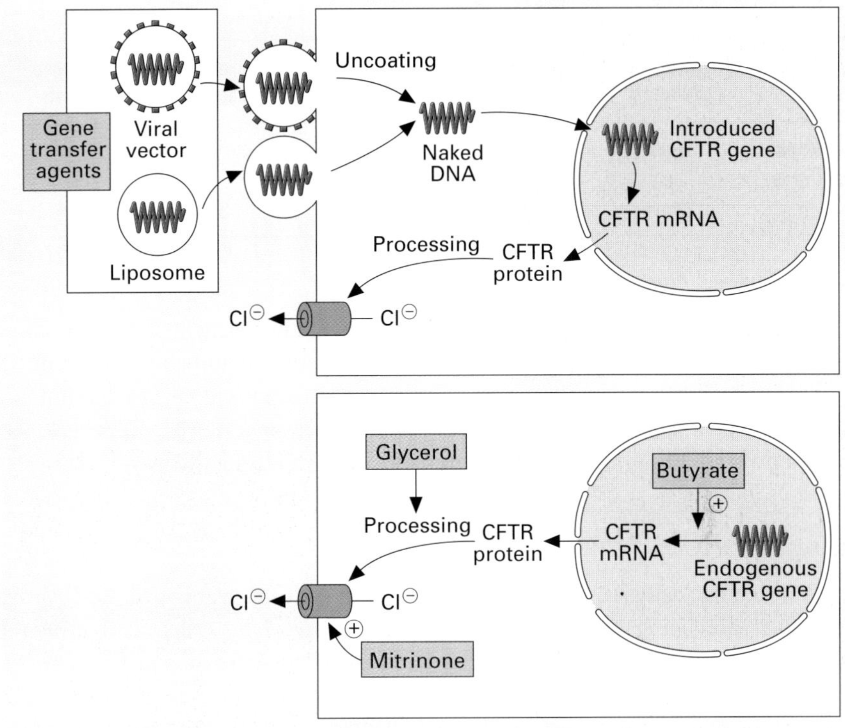

Fig. 7 Strategies to enhance the activity of the CFTR protein in patients with cystic fibrosis. These include gene therapy, with the CFTR gene delivered to the airways epithelial cell in either a modified virus or a liposome, and various chemicals that increase CFTR synthesis (butyrate), protect it during processing (glycerol, a chemical 'chaperone'), or enhance the activity of the chloride channel. GTA, Gene transfer agent.

order to reduce host reactions, and non-viral chemists adding proteins to enhance efficiency, the two technologies may eventually converge.

The clinical trials of gene therapy that are completed or in progress are summarised in Table 1. Adenoviral vectors can initially produce CFTR mRNA levels that are approximately 5% of endogenous levels in normal subjects; this may be adequate but gene transfer becomes progressively less efficient with repeated dosing. Adeno-associated viral vectors can partially correct the chloride channel defect, but the results of repeated dosing are as yet unknown. Liposome-protected complexes can achieve up to 25% correction of the chloride transport defect, but do not improve sodium channel function. The only study that administered these complexes to the lung reported a transient febrile reaction, which may have been due to the high dose of bacteria-derived DNA. All studies, irrespective of the vector, have shown only transient (1–2 weeks) expression of the therapeutic gene.

Current research is concentrating on optimising gene transfer, by modifying the vectors and by circumventing *in vivo* barriers. The longer-term goal is to develop

Table 1 Clinical trials of gene therapy in CF. The percentages of patients that had evidence of successful gene transfer and of phenotypic improvement.

Vector	Route of delivery	Number of subjects	Induction of CFTR mRNA	Improved ion transport	Adverse events
Adenovirus	Nose	45	45%	34%	4%
Adenovirus	Lung	73	37%	—	30%
Liposome	Nose	46	45%	35%	0%

systems that deliver the gene together with its regulatory elements, and so allow physiological control of gene expression. These problems will probably be overcome, but it is impossible to guess how long effective gene therapy will take to develop.

Systemic gene therapy or local delivery to bile duct, pancreas or gut have so far received little attention in CF, as the dominant problem is lung disease.

Ion transport therapy

Many available drugs modulate chloride and sodium transport, and three approaches are being explored to develop new topical or systemic treatments (Fig. 7 and Table 2). The first approach attempts to increase the function of the mutant CFTR, the second to stimulate alternative chloride channels, and the third to reduce the enhanced sodium absorption from the airways mucus. The function of mutant CFTR can be enhanced by stimulating protein production with phenylbutyrate; alternatively, agents such as glycerol may act as chemical 'chaperones' and overcome the trafficking defect resulting from the ΔF 508 mutation. Finally, agents such as xanthines or milrinone may increase the chloride transport capacity of any mutant CFTR that reaches the membrane. So far, only phenylbutyrate has been assessed in a clinical trial, with encouraging results. Chloride transport through alternative (calcium-dependent) channels can be enhanced by bradykinin, ATP or UTP; a programme to develop nebulised UTP for clinical use in under way.

Finally, the channels that allow Na^+ ions to enter the epithelium can be blocked with amiloride delivered topically to the airways. Unfortunately, the initially encouraging clinical reports have not been borne out by more extensive trials. Longer-acting amiloride analogues (eg benzamil), or combination therapy for both sodium and chloride channel defects, may be more effective.

Anti-inflammatory drugs

Three approaches have been proposed: corticosteroids, ibuprofen and anti-elastases. Prednisolone (2 mg/kg/day) slows the decline in lung function, but at the expense of unacceptable side-effects. Inhaled corticosteroids are theoretically attractive and are currently being evaluated. The non-steroidal anti-inflammatory drug ibuprofen has been evaluated in 85 CF patients in a placebo-controlled trial lasting 4 years.

Table 2 Treatments to modify the course of cystic fibrosis

Enhancing the action of CFTR

- *Gene therapy with exogenous CFTR*

Increase synthesis of endogenous CFTR

- Butyrate, phenylbutyrate

Decrease CFTR degradation during processing

- Glycerol

Increase Cl^- channel activity of CFTR protein

- Milrinone
- Xanthines

Down-regulate apical membrane Na^+ channel

- Amiloride
- Benzamil

Anti-inflammatory drugs

- Corticosteroids
- Ibuprofen
- Elastase inhibitors (eg a_1-antitrypsin)

Mucolytic agents

- DNase
- Gelsolin
- Nacysteline

Progression of lung disease was slowed in children aged under 13 years who had mild disease, but no benefit was detectable in older patients. These results need to be confirmed and extended in larger numbers of patients with a wider range of disease severity.

Anti-elastase agents include human alpha 1 antitrypsin (derived from donated blood or from transgenic sheep) and various recently developed drugs with systemic activity. The latter include pentoxifylline which, in a single small clinical study, reduced sputum elastase levels and achieved borderline improvements in some measures of lung function.

Established treatments

Physiotherapy, adequate nutrition and antibiotics are the cornerstones of treatment of CF lung disease. Self-administered postural drainage with the forced expiratory manoeuvre remains the best way to clear secretions; the continuing stream of new mechanical devices may improve the financial health of their inventors but does little for CF patients. Nutritional advice is important; the main change in recent years is a trend towards earlier use of gastrostomy feeding.

Antimicrobial agents

Antibiotic therapy for pulmonary exacerbations is usually given for 10–14 days, guided by bacterial antibiotic sensitivities. Monotherapy is probably adequate for *Staphylococcus aureus* infection, whereas two drugs should be given together for *Pseudomonas aeruginosa* to limit the development of antibiotic resistance. The pseudomonad *Burkholderia cepacia* remains an important challenge, as its carriage accelerates the decline in pulmonary function and it is sensitive to few antibiotics; the most useful are ceftazidime, temocillin, trimethoprim and chloramphenicol.

The Copenhagen centre promotes the use of nebulised colomycin when *Pseudomonas* is first isolated, to try to delay colonisation; many centres have since adopted this approach. More contentious, however, is their policy of regular 3-monthly courses of systemic anti-pseudomonal antibiotics once colonisation is established. A recent UK study failed to show benefit from such treatment, which is also time-consuming and expensive. On the other hand, the value of anti-pseudomonal antibiotics given regularly by nebuliser has been confirmed in several studies and a recent meta-analysis (Fig. 8), and is probably better than regular intravenous treatment.

The value of regular anti-staphylococcal therapy has not been adequately tested, with one small study showing benefit which was not confirmed by a recently reported larger study. In order to rationalise antimicrobial approaches to CF, a Cochrane Centre has recently been established to evaluate evidence-based data.

Mucolytic drugs

DNase improves lung function by 10–15% within weeks and by 5% after six months, and also marginally reduces the frequency of pulmonary infections. Other mucolytic drugs such as gelsolin and nacysteline show some promise but have not yet been fully evaluated. DNase costs about £8000 per annum and most centres have drawn up protocols to establish which patients show worthwhile objective and subjective

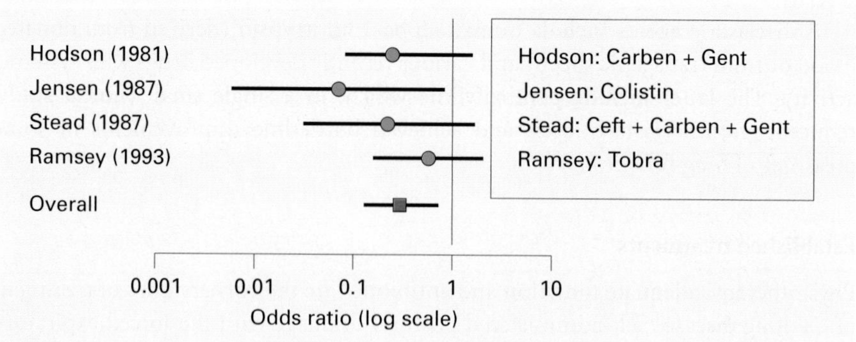

Fig. 8 Meta-analysis of the effects of various nebulised antibiotics used prophylactically in reducing infective exacerbations that required systemic antibiotic treatment. Similar improvements have also been shown for FEV_1 and *Pseudomonas* load (Data from [2]). Carben, carbenicillin; Ceft, ceftazidione; Gent, gentamicin, Tobra, tobramycin.

improvements before recommending long-term use. The ideal dosing and timing of DNase remains unclear; some patients limit its use to symptomatic episodes, while others claim benefit from doubling the dose during exacerbations.

Lung transplantation

Around 1000 patients with CF worldwide have now received a lung transplant. The survival averages 70% at 1 year and 50% at 3 years, comparable to that for other indications (Fig. 9). At present, the chief problems are a shortage of donor lungs, long-term graft failure (chiefly from obliterative bronchiolitis), and the choice of optimal timing and selection of recipients. Both lungs are needed in CF, whereas single-lung transplantation is adequate for most other diseases; even if all suitable donor lungs were identified and donated, there would be enough for only 50% of CF patients. The possibility of animal organ donation is the subject of much research and debate but remains a distant prospect. Graft failure remains a problem, and appears to be due to inadequate immunosuppression. More intensive immunosuppression and new drugs are currently being evaluated. Until all these problems are solved, the terminal management of CF will remain very difficult; an aggressive approach is appropriate for those fortunate enough to receive a transplant but may increase suffering for those who do not.

□ THE FUTURE

The outlook for people with CF continues to improve, with median survival now approaching 32 years (Fig. 10). This is likely to continue due to more precise application of conventional treatment and the development of practical gene- or

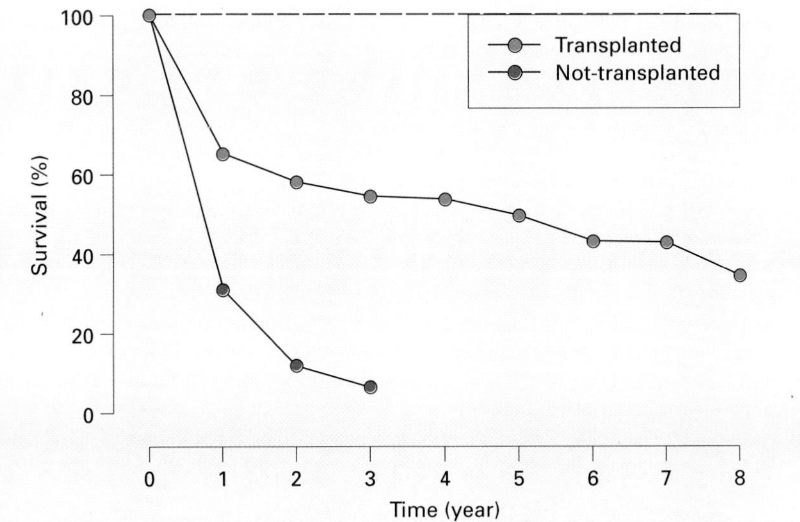

Fig. 9 Actuarial survival plot of patients who received lung transplants versus others who did not.

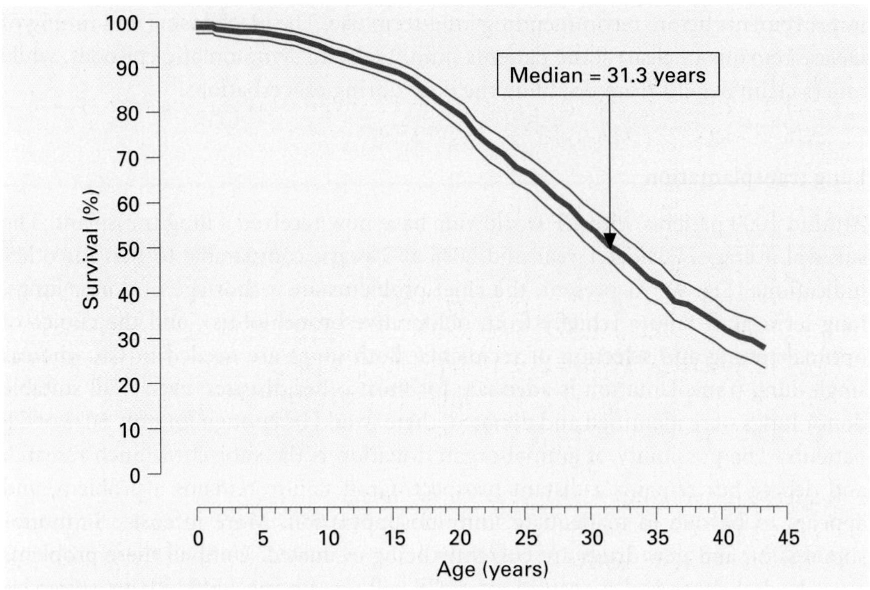

Fig. 10 Actuarial survival plot for all cystic fibrosis patients on the National CF Patient Registry of the Cystic Fibrosis Foundation, 1996

ion-transport therapy. Nevertheless, cystic fibrosis remains a devastating condition for both the individual and his or her family and there is still a long way to go.

REFERENCES

1 Brock DJH. Prenatal screening for CF: 5 years experience reviewed. *Lancet* 1996; **347**: 148–50.

2 Mukhopadhyay S, Singh M, Carter JI *et al.* Nebulised antipseudomonal antibiotic therapy in CF: a meta-analysis of benefits and risks. *Thorax* 1996; **51**: 364–8.

FURTHER READING

Rosenstein BJ, Zeitlin PL. Cystic Fibrosis. *Lancet* 1998; **351**: 277–82.

Wicklen B, Wiley V, Sherry G, Bayliss U. Neonatal screening for CF: a comparison of two strategies for case detection in 1.2 million babies *Pediatr* 1995; **127**: 965–70.

Smith JJ, Travis SM, Greenberg EP, Welsh MJ. Cystic fibrosis airway epithelia fail to kill bacteria because of abnormal airway surface fluid. *Cell* 1996; **85**: 229–36.

Davies JC, Stern M, Dewar AM, Caplen NJ, *et al.* CFTR gene transfer reduces the binding of *Ps. aeruginosa* to CF respiratory epithelium. *Am J Respir Cell Mol Biol* 1997; **16**: 657–63.

Alton EWFW, Geddes DM, Gill DR *et al.* Towards gene therapy for cystic fibrosis: a clinical progress report. *Gene Ther* 1998; **5**: In press.

Rubenstein RC, Egan ME, Zeitlin PL. *In vitro* pharmacologic restoration of CFTR-mediated chloride transport with sodium 4-phenylbutyrate in CF epithelial cells. *J Clin Invest* 1997; **100**: 2457–65.

Konstan MW, Byard PJ, Hoppel CL, Davis PB. Effect of high dose ibuprofen in patients with cystic fibrosis. *N Engl J Med* 1995; **332**: 848–54.

Fuchs HJ, Borowitz DS, Christiansen DM, Morris EM, Nash ML. Effect of aerosolised recombinant DNase on exacerbations of respiratory symptoms in patients with CF. *N Engl J Med* 1994; **331**: 637–42.

Egan TM, Detterbeck FC, Mill MR, Paradowski LJ. Improved results of lung transplantation for patients with CF. *J Thorac Cardiovasc Surg* 1995; **109**: 224–34.

☐ MULTIPLE CHOICE QUESTIONS

1 The ΔF of 508 mutation:
 (a) Is rare in North American CF populations
 (b) Fails to traffic to the cell membrane
 (c) Is associated with pancreatic sufficiency
 (d) Can transport chloride if it reaches the cell membrane
 (e) Is associated with thrombocytosis

2 Local concentration of sodium chloride alters:
 (a) Defensin activity
 (b) Bacterial adherence
 (c) Neutrophil elastase activity
 (d) Submucosal gland secretion
 (e) Lysozymal bacterial killing

3 Adenoviral vectors
 (a) Are more efficient *in vitro* than *in vivo*
 (b) Integrate into the host chromosome
 (c) Show reduced gene transfer on repeat application
 (d) Are more efficient if combined with plasmid DNA
 (e) Can be nebulised to the airways

4 Chloride transport in CF is altered by:
 (a) Pentoxifylline
 (b) Aminophylline
 (c) UTP
 (d) Bradykinin
 (e) Amiloride

5 *Burkholderia cepacia* in CF
 (a) Is associated with accelerated decline in lung function
 (b) Contraindicates gastrostomy feeding
 (c) Is usually resistant to tetracycline
 (d) Is usually sensitive to colomycin
 (e) Is commonly acquired from nebuliser

ANSWERS

1a False	2a True	3a True	4a False	5a True
b True	b False	b False	b False	b False
c False	c False	c True	c True	c True
d True	d False	d False	d True	d False
e False	e True	e True	e False	e False

The Lumleian Lecture

C-reactive protein and amyloidosis: from proteins to drugs?

Mark B Pepys

> *'Caldwellus, qui, ut de repub. Bene meretur, adscito in partem honoris Barone Lumleio, lectionem chirurigicam, honesto salario, in Medicorum Collegio Londini a Thoma Linacro fundato, instituit.'*

> 'Caldwell, as an act of generosity to the public, instituted, along with Lord Lumley, a lecture in surgery endowed with a proper salary, in the College of Physicians in London which had been founded by Thomas Linacre.'

Caldwell was 'renowned for his singular erudition... one and the same day admitted as Member, Fellow and Censor.' 'He was responsible for instituting lectures in surgery, and this is highly appropriate, since the best way to learn how to heal comes through contemplating Nature and her clever methods of healing those illnesses that can be experienced directly. Caldwell was very learned and did not want the original base of medical science to be separated from current practice.'

Richard Caldwell, who founded this, the oldest named College lecture, in 1582, was clearly an early practitioner of evidence-based medicine! William Harvey's Lumleian Lectures, in which he demonstrated the circulation of the blood, were a hard act to follow but in the past 160 years the subjects have included cardiovascular disease and atherosclerosis, dementia, nephritis and rheumatic diseases. Here I describe the structure and function of proteins involved in all these disorders and the elucidation of pathophysiological mechanisms, leading to identification of new potential therapeutic targets.

☐ PENTRAXINS

The pentraxins are a family of phylogenetically conserved normal plasma proteins [1]. The two human members of the family are C-reactive protein (CRP), the classical acute phase protein, and serum amyloid P component (SAP), named for its universal presence in the pathological protein deposits known as amyloid. Both molecules are structurally invariant in man and no deficiency or polymorphism of either has yet been reported. Although they are closely related to each other, they are quite distinct but share a capacity for calcium dependent ligand binding which underlies their functional properties. They also share very similar structural organisation, each being composed of five protomers non-covalently associated in a disc-like configuration with cyclic pentameric symmetry (Fig. 1), hence the name

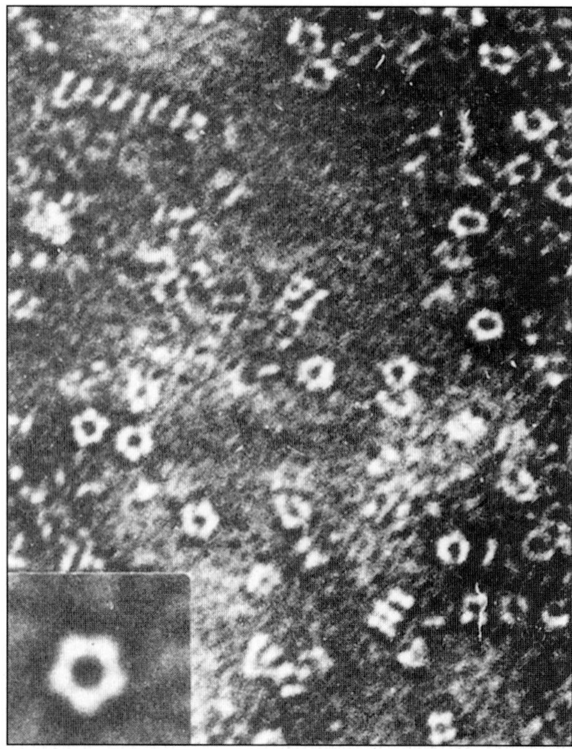

Fig. 1 Electron microscopic appearance of serum amyloid P component (SAP) (negative staining). Typical field including pentagonal rings and linear stacks. Magnification × 590,000. Inset: face view of single molecule from same field obtained by rotational integration; maximum diameter 8.3 nm. (From Pepys *et al.* [2] with kind permission of The Lancet Ltd.)

pentraxin derived from the Greek for 'five berries'. Since I gave the College's Goulstonian Lecture on this subject, in 1982, the structures of both molecules, alone and in calcium dependent complexes with their respective specific ligands, have been solved at atomic resolution by x-ray crystallography [3,4,5] (Fig. 2). The tertiary fold, that is the underlying molecular architecture, of CRP and SAP is a flattened β-jellyroll, and is unexpectedly shared by a number of other, diverse proteins from plants, animals and bacteria. These proteins have no amino acid sequence homology but they all bind to specific carbohydrates, and we have named the group the 'lectin fold' superfamily.

□ C-REACTIVE PROTEIN

CRP was the first plasma protein recognised as an acute phase reactant and is the best objective marker for quantitative monitoring of the acute phase response in clinical medicine. The normal concentration is less than 3 mg/l but can rise to over 500 mg/l in the acute phase response. It is a non-glycosylated protein, secreted and catabolised only by hepatocytes [6]. Its synthesis is under transcriptional control,

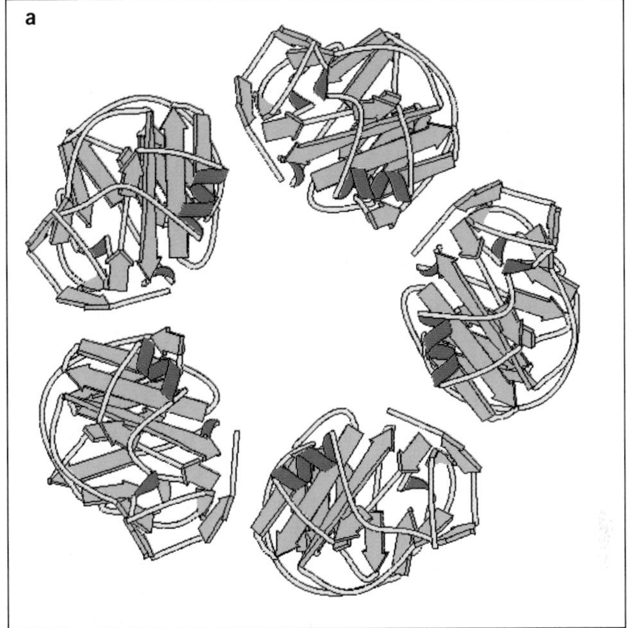

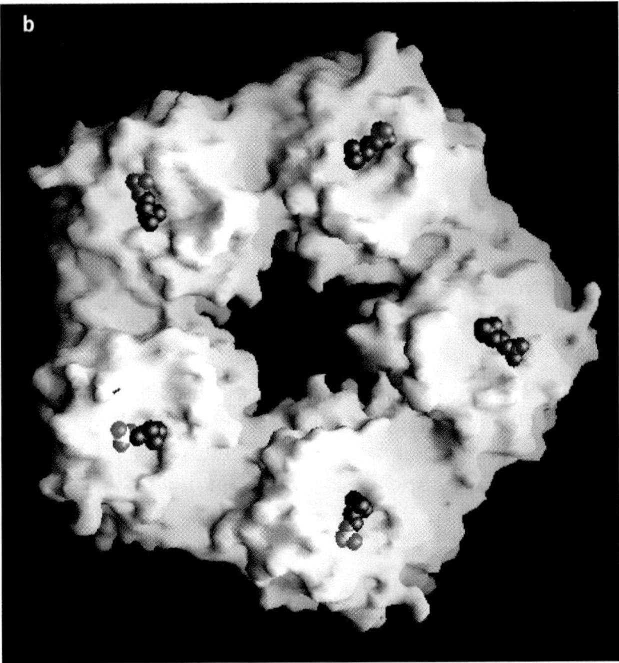

Fig. 2 (a) Crystallographic structure of fully calcified human CRP at 2.5 Å resolution displayed in MOLSCRIPT, showing the flattened β-jellyroll fold of the protomers and their pentameric assembly; β-strands in green, α-helices in red. **(b)** CRP pentamer from the crystal structure at 2.5 Å resolution, viewed face-on and displayed as a GRASP representation with the positions of the five bound molecules of phosphocholine indicated. (From Thompson *et al.* [5] by permission of *Structure*.)

regulated by cytokines, especially interleukin-6. The plasma half-life of CRP is about 19 hours under all normal and pathological conditions that have been investigated, so the secretion rate of CRP is the sole determinant of its plasma concentration [7].

CRP was so named because of its interaction with pneumococcal somatic C-polysaccharide, in which it specifically recognises phosphocholine. CRP also binds phosphoethanolamine and a range of other phosphate monoesters. Once bound to macromolecular ligands, CRP is an efficient activator of the classic complement pathway and engages the opsonic and pro-inflammatory effector functions of complement. In experimental model systems, CRP powerfully confers resistance to pneumococcal infection [8] and, given the wide distribution of phosphocholine among micro-organisms, including bacteria such as *Haemophilus influenzae*, fungi such as *Aspergillus*, and various parasitic worms, it is likely that CRP contributes to innate host resistance to infection. CRP may also protect against the toxicity of Gram negative bacterial lipopolysaccharide. On the other hand, CRP also binds to autologous constituents, including plasma membranes of damaged cells, exposed small nuclear ribonucleoprotein particles, and platelet activating factor, an important pro-inflammatory mediator. Aggregated CRP selectively binds plasma low density and very low density lipoproteins [9]. CRP may thus have important normal, and potentially pathophysiological, functions related to its interactions with autologous ligands. Two other contrasting actions of CRP have been described that may not necessarily be effected via its ligand binding property. First, CRP enhances production by macrophages of tissue factor, the initiator of the extrinsic pathway of blood coagulation, and CRP may thus potentially be a pro-coagulant. Second, in models of lung inflammation CRP reduces polymorph motility and chemotaxis with anti-inflammatory consequences.

□ SERUM AMYLOID P COMPONENT

SAP is a constitutive plasma glycoprotein in man, circulating at a rather tightly controlled concentration of about 30 mg/l, with a plasma half-life of about 24 hours. It is synthesised and catabolised exclusively by hepatocytes [6]. There is a single, invariant, typical complex biantennary oligosaccharide attached to each SAP protomer. Uniquely in man (ie in no other species studied so far) SAP is also an extracellular matrix constituent, located in the glomerular basement membrane and the microfibrillar mantle of elastic fibres throughout the body.

SAP is a lectin with calcium dependent binding specificity for particular anionic carbohydrates, including cyclic pyruvate acetals, heparan sulphate and dermatan sulphate glycosaminoglycans. It also specifically binds phosphoethanolamine but, unlike CRP, not phosphocholine. SAP is so named because of its presence in amyloid deposits where it is calcium dependently bound to the amyloid fibrils, and SAP binds *in vitro* to such fibrils produced from pure non-glycosylated precursor proteins [10]. Aggregated SAP selectively binds fibronectin and C4-binding protein from whole serum. Finally, SAP is the single protein in whole plasma that shows specific calcium dependent binding *in vitro* to DNA, chromatin and nucleosomes, and this also occurs *in vivo* when chromatin is exposed in or on necrotic and apoptotic cells. The interaction with native long chromatin is very avid and displaces histone H1 so that the otherwise insoluble chromatin becomes soluble at physiological pH and ionic strength [11]. Furthermore, the DNA within the SAP-chromatin complex is protected from cleavage by polymorphs and macrophages.

The diverse range of binding reactivities of SAP suggest a variety of possible *in vivo* functions. We have long believed that the universal association with amyloid deposits reflects involvement in pathogenesis of amyloidosis. Similarly the remarkable avidity and functional effects of the SAP-chromatin interaction indicated likely participation of SAP in normal *in vivo* handling of chromatin from dead cells. The lectin binding of SAP to some bacteria hinted at a possible contribution to innate resistance to infection.

□ AMYLOID

Amyloidosis is the extracellular deposition of normally soluble autologous proteins as abnormal insoluble fibrils in the tissues. The different types of amyloid are named according to the fibril protein type (eg 'AL' from A:amyloid, L:monoclonal immunoglobulin light chain; 'AA' from A:amyloid, A:amyloid A protein) (Tables 1, 2) [12]. The deposits are rich in glycosaminoglycans and always contain SAP bound to the fibrils. Amyloid deposits tend to persist and accumulate, leading to structural and functional damage, tissue and organ dysfunction, disease, and usually death. Amyloidosis is usually diagnosed histologically on biopsy or autopsy material, but only if the possibility is considered and the correct histochemical stains are performed with sufficient expertise (Fig. 3). It has therefore been perceived as a very rare condition. However, lately it has been recognised that amyloid deposition is actually a very common pathological process. Focal deposits in various tissues are

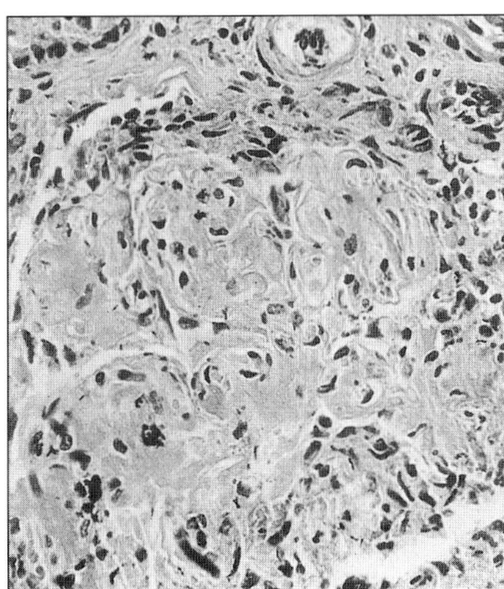
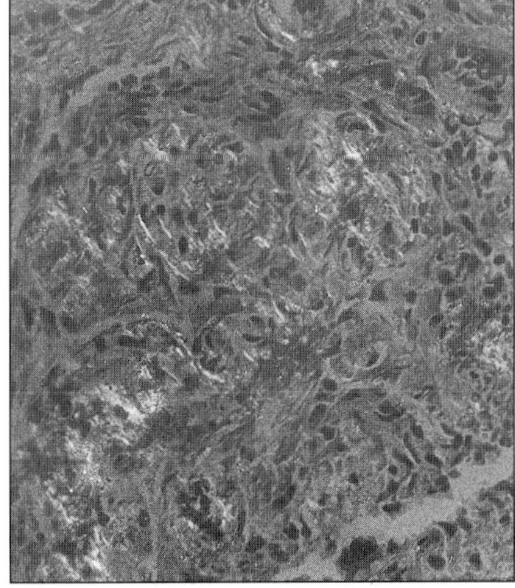

Fig. 3 Renal glomerular amyloid deposits stained with Congo Red in a case of AA amyloidosis complicating renal adenocarcinoma. Left: normal illumination. Right: polarised light showing pathognomonic birefringence (× 400).

Table 1 Acquired amyloidosis syndromes.

Clinical syndrome	Fibril protein
Systemic AL amyloidosis, associated with immunocyte dyscrasia, myeloma, monoclonal gammopathy, occult dyscrasia	AL fibrils derived from monoclonal immunoglobulin light chains
Local nodular AL amyloidosis (skin, respiratory tract, urogenital tract, etc) associated with focal immunocyte dyscrasia	AL fibrils derived from monoclonal immunoglobulin light chains
Reactive systemic AA amyloidosis, associated with chronic active diseases	AA fibrils derived from serum amyloid A protein (SAA)
Senile systemic amyloidosis	Transthyretin (TTR) derived from plasma TTR
Focal senile amyloidosis: atria of the heart	Atrial natriuretic peptide
brain	β-protein
joints	Not yet characterised
seminal vesicles	Not yet characterised
prostate	β_2-microglobulin
Alzheimer's disease, dementia in Down's syndrome, sporadic cerebral amyloid angiography	Aβ derived from β-amyloid protein precursor (APP)
Sporadic Creutzfeldt-Jakob disease, kuru (transmissible spongiform encephalopathies, prion diseases)	Prion protein (PrP) derived from prion protein precursor
Type II diabetes mellitus	Islet amyloid polypeptide (IAPP), amylin, derived from its precursor protein
Endocrine amyloidosis, associated with APUDomas	Peptide hormones or fragments thereof (eg precalcitonin in medullary carcinoma of thyroid)
Haemodialysis associated amyloidosis; osteoarticular or systemic	β_2-microglobulin derived from high plasma levels
Primary localised cutaneous amyloid (macular, papular)	? Keratin derived
Ocular amyloid (cornea, conjunctiva)	Not yet characterised
Orbital amyloid	Not yet characterised; AH derived from monoclonal immunoglobulin heavy chains in one case

universally associated with 'normal' ageing and may cause clinical disease, in particular heart failure in senile cardiac amyloidosis. More importantly, amyloid deposits are hallmark features of the cerebral neuropathology of Alzheimer's disease, and of the pathology of the islets of Langerhans in type II, maturity onset, diabetes mellitus. Other common types of amyloidosis include the predominantly osteoarticular deposits of β_2-microglobulin occurring in patients on haemodialysis for end stage renal failure, systemic monoclonal immunoglobulin light chain (AL) amyloidosis which is responsible for 1:2,000–1:1,000 of all deaths in the UK, and systemic reactive (AA) amyloidosis complicating chronic inflammatory diseases such as rheumatoid arthritis, juvenile arthritis and Crohn's disease.

Table 2 Hereditary amyloidosis syndromes.

Clinical syndrome	Fibril protein
Predominant peripheral nerve involvement, familial amyloid polyneuropathy (FAP). Autosomal dominant	Transthyretin (TTR) genetic variants (most commonly Met30, but over 50 others described)
Predominant peripheral nerve involvement, FAP. Autosomal dominant	Apolipoprotein AI (apoAI) N-terminal fragment of genetic variant Arg26
Predominant cranial nerve involvement with lattice corneal dystrophy. Autosomal dominant	Gelsolin, fragment of genetic variant Asn187 or Tyr187
Prominent visceral involvement without neuropathy. Autosomal dominant	ApoAI, N-terminal fragment of genetic variant Arg26, Arg50, Arg60 or deletion variants Lysozyme genetic variant Thr56 or His67 Fibrinogen α-chain genetic variants Leu554, Val526 and others Other proteins/variants may well exist
Predominant cardiac involvement, no clinical neuropathy. Autosomal dominant	TTR genetic variants Thr45, Ala60, Ser84, Met111, Ile122
Hereditary cerebral haemorrhage with amyloidosis (cerebral amyloid angiopathy). Autosomal dominant	
Icelandic type (with major asymptomatic systemic amyloid)	Cystatin C, fragment of genetic variant Glu68
Dutch type	β-protein derived from genetic variant APP Gln693
Familial Alzheimer's disease	Aβ derived from genetic variant APP Ile717, Phe717, Gly717 and others Aβ derived from wild type APP in presence of presenilin mutations
Familial dementia; probable Alzheimer's disease	β-protein derived from genetic variant APP Asn70, Leu671
Familial Creutzfeldt-Jakob disease, Gerstmann-Sträussler-Scheinker syndrome (hereditary spongiform encephalopathies, prion diseases)	Prion protein (PrP) derived from genetic variants of PrP precursor protein 51–91 insert, Leu102, Val117, Asn178, Lys200
Familial Mediterranean fever. Autosomal recessive	AA derived from SAA
Muckle-Wells syndrome of nephropathy, deafness, urticaria, limb pain	AA derived from SAA
Cardiomyopathy with persistent atrial standstill	Not yet characterised
Cutaneous deposits (bullous, papular, pustulodermal)	Not yet characterised

Different proteins form amyloid fibrils in the different types of amyloidosis but the ultrastructural morphology of the fibrils is always remarkably similar (Fig. 4). X-ray fibre diffraction reveals that all amyloid fibrils share a common core structure consisting of a β-sheet helix with the long axes of the β-strands lying perpendicular to the fibre long axis [14,15]. The degree of similarity is extraordinary given the great diversity of the protein precursors of amyloid fibrils, which do not share amino acid

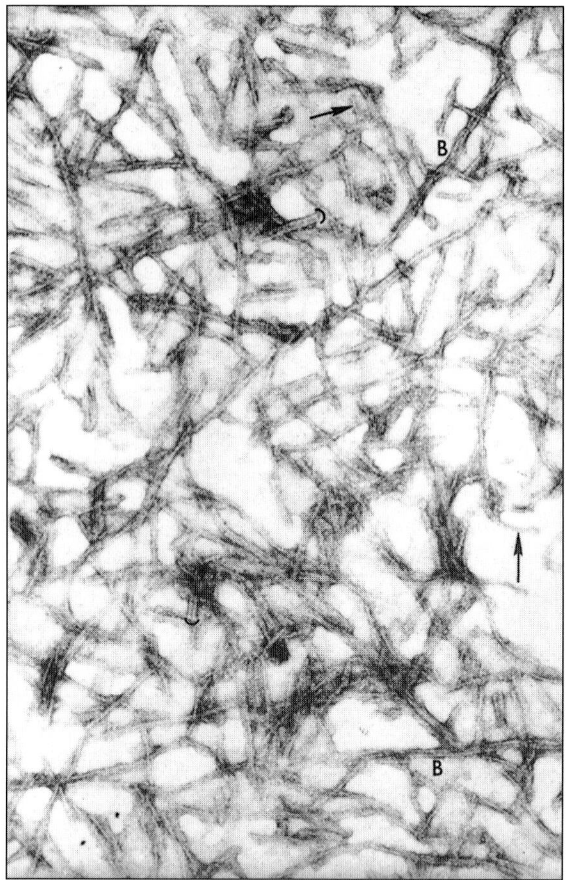

Fig. 4 Isolated purified amyloid fibrils negatively stained with phosphotungstic acid. Arrows point to single filaments. Most filaments are paired and end together (half circles). There are also some thicker bundles (B) in which filaments are twisting around each other (× 64,000). (From Franklin EC *et al.* [13] with permission of *Advances in Immunology*.)

sequence homology, subunit composition or tertiary fold. Amyloid fibrillogenesis thus involves dramatic unfolding of precursor proteins followed by refolding and stabilisation in the characteristic common cross-β fold.

□ INHIBITION OF FIBRILLOGENESIS AND THE LYSOZYME MODEL

Since amyloidogenesis of all different precursor proteins converges on such a similar final product, it is likely that the penultimate intermediates on the different refolding pathways may also be similar. The use of small molecule drugs to stabilise such late intermediates, thereby preventing formation of amyloid fibrils, is an attractive therapeutic strategy because a single agent could be applicable across the whole range of amyloid related diseases. The alternative approach of stabilising the native structures of the different precursors, to prevent the original unfolding, is also conceivable but would probably require different drugs for each type of amyloid and, in the case of monoclonal AL amyloid, possibly even for each patient. Unfortunately, although the high resolution crystal structures are known for several amyloid fibril precursor proteins, including β_2-microglobulin and transthyretin, there is little detailed information on their folding pathways. We were therefore very excited in 1993 to discover that lysozyme was the amyloid fibril protein in two kindreds under our care for autosomal dominant hereditary amyloidosis [16]. This is a rare syndrome in which the amyloid fibrils are derived in different families from different variant proteins usually encoded by point mutations. Our finding of lysozyme as a hereditary amyloid protein led to identification of the first two mutations to be described in the human lysozyme gene, but more importantly was of interest because both the native structure and folding pathways of lysozyme have been so exhaustively studied.

We expressed the two amyloidogenic lysozyme variants, Ile56Thr and Asp67His, *in vitro* and found that they were markedly less stable than wild type lysozyme [17]. Furthermore, they spontaneously aggregated and formed typical amyloid fibrils *in vitro*, as they do *in vivo*. Characterisation of the intermediates showed that they populated partly unfolded states in which amide groups lost the protection against deuterium exchange conferred by the mature fully folded structure. The main elements of secondary structure were retained although the tertiary fold was lost, and hydrophobic interactions were much enhanced. These are characteristics of so-called molten globule intermediates, and we presume that these tend to form intermolecular aggregates that stabilise a predominantly β-sheet amyloid fibril structure. Interestingly, it was also possible, using concentrated guanidine, a powerful chaotropic solvent, to dissolve otherwise insoluble, totally enzymatically inactive, *ex vivo* lysozyme amyloid fibrils, and then refold them to form native, fully enzymatically active lysozyme. Although this surprising demonstration of the remarkable plasticity of protein folding *in vitro* is not of direct therapeutic relevance, further analysis of the lysozyme model should assist future rational design and improvement of drugs capable of inhibiting fibrillogenesis.

□ TREATMENT AND PREVENTION OF AMYLOIDOSIS

Over the past 11 years we have developed and implemented the use of radiolabelled human SAP as a specific quantitative *in vivo* scintigraphic tracer for diagnosis and monitoring of systemic amyloidosis (Fig. 5) [18,19]. This safe, non-invasive procedure has been highly informative about the natural history and response to treatment of all forms of systemic amyloid, and has transformed our approach to management. In particular we have found that treatments that effectively suppress production of amyloid fibril precursor proteins halt the progressive accumulation of amyloid deposits and in many cases are associated with amyloid regression, improved organ function and survival (Fig. 6) [20]. Amyloid deposits are evidently turning over, their net size reflecting the balance of deposition and regression. The usual clinical impression of inexorable progression of amyloidosis actually reflects the progressive and usually incurable nature of the underlying primary conditions

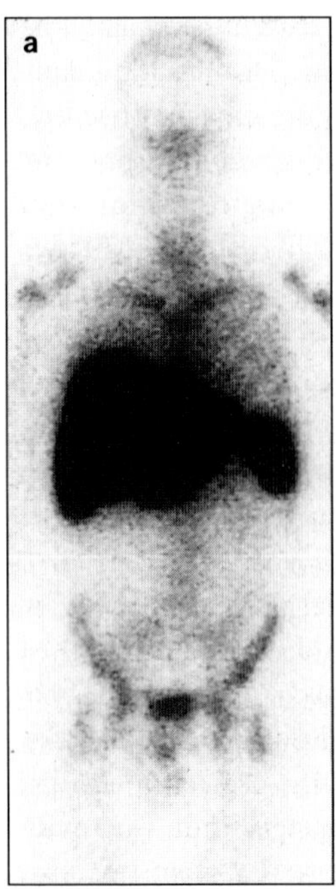

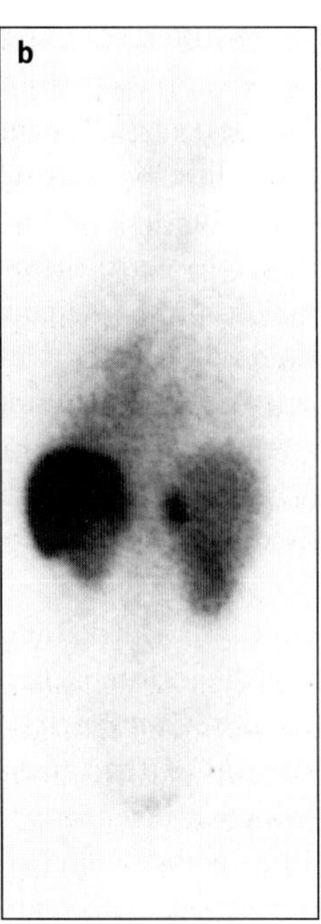

Fig. 5 ^{123}I-SAP scintigraphy in two young adults with systemic amyloidosis. **(a)** anterior whole body scan of a 26 year-old man showing uptake of tracer into substantial liver, spleen and bone marrow amyloid, a distribution diagnostic of systemic AL amyloidosis. **(b)** posterior whole body scan showing AA amyloid deposits in the spleen, adrenals and kidneys of a 34 year-old woman with rheumatoid arthritis.

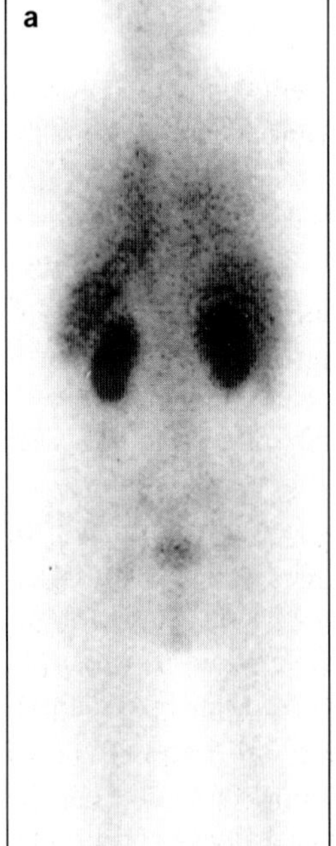

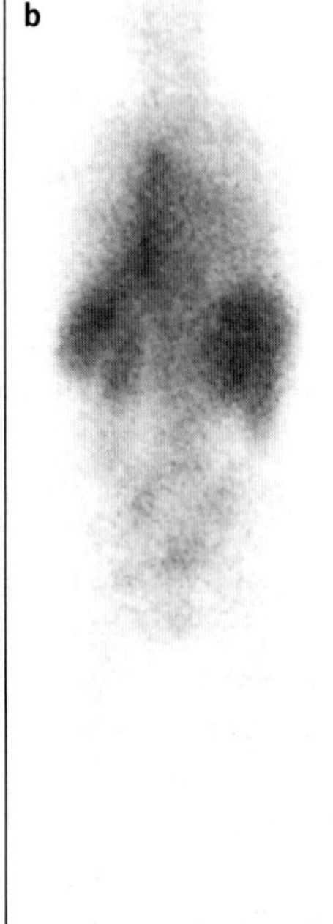

Fig. 6 Serial posterior whole body SAP scans in a man who presented with nephrotic syndrome and renal impairment due to systemic AL amyloidosis. The renal amyloid deposits visualised at presentation **(a)** had regressed substantially three years later **(b)** following 'VAD' chemotherapy associated with recovery of normal renal function. The other parts of the images represent the normal blood-pool background signal, the level of which is inversely proportional to the whole body load of amyloid.

that are complicated by amyloidosis. However, new and aggressive approaches to therapy, such as cytotoxic anti-inflammatory drugs in chronic rheumatic inflammation causing AA amyloid, radical chemotherapy including autologous stem cell transplantation for monoclonal gammopathy causing AL amyloid, and liver transplantation for hereditary transthyretin amyloid, all lead to impressive amyloid regression and prolonged survival. Unfortunately these treatments do not always work and there are many forms of amyloid in which such approaches are neither possible now nor likely to become feasible in future.

An alternative approach to therapy is the development of drugs to inhibit amyloid fibrillogenesis, as discussed above in relation to the lysozyme model, but no pharmaceutical products are yet available.

The third avenue involves strategies to promote regression of amyloid deposits. Although the mechanisms by which amyloid deposits are cleared are not known, they presumably involve degradation of the fibrils and associated molecules by macrophages and/or parenchymal cells. Our scintigraphic studies with radiolabelled SAP have shown unequivocally that amyloid deposits are cleared *in vivo* if the supply of fibril precursor proteins is suppressed, and isolated *ex vivo* amyloid fibrils are degradable *in vitro* by proteolytic enzymes and phagocytic cells. Thus, although the cross-β core structure of amyloid fibrils certainly is very stable, it is not indestructible, and a critical question about amyloidosis is why the deposits persist. Substantial extracellular matrix structures, including fibrous tissue, cartilage and bone, are rapidly remodelled during growth, development and wound healing. Why does this not happen with amyloid deposits composed exclusively of autologous macromolecules, albeit in an abnormal configuration?

□ THE SAP HYPOTHESIS

Our early work on circulating SAP levels in mice with experimental amyloidosis first indicated that SAP production might be related to pathogenesis of amyloidosis. Subsequently many strands of evidence have supported this idea, and especially the concept that SAP may contribute to persistence of amyloid fibrils *in vivo* [21]. When we originally identified the cyclic pyruvate acetal of galactose as a specific calcium dependent ligand for SAP, and showed that it could dissociate SAP out of amyloid deposits *in vitro*, we suggested that this might be an approach to therapy of amyloidosis [22].

SAP is universally present in amyloid deposits, bound to the fibrils (Fig. 7), and is identical to the circulating protein. Although it remains in dynamic equilibrium with the blood and extravascular fluid pool, SAP persists for prolonged periods in amyloid, compared with its rapid turnover in the plasma, and it is not catabolised until it returns to the blood. This may reflect the fact that SAP is taken up and catabolised only by hepatocytes. Also, under physiological conditions SAP itself is extremely resistant to proteolysis. I have therefore proposed that binding of SAP must stabilise amyloid fibrils, first on thermodynamic grounds as a simple result of binding itself. Second, coating with autologous unaltered SAP is likely to mask the abnormal protein conformation of the fibrils. Third, the proteinase resistance of SAP

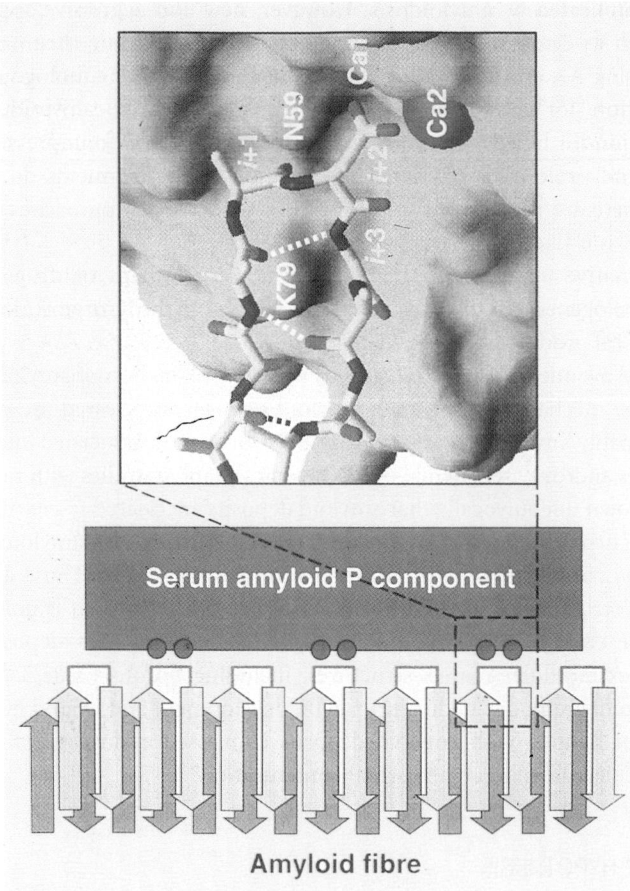

Fig. 7 Model of binding of SAP to the common cross-β core structure of amyloid fibrils, as predicted by Pepys [21]. Above: docking of a single type I G-bulged β-turn with an aspartic residue in position i+2, represented as a ball and stick model, into the calcium-dependent SAP ligand binding site, displayed as a GRASP representation. Below: diagram of face-on binding of SAP oligomer to multiple β-turns along the length of an amyloid fibril. (Courtesy of E Hohenester.)

may further protect the fibrils from degradation. Finally, in both the mouse and the Syrian hamster models of experimental AA amyloidosis, there is an excellent correlation between SAP production and development of amyloid.

More recently we have shown that binding of SAP to amyloid fibrils *in vitro* does indeed protect them from proteolytic digestion by macrophages and even by aggressive mammalian digestive or microbial proteinases [23]. Furthermore, in mice with targeted deletion of the SAP gene and therefore complete deficiency of SAP, the deposition of experimental AA amyloid is delayed and reduced in quantity [24]. Amyloid does eventually form in the SAP knockout mice, but this is not surprising as amyloid fibrils can be produced *in vitro* from their pure precursor proteins and there is no evidence that SAP or any other additional molecule is required for amyloid fibrillogenesis. Nevertheless our findings in SAP deficient mice powerfully support our therapeutic strategy of seeking compounds capable of inhibiting binding of SAP to amyloid fibrils *in vivo*, and of dissociating SAP that is already bound. The SAP hypothesis predicts that such treatment should accelerate regression of amyloid deposits, and the increment may not need to be very great for the balance between deposition and clearance of amyloid to be favourably shifted toward regression.

In collaboration with F Hoffmann-La Roche Ltd we have identified and developed compounds that inhibit SAP-fibril binding *in vitro* and *in vivo*. Infusion of these compounds completely dissociates SAP from the amyloid deposits (Figs 8, 9). It is not technically feasible to assess amyloid regression in this mouse model, but preparations are proceeding for trials of the lead compound in man early in 1999.

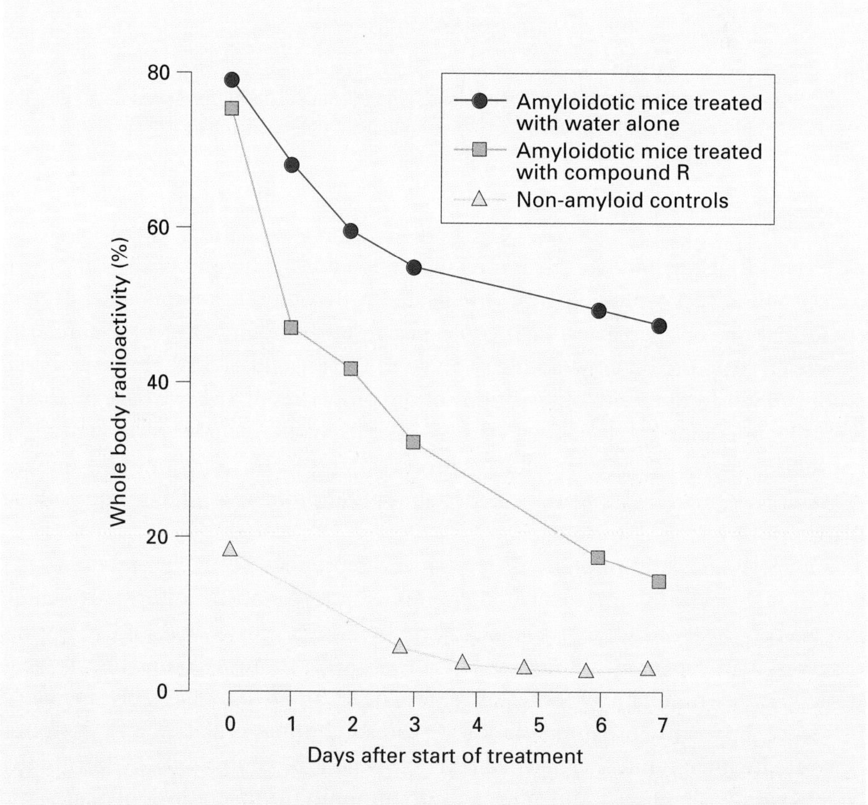

Fig. 8 Effect *in vivo* of Roche SAP inhibitor on retention of ^{125}I-human SAP tracer in mouse AA amyloid deposits. All mice received the same tracer dose 24 hours before starting treatment, in order to load their deposits with labelled SAP. Control non-amyloid mice retained little tracer and rapidly cleared it completely. Amyloidotic mice retained about 80% of the injected dose and in those treated with water alone the whole body clearance had a half-time of about three days. Mice receiving compound R cleared the tracer much more rapidly, approaching background levels by seven days.

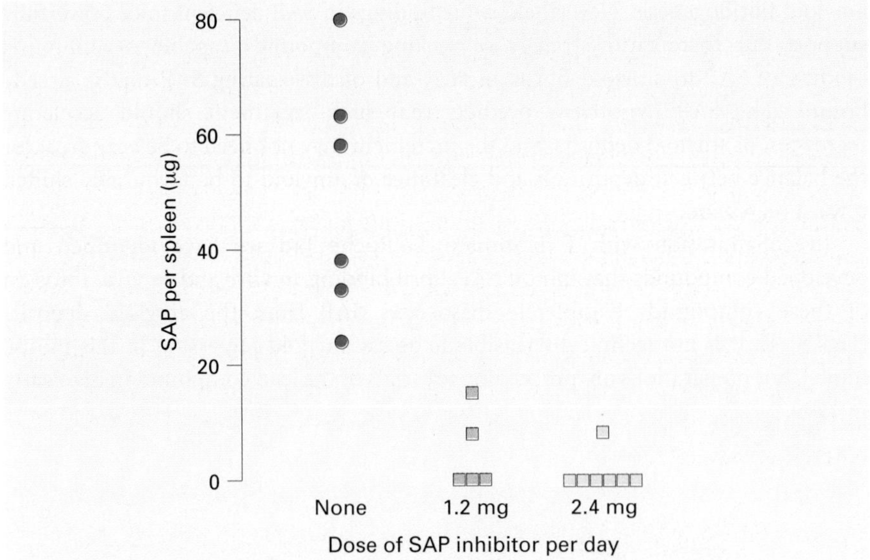

Fig. 9 Effect of Roche SAP inhibitor on mouse SAP in splenic amyloid deposits. Mice with AA amyloidosis received compound R or water alone by continuous infusion for seven days, and the SAP content of their spleens was then measured. Each point represents an individual animal.

□ NORMAL FUNCTIONS OF SAP

Involvement in amyloidogenesis is obviously not a normal function of SAP. It might conceivably reflect a physiological role related to recognition of abnormal protein conformations or aggregates, or it could just result from an 'accidental' similarity between a structure on amyloid fibrils and a normal ligand of SAP. However, based on our *in vitro* and *ex vivo* observations of the properties of SAP, we have predicted that the physiological functions of SAP are likely to include participation in appropriate handling of extracellular chromatin and DNA, contributing to innate resistance to microbial infection, and stabilisation/protection of the extracellular matrices of which SAP forms a part.

Our SAP knockout mice grow, develop and reproduce normally, and deficiency of SAP is thus clearly not a lethal defect. This model cannot be informative about functions of SAP in the extracellular matrix because SAP is only found in normal tissues in man. However, among a cohort of 113 SAP –/– mice, comprising approximately equal numbers of both sexes, we have found a remarkably increased incidence and titre of autoantibodies against chromatin, DNA and histones, compared with age and sex matched SAP +/+ wild type controls. The control mice spontaneously developed anti-nuclear autoimmunity in up to 28% of males and 54% of females by eight months, and immune complex glomerulonephritis in 2% of males and 9% of females. However, the incidence and titre of autoantibodies to all the antigens tested was much greater ($p < 0.0001$) in the SAP –/– animals, reaching 65% in males and 82% in females. Furthermore, glomerulonephritis was present in 4% of males and a remarkable 42% of females ($p < 0.01$ compared with wild type).

In contrast there were no tissue specific or non-chromatin anti-nuclear autoantibodies in any mice, indicating no global breakdown in tolerance.

There is a genetic and female sex predisposition to systemic lupus erythematosus (SLE) in man and the mouse, as seen in the 129sv x C57Bl/6 background we have studied so far. However, the dramatically higher incidence of immune complex glomerulonephritis associated with higher incidence and titres of autoantibodies to chromatin, DNA and histones in SAP –/– mice demonstrates that SAP has an important normal function in handling chromatin *in vivo*, preventing autoimmunisation and its pathological consequences.

SAP seems also to contribute to host defence against infection. For example, intraperitoneal infection with a dose of *Salmonella typhimurium* that killed 60% of wild type SAP +/+ mice by day 13 was fatal by day 7 in 90% of age and sex matched SAP deficient animals. Work to elucidate the involvement and mode of action of SAP in this and other infections is actively in progress, together with further studies of the SAP-chromatin interaction.

□ NORMAL FUNCTIONS OF CRP

There is good experimental evidence that CRP contributes to defence against infections caused by micro-organisms to which it can bind. In addition, CRP is likely to participate in the handling *in vivo* of autologous cellular and tissue constituents to which it binds. For example, although human CRP does not bind to chromatin under physiological conditions, it does bind specifically to small nuclear ribonucleoproteins. Antibodies to these particles cross-react with DNA, and they may be important autoantigens in human SLE. The acute phase response of CRP to disease flares is defective in SLE, and it is therefore possible that CRP may function to prevent autoimmunisation in man, in a manner similar to that shown for SAP in the mouse knockout model. The capacity of CRP to bind platelet activating factor and to down-regulate polymorph infiltration suggests that it may also serve as a modulator of inflammation.

□ CRP AS A MEDIATOR OF PATHOGENESIS

Injection of C-polysaccharide into the skin of individuals with high levels of circulating CRP elicits erythema, oedema and induration, resembling immune complex lesions. Serum CRP concentrations generally correspond closely to the extent and activity of inflammation and tissue damage in diseases associated with an acute phase response. Since CRP can bind to many ligands exposed in damaged cells, and can then activate complement, it is likely that in some circumstances CRP may enhance tissue damage. CRP may also promote coagulation through its capacity to stimulate tissue factor production.

□ CRP AND ATHEROTHROMBOSIS

A striking predictive association has lately emerged between serum CRP values and subsequent coronary events. This was first noted in patients admitted to hospital with severe unstable angina [25] and in outpatients with both stable and unstable angina [26], but the association holds as well for completely asymptomatic individuals [27,28]. Individuals in the top quintile of the CRP distribution have a two to five fold increased risk of a future coronary event. Similar associations seem to hold for cerebrovascular and peripheral vascular disease [29]. These remarkable observations clearly show a relationship between inflammation and thrombotic complications of atherosclerosis, though the acute phase responses involved are very modest, and the CRP values largely fall within the range previously considered normal. Perhaps the increased CRP production simply reflects the inflammatory nature of atherosclerosis itself and its extent. Alternatively, CRP synthesis may be stimulated by intercurrent low grade infections which are known to be risk factors for atherothrombosis. Whatever the stimuli, it is intriguing to consider whether CRP itself might contribute to atherogenesis, via its interaction with low density lipoprotein, and to clotting, via its stimulation of tissue factor production. For example, it has long been recognised that a substantial proportion of myocardial infarctions are immediately preceded by acute infections or other disorders likely to be associated with an acute phase response [30]. Furthermore, once myocardial infarction has occurred, CRP production is maximally stimulated, CRP is deposited in the damaged tissue and may then enhance inflammation and lesion size, especially by activating complement. Indeed, there is a significant association between the peak serum CRP concentration after myocardial infarction and short- and long-term prognosis [31,32].

□ PROTEINS TO DRUGS

I have discussed several strands of investigation of protein structure and function that suggest possible new avenues for therapeutic drug intervention in important diseases.

Inhibitors of the protein misfolding that underlies amyloid fibrillogenesis could control systemic amyloidosis and conceivably contribute to management of disorders associated with local amyloid deposition, including Alzheimer's disease and type II diabetes.

The pentraxins, CRP and SAP, are phylogenetically ancient and highly conserved proteins which are invariant in man and for which no deficiency states have yet been described. This strongly suggests that they have very important normal functions of sufficient survival value to have persisted in evolution. In the case of SAP we have now demonstrated such functions: chromatin binding to prevent autoimmunisation and a role in host defence against bacterial infection. In the case of CRP there is good evidence for a role in host defence against bacteria, and presumptive evidence of beneficial functions with respect to autologous ligands. However, evolution, driven by natural selection, is 'blind' to the fate of individuals after they have reproduced. There is therefore no reason why molecules, processes or functions that are of survival value up to the reproductive age may not have significant adverse effects later in life. SAP definitely contributes to the pathogenesis of amyloidosis and is an attractive target for drug therapy, the potential efficacy of which we shall soon be able to assess directly. Increased CRP production predicts myocardial infarction and other atherothrombotic events, and may enhance both ischaemic and non-ischaemic tissue damage across the whole spectrum of diseases characterised by major acute phase responses. Compounds able to block binding by CRP to its various autologous ligands may thus have wide-ranging applications. Availability of the crystallographic structures of CRP and its specific ligand complex should assist design of such drugs.

ACKNOWLEDGEMENTS

I thank my past and present colleagues in the Immunological Medicine Unit of the former Royal Postgraduate Medical School, now Imperial College School of Medicine, for their scientific excellence and industry, and our many collaborators especially in Birkbeck College London, Cambridge, Oxford, Rome and Basel, as well as at the Hammersmith. The work described here would not have been possible without their many essential contributions. I also gratefully acknowledge the generous financial support of the Medical Research Council, the Wellcome Trust, the Arthritis and Rheumatism Council, the Maurice Wohl Charitable Foundation and F Hoffmann-La Roche Ltd. Finally, I thank Professor Martin Goodman for the expert translation of the sixteenth century Latin of *Munk's Roll.*

REFERENCES

1 Pepys MB, Baltz ML. Acute phase proteins with special reference to C-reactive protein and related proteins (pentaxins) and serum amyloid A protein. *Adv Immunol* 1983; **34**: 141–212.

2 Pepys MB, Dash AC. Isolation of amyloid P component (protein AP) from normal serum as a calcium-dependent binding protein. *Lancet* 1977; **i**: 1029–31.

3 Emsley J, White HE, O'Hara BP, *et al.* Structure of pentameric human serum amyloid P component. *Nature* 1994; **367**: 338–45.

4 Shrive AK, Cheetham GMT, Holden D, *et al.* Three-dimensional structure of human C-reactive protein. *Nature Struct Biol* 1996; **3**: 346–54.

5 Thompson D, Pepys MB, Wood SP. The physiological structure of human C-reactive protein and its complex with phosphocholine. *Structure* 1999; **7**: 169–77.

6 Hutchinson WL, Noble GE, Hawkins PN, Pepys MB. The pentraxins, C-reactive protein and serum amyloid P component, are cleared and catabolised by hepatocytes *in vivo*. *J Clin Invest* 1994; **94**: 1390–6.

7 Vigushin DM, Pepys MB, Hawkins PN. Metabolic and scintigraphic studies of radioiodinated human C-reactive protein in health and disease. *J Clin Invest* 1993; **91**: 1351–7.

8 Yother J, Volanakis JE, Briles DE. Human C-reactive protein is protective against fatal *Streptococcus pneumoniae* infection in mice. *J Immunol* 1982; **128**: 2374–6.

9 Pepys MB, Rowe IF, Baltz ML. C-reactive protein: binding to lipids and lipoproteins. *Int Rev Exp Pathol* 1985; **27**: 83–111.

10 Pepys MB, Booth DR, Hutchinson WL, *et al.* Amyloid P component: a critical review. *Amyloid: Int J Exp Clin Invest* 1997; **4**: 274–95.

11 Butler PJG, Tennent GA, Pepys MB. Pentraxin-chromatin interactions: serum amyloid P component specifically displaces H1-type histones and solubilizes native long chromatin. *J Exp Med* 1990; **172**: 13–18.

12 Tan SY, Pepys MB. Amyloidosis. *Histopathology* 1994; **25**: 403–14.

13 Franklin EC, Zucker-Franklin D. Current concepts of amyloid. *Adv Immunol* 1972; **15**: 249.

14 Eanes ED, Glenner GG. X-ray diffraction studies on amyloid filaments. *J Histochem Cytochem* 1968; **16**: 673–7.

15 Sunde M, Serpell LC, Bartlam M, *et al.* Common core structure of amyloid fibrils by synchrotron X-ray diffraction. *J Mol Biol* 1997; **273**: 729–39.

16 Pepys MB, Hawkins PN, Booth DR, *et al.* Human lysozyme gene mutations cause hereditary systemic amyloidosis. *Nature* 1993; **362**: 553–7.

17 Booth DR, Sunde M, Bellotti V, *et al.* Instability, unfolding and aggregation of human lysozyme variants underlying amyloid fibrillogenesis. *Nature* 1997; **385**: 787–93.

18 Hawkins PN, Myers MJ, Lavender JP, Pepys MB. Diagnostic radionuclide imaging of amyloid: biological targeting by circulating human serum amyloid P component. *Lancet* 1988; **i**: 1413–18.

19 Hawkins PN, Pepys MB. Imaging amyloidosis with radiolabelled SAP. *Eur J Nucl Med* 1995; **22**: 595–9.

20 Hawkins PN. The diagnosis, natural history and treatment of amyloidosis. The Goulstonian Lecture 1995. *J R Coll Physicians Lond* 1997; **31**: 552–60.

21 Pepys MB. Amyloid P component: structure and properties. In: Marrink J, van Rijswijk MH (Eds). *Amyloidosis.* Dordrecht: Martinus Nijhoff, 1986: 43–50.

22 Hind CRK, Collins PM, Caspi D, Baltz ML, Pepys MB. Specific chemical dissociation of fibrillar and non-fibrillar components of amyloid deposits. *Lancet* 1984; **ii**: 376–8.

23 Tennent GA, Lovat LB, Pepys MB. Serum amyloid P component prevents proteolysis of the amyloid fibrils of Alzheimer's disease and systemic amyloidosis. *Proc Natl Acad Sci USA* 1995; **92**: 4299–303.

24 Botto M, Hawkins PN, Bickerstaff MCM, *et al.* Amyloid deposition is delayed in mice with targeted deletion of the serum amyloid P component gene. *Nature Med* 1997; **3**: 855–9.

25 Liuzzo G, Biasucci LM, Gallimore JR, *et al.* The prognostic value of C-reactive protein and serum amyloid A protein in severe unstable angina. *N Engl J Med* 1994; **331**: 417–24.

26 Haverkate F, Thompson SG, Pyke SDM, Gallimore JR, Pepys MB. Production of C-reactive protein and risk of coronary events in stable and unstable angina. *Lancet* 1997; **349**: 462–6.

27 Kuller LH, Tracy RP, Shaten J, Meilahn EN. Relation of C-reactive protein and coronary heart disease in the MRFIT nested case control study. *Am J Epidemiol* 1996; **144**: 537–47.

28 Ridker PM, Cushman M, Stampfer MH, *et al.* Inflammation, aspirin, and the risk of cardiovascular disease in apparently healthy men. *N Engl J Med* 1997; **336**: 973–9.

29 Ridker PM, Cushman M, Stampfer MJ, *et al.* Plasma concentration of C-reactive protein and risk of developing peripheral vascular disease. *Circulation* 1998; **97**: 425–8.

30 Spodick DH. Inflammation and the onset of myocardial infarction. *Ann Intern Med* 1985; **102**: 699–702.

31 Pietilä KO, Harmoinen AP, Jokiniitty J, Pasternack AI. Serum C-reactive protein concentration in acute myocardial infarction and its relationship to mortality during 24 months of follow-up in patients under thrombolytic treatment. *Eur Heart J* 1996; **17**: 1345–9.

32 Ueda S, Ikeda U, Yamamoto K, *et al.* C-reactive protein as a predictor of cardiac rupture after acute myocardial infarction. *Am Heart J* 1996; **131**: 857–60.

Prion diseases of man and other species

Glenn C Telling

☐ INTRODUCTION

The prion diseases, otherwise referred to as transmissible spongiform encephalopathies (TSEs), are transmissible neurodegenerative diseases of the central nervous system (CNS). They include bovine spongiform encephalopathy (BSE), scrapie of sheep and goats, and kuru and Creutzfeldt-Jakob disease (CJD) in humans (Table 1). Because they are transmissible, it was previously believed that these diseases were caused by viruses or unconventional infectious agents containing a nucleic acid genome. Indeed, until relatively recently, they were classified as 'slow viral infections'. However, the infectious agent is unusual in that, unlike conventional pathogens, it is extremely resistant to treatments that modify or destroy nucleic acids, notably high temperatures, formaldehyde treatment and ultraviolet radiation. The prevailing view now endorses the previously heretical notion that these diseases are caused by subcellular pathogens called 'prions', which are defined as small proteinaceous infectious particles, which survive procedures that modify nucleic acids [1]. In recent years, the prion diseases have taken centre stage in public awareness, initially because of the emergence of BSE which was first diagnosed in April 1985 and subsequently reached epidemic proportions in the UK (Fig. 1). The epidemic affected more than 170,000 cattle and reached a peak in the early 1990s, with an annual incidence of almost 40,000 cases (~1% of all cows in the UK); numbers of affected animals now appear to be declining, following a comprehensive cull of all cattle over 30 months and prohibition of the previously widespread practice of feeding cattle with bovine offal supplements.

At the same time, human prion diseases acquired prominence. First, rare cases of CJD were identified in people who had been treated with human cadaveric products derived from CNS (growth hormone and dura mater grafts). Second, and more alarming, several cases of a CJD-like neurodegenerative disease were reported in patients who were decades younger than the usual age of onset of CJD. It was suspected that this 'new variant' CJD (vCJD) was caused by exposure to BSE through eating contaminated meat products, and there is now convincing evidence that vCJD is due to the interspecies transmission of the infectious agent that causes BSE in cattle.

These issues highlight the crucial importance of understanding how prions replicate, as well as the factors determining prion strains and the barriers that limit their transmission to other species. These properties are beginning to be elucidated by studies with transgenic mice which have provided crucial information about the key role of the primary structure of the prion protein (PrP) and the conformation of its infectious isoform (PrP^{Sc}).

Table 1 The animal and human prion diseases (transmission spongiform encephalopathies).

Animal Prion Diseases

Disease	**Host**	**Aetiology**
Scrapie	Sheep and goats	Thought to involve both horizontal and vertical transmission
Transmissible mink encephalopathy	Captive mink	Probably food-borne, though the origin of infectious prions is uncertain
Chronic wasting disease	Captive and free-ranging mule deer and Rocky Mountain elk	Possibly food-borne, though there is evidence for horizontal transmission
Bovine spongiform encephalopathy	Cattle	Food-borne in the form of contaminated meat and bone meal
Feline spongiform encephalopathy	Domestic and zoo cats (eg cheetah)	BSE contaminated feed
Exotic ungulate encephalopathy	Captive bovidae (eg nyala)	BSE contaminated feed

Human Prion Diseases

Disease	**Incidence**	**Aetiology**	**Age of onset/incubation period and duration of illness**
Sporadic CJD	One per million population	Unknown but hypotheses include somatic mutation or spontaneous conversion of PrP^{C} into PrP^{Sc}	Age of onset is usually in the 45–75 year age group with peak onset between 60–65. 70% of cases die in under 6 months
Familial CJD, GSS, FFI	10–20% of human prion disease cases	Autosomal dominant *PRNP* mutation	Average age of onset for GSS is 45 years with a 5-year mean duration of illness
Kuru (1957–1982)	>2500 cases among the Fore in Papua New Guinea	Infection through ritualistic cannibalism	Incubation periods range from 60 to 360 months with duration of illness between 3 and 12 months
Iatrogenic CJD	About 80 cases to date	Infection from contaminated human growth hormone, HGH human gonadotrophin, depth electrodes, corneal transplants, dura mater grafts, neurosurgical procedures	Incubation periods of HGH cases range from 4 to 30 years with a duration of illness between 6 and 18 months
New Variant CJD	>30 young adults in the UK and France	Infection by BSE prions	Mean age of onset is 26 years with a mean duration of illness of 14 months

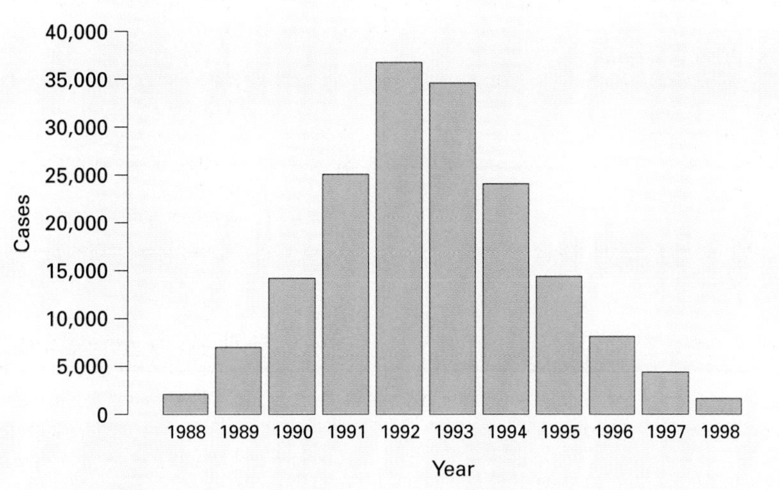

Fig. 1 Annual incidence of confirmed cases of BSE. Bovine spongiform encephalopathy (BSE), often referred to as 'mad cow disease' was first diagnosed in April 1985. The epidemic, which has affected over 170,000 cattle in the UK, reached its peak in 1992 when over 1000 cases a week were diagnosed. The average incubation period of BSE is 5 years, and only very rarely do animals under 3 years of age display symptoms. This suggests that cattle in Great Britain first became infected in the early 1980s. It has been estimated that up to 1 million cattle were infected with BSE. Epidemiological studies point to contaminated offal, used in the manufacture of meat and bone meal (MBM) and fed to cattle, as the source of prions responsible for BSE. In July 1988 a ban on feeding ruminant-derived protein to ruminants was introduced to break the cycle of infection via feed. Since then the number of cases has decreased and there are now around 100 new BSE suspect cases a week. The specified bovine offals (SBO) ban was introduced in the UK in 1989 to prevent inclusion in the human food chain of bovine tissues thought to contain the highest titre of prions. These included tissues from the lymphoreticular system (LRS) and the CNS, namely brain, spinal cord, tonsil, thymus, spleen and intestine.

□ NEUROPATHOLOGICAL FEATURES OF PRION DISEASES

The prion diseases share a number of characteristic clinical and neuropathological features. All these diseases have long incubation times, ranging from months to years, and there is no well defined response to infection by the immune system. The brains of patients or animals with prion diseases frequently show no obvious macroscopic damage, but microscopic examination of the CNS reveals typical neuropathological abnormalities, notably:

- Neuronal degeneration and neuronal loss, giving the grey matter a microvacuolated or 'spongiform' appearance (Fig. 2)
- Severe astrocytic gliosis, which is often out of proportion to the degree of nerve cell loss
- Deposition of amyloid in plaques, although an inconstant feature, occurs in some examples of prion disease such as kuru and vCJD (Fig. 2).

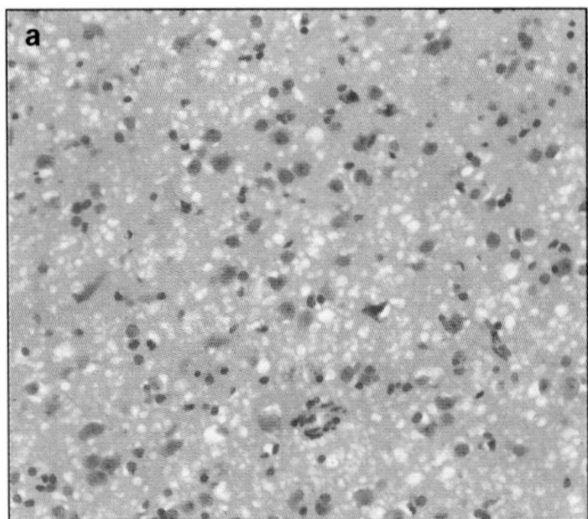

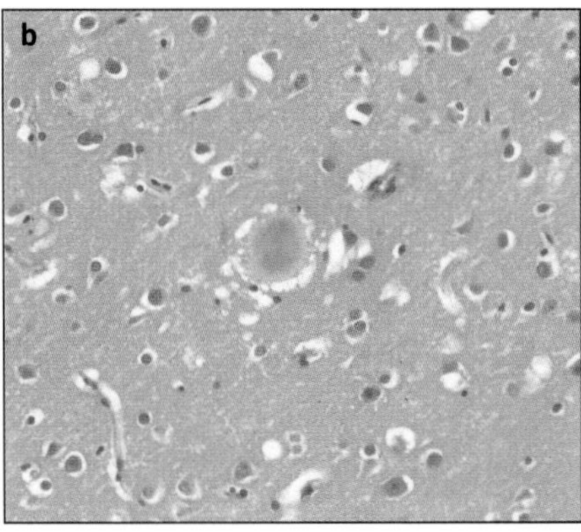

Fig. 2 (a) Frontal cortex from a 65 year old male with sporadic CJD showing widespread spongiform change with numerous small vacuoles in the grey matter. There is also extensive neuronal loss and astrocytosis. **(b)** Frontal cortex from a 27 year old female with new variant CJD, showing a characteristic florid plaque (centre) composed of a central amyloid core surrounded by a halo of spongiform change. The grey matter elsewhere shows only patchy spongiform change, and neuronal loss and astrocytosis are less pronounced than in (a). (Haematoxylin and Eosin stains. Figures courtesy of Dr James Ironside.)

□ THE PRION HYPOTHESIS

The unifying hallmark of the prion diseases is the involvement of the prion protein (PrP), which exists in at least two conformational states that have markedly different physicochemical properties. PrP is a sialoglycoprotein expressed in a number of tissues including brain, lung, heart, kidney and spleen. The normal form of the protein is found in the brains of both infected and uninfected animals, which is sensitive to protease treatment and soluble in detergents; it is referred to as PrP^{C}. PrP^{C} is attached to the external cell surface by a glycosyl-phosphatidylinositol (GPI) anchor. By contrast, the disease-associated isoform, PrP^{Sc}, is found only in the brains of infected animals and is partly resistant to protease treatment and insoluble in detergents. Protease cleavage of the N-terminal 66 or so amino acids of PrP^{Sc} yields a protease-resistant core referred to as PrP27–30. The structure of murine PrP is shown in Figs 3 and 4.

While the precise molecular structure of the prion still eludes definitive characterisation, considerable evidence argues that prions are composed of infectious PrP^{Sc} molecules and that prions propagate by PrP^{Sc} coercing PrP^{C} to adopt the infectivity-associated conformation (see Fig. 5) [4]. This model is supported by structural studies which show that PrP^{C} has a high α-helical content and is virtually devoid of the β-sheet structure, whereas PrP^{Sc} has a high β-sheet content [5]. Nuclear magnetic resonance (NMR) spectroscopy has been used to characterise the three-dimensional structures of recombinant mouse PrP (residues 121–231) [6] and Syrian hamster PrP (residues 29–231) [7]. These studies show that the C-terminal portion is globular and consists of three α-helices (designated H1, H2 and H3) separated by two short sections which form a β-pleated sheet, while the N-terminal region is largely unstructured (see Fig. 4).

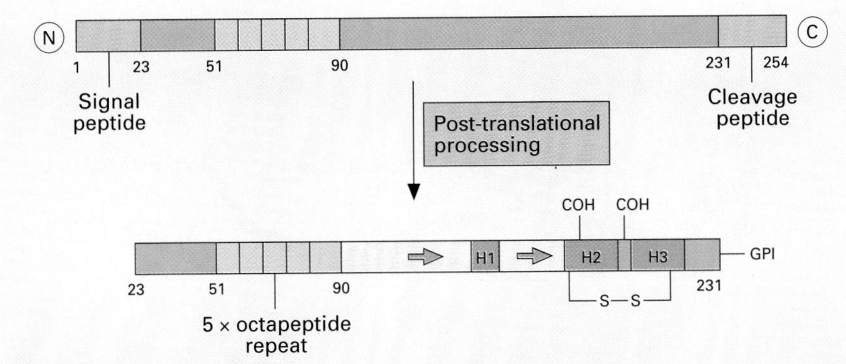

Fig. 3 Structural features of the prion protein. The mouse PrP gene encodes a 254 amino acid residue translation product which is processed by removal of an amino-terminal signal peptide of 22 amino acids and a carboxy-terminal hydrophobic peptide of 23 amino acids, both shown in blue. After cleavage of the carboxy terminal peptide a glycosylphosphatidylinositol (GPI) anchor is added. The three α-helices (designated H1, H2 and H3 or A, B and C) and two short sections forming a β-pleated sheet (represented as arrows) which have been identified by NMR spectroscopy of recombinant PrP are shown in yellow. In recombinant mouse PrP, H1 extends from amino acid residue 143 to amino acid residue 153, H2 from residue 175 to residue 192, and H3 from residue 199 to residue 218, while the two regions making up the β-pleated sheet extend from residues 127 to 130 and residues 160 to 163 (mouse PrP numbering). The amino-terminal portion of the molecule appears to be largely unstructured and contains a tandem array of 5 octapeptide repeats between codons 51 and 90 which are represented by black boxes. Asn-linked oligosaccharides are attached at residues 180 and 196 and H2 and H3 are connected by a disulphide bond that joins codons 178 and 213. Protease cleavage of the amino-terminal 66, or so, amino acides of PrP^{Sc} gives rise to a protease-resistant core represented by PrP27–30 which is shown in grey.

□ PATHOGENESIS

While detection of PrP^{Sc} in brain material by immunohistochemical or immunoblotting techniques is considered to be diagonistic of prion disease, certain examples of natural and experimental prion disease occur without accumulation of detectable protease resistant PrP^{Sc} and the time course of neurodegeneration is not equivalent to the time course of PrP^{Sc} accumulation in mice expressing lower than normal levels of PrP^{C} [8]. Moreover, PrP^{Sc} is not toxic to cells that do not express PrP^{C} [9]. Thus, it appears that accumulation of PrP^{Sc} may not be the sole cause of pathology in prion diseases. An alternative mechanism of PrP-induced neuronal degeneration has been suggested from recent studies of mutant forms of PrP that disrupt the regulation of PrP biogenesis in the endoplasmic reticulum [10].

As PrP^{C} is the source of PrP^{Sc}, this model predicts that elimination of PrP^{C} would abolish prion replication. To test this hypothesis, PrP 'knockout' mice were generated by disrupting the *Prnp* locus through homologous recombination in embryonic stem cells [11]. The homozygous ($Prnp^{0/0}$) knockout mice fail to express PrP^{C}. These mice do not develop the characteristic clinical and neuropathological symptoms of scrapie after inoculation with mouse prions, and do not propagate infectivity [12].

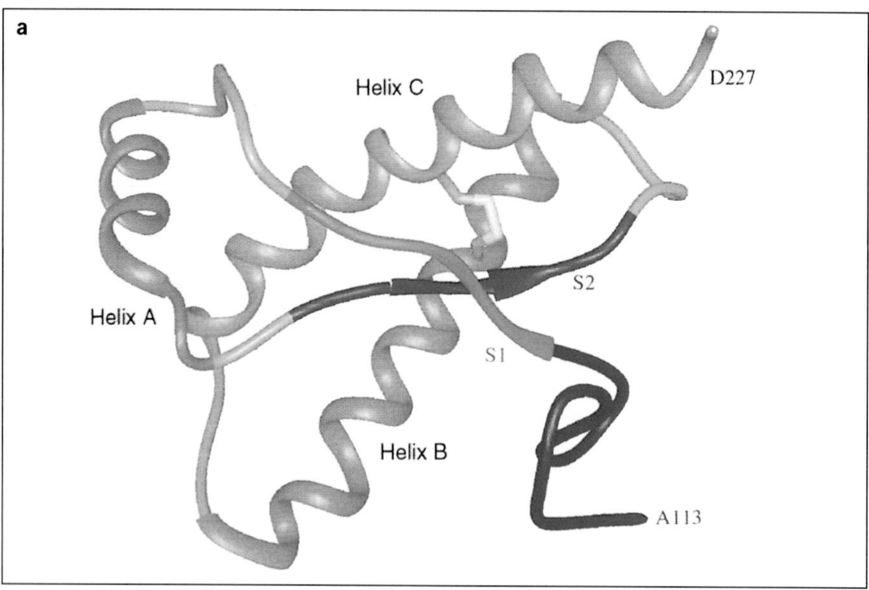

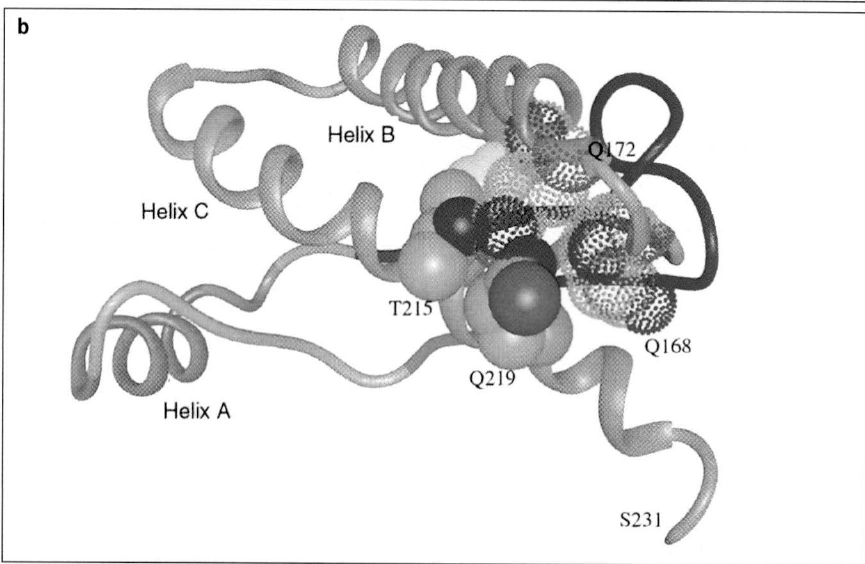

Fig. 4 (a) NMR Structure of Syrian hamster (SHa) recombinant (r). Presumably, the structure of the ∝ helical form of rPrP(90–231) resembles that of PrP^c. rPrP(90–231) is viewed from the interface where PrP^{Sc} is thought to bind to PrP^c. Colour scheme ∝ helices A (residues 144–157), B (172–193), and C (200–227). In pink: disulphide between cys-179 and Cys-214 in yellow; conserved hydrophobic region composed of residues 113–126 in red; loops in grey; residues 129–134 in green encompassing strand S1 and residues 159–166 in blue encompassing strand S2; the arrows span residues 129–131 and 161–163 as these show a clear resemblance to β sheets [2]. **(b)** NMR structure of rPrP(90–231) is viewed from the interface where protein X is thought to bind to PrPc. Protein X appears to bind to the side chains of residues that form a discontinuous epitope: some amino acids are in the loop composed of residues 165–171 and at the end of helix β (Gln-168 and Gln-172 with a low density van der Waals rendering) while others are on the surface of helix C (Thr-215 and Gln-219 with a high density van der Waals rendering) [3]. (Figures courtesy of Professor Stanley Prusiner. Reproduced by permission of National Academy of Sciences USA. ©1997.)

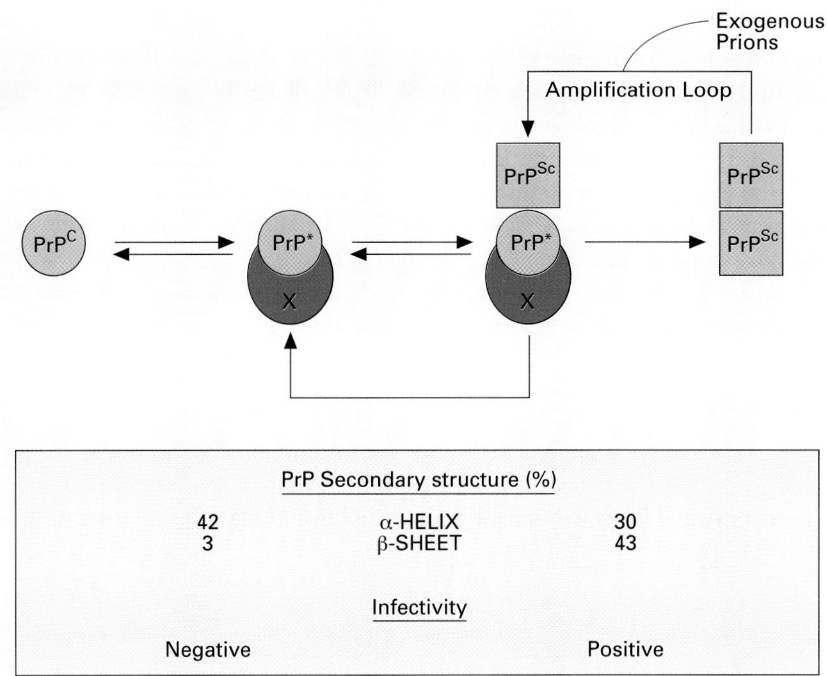

Fig. 5 Prion replication. The prion protein (PrP) exists in at least two different conformational states: PrP^{C} which has a high content of α-helix and PrP^{Sc} which is rich in β-pleated sheet. It has been suggested that PrP^{C} exists in equilibrium with PrP* [4] that is bound to an ancillary factor, referred to as 'protein X' [39]. In the 'protein only' model of prion replication, the PrP*-protein X complex interacts with PrP^{Sc} which unduces a conformational change in PrP*. The end result is two molecules of PrP with the infectious PrP^{Sc} conformation which are free to induce conformational changes in additional PrP* molecules during the infectious cycle.

□ ROLE OF PrP^{C} FROM GENE-TARGETED MICE

Gene targeted *Prnp*$^{0/0}$ mice have also been studied to probe the normal function of PrP^{C}. Two independently generated lines of gene-targeted *Prnp*$^{0/0}$ developed normally and appeared to suffer no gross phenotypic abnormalities [11,13]. The relative normality of these PrP null mice could result from effective adaptive changes during development. However, cerebellar Purkinje cell degeneration has been reported in a third line of *Prnp*$^{0/0}$ mice [14] and several other phenotypic defects are being investigated in *Prnp*$^{0/0}$ mice including altered circadian rhythms and sleep patterns [15], alterations in superoxide dismutase activity (SOD-1) [16] and defects in copper metabolism [17]. Electrophysiological studies demonstrated that $GABA_{A}$ receptor-mediated inhibition and long-term potentiation were impaired in hippocampal slices from *Prnp*$^{0/0}$ mice [18,19] and calcium-activated potassium currents were disrupted [20]. These abnormalities of synaptic inhibition are reminiscent of the neurophysiological defects seen in patients with CJD and scrapie infected mice [18].

☐ HUMAN PRION DISEASES

The majority of cases of human prion disease occur sporadically as CJD, but approximately 10–20% of cases occur in families and display an autosomal dominant mode of inheritance. The epidemiological and clinical features of these diseases are summarised in Table 2. From this it is apparent that there is considerable variation, in both the extent and the nature of CNS involvement, and particularly in the neurological manifestations. Detailed clinical and pathological descriptions are beyond the scope of this chapter, and are referenced in the recent review by Haywood [21]. However, the example of new variant CJD merits discussion, because it illustrates important aetiolgoical principles that apply to human prion diseases.

New variant CJD

While all forms of human prion disease are experimentally transmissible, the acquired forms have until recently been confined to rare and unusual situations, such as treatment with growth hormone extracted from cadaver pituitaries, the use

Table 2 Clinical and pathological features of human prion diseases (full references in Haywood [21]).

Disease	Neuropathological features	Clinical features
Sporadic CJD	• Amyloid plaques in 10% of cases • Characteristic EEG pattern	• Onset 30–80 (median 60 y) • Intellectual deterioration • Myoclonus • Variable cerebellar, oculomotor dysfunction • Death in <12 months
Familial CJD		• Earlier onset (variable) • Longer survival (variable) compared with sporadic CJD
New variant CJD	• 'Florid' amyloid plaques	• Onset 16–40 (median 26 y) • Behavioural and psychiatric disturbances • Cerebellar ataxia • Peripheral sensory neuropathy • Death usually >12 months
Gertsmann-Straussler-Scheinker syndrome	• Amyloid plaques	• Early onset • Cerebellar dysfunction • Pyramidal motor dysfunction • Intellectual deterioration
Fatal Familial insominia	• Thalamic involvement	• Insomnia • Autonomic dysfunction • Motor dysfunction
Kuru	• Amyloid plaques	• Cerebellar ataxia • Pyramidal motor dysfunction • Intellectual deterioration • Death in<12 months

of dura mater implants, or stereotaxis with contaminated intracerebral EEG electrodes. Moreover, sporadic CJD is extremely rare in individuals under 30 years of age. Thus, the appearance of CJD in teenagers and young adults in the UK in the mid-1990s, during the BSE epidemic, caused considerable concern that these cases might have been acquired by exposure to BSE. By March 1996, additional CJD cases had been reported in young adults and teenagers [22], and it became clear that all showed unusual neuropathological features, notably extensive amyloid plaques reminiscent of kuru pathology but generally absent from typical sporadic CJD. These cases were termed 'new variant' CJD. In the past three years, more than 30 cases of vCJD have been reported in the UK, mainly in teenagers and young adults, with a single case described in France [23].

All reported cases of vCJD have occurred in individuals who were homozygous (Met/Met) at codon 129 [24] (see below). Transmission of BSE to three macaques produced disease with neuropathological features similar to those reported for cases of vCJD in humans [25]. Recent strain typing experiments have demonstrated that vCJD has similar properties to BSE [26–28]; suggesting that vCJD is acquired by exposure to BSE prions.

☐ SUSCEPTIBILITY TO PRION DISEASES: INSIGHTS FROM THE PRP GENE

Attempts to understand the genetic factors in familial prion diseases, as well as individual susceptibility to these disorders, has focused attention on the PrP gene in various experimental animals and on its human homologue, *PRNP*, which is located on chromosome 20. An early finding was the discovery of genetic linkage between the PrP gene and the incubation times for scrapie in mice, which suggested that similar factors might operate for the inherited human prion diseases. To date, 20 different non-conservative mutations have been identified within the coding sequence of *PRNP* that segregate with certain dominantly inherited neurodegenerative disorders (Fig. 6). These include missense point mutations and insertions of additional octapeptide repeats. Five of these mutations have been genetically linked to loci controlling familial CJD, Gertsmann-Straussler-Scheinker syndrome (GSS) and fatal familial insomnia (FFI), all of which are inherited human prion diseases that can be transmitted to experimental animals.

In addition to these mutations, the PrP coding sequence is polymorphic at a number of amino acid residues and for a deletion of a single octapeptide repeat. While these polymorphisms do not appear to be associated with clinical disease, the polymorphism at residue 129 influences susceptibility to CJD (see below). Codon 129 encodes either methionine (Met) or valine (Val) (Fig. 6) [29], and homozygosity for either amino acid has been reported to predispose individuals to the development of both sporadic CJD [30] and iatrogenic CJD [31]. There is also crucial interplay between residue 129 and the pathogenic mutations which has a dramatic impact on the clinical and pathological phenotypes. For example, a mutation at position 178 that changes aspartic acid (Asp) to asparagine (Asn) is linked to either FFI or a subtype of familial CJD depending on whether Met or Val respectively is encoded at position 129 on the mutant allele [32].

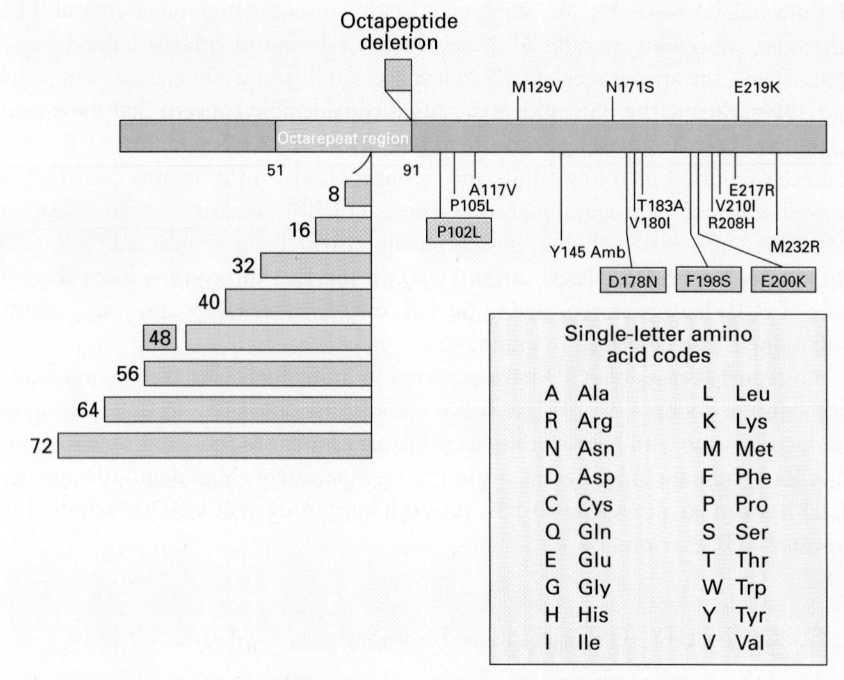

Fig. 6 Pathogenic mutations and polymorphisms in the human prion protein gene. The 253 amino acid residue coding sequence of the gene is represented as an extended rectangle. The pathogenic mutations associated with human prion disease are shown below. These consist of 8, 16, 32, 40, 48, 56, 64 and 72 amino acids insertions within the octarepeat region between codons 51 and 91, and point mutations causing non-conservative missense amino acid substitutions. Point mutations are designated by the wild-type amino acid preceding the codon number, followed by the mutant residue, using single-letter amino acid conventions (panel). The mutations for which genetic linkage with familial CJD, GSS and FFI have been established are shown in bold type in boxes. Deletion of a single octapeptide repeat is not associated with disease. Other polymorphisms found at codons 129, 171 and 219 are also shown above the coding sequence.

Insights from transgenic mice

To understand how a mutation in the PrP gene could result in a disease that was both inherited and infectious, transgenic mice were generated that expressed a proline (Pro) to leucine (Leu) mutation at codon 101 of mouse PrP; this is equivalent of the Pro→Leu substitution at codon 102 of the human *PRNP* gene which is associated with GSS (see Fig. 6). These mice spontaneously developed clinical and neuropathological symptoms similar to mouse scrapie at between 150 and 300 days of age [33,34], while transgenic mice overexpressing wild-type mouse PrP at equivalent levels did not develop disease [34]. The *de novo* generation of prions was confirmed by demonstrating that infectivity from the brains of these spontaneously sick mice could be serially propagated to indicator mice that expressed low levels of the mutant protein [34,35]. These findings suggest that the disease-associated mutations destabilise the structure of PrP^{C}, causing it spontaneously to adopt the infectious PrP^{Sc} conformation.

Species barriers and prion strains

Two features of the biology of these diseases account for prion variation, and have important implications for their transmission to man. These are the 'species barrier', ie the difficulty with which prions from one species can cause disease in another, and the existence of various strains of prions.

Species barriers

The initial passage of prions between species is associated with a prolonged incubation time and with only a few animals developing illness. With subsequent passage in the same species, all the animals become ill after greatly shortened incubation times.

Transgenic techniques are helping to elucidate the nature of the species barrier. Certain barriers have been successfully overcome by expressing PrP genes from other species, or artificially engineered hybrid PrP genes in transgenic mice. For instance, wild-type mice are normally resistant to infection with Syrian hamster prions. However, expression of Syrian hamster PrP^C in transgenic mice, referred to as Tg(SHaPrP) mice, conferred susceptibility to Syrian hamster prion infection [36], indicating that this particular barrier had been overcome. These and subsequent studies [37] indicated that disease transmission is facilitated when elements of the primary structure of host-encoded PrP^C and PrP^{Sc} in the inoculum are identical.

The infrequent transmission of human prion disease to rodents has also been cited as an example of the species barrier. Based on the results with Tg(SHaPrP) mice, it was expected that the species barrier to human prion propagation could similarly be abrogated in transgenic mice that expressed human PrP. However, transmission of human prion disease was generally no more efficient in Tg(HuPrP) mice, transgenic mice expressing human PrP^C on wild-type background, than in non-transgenic mice [38]. By contrast, propagation of human prions was highly efficient in transgenic mice expressing a chimaeric mouse-human PrP gene, referred to as Tg(MHu2M) [38,39]. The barrier to CJD transmission in Tg(HuPrP) mice was abolished when HuPrP was expressed in PrP-knockout ($Prnp^{0/0}$) mice; this demonstrated that mouse PrP^C inhibited the transmission of prions to Tg mice expressing human PrP^C, but not to those expressing chimeric PrP [39]. To explain these and other data, it was suggested that the most likely mediator of this inhibition is an auxiliary non-PrP molecule, provisionally designated protein X, which is thought to participate in the formation of prions by interacting with the C-terminal region of PrP^C to facilitate its conversion in to PrP^{Sc} [39].

Strains of prions

Like other infectious agents, prions exist as different strains with well defined, heritable properties that include incubation time and CNS pathology in inbred strains of mice. In the face of convincing evidence that vCJD is caused by human exposure to BSE, the issue of prion strains has acquired very practical consequences. Recent work indicates that prion strain information is encoded within the conformation of PrP^{Sc}, thus providing a mechanism for both the generation and the propagation of prion strains.

Two strains of prion disease in mink (transmissible mink encephalopathy), referred to as hyper (HY) and drowsy (DY), which produced different clinical symptoms and incubation periods in Syrian hamsters, showed different resistance to proteinase K digestion and altered amino-terminal proteinase K cleavage sites [40], suggesting that different strains might represent different conformational states of PrP^{Sc}. Evidence supporting the concept the conformation of PrP^{Sc} functions as a template in directing the formation of nascent PrP^{Sc} has emerged from transmission studies of inherited human prion diseases in transgenic mice. The mutant prion proteins expressed by patients with FFI and fCJD (see Fig. 6) have different PrP conformations, reflected in altered proteinase K cleavage sites; exposure to this enzyme generates protease resistant PrP^{Sc} molecules with molecular weights of 19 kDa in FFI and 21 kDa in inherited and sporadic CJD [41]. Extracts from the brains of FFI and CJD patients transmit disease to transgenic mice and induce the formation of the 19 kDa PrP^{Sc} and 21 kDa PrP^{Sc}, respectively [42]. On subsequent passage, these characteristic molecular species persist, but no incubation times diverge for the FFI and fCJD prions (Telling and Prusiner, unpublished observations). This suggests that mutant prion proteins with different primary structures produce distinct prion strains, and that different tertiary structures of PrP^{Sc} can be imparted upon a single PrP^{C} by conformational templating. Studies of established mouse and Syrian hamster prion strains in transgenic mice suggest that the diversity of prion strains may be limited to a finite constellation of PrP^{Sc} conformations that can be adopted by the primary structure of PrP in the host [43].

Other studies have shown that different sporadic and iatrogenic CJD cases associated with specific codon 129 genotypes can be typed according to PrP^{Sc} fragment sizes generated by proteinase K [27,44]. These banding patterns are also maintained upon experimental transmission to transgenic mice, except when mismatches occur between PrP^{Sc} in the inoculum and PrP^{C} in the recipient mice. A characteristic banding pattern of PrP^{Sc} found in vCJD patients and BSE infected animals distinguishes vCJD PrP^{Sc} from the patterns observed in classical CJD [27,28].

□ CONCLUSIONS

Our knowledge of prion diseases in man and other species has expanded rapidly in the past few years, through a multidisciplinary approach that has combined the skills of molecular biologists, neurologists, epidemiologists and public health physicians. It is to be hoped that this new knowledge will ultimately be translated into clinical benefits for the patients affected by these devastating diseases.

□ ACKNOWLEDGEMENTS

The author would like to thank Dr James Ironside, National Creutzfeldt-Jakob Disease Surveillance Unit, Edinburgh, and Professor Stanley Prusiner, University of California, San Francisco, for kindly supplying figures for this chapter.

REFERENCES

1 Prusiner SB. Novel proteinaceous infectious particles cause scrapie. *Science* 1982; **216**: 136–44.

2 James TL, Liu H, Ulyanov NB, *et al.* Solution structure of a 142-residue recombinant prion protein corresponding to the infectious fragment of the scrapie isoform. *Proc Natl Acad Sci USA* 1997; **94**: 10086–91.

3 Kaneko K, Zulianello L, Scott M, *et al.* Evidence for protein x binding to a discontinuous epitope on the cellular prion protein during scrapie prion propagation. *Proc Natl Acad Sci USA* 1997; **94**: 10069–74.

4 Cohen FE, Pan K-M, Huang Z, *et al.* Structural clues to prion replication. *Science* 1994; **264**: 530–1.

5 Pan K, Baldwin MA, Nguyen J, *et al.* Conversion of α-helices into β-sheets features in the formation of the scrapie prion proteins. *Proc Natl Acad Sci USA* 1993; **90**: 10962–6.

6 Riek R, Hornemann S, Wider G, Billeter M, Glockshuber R, Wuthrich K. NMR structure of the mouse prion domain PrP (121–231). *Nature* 1996; **382**: 180–2.

7 James TL, Liu H, Ulyanov NB, *et al.* Solution structure of a 142-residue recombinant prion protein corresponding to the infectious fragment of the scrapie isoform. *Proc Natl Acad Sci USA* 1997; **94**: 10086–91.

8 Bueler H, Raeber A, Sailer A, *et al.* High prion and PrP^{Sc} levels but delayed onset of disease in scrapie-inoculated mice heterozygous for a disrupted PrP gene. *Mol Med* 1995; **1**: 19–30.

9 Brandner S, Osenmann S, Raeber A, *et al.* Normal host prion protein necessary for scrapie-induced neurotoxity. *Nature* 1996; **379**: 339–43.

10 Hegde RS, Mastrianni JA, Scott MR, *et al.* A transmembrane form of the prion protein in neurodegenerative disease. *Science* 1998; **279**: 827–34.

11 Bueler H, Fischer M, Lang Y, *et al.* Normal development and behaviour of mice lacking the neuronal cell-surface PrP protein. *Nature* 1992; **356**: 577–82.

12 Bueler H, Aguzzi A, Sailer A, *et al.* Mice devoid of PrP are resistant to scrapie. *Cell* 1993; **73**: 1339–47.

13 Manson JC, Clarke AR, Hooper ML, *et al.* 129/Ola mice carrying a null mutation in PrP that abolishes mRNA production are developmentally normal. *Mol Neurobiol* 1994; **8**: 121–7.

14 Sakaguchi S, Katamine S, Nishida N, *et al.* Loss of cerebellar Purkinje cells in aged mice homozygous for a disrupted PrP gene. *Nature* 1996; **380**: 528–31.

15 Tober I, Gaus SE, Deboer T, *et al.* Altered circadian activity rhythms and sleep in mice devoid of prion protein. *Nature* 1996; **380**: 639–42.

16 Brown DR, Schulz-Schaeffer WJ, Schmidt B, Kretzschmar HA. Prion protein-deficient cells show altered response to oxidative stress due to decreased SOD-1 activity. *Exp Neurol* 1997; **146**: 104–12.

17 Brown DR, Qin K, Herms JW, *et al.* The cellular prion protein binds copper *in vivo. Nature* 1997; **390**: 684–7.

18 Collinge J, Whittington MA, Sidle KCL, *et al.* Prion protein is necessary for normal synaptic function. *Nature* 1994; **370**: 295–7.

19 Whittington MA, Sidle KCL, Gowland I, *et al.* Rescue of neurophysiological phenotype seen in PrP null mice by transgene encoding human prion protein. *Nature Genetics* 1995; **9**: 197–201.

20 Colling SB, Collinge J, Jefferys JGR. Hippocampal slices from prion protein null mice: disrupted Ca^{2+}-activated K^{+} currents. *Neurosci Lett* 1996; **209**: 49–52.

21 Haywood AM. Transmissible spongiform encephalopathies. *N Engl J Med* 1997; **337**: 1821–8.

22 Will RG, Ironside JW, Zeidler M, *et al.* A new variant of Creutzfeldt-Jakob disease in the UK. *Lancet* 1996; **347**: 921–5.

23 Chazot G, Broussolle E, Lapras CI, *et al.* New Variant of Creutzfeldt-Jakob disease in a 26-year-old French man. *Lancet* 1996; **347**: 1181.

24 Collinge J, Beck J, Campbell T, Estibeiro K, Will RG. Prion protein gene analysis in new variant cases of Creutzfeldt-Jakob disease. *Lancet* 1996; **348**: 56.

25 Lasmézas CI, Deslys J-P, Demaimay R, *et al.* BSE trasmission to macaques. *Nature* 1996; **381**: 743–4.

26 Bruce ME, Will RG, Ironside JW, *et al.* Transmissions to mice indicate that 'new variant CJD is caused by the BSE agent. *Nature* 1997; **389**: 498–501.

27 Collinge J, Sidle KCL, Meads J, Ironside J, Hill AF. Molecular analysis of prion strain variation and the aetiology of 'new variant' CJD. *Nature* 1996; **383**: 685–90.

28 Hill AF, Desbruslais M, Joiner S, *et al.* The same prion strain causes vCJD and BSE. *Nature* 1997; **389**: 448–50.

29 Owen F, Poulter M, Collinge J, Crow TJ. A codon 129 polymorphism in the PRIP gene. *Nucleic Acids Res* 1990; **18**: 3103.

30 Palmer MS, Dryden AJ, Hughes JT, Collinge J. Homozygous prion protein genotype predisposes to sporadic Creutzfeldt-Jakob disease. *Nature* 1991; **352**: 340–2.

31 Collinge J, Palmer MS, Dryden AJ. Genetic predisposition to iatrogenic Creutzfeldt-Jakob disease. *Lancet* 1991; **337**: 1441–2.

32 Goldfarb LG, Petersen RB, Tabaton M, *et al.* Fatal familial insomnia and familial Creutzfeldt-Jakob disease: disease phenotype determined by a DNA polymorphism. *Science* 1992; **258**: 806–8.

33 Hsiao KK, Scott M, Foster D, *et al.* Spontaneous neurodegeneration in transgenic mice with mutant prion protein. *Science* 1990; **250**: 1587–90.

34 Telling GC, Haga T, Torchia M, *et al.* Interactions between wild-type and mutant prion proteins modulate neurodegeneration in transgenic mice. *Genes Dev* 1996; **10**: 1736–50.

35 Hsiao KK, Groth D, Scott M, *et al.* Serial transmission in rodents of neurodegeneration from transgenic mice expressing mutant prion protein. *Proc Natl Acad Sci USA* 1994; **91**: 9126–30.

36 Scott M, Foster D, Mirenda C, *et al.* Transgenic mice expressing hamster prion protein produce species-specific scrapie infectivity and amyloid plaques. *Cell* 1989; **59**: 847–57.

37 Prusiner SB, Scott M, Foster D, *et al.* Transgenetic studies implicate interactions between homologous PrP isoforms in scrapie prion replication, *Cell* 1990; **63**: 673–86.

38 Telling GC, Scott M, Hsiao KK, *et al.* Transmission of Creutzfeldt-Jakob disease from humans to transgenic mice expressing chimeric human-mouse prion protein. *Proc Natl Acad Sci USA* 1994; **91**: 9936–40.

39 Telling GC, Scott M, Mastrianni J, *et al.* Prion propagation in mice expressing human and chimeric PrP transgenes implicates the interaction of cellular PrP with another protein. *Cell* 1995; **83**: 79–90.

40 Bessen RA, Marsh RF. Biochemical and physical properties of the prion protein from two strains of the transmissible mink encephalopathy agent. *J Virol* 1992; **66**: 2096–101.

41 Monari L, Chen SG, Brown P, *et al.* Fatal familial insomnia and familial Creutzfeldt-Jakob disease: different prion proteins determined by a DNA polymorphism. *Proc Natl Acad Sci USA* 1994; **91**: 2839–42.

42 Telling GC, Parchi P, DeArmond SJ, *et al.* Evidence for the conformation of the pathologic isoform of the prion protein enciphering and propagating prion diversity. *Science* 1996; **274**: 2079–82.

43 Scott MR, Groth D, Tatzelt J, *et al.* Propagation of prion strains through specific conformers of the prion protein. *J Virol* 1997; **71**: 9032–44.

44 Parchi P, Castellani R, Capellari S, *et al.* Molecular basis of phenotypic variability in sporadic Creutzfeldt-Jakob disease. *Ann Neurol* 1996; **39**: 669–80.

Investigation and early management of meningococcal disease

Keith AV Cartwright

☐ INTRODUCTION

Neisseria meningitidis is a fastidious Gram-negative diplococcus which colonises man. It is not found in the environment or in animals. Meningococci are harboured in the posterior nasopharynx, passing from person to person only with difficulty. Carriage rates average 10%, peaking in late teenage (Fig. 1). Most strains have little or no invasive potential and probably help to boost immunity. Meningococci have a uniquely high capacity to shed endotoxin-rich outer membrane vesicles or 'blebs' (Fig. 2), which are highly toxic to small blood vessels and produce the characteristic haemorrhagic rash. Disease attack rates are highest in infants, but there is a secondary peak in late teenage and early adulthood, associated with the peak of nasopharyngeal carriage and acquisition (Fig. 1). If invasive disease occurs, it does so normally within a few days of acquisition of a new, virulent strain.

☐ EPIDEMIOLOGY

Serogroups are defined by variations in the capsular polysaccharide; only serogroups A, B and C commonly invade immunocompetent individuals. Serogroup A disease, the most important worldwide, is rare in the UK. Serogroup B strains have predominated in this country over the past 15–20 years, causing

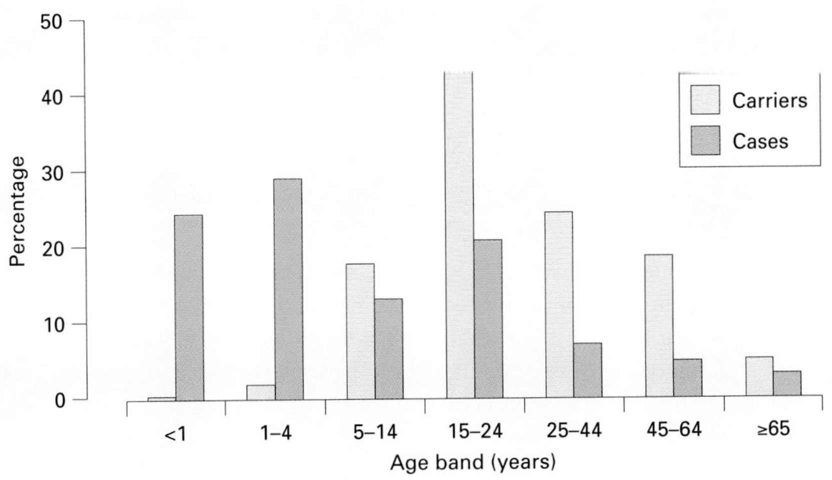

Fig. 1 Percentage of meningococcal cases and carriers within age groups.

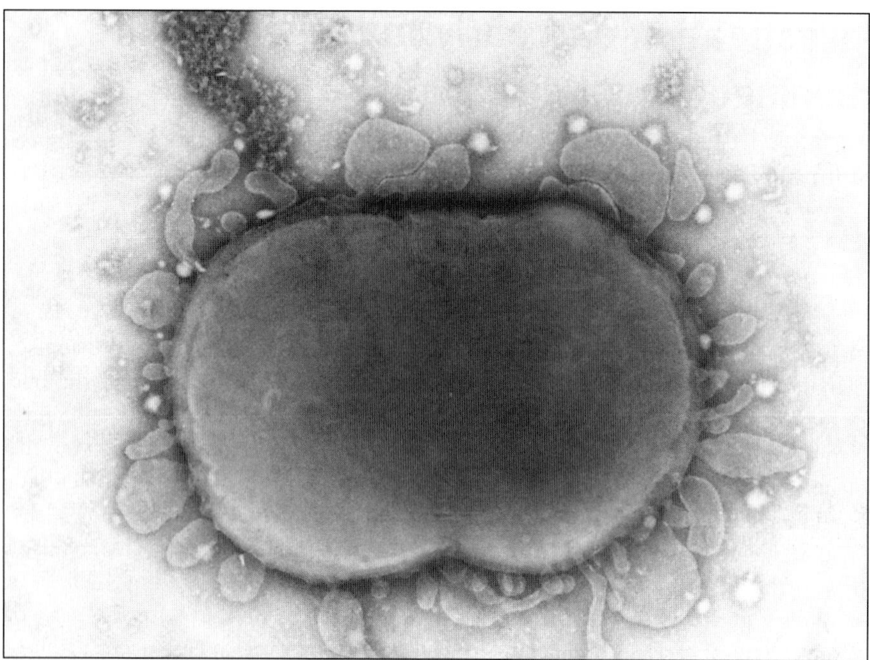

Fig. 2 *Neisseria meningitidis*, showing meningococcal 'blebbing'. (Photomicrograph by courtesy of Dr Barry Dowsett, Centre for Applied Microbiology and Research, Porton Down.)

60–75% of cases, with most others caused by serogroup C. Recently, the proportion of serogroup C cases has been unusually high (up to 45%), with an associated increase in the proportion of affected teenagers and adults and a higher prevalence of clusters and outbreaks in schools and universities. Overall attack rates are currently high (Fig. 3); provisional data from the Office for National Statistics indicate more than 2,600 notified cases and 242 deaths (9.3% case fatality rate) in England and Wales in 1997. Mortality is lowest in those aged 5–9 years, with higher rates in infants and those aged over 25. Thereafter, mortality rates rise progressively with age. The true case fatality rate is somewhat lower than the 9% suggested by last year's report, since fatal cases are notified more efficiently than survivors. Disease attack rates are highest in the winter, peaking in December and January.

□ CLINICAL PRESENTATIONS

Meningococcal infection presents most frequently as meningitis (80–85% of cases), which has a fatality rate of about 2–4%; the remainder have septicaemia without meningitis, which is associated with a case fatality rate of 20–40%. Most, if not all, cases of meningococcal disease are thought to be bacteraemic. Permanent sequelae are less frequent after meningococcal than after pneumococcal or *Haemophilus influenzae* meningitis, but deafness and/or neurodevelopmental delay occur in 5–8%; survivors of septicaemia who have severely ischaemic limbs may require amputation. A few patients may present with other focal pyogenic infections such as

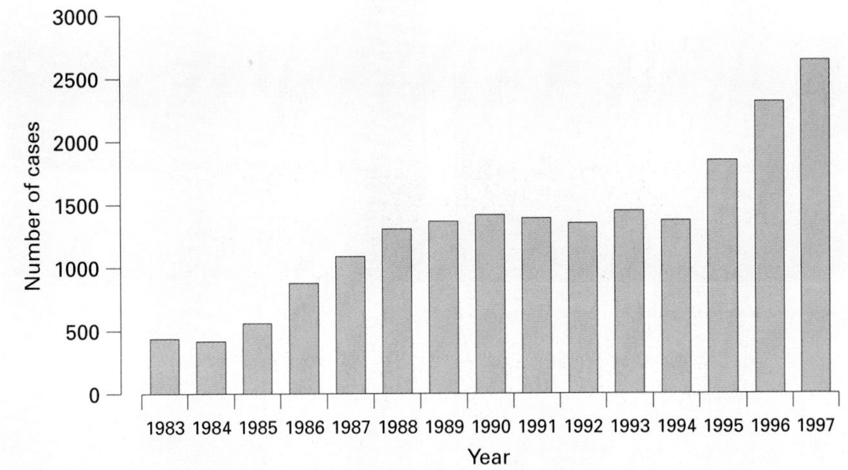

Fig. 3 Notifications of meningococcal disease, England & Wales, 1983–97. (Data from Office for National Statistics; data for 1997 are provisional.)

conjunctivitis, septic arthritis or pneumonia, the latter being associated particularly with serogroup Y strains. Chronic meningococcal septicaemia is now rare (1%).

☐ STRATEGIES FOR PREVENTION

Highly effective conjugated vaccines for serogroup C disease are now imminent and should be introduced in 1999–2000, whilst vaccines for serogroup B disease may be available within 5–10 years. The current imperative is therefore to optimise clinical management while vaccines are awaited, in order to minimise mortality and morbidity.

☐ PRE-HOSPITAL MANAGEMENT

Diagnosis

Early symptoms are non-specific, resembling those of influenza. It may be impossible to diagnose early meningococcal infection until severe symptoms or a rash develop (Fig. 4). Haemorrhagic rashes that do not fade under pressure are the hallmark of meningococcal infection, but are often preceded by less characteristic macular, blanching rashes distributed either locally or widely. There may be no rash at all. Most patients sicken progressively over 24–48 hours, but exceptional cases become moribund within a few hours. Rapid recognition and management are therefore vital.

Awareness of the symptoms and prompt resort to medical attention are the patient's best defences. Patients and parents should trust their instincts in seeking help, and general practitioners should be responsive, maintaining a high degree of suspicion and being prepared to visit and examine patients more than once. A

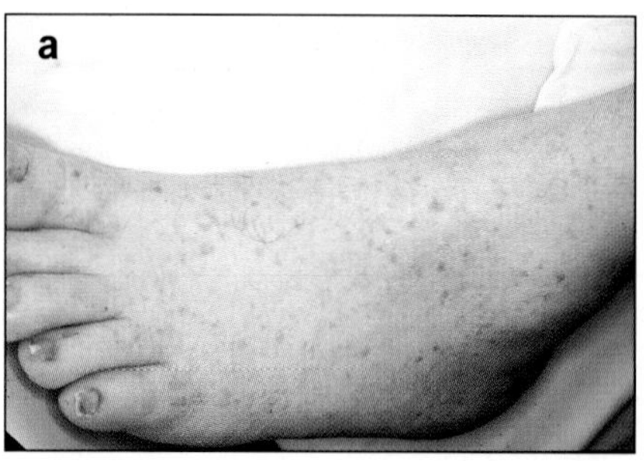

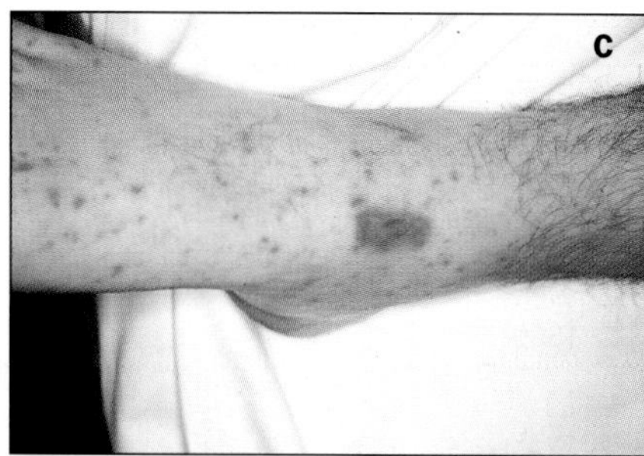

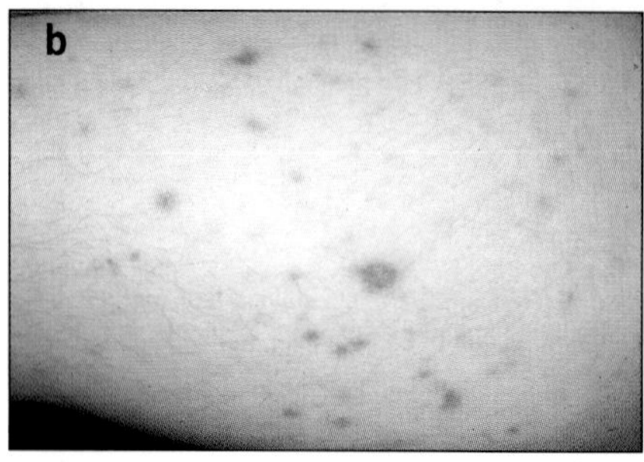

Fig. 4 Meningococcal infection: **(a)** early, fading rash; **(b)** more advanced, petechial rash; **(c)** purpuric rash.

common error is to fail to examine the entire skin surface carefully; the rash may at first be scanty and in an inaccessible location such as groin or axilla. Early rashes are harder to detect in dark-skinned people; careful examination of the conjunctivae may reveal petechiae.

Pre-admission benzylpenicillin

The first doctor to suspect either bacterial meningitis or meningococcal septicaemia should administer a dose of benzylpenicillin by the intramuscular or (better) intravenous route, followed by immediate transfer to hospital [1] (Table 1). Recommended dosages are 300 mg for children aged under 1 year, 600 mg for children aged 1–9 years, and 1,200 mg for children aged 10 years or more and adults. Benzylpenicillin should not be given to patients who have suffered anaphylactic reactions to penicillins, but should otherwise be administered if there is a history of allergy; only 3% of such cases have IgE antibodies to penicillin. Alternative agents for immediate empirical therapy in patients with a history of penicillin anaphylaxis are: chloramphenicol 25 mg/kg in children under 12 years and 1,200 mg in children aged 12 years or more and adults; cefotaxime 25 mg/kg for neonates, 50–75 mg/kg for children under 12 years and 1,000 mg for children aged 12 years or more and adults.

☐ INPATIENT MANAGEMENT

Initial evaluation

Infection generally progresses so rapidly that the diagnosis is usually established swiftly in hospital. If meningococcal disease or bacterial meningitis is suspected and

Table 1 Effect of pre-admission benzylpenicillin on mortality.

	Treated			Untreated			Total		
Study	**Survived**	**Died**	**(%)**	**Survived**	**Died**	**(%)**	**Survived**	**Died**	**(%)**
5 UK centres, 1982–91	123	6	(4.7)	317	41	(11.5)	440	47	(9.7)
New Zealand, 1993–95	111	2	(1.8)	254	22	(8.0)	365	24	(6.2)
UK (Wessex), 1990–93)	13	0	(0)	52	3	(5.8)	65	3	(4.6)
Denmark, 1980–89	19	6	(24.0)	69	4	(5.5)	88	10	(10.2)
Total	*266*	*14*	*(5.0)*	*692*	*70*	*(9.2)*	*958*	*84*	*(8.1)*

Summary of data from all studies: χ^2 4.8, p = 0.03.

parenteral antibiotic treatment has not been commenced, blood should be sampled for culture and a dose of benzylpenicillin, cefotaxime or ceftriaxone administered immediately (see below). Other investigations can then follow.

Several prognostic scoring systems for meningococcal sepsis have been developed and evaluated, based on factors associated with a poor outcome (Table 2). That most widely used in the UK is the Glasgow Meningococcal Disease Prognostic Score [2], originally evaluated in children and utilising easily measured parameters; other systems are applicable to patients of all ages [3]. Careful recording of data from the time of admission and objective assessment of severity of illness are helpful in immediate management, predicting outcome and evaluating the effect of interventions, and are also invaluable for later audit.

Dexamethasone

Dexamethasone [4] has been used as adjunctive therapy in meningococcal infections, but its use in meningococcal septicaemia without meningitis and its place in meningococcal meningitis remain controversial. Dexamethasone reduces neuronal tissue damage by blocking the microbe-induced inflammatory cascade within the subarachnoid space at various points, resulting in reduction of blood-brain barrier permeability, meningeal inflammation and cerebral oedema. Benefical effects of dexamethasone as measured by neurological outcome have been best assessed in *H. influenzae* meningitis in infants and children. Several studies of bacterial meningitis have shown that dexamethasone reduces the incidence of neurological sequelae, particularly deafness, but only when administered with, or soon after, the first dose of parenteral antibiotic. It should not be given outside hospital. Since the mechanism of deafness in meningitis is thought to be common to all bacterial pathogens, and since short-term administration of dexamethasone is only rarely accompanied by adverse effects, its use can be considered in adults with

Table 2 Factors associated with a poor outcome in meningococcal sepsis.

- Short duration of symptoms
- Lack of meningism
- Established or incipient shock
  - hypotension
  - skin/rectal temperature difference >3°C
- Extensive or progressive purpura
- Low or falling white blood cell or platelet count
- Coma or deteriorating conscious level
- Focal neurological signs
- Intractable fitting

meningococcal meningitis. Large prospective studies in meningococcal meningitis have not been carried out to date.

Investigations

These are outlined in Table 3 [5].

Blood cultures

Blood cultures are positive in only one-half of untreated patients and almost always negative after starting parenteral antibiotic treatment. The intensity of bacteraemia is highly variable and is correlated with the severity of rash and ultimately with outcome.

Examination of cerebrospinal fluid

If meningococcal meningitis is suspected, microscopy and/or culture of

Table 3 Microbiological investigation of suspected meningococcal infection.

- Blood cultures
- Blood sample for PCR* (EDTA, the preferred specimen, or heparin sample)
- CSF (if lumbar puncture not contraindicated)
  For microscopy, culture, PCR, antigen detection
- Throat swab*
- Paired serum samples
  Rising antibody titre in convalescent sample
- Aspirate from rash
  For microscopy, culture and PCR

*Of particular value if parenteral antibiotics have already been administered.

cerebrospinal fluid (CSF) are the investigations most likely to confirm the diagnosis (83% of cases in one recent series) [6]. It may take an hour or more for bactericidal concentrations of antibiotics to be achieved in CSF, so culture will often be positive even when lumbar puncture is undertaken after antibiotics have been started [1]. Examination of CSF is indicated if there is a reasonable possibility that infection may be due to another bacterium (such as a penicillin-resistant pneumococcus) or that symptoms may not be attributable to meningitis at all (Fig. 5).

However, lumbar puncture is inherently unsafe. It may cause clinical deterioration if performed in incipient septic shock. Brainstem herniation (coning), which is generally fatal, follows lumbar puncture in approximately 0.5% of cases with suspected meningococcal meningitis [6]; without prospective studies, it cannot be determined whether the disease itself or the investigation causes coning. CSF examination shows no abnormality in meningococcal septicaemia and, in a recent review of 120 patients with suspected meningococcal meningitis whose CSF subsequently grew meningococci, 8% showed no abnormality on first examination [6]. Therefore, antibiotic treatment must never be withheld on the basis of a normal initial CSF.

There are several contraindications to lumbar puncture in suspected meningococcal infection (Table 4). Although undoubtedly a valuable investigation, there must be rigorous appraisal of risk and benefit on each occasion its use is contemplated. The development of highly sensitive polymerase chain reaction (PCR) tests

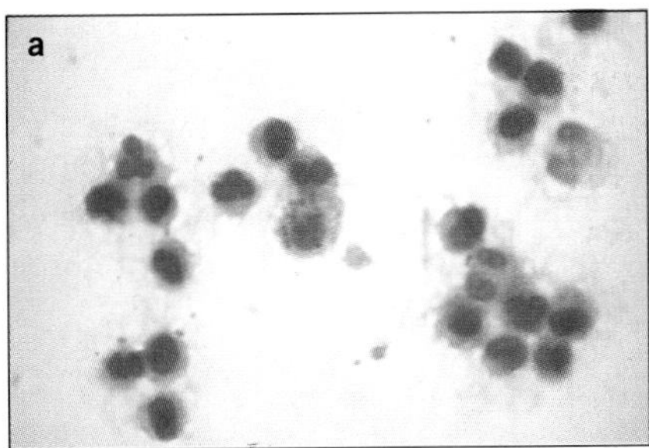

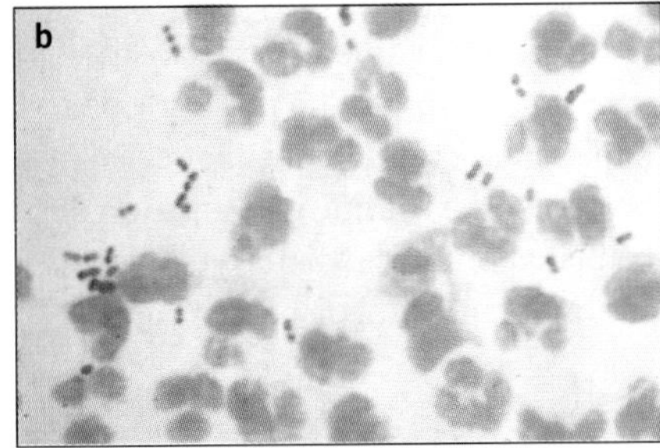

Fig. 5 (a) Meningococcal meningitis with Gram negative diplococci. **(b)** Pneumococcal meningitis with Gram-positive diplococci.

Table 4 Contraindications to lumbar puncture in patients with suspected meningococcal infection (after Wylie *et al* [6]).

- Confident clinical diagnosis
- Drowsiness or impairment of consciousness
  - Glasgow coma scale score of <13, or deteriorating scores
- Other signs of raised intracranial pressure
  - Marked instability of blood pressure or heart rate
- Focal neurological signs
- Impending or established septic shock
- Infection at planned lumbar puncture site

to detect meningococcal and pneumococcal infection means that lumbar puncture in suspected bacterial meningitis may now sometimes be deferred to allow the patient's clinical condition to stabilise.

PCR amplification of meningococcal DNA

PCR tests for meningococcal DNA in blood and CSF have transformed the investigation of suspected meningococcal infection. Part of the first blood sample (which may be taken into either EDTA or heparin) should be reserved for PCR testing, which is available throughout the UK and Eire via national reference units (details given below after 'Further Reading'). In the UK, samples are first screened with a sensitive assay and positives confirmed with a second, highly specific assay. The confirmatory assay is based on the *siaD* gene which determines the meningococcal serogroup, thereby providing invaluable information for management of contacts and of clusters.

Meningococcal DNA is cleared rapidly from the circulation, but far less swiftly from the CSF; accordingly, the PCR blood assay may become negative within 12–24 hours after starting antibiotic treatment, but remains positive in CSF for 48 hours or more. PCR testing must therefore be carried out on the first blood and/or CSF samples collected.

Throat swab

A throat swab (or a pernasal swab if the patient is unable to cooperate) passed straight back on to the posterior pharyngeal wall yields meningococci in about 50% of patients, a rate largely unaffected by prior antibiotic therapy. A throat swab should be part of the routine investigation of suspected meningococcal infection and should be plated out immediately. In over 95% of cases, meningococci isolated from throat swabs are indistinguishable from the strain causing systemic infection.

Other investigations

Aspiration of tissue fluid from haemorrhagic skin lesions is simple and gives good chances of positive culture and/or microscopy [7]. A purpuric skin lesion is pinched between finger and thumb to exclude circulating blood. The lesion is scraped, 'picked' or punctured with a sterile hypodermic needle (25G) or the point of a fine scalpel blade. A little more pressure is applied to squeeze out a drop of tissue fluid and blood which is then smeared on a glass slide. Several small smears of 3–4 mm are better than one large one. These are then fixed in methanol and stained with Giemsa stain (organisms stain blue-black) or Gram stain (organisms stain pink-red). Tissue fluid can also be plated directly on to chocolate agar for culture. PCR testing can also be used on skin aspirates.

Meningococcal infection can be diagnosed retrospectively by demonstrating a rising antibody titre between acute and convalescent serum samples; the latter are best collected 2–3 weeks after the onset of infection.

Antibiotic treatment

Table 5 shows the main options. Cefotaxime or ceftriaxone are widely employed for the empirical antibiotic treatment of suspected bacterial meningitis and meningococcal septicaemia. Cefuroxime is inferior. Once meningococcal infection has been confirmed, benzylpenicillin should be substituted. It is highly active (no resistance has been reported in the UK), cheap, exerts minimum selection pressure, and has acquired familiarity through decades of clinical experience. Chloramphenicol is an alternative in patients allergic to penicillins and cephalosporins.

Antibiotic treatment of uncomplicated meningococcal infection is normally for 5–7 days, with more severe infections generally treated for 10–14 days. If the patient has meningitis, full antibiotic doses should be sustained throughout the treatment period since penetration of penicillins and cephalosporins into the subarachnoid space diminishes as inflammation of the blood-brain barrier subsides.

Benzylpenicillin and cefotaxime do not reliably clear meningococci from the nasopharynx, and all patients should be given prophylactic rifampicin or ciprofloxacin at, or just before, discharge from hospital. Prophylaxis is not required in patients treated with ceftriaxone, as this drug reliably clears nasopharyngeal carriage.

Monitoring progress

Meningococcal infection evolves rapidly, and patients should be re-evaluated frequently until stable. Progressive rash, low or falling white blood cell or platelet count, unstable or deteriorating conscious level, persistent fitting, incipient or progressive shock, or worsening disseminated intravascular coagulation all indicate the need for continued aggressive management.

Sick patients are best managed in an intensive care unit, as multisystem support may be required. The mainstays of treatment are early elective ventilation and circulatory support with rapid, monitored fluid replacement (initially mainly colloid) and inotropes. Many patients with severe meningococcal sepsis also suffer major disruptions of haemostasis and also of renal and hepatic function.

Several new therapies for meningococcal septic shock have been described but have not yet been rigorously evaluated. These include, in the past few years, haemodiafiltration, extracorporeal membrane oxygenation (ECMO), protein C and

Table 5 Antibiotic treatment of meningococcal infection.

Empirical antibiotic treatment of suspected meningococcal infection		
Cefotaxime	2 g × 6–8 hourly	intravenous
Ceftriaxone	2 g × 12 hourly	intravenous
Once meningococcal disease is confirmed		
Benzylpenicillin	1.2–2.4 g × 4 hourly	intravenous
Chemoprophylaxis prior to discharge from hospital		
Rifampicin	600 mg bd for 2 days	oral
Ciprofloxacin	500 mg stat	oral

recombinant bactericidal permeability-increasing protein [8]. Protein C suppresses intravascular coagulation by inactivating cofactors in thrombin production and by simultaneously promoting fibrinolysis. It is also thought to modulate the inflammatory response to bacterial infection through an interaction with specific receptors on mononuclear phagocytes and on epithelial cells. Recombinant bactericidal permeability-increasing protein is at present the subject of a multicentre prospective blinded trial. Centoxin, a monoclonal anti-endotoxin antibody, has been shown to be ineffective in meningococcal septicaemia.

□ OTHER ASPECTS OF MANAGEMENT

Patients with invasive meningococcal infection should be nursed in isolation for the first 24 hours, and attendants should wear a mask. Thereafter, except for very rare cases of meningococcal pneumonia, patients can be nursed safely on the open ward. Relatives living with the patient prior to admission do not need to be excluded during isolation nursing. Sick patients, and all those with meningitis, benefit from being nursed in a quiet environment, such as a side room.

The vast majority of adults, including health care staff, are immune to meningococcal infection, and the risk of transmission of infection to medical and nursing staff is extremely low. Chemoprophylaxis (eg rifampicin) is only indicated for those who have carried out mouth-to-mouth resuscitation.

Patients infected with meningococci of serogroups other than A, B or C (most frequently Y, W-135 or X) should be investigated to exclude the possibility of an inherited deficiency of a late complement component (C5 to C9), as should those experiencing a second attack of meningococcal infection.

Notification and prophylaxis of contacts

About 5% of meningococcal disease cases are secondary, ie acquired from another case rather than from an asymptomatic carrier. Chemoprophylaxis is therefore required for close family contacts of cases. Stocks of rifampicin and ciprofloxacin can be kept on one or two wards in the hospital (eg the intensive care unit) and issued, together with detailed information on the symptoms of meningococcal infection, to relatives accompanying the patient to hospital. Those receiving rifampicin should be warned that it colours urine and contact lenses red, and may interfere with oral contraception; a pharmacist should be involved in selecting appropriate chemoprophylactic antibiotics and in giving information and advice.

Suspected or confirmed cases of meningococcal disease must be notified to the proper officer; in England and Wales, this is the Consultant in Communicable Disease Control (CCDC), and in Scotland the Consultant in Public Health Medicine (CPHM). The CCDC or CPHM have statutory responsibility for identification and management of contacts. As secondary cases often follow quickly after primary cases, admitting doctors must give notification of all suspected or confirmed cases of meningococcal infection immediately by telephone.

□ AFTER-EFFECTS

All patients should have at least one follow-up outpatient appointment to check for hearing loss and other residual effects. Headaches, lethargy, tearfulness and depression are common for weeks or months after the acute episode. Reassurance that full recovery is to be expected is helpful. The National Meningitis Trust (helpline 0345 538118) offers information, advice and support, and may also make grants to patients and relatives suffering financial hardship.

□ AUDIT

Accurate, structured recording of clinical and laboratory data facilitates audit of management and outcome of meningococcal infection. Regular audit is strongly recommended. A checklist of standards suitable for clinical audit is available on request from the author (telephone 01452 305334; e-mail: kcartwright@phls.co.uk).

REFERENCES

1 Cartwright K, Reilly S, White D, Stuart J. Early treatment with parenteral penicillin in meningococcal disease. *Br Med J* 1992; **305**: 143–7.

2 Sinclair JF, Skeoch CH, Hallworth D. Prognosis of meningococcal septicaemia. *Lancet* 1987; **ii**: 38.

3 Barquet N, Domingo P, Cayla JA, *et al.* Prognostic factors in meningococcal disease. *J Am Med Assoc* 1997; **278**: 491–6.

4 Kaplan SL. Adjuvant therapy in meningitis. *Adv Pediatr Infect Dis* 1995; **10**: 167–86.

5 Kaczmarski EB, Cartwright KAV. Control of meningococcal disease: guidance for microbiologists. *Commun Dis Rep Rev* 1995; **5**: R196–8.

6 Wylie PAL, Stevens D, Drake W, *et al.* Epidemiology and clinical management of meningococcal disease in west Gloucestershire: retrospective, population based study. *Br Med J* 1997; **315**: 774–9.

7 van Deuren M, van Dijke BJ, Koopman RJJ, *et al.* Rapid diagnosis of acute meningococcal infections by needle aspiration or biopsy of skin lesions. *Br Med J* 1993; **306**: 1229–32.

8 Giroir BP, Quint PA, Barton P, *et al.* Preliminary evaluation of recombinant amino-terminal fragment of human bactericidal/permeability-increasing protein in children with severe meningococcal sepsis. *Lancet* 1997; **350**: 1439–43.

FURTHER READING

Quagliarello V, Scheld WM. Bacterial meningitis: pathogenesis, pathophysiology and progress. *N Engl J Med* 1992; **327**: 864–72.

Sigurdardottir B, Bjornsson OM, Jonsdottir KE, *et al.* Acute bacterial meningitis in adults. *Arch Intern Med* 1997; **157**: 425–43.

A Working Group of the British Infection Society is currently finalising guidelines on the investigation, diagnosis, treatment and secondary prevention of adult bacterial meningitis in patients with normal immunity. The guidelines will be published shortly in the *Journal of Infection.*

National reference units

England & Wales: Meningococcal Reference Unit, Public Health Laboratory, Withington Hospital, Manchester M20 8LR (tel: 0161 291 4628)

Scotland: Scottish Meningococcus and Pneumococcus Reference Laboratory (SMPRL), Department of Laboratory Medicine, Ruchill Hospital, Glasgow G20 9NB (tel: 0141 946 7120 ext 1337)

Ireland: Meningococcal Reference Laboratory, Children's Hospital, Temple Street, Dublin 1, Eire (tel: 00 353 1 809 5432)

☐ MULTIPLE CHOICE QUESTIONS

1 Meningococci:
(a) Can be acquired from contaminated water
(b) Can be acquired from household pets
(c) Are not easily transmissible
(d) Shed very large amounts of endotoxin
(e) If they are going to do so, will usually cause disease within a few days of colonising a new host

2 Meningococcal disease in the UK:
(a) Is caused predominantly by strains of serogroup B
(b) Caused more than 200 deaths in 1997
(c) In adults, case fatality rates increase with age
(d) Peaks in the autumn
(e) Should be notified by telephone to the CCDC or CPHM

3 Meningococcal septicaemia:
(a) Is the commonest clinical presentation
(b) Is associated with a case fatality rate of ≥20%
(c) May be difficult to distinguish at first from influenza
(d) May present with a blanching, maculopapular skin rash
(e) Usually causes a polymorph cellular response in CSF

4 In meningococcal disease:
(a) Blood cultures are nearly always positive in previously untreated patients
(b) Coning may follow lumbar puncture in 0.5% of those with meningitis
(c) If initial examination of CSF reveals no abnormality, parenteral antibiotics should be withheld pending results of other tests
(d) Culture of meningococci from throat swabs is largely unaffected by prior antibiotic therapy
(e) PCR testing can be carried out on blood, CSF and skin aspirate

5 Patients with severe meningococcal sepsis:
(a) Should be nursed in isolation for 48–72 hours
(b) Should be treated with dexamethasone 0.6 mg/kg/day for 2 days
(c) Early and elective ventilation should be considered
(d) Initial correction of circulating fluid depletion should be principally with crystalloid

(e) Should be treated with rifampicin or ciprofloxacin prior to discharge from hospital

ANSWERS

1	2	3	4	5
1a False	2a True	3a False	4a False	5a False
b False	b True	b True	b True	b False
c True	c True	c True	c False	c True
d True	d False	d True	d True	d False
e True	e True	e False	e True	e True

Is HIV now treatable?

Michael Barry, David Back and Alasdair Breckenridge

□ INTRODUCTION

The first recognised cases of the acquired immunodeficiency syndrome (AIDS) occurred in 1981, with reports of *Pneumocystis carinii* pneumonia and Kaposi's sarcoma in homosexual men. Since then, infection with the causative organism, human immunodeficiency virus (HIV-1), has reached pandemic proportions. A recent review from the joint United Nations programme on HIV/AIDS (UNAIDS) and the World Health Organization shows that rates of transmission of HIV have been grossly underestimated worldwide. Over 30 million adults and children are now believed to be infected with HIV and, if current transmission rates hold, the total number of people with HIV could reach 40 million by the year 2000 (Fig. 1) [1]. In the UK, 30,162 HIV infections, 14,719 cases of AIDS and 10,663 deaths from AIDS had been reported to the Public Health Laboratory Service up to September 1997 [2]. Over 80% of HIV infections in the UK were acquired through sexual contact, predominantly sex between men (69%) (see Fig. 2).

Our approach to the treatment of patients infected with HIV has changed significantly over the past two years. This follows a number of recent advances which include a better understanding of HIV pathogenesis and replication, the development of new techniques for sensitive and accurate quantitation of HIV-1 RNA in plasma, the availability of newer antiretroviral agents, and the demonstration that combination therapy is more effective than monotherapy. These advances and their influence on the clinical management of HIV disease are reviewed in this chapter.

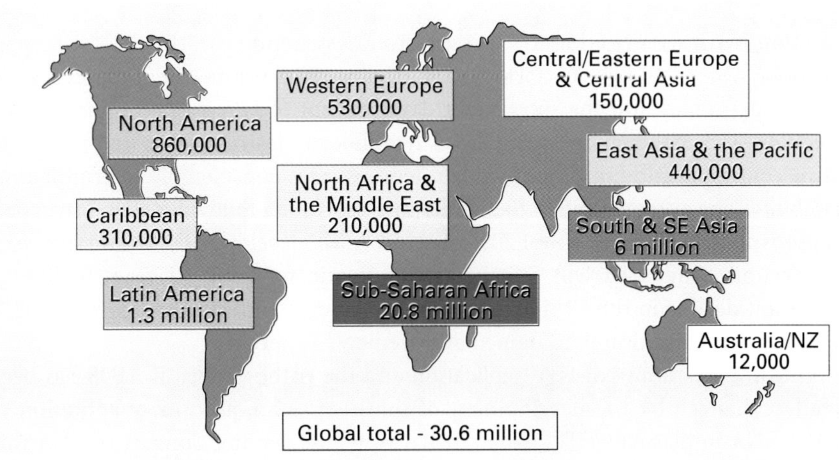

Fig. 1 Estimated number of persons living with HIV/AIDS at the end of 1997 [1].

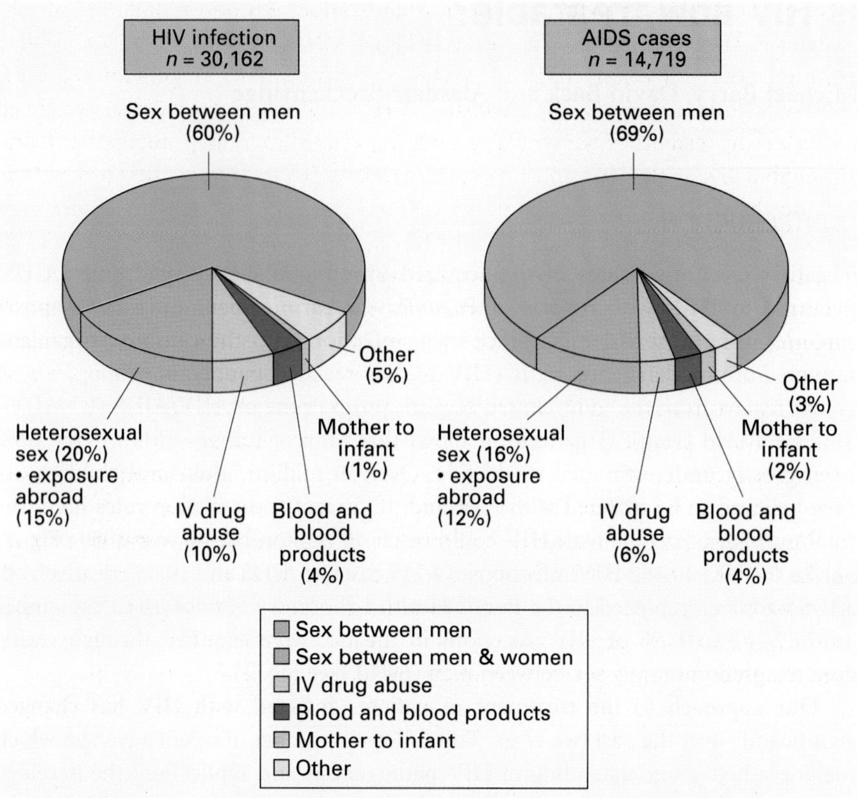

Fig. 2 Causes of exposure resulting in HIV infection (left) and AIDS (right) in cases reported in the UK to the end of September 1997 [2] (IV = intravenous).

□ HIV PATHOGENESIS AND REPLICATION

Infection with HIV-1 initiates progressive destruction of the CD4 (helper) T lymphocyte. The rate of CD4 T cell decline determines the progression of immunodeficiency and the subsequent development of HIV-related opportunistic infections and malignancies [3]. CD4 T lymphocyte destruction is due mainly to active viral replication, a process which demonstrates considerable interindividual variability. The average time to the development of AIDS following HIV-1 infection is approximately 10 years; about 20% of subjects will develop AIDS within five years of infection, while 5% will remain asymptomatic for over 10 years without a significant decline in the CD4 T cell count. In patients with slowly progressive HIV disease, viral replication is contained at extremely low levels.

Our understanding of HIV replication and the pathogenesis of AIDS has been greatly enhanced by the development of sensitive techniques for quantitation of HIV-1 RNA in plasma. (HIV-1 is a retrovirus, whose genome consists of RNA that is transcribed by reverse transcriptase into DNA, which then becomes integrated into the host's DNA.) Methodology such as target amplification (eg quantitative reverse transcriptase polymerase chain amplification; Amplicor Roche Molecular Systems, US) enables the determination of HIV-1 RNA levels as low as 20 copies/ml, although the detection limit of assays in clinical use is generally around 400 copies/ml. In general, the quantity of HIV-1 RNA in the plasma accurately indicates the extent of virus replication, especially in lymophoreticular tissue, although active replication in some compartments (eg the central nervous system) may not be reflected by the plasma HIV RNA levels. Plasma HIV RNA may show marked variation, depending on the stage of infection. Primary HIV infection (the initial stage of the disease with enhanced viral replication and dissemination in lymphoid tissue), may produce plasma HIV RNA concentrations in excess of 10^7 copies/ml. After approximately six months, the emergence of an immune response results in a steady-state level – the so-called viral load 'set point' – which varies between patients but usually lies between 10^3 and 10^5 copies/ml of HIV RNA (Fig. 3). This viral load set point may remain stable for many years, but HIV RNA levels eventually increase, with a deterioration in immune function and the development of opportunistic infections and neoplasms.

We now know that the course of HIV infection is a dynamic process that depends on the balance between CD4 T cell production and the destruction of these cells mediated by viral replication. It has been estimated that 10^8 virus particles must be produced each day to maintain steady state. The measurement of HIV RNA at steady state (set point) is of significant prognostic value [4]. A clear relationship has been

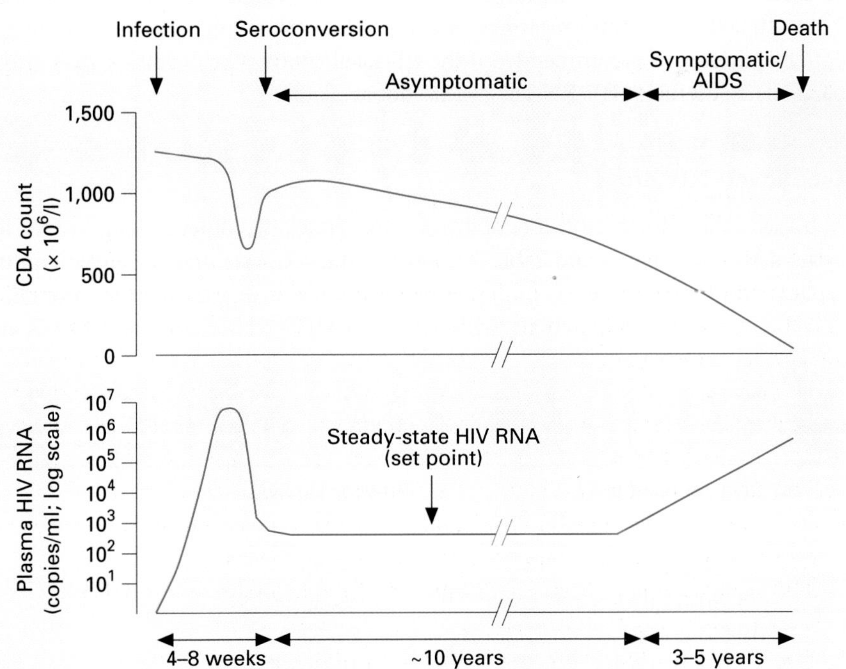

Fig. 3 Plasma HIV RNA and CD4 T lymphocyte count during the course of HIV infection.

shown between disease progression and death and increasing concentrations of plasma HIV RNA (Table 1). By contrast, baseline CD4 T cell counts have little discriminatory value in predicting disease progression, except when counts fall below 320 × 10^6/l. The prognostic independence of viral load from the CD4 count is demonstrated by findings from patients with CD4 counts greater than 500 × 10^6/ml: 50% of those with HIV RNA levels greater than 10,900 copies/ml died within six years, compared with only 5% of those whose HIV RNA levels were below this level.

These observations have provided the foundations for recent guidelines for initiation of antiretroviral therapy in HIV disease. The aim of treatment, stated by the International AIDS Society-USA Panel in June 1997, is to reduce and maintain plasma HIV RNA levels to less than 400 copies/ml [5].

□ ANTIRETROVIRAL THERAPY

Indications for treatment

Most clinicians now agree that antiretroviral therapy should be introduced early, before substantial immunodeficiency develops (see Table 2). As the onset of HIV-related symptoms (eg recurrent oral candidiasis, chronic fever, weight loss) is a strong predictor of further progression to HIV-related opportunistic infections, all patients with symptomatic HIV disease should be treated. Since the availability of HIV RNA assays, various guidelines on initiation of anti-HIV therapy have been published, the most recent in June 1997 [5]. Treatment with anti-HIV drugs is now advised for all patients with plasma HIV RNA concentrations greater than 5,000–10,000 copies/ml, regardless of the CD4 cell count. For asymptomatic patients, therapy is recommended if the CD4 cell count is below 500 × 10^6/l; this is particularly useful if HIV RNA assays are not available.

Specific anti-HIV drugs

At present, there are three classes of drugs which attack two different stages of the life cycle of HIV (see Fig. 4 and Table 3). Reverse transcriptase, the key enzyme in the replication of retroviruses, is inhibited by nucleoside analogues such as zidovudine (ZDV), first used to treat patients with AIDS and AIDS-related complex in 1987, and

Table 1 Relationship between steady-state ('set point') plasma HIV RNA levels and 10-year mortality.

HIV RNA set point level (copies/ml)	10-year survival (%)
<5,260	65–70
5,261–12,890	45–50
12,891–37,020	25–30
>37,020	10–20

Note: 'set point' occurs 6–12 months after initial infection.

Table 2 Recommendations for initiation of antiretroviral therapy in patients with HIV [5].

Therapy is recommended in:

- All patients with HIV-related symptoms
- All patients with HIV RNA levels >5,000 copies/ml
- Patients with rapidly declining CD4 T lymphocyte counts (eg fall exceeding 300 × 10^6/l over 12 months)

Consider therapy at:

- Any CD4 T-lymphocyte count level, especially if <500 × 10^6/l

Treatment may be deferred if:

- CD4 count is stable between 350–500 × 10^6/l and plasma HIV RNA levels are <5,000 copies/ml

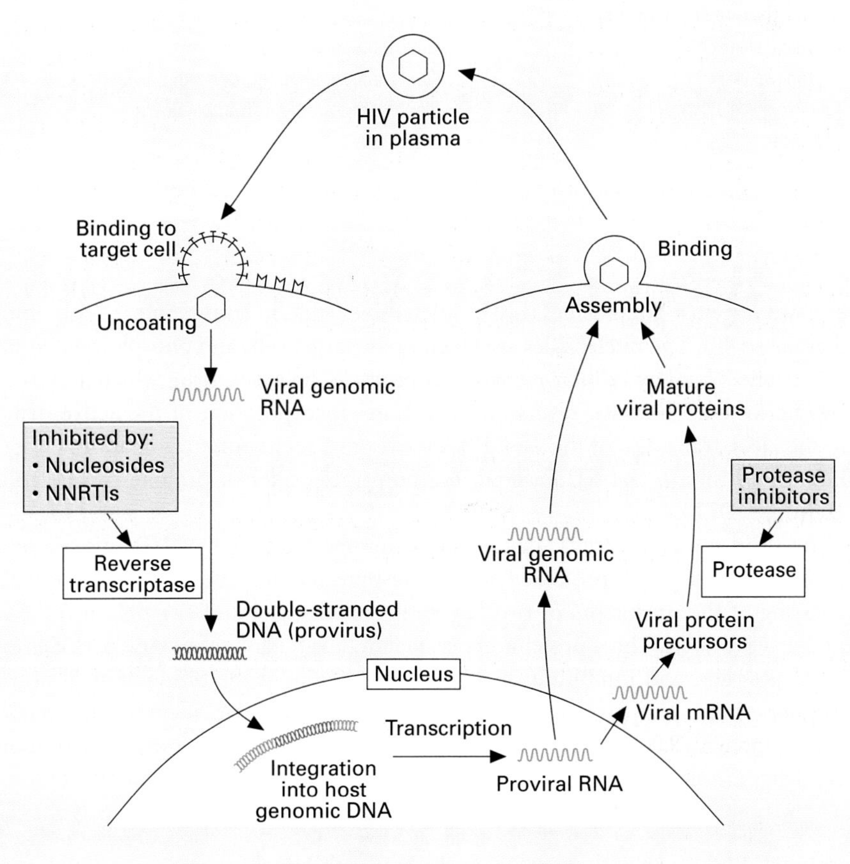

Fig. 4 Life cycle of HIV (NNRTI = non-nucleoside reverse transcriptase inhibitor; for explanation of drug abbreviations see Table 3).

Table 3 Currently available anti-HIV drugs and their major side effects.

Anti-HIV drugs	Major side effects
Inhibitors of reverse transcriptase (inhibit retrovirus replication)	
Nucleosides:	
• Zidovudine (ZDV)	• Anaemia, neutropenia, headache, insomnia
• Didanosine (ddI)	• Peripheral neuropathy, pancreatitis
• Zalcitabine (ddC)	• Peripheral neuropathy, mucocutaneous ulceration
• Lamivudine (3TC)	• Peripheral neuropathy
• Stavudine (d4T)	• Peripheral neuropathy
Non-nucleosides (NNRTIs):	
• Nevirapine (NVP)	• Skin rash
• Delavirdine (DEL)	• Skin rash, neutropenia
Protease inhibitors (produce non-infective viral particles):	
• Saquinavir (SQV)	• Gastrointestinal upset
• Ritonavir (RIT)	• Gastrointestinal upset, perioral paraesthesia
• Indinavir (IND)	• Nephrolithiasis, hyperbilirubinaemia
• Nelfinavir (NEL)	• Diarrhoea

NNRTI = non-nucleoside reverse transcriptase inhibitor.

the newer agents didanosine (ddI), zalcitabine (ddC), lamivudine (3TC) and stavudine (d4T). The nucleosides are taken up by target cells and phosphorylated to the 5'-triphosphate by cellular enzymes to produce the active drug which acts as a substrate for, and inhibits, reverse transcriptase. Incorporation of the active drug into the DNA transcript of the viral RNA leads to its premature termination. Other inhibitors of reverse transcriptase are the non-nucleosides nevirapine (NVP) and delavirdine (DEL).

The third group of drugs now available for the treatment of HIV disease are inhibitors of the HIV protease enzyme responsible for the post-translational processing of the precursors of two key viral proteins, gag and gag-pol, into their functional products. These proteins are crucial in the attachment of viral particles to their target cells, and inhibition of this enzyme results in the production of non-infectious virus. The protease inhibitors currently available include saquinavir (SQV), ritonavir (RIT), indinavir (IND) and nelfinavir (NEL). The sites of action of these drugs are shown in Fig. 4.

Combination therapy with reverse transcriptase inhibitors

ZDV used alone was shown to decrease mortality and the frequency of opportunistic infections, in HIV patients with advanced disease. Unfortunately, however, its beneficial effects were not sustained, due in part to the emergence of ZDV-resistant viral strains. Combination therapy using ZDV with other nucleoside analogues was tried, as synergistic anti-HIV effects had been demonstrated *in vitro*, and the potential to delay the emergence of resistant virus and sustain antiviral efficacy was supported by surrogate marker changes from a number of short-term studies. A number of large-scale, double-blind randomised trials were then undertaken to investigate the potential benefits of combination therapy with nucleoside analogues in HIV-infected adults. These include ACTG 175 initiated in 1991, Delta and CPCRA (1992) and the CAESAR trial (1995). The preliminary results of ACTG 175 and Delta, published in 1995, demonstrated unequivocal beneficial effects of combination therapy and thus brought to an end the era of monotherapy. The key findings from these trials are discussed below and summarised in Table 4.

Randomised trials of combination therapy with reverse transcriptase inhibitors

ACTG 175 [6] compared monotherapy using either zidovudine (ZDV) 600 mg/day or didanosine (ddI) 400 mg/day, with combination therapy including ZDV plus ddI or ZDV plus ddC 2.25 mg/day. The incidence of an AIDS defining event or death was 16% for ZDV monotherapy, 11% for ZDV + ddI, 12% with ZDV + ddC, and 11% for ddI monotherapy, with statistically significant improvements over ZDV alone in each of the two ddI groups. Similarly, the mortality rate was significantly reduced in patients treated with ZDV + ddI (5%), ddI (5%) but not ZDV + ddC (7%) when

Table 4 Randomised, double-blind controlled trials of monotherapy versus combination therapy using reverse transcriptase inhibitors. For explanation of drug abbreviations, see Table 3.

	ACTG 175	**Delta***	**CAESAR**	**CPCRA**
Patients	2,467	3,207	1,840	1,102
Median follow-up (weeks)	143	120	52	140
CD4 cells ($\times 10^6$/l)	200–500	<350	25–250	<200
Treatment	ZDV+ddI ZDV+ddC ddI ZDV	ZDV+ddI ZDV+ddC ZDV	Current treatment+: placebo 3TC 3TC+loviride†	ZDV+ddI ZDV+ddC ZDV
Reduction in mortality	ZDV+ddI (43%) ddI (46%)	ZDV+ddI (30%) ZDV+ddC (19%)	Current treatment +3TC (50%)	No significant change
Reduced progression to AIDS or death**	ZDV+ddI (32%) ddI (26%)	ZDV+ddI	Current treatment +3TC (55%)	No significant change

* The Delta trial was subdivided into Delta-1 and Delta-2 according to whether patients had not or had previously been treated with ZDV.
† Loviride is a non-nucleoside reverse transcriptase inhibitor (NNRTI) which was withdrawn from the market due to limited efficacy.
** This percentage accounts for both the number of patients who died and the number of patients who developed an AIDS-defining illness, eg Kaposi's sarcoma.

compared with ZDV monotherapy (9%). Subgroup analysis demonstrated that for patients previously untreated with antiretroviral agents, combinations of ZDV + ddI or ZDV + ddC or ddI monotherapy were superior to ZDV alone; for patients who had been treated with antiretroviral therapy, a change to ZDV + ddI or ddI monotherapy was beneficial.

The European-Australian Delta study [7] compared ZDV (600 mg/day) with ZDV 600 mg + ddI 400 mg daily or ZDV 600 mg + ddC 2.25 mg daily. For patients without prior ZDV therapy (Delta 1), the mortality among patients treated with ZDV alone was 21%, significantly higher than for ZDV + ddI (13%) and ZDV + ddC (15%). For previously ZDV-treated patients (Delta 2), mortality was 35% for ZDV, 28% for ZDV + ddI and 33% for ZDV + ddC; only the ZDV + ddI combination significantly reduced mortality. Overall, the Delta trial demonstrated significant reductions in mortality with combinations of ZDV + ddI and ZDV + ddC, when compared with ZDV monotherapy.

The CAESAR trial [8] (based in Canada, Australia, Europe and South Africa) compared the efficacy of the nucleoside 3TC + loviride (LOV) versus placebo when added to existing ZDV-containing regimens. There were 50–55% reductions in disease progression or death in the 3TC-containing arms compared with placebo, clearly demonstrating the benefits of adding 3TC to ZDV.

In *the CPCRA study* (Community Programs for Clinical Research on AIDS) [9], patients with AIDS or fewer than 200 × 10^6/l CD4 cells were randomised to receive ZDV 600 mg/day, ZDV 600 mg + ddI 400 mg daily, or ZDV 600 mg + ddC 2.25 mg daily. During follow-up, there was either disease progression or death in 65% of patients treated with ZDV alone, 62% of patients treated with ZDV + ddI and 63% for ZDV + ddC. Similarly, there were no significant differences in mortality between the three groups (ZDV alone 51%, ZDV + ddI 48%, ZDV + ddC 49%). It is important to note that these subjects were selected to have advanced HIV disease, with a median CD4 count between 87 and 102 × 10^6/l; over 30% had an AIDS-defining illness and approximately 77% had received prior treatment with ZDV.

Overall, these large randomised trials yielded several useful conclusions. The combination of ZDV + ddI or ZDV + ddC is superior to ZDV alone for patients without prior antiretroviral therapy, and for asymptomatic patients with CD4 counts less than 500 × 10^6/l, with the important exception of subjects with advanced disease, in whom there was no clear benefit of combination therapy. For ZDV-experienced patients, the addition of ddI or 3TC will reduce mortality and disease progression to AIDS. As a result of these trials the International AIDS Society-USA Panel recommended in July 1996 that the combinations of ZDV + ddI, ZDV + ddC and ZDV + 3TC should be used for initial therapy of HIV disease [10].

Protease inhibitors

Further progress in the treatment of HIV infection followed the introduction of the protease inhibitors in 1996. These drugs are potent anti-HIV agents: for example, RIT produced a 1.7 log-unit reduction in plasma HIV RNA, similar to that produced by ZDV + 3TC. A recent study of 1,090 patients with advanced HIV disease (mean

CD4 count of 30 × 10^6/l) demonstrated that RIT reduced disease progression (by 41%) and mortality (by 25%) when added to existing therapy with two nucleoside analogues [11]. Moreover, triple therapy with two nucleosides (ZDV and ddC) and SQV (protease inhibitor) reduced HIV replication and increased CD4 cell counts to a greater extent when compared with either ZDV + ddC or ZDV + SQV [12]. Similarly, the triple combination ZDV + 3TC + IND had greater antiviral efficacy than ZDV + 3TC, and reduced plasma HIV RNA to below 500 copies/ml in 90% of patients with CD4 counts ranging from 50 to 400 × 10^6/l and initial HIV RNA levels of more than 20,000 copies/ml [13]. None of the patients treated with ZDV + 3TC achieved this target.

Recent work has confirmed, on the basis of clinical end-points, the superiority of three-drug combinations. Treatment with ZDV + 3TC + IND significantly slowed the progression of HIV disease in patients with a CD4 count less than 200 × 10^6/l compared to ZDV + 3TC, significantly reducing both the percentage of patients with disease progression to AIDS or death (6% vs 11%) and mortality (1.4% vs 3.1%) [14].

Antiretroviral regimens

The initial regimen recommended by the International AIDS Society-USA Panel (June 1997) as most likely to reduce and maintain plasma HIV RNA levels below the level of detection (ie less than 400 copies/ml) consists of two nucleoside analogues plus a protease inhibitor with high *in vivo* potency [5].

Some potential combinations are shown in Table 5. Certain rules should be observed. When two nucleosides are combined, they should not have overlapping toxicities (see Table 3) or be activated by similar phosphorylation pathways as they would then compete for the same enzymes. Combinations including ZDV + d4T and 3TC + ddC should therefore be avoided. All initial regimens should include either ZDV or d4T which cross the blood-brain barrier to a greater extent than other anti-HIV drugs. The possibility of cross-resistance must also be taken into consideration. The development of ZDV resistance – which appears to be an independent risk factor for disease progression – may be delayed by concurrent treatment with 3TC; the combination of ZDV + 3TC is therefore an attractive option. On the other

Table 5 Initial antiretroviral therapy.

• 2 Nucleoside analogues with a protease inhibitor				
ZDV		ddI		IND
	+	ddC	+	NEL
d4T		3TC		RIT
• 2 Nucleoside analogues with a non-nucleoside reverse transcriptase inhibitor				
ZDV		ddI		NVP
	+	ddC	+	
d4T		3TC		DEL

For explanation of drug abbreviations, see Table 3.

hand, early use of 3TC may limit the future efficacy of both ddC and ddI, and ZDV + ddI may thus also be used as initial therapy. Recently, d4T + ddI has been demonstrated to be a potent nucleoside combination.

Similar considerations apply when choosing which protease inhibitor to include in a triple therapy regimen. Pharmacokinetic issues include bioavailability, tolerability and drug interactions [15]. The bioavailability of RIT (75%), IND (13–70%) and NEL (17–47%) is satisfactory, whereas the soft gelatin preparation of SQV is only 4% bioavailable and results in very low SQV plasma levels in some patients. Tolerability is also important: a discontinuation rate of 28% has been described for RIT (due to the high incidence of side effects, ie fever, weight loss, gastrointestinal disturbance), compared with 10% for SQV and 5% for IND. The protease inhibitors may inhibit the enzyme cytochrome P450 (CYP P450), so interactions may occur with other drugs metabolised by CYP P450. Some frequently used for the treatment of patients with HIV include other protease inhibitors, macrolide antibiotics and azole antifungal agents. RIT is a potent inhibitor of CYP P450, and its potential for drug interactions may limit its use. The development of cross-resistance among the protease inhibitors must also be considered. Use of IND may select for cross-resistance to RIT and vice versa. Although triple therapy with two nucleosides and a protease inhibitor is the regimen of choice, the recommended alternative is a combination of two nucleosides plus a non-nucleoside reverse transcriptase inhibitor (NNRTI). Use of currently available NNRTIs is maximised when combined with other drugs in patients previously untreated with antiretroviral drugs. The NNRTIs have good bioavailability (eg NVP (90%) and DEL (85%)), and are extensively metabolised by CYP P450. Drug interactions are likely to occur if prescribed together with protease inhibitors, as NVP is an inducer and DEL an inhibitor of CYP P450. Patients who are not candidates for triple therapy but are at high risk of disease progression should begin with dual nucleoside therapy, for example, ZDV + 3TC.

Alternative antiretroviral regimens for treatment failure

Indications of treatment failure include a lack of initial virological response, return of plasma HIV RNA to pretreatment levels, declining CD4 count or clinical progression. In patients who have achieved viral load reduction to below the conventional limit of detection (400 copies/ml), a subsequent increase in plasma HIV RNA to greater than 2,000–5,000 copies/ml is an indication to change therapy. For those who had a significant decrease in plasma HIV RNA initially, but not to below 400 copies/ml, a rise to greater than 5,000–10,000 copies/ml should indicate a treatment change. A triple-therapy regimen will generally reduce HIV RNA within 2–4 weeks. However, patients with a high pretreatment viral load may not achieve maximal suppression until 12–24 weeks after commencing therapy, and care must therefore be taken not to abandon a given regimen too early.

The guiding principle when changing therapy is to change all three drugs, or at least to include a minimum of two new drugs in the revised regimen. The addition of a single drug to a regimen which has failed is strongly discouraged; it is considered equivalent to sequential monotherapy, and is likely to facilitate the rapid emergence of viral resistance. The best alternative protease inhibitor after the failure of an initial regimen including one of these agents is unknown. Cross-resistance between IND and RIT is almost complete, and use of one will limit the subsequent use of the other, but the use of either drug may not select for cross-resistance to NEL. An NNRTI is unlikely to produce undetectable HIV RNA levels in patients previously exposed to antiretroviral drugs. One alternative is the combination of the protease inhibitors RIT + SQV, with a reduced dose of SQV as its metabolism is inhibited by RIT. Examples of alternative antiretroviral therapy following treatment failure are shown in Table 6.

Table 6 Alternative antiretroviral regimens for treatment failure.

Regimen	
Initial	**Alternative**
ZDV + ddI + IND	d4T + 3TC + NLF d4T + 3TC + NVP RIT + SQV + 3TC
ZDV + 3TC + IND	d4T + ddI + NLF d4T + ddI + NVP RIT + SQV + d4T
d4T + 3TC + IND	ZDV + ddI + NLF ZDV + ddI + NVP RIT + SQV + ZDV
ZDV + ddI + NVP	d4T + 3TC + IND ZDV + 3TC + IND

For explanation of drug abbreviations, see Table 3.

□ CONCLUSION

When treating patients with HIV disease, the aim is maximal suppression of HIV replication for as long as possible. The ability to determine plasma HIV RNA and the availability of new potent anti-HIV drugs facilitate this aim. The current standard of care for HIV patients is a three-drug combination consisting of two nucleoside analogues plus a protease inhibitor. As a result of the recent changes outlined above, there are now fewer HIV-related deaths and opportunistic infections, in addition to a reduction in hospital admissions and lengths of stay in the USA and Europe.

However, 90% of people with HIV infection live in the developing world and have little or no access to these expensive antiretroviral drugs. This would partly explain recent estimates that 2.3 million people died of AIDS in 1997 – a 50% increase over 1996. Current antiretroviral therapy enables us to treat HIV infection, but does not provide a cure. In view of the limited availability of these drugs to many millions of patients, much work needs to be done.

REFERENCES

1 Report on the Global HIV/AIDS epidemic. UNAIDS Global HIV/AIDS and STD. Surveillance Report, 1997: 1–21.

2 AIDS/HIV Quarterly Surveillance Table, UK (date to end September 1997). *PHLS AIDS Centre Report* 1997; **37**: 1–30.

3 Feinberg M. Changing the natural history of HIV disease. *Lancet* 1996; **348**: 239–46.

4 Mellors JW, Rinaldo CR, Gupta P, *et al.* Prognosis in HIV-1 infection predicted by the quantity of virus in plasma. *Science* 1996; **272**: 1167–70.

5 Carpenter CCJ, Fiscl MA, Hammer SM, *et al.* Antiretroviral therapy for HIV infection in 1997. *JAMA* 1997; **277**: 1962–9.

6 Hammer SM, Katzenstein DA, Hughes MD, *et al.* A trial comparing nucleoside monotherapy with combination therapy in HIV infected adults with CD4 cell counts from 200–500 per cubic millimeter. *N Engl J Med* 1996; **335**: 1081–90.

7 Delta Coordinating Committee. DELTA; a randomised double blind controlled trial comparing combinations of zidovudine plus didanosine or zalcitabine with zidovudine alone in HIV infected individuals. *Lancet* 1996; **348**: 283–91.

8 Caesar Coordinating Committee. Randomised trial of addition of lamivudine plus loviride to zidovudine-containing regimens for patients with HIV-1 infection: the CAESAR trial. *Lancet* 1997; **349**: 1413–21.

9 Saravolatz LD, Winslow DL, Collins G, *et al.* Zidovudine alone or in combination with didanosine or zalcitabine in HIV infected patients with the acquired immunodeficiency syndrome or fewer than 200 CD4 cells per cubic millimeter. *N Engl J Med* 1996; **335**: 1099–106.

10 Carpenter CCJ, Fisol MA, Hammer SM, *et al.* Antiretroviral therapy for HIV infection in 1996. *JAMA* 1996; **276**: 146–54.

11 Cameron DW, Heath-Chiozzi M, Kravcik S, *et al.* Prolongation of life and prevention of AIDS complications in advanced HIV immunodeficiency with ritonavir, update. XI international Conference on AIDS, Vancouver July 7–12, 1996 (abstract Mo. B 411).

12 Collier AC, Coombs RW, Schoenfeld DA, *et al.* Treatment of human immunodeficiency virus infection with saquinavir, zidovudine and zalcitabine. *N Engl J Med* 1996; **334**: 1011–7.

13 Gulick RM, Mellors JW, Havlir D, *et al.* Treatment with indinavir, zidovudine and lamivudine in adults with human immunodneficiency virus infection and prior antiretroviral therapy. *N Engl J Med* 1997; **337**: 734–9.

14 Hammer SM, Squires KE, Hughes MD, *et al.* A controlled trial of two nucleoside analogues plus indinavir in persons with human immunodeficiency virus infection and CD4 cell counts of 200 per cubic millimeter or less. *N Engl J Med* 1997; **337**: 725–33.

15 Barry M, Gibbons S, Back D, Mulcahy F. Protease inhibitors in patients with HIV disease: clinically important pharmacokinetic onsiderations. *Clin Pharmacokinetics* 1997; **32**: 194–209.

□ MULTIPLE CHOICE QUESTIONS

1 Plasma HIV RNA (copies/ml):
- (a) Accurately reflects the extent of viral replication
- (b) Levels are constant throughout all stages of HIV disease
- (c) May be in excess of 10^7 copies/ml during primary HIV
- (d) Will frequently lie between 10^3 and 10^5 copies/ml at steady state
- (e) At steady state is of significant prognostic value

2 The following are useful in predicting disease progression in HIV patients:
 (a) Baseline CD4 T cell count
 (b) CD4 counts >500 × 10^6/l
 (c) Plasma HIV RNA levels
 (d) Onset of HIV-related symptoms
 (e) Rapidly falling CD4 T cell count

3 Antiretroviral therapy is indicated for patients with:
 (a) Plasma HIV RNA levels >5,000–10,000 copies/ml
 (b) Symptomatic HIV disease
 (c) Rapidly declining CD4 T cell counts
 (d) CD4 T cell counts >500 × 10^6/l and plasma HIV RNA levels <5,000 copies/ml
 (e) HIV seroconversion illness

4 The following drugs inhibit the HIV reverse transcriptase enzyme:
 (a) Zidovudine
 (b) Saquinavir
 (c) Nevirapine
 (d) Nelfinavir
 (e) Lamivudine

5 When treating patients with HIV disease:
 (a) Combination therapy is preferable to monotherapy
 (b) The combination of zidovudine and stavudine should be avoided
 (c) The efficacy of antiretroviral therapy is maximised when prescribed for patients with advanced disease
 (d) Non-nucleoside reverse transcriptase inhibitors are best reserved for antiretroviral-experienced patients
 (e) Cross-resistance among the protease inhibitors is not considered to be a problem

ANSWERS

1a True	2a False	3a True	4a True	5a True
b False	b False	b True	b False	b True
c True	c True	c True	c True	c False
d True	d True	d False	d False	d False
e True	e True	e True	e True	e False

The Watson-Smith Lecture
Intestinal stem-cell repertoire: from normal gut development to the origins of colonic cancer

Nicholas A Wright

☐ INTRODUCTION

Stem cells lay down the many cell lineages which form tissues and organs during embryonic life, and are responsible for the continued production of cells in tissues where *constant renewal* is a feature, notably bone marrow and epithelia. The study of *epithelial* stem cells is important, not only because epithelia cover most of the body's surface and line its cavities, but also because most human tumours derive from epithelial tissues and stem cells are intimately involved in carcinogenic mechanisms.

One of the more important characteristics claimed for intestinal stem cells is *pluripotentiality*, or the ability to give rise to cells of more than one lineage. Until comparatively recently, direct evidence for pluripotent stem cells in the gut was lacking, and even now there is little or no idea of the mechanisms which decide cell fate in gut epithelia. Pluripotentiality may have practical therapeutic importance as well as theoretical interest. For example, introducing a gene into an epithelial sheet to correct an inherited defect (such as transfection of the cystic fibrosis transmembrane conductance regulator (CFTR) into the pseudostratified epithelium of the tracheo-bronchial tree; see chapter 27) will have little lasting effect if the cells targeted are merely transit cells destined for early elimination; by contrast, targeting of the stem cell would ensure persistence of the gene in the epithelium.

☐ BASIC CONCEPTS: STEM CELLS AND EPITHELIAL RENEWAL

The renewal systems of gastrointestinal epithelia are based upon tubules of various types. The simplest tubule design is the crypt of the colon, which is closed at one end while the other opens on to the luminal surface (Fig. 1a). The arrangement in the small intestine is similar, but here the surface bears projections (villi), covered with a single layered sheet of epithelium continuous with the underlying crypts (Fig. 1b). In the stomach, longer tubules (gastric glands) open on to the surface as foveolae (Fig. 1c).

An important first concept is that stem cells in the gut are located in specific sites that mark the origin of the cell flux. In the small intestinal crypt, cells migrate from the base of the crypt and emerge on to the villi; consequently, the basal crypt cells (or a subset of these) are candidate stem cells. In the gastric gland, the kinetic arrangements are quite different; cell proliferation is confined to the upper-middle

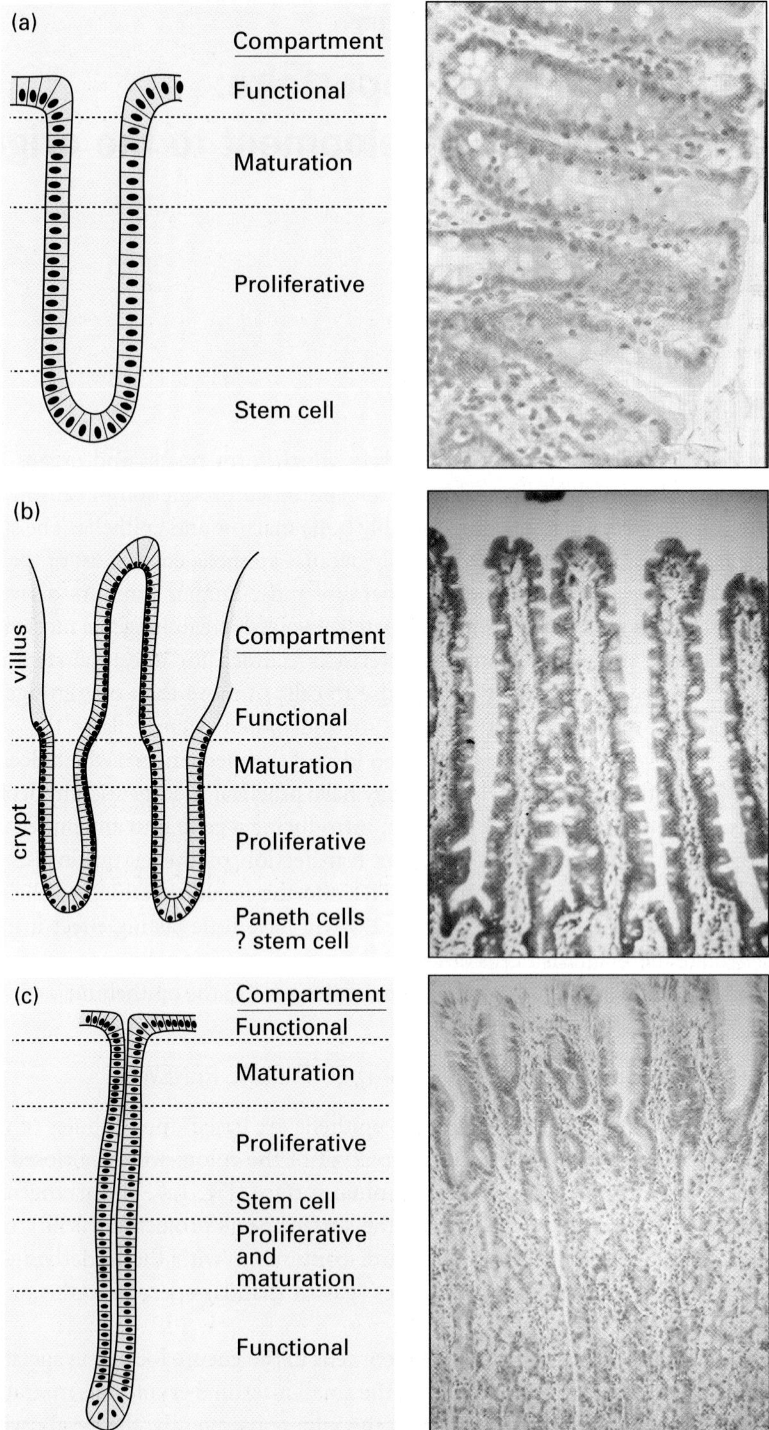

Fig. 1 Histological appearance and organisation of **(a)** the colon; **(b)** the small intestine; **(c)** the acid-secreting gastric mucosa.

portion of the tubule (where candidate stem cells may reside) and cells are thought to migrate bi-directionally to supply both the gastric surface and the base of the tubule. In the colon, there is evidence for both basally sited stem cells in some areas and, more recently, for bi-directional migration from stem cells in the middle of the crypt, as in the gastric glands.

Another key proposal is that stem cells are scarce within the tubules. The actual number of stem cells in each tubule remains uncertain, but many studies indicate that the clonogenic population of cells capable of regenerating a crypt (eg after severe irradiation damage) is small compared with the total number of proliferating cells in the crypt. Moreover, experiments with mutagens, which induce phenotypic changes in colonic and small intestinal crypts, can best be explained by mutations induced in a single, or a very small number, of stem cells (see below).

This chapter will explore the characteristics of stem cells as exemplified in the gastrointestinal tract, and will emphasise the wide functional repertoire of gut stem cells. I hope to demonstrate that:

- Gut stem cells give rise to all intestinal cell lineages.
- Gut stem cells can be induced in certain circumstances to develop 'reparative' lineages, which produce a series of 'trefoil' peptides that promote mucosal repair.
- In both the developing and adult gut, stem cells are responsible for the growth of new crypts and glands.
- Stem cells play a role in the development of colonic cancer.

CELL LINEAGES IN THE GUT EPITHELIUM ARE DERIVED FROM PLURIPOTENTIAL STEM CELLS

Several lines of evidence support the view that stem cells can give rise to multiple lineages. The first is the *in vitro* differentiation of transformed human colorectal cells.

Pluripotential colorectal carcinoma cell lines

Neoplastic proliferations rarely consist of one cell type, and this has led to the erroneous but often-cited conclusion that, since tumours are held to be monoclonal in origin, the contained cell lineages must be the progeny of a single stem cell. On the other hand, valid experiments have attempted to show that malignant cells derived from colorectal carcinomas can differentiate into the several cell lineages found in the normal colonic crypt. The most convincing report, by Cox and Pierce [1], claimed that putatively single cells from a rat colonic adenocarcinoma injected subcutaneously into mice occasionally gave rise to tumours which showed all colonic cell lineages. Kirkland [2] addressed this question in the human HRA19 cell line, derived from a moderately well-differentiated colorectal carcinoma. In culture, HRA 19 cells form a polarised monolayer of epithelial cells and displaying neuroendocrine differentiation, with positive immunostaining for specific markers of endocrine cells

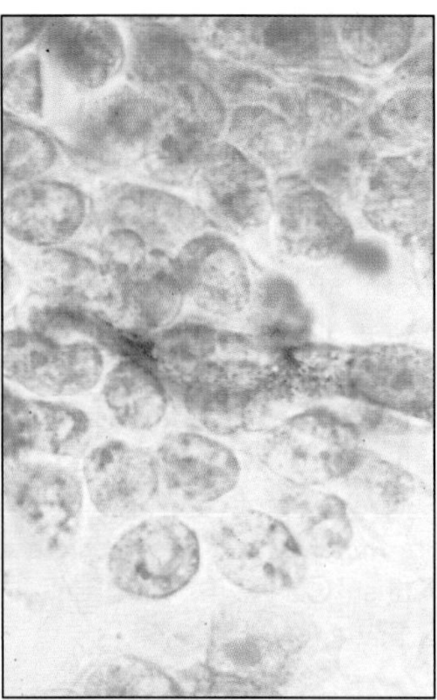

Fig. 2 An endocrine cell, immunostained with chromogranin A, growing in a culture of HRA-19 cells. Note the typical bipolar morphology. (Courtesy of Dr Susan Kirkland.)

such as chromogranin A (Fig. 2). Single cells were selected with a Pasteur pipette, confirmed by direct observation, and grown in culture together with 'feeder cells' (lethal-irradiated fibroblasts) to promote growth. To ensure the single-cell origin of the cloned cell line, the cloning procedure was repeated. Sizeable tumours formed four months after grafting these cloned epithelial cells into the subcutaneous tissue of the nude mouse (Fig. 3a). These tumours contained both columnar and goblet cells (Fig. 3b), together with typical triangular neuroendocrine cells identified by their positive argentophil (Grimelius) reaction (Fig. 3c) and chromogranin A immunostaining (Fig. 3d). The human origin of these endocrine cells was confirmed using double-labelling with the Grimelius stain and the Hoechst dye 1068 [2], which enables mouse cells to be clearly distinguished from human cells. Thus, a single epithelial cell, albeit malignant, can give rise to all cell types seen in the colorectal epithelium.

Allophenic tetraparental chimaeric mice

In this technique, two strains of mice are selected, one of which bears a marker specific for the tissue of interest. Fertilised zygotes from each strain are treated with pronase and, on incubation, form a single zygote. These chimaeric zygotes are introduced into the uterus of a pseudopregnant female (previously mated with a vasectomised male), and the resulting pups are chimaeras of the two strains selected. The origins of the intestine can be studied, thanks to a polymorphism at the *Dlb-1* locus (on chromosome 1) which affects the lectin-binding capacity of the intestinal epithelium: mice of the C57BL strains bind *Dolichos biflorus* agglutinin (DBA) (a lectin which selectively recognises the N-acetylgalactosamine residues present in

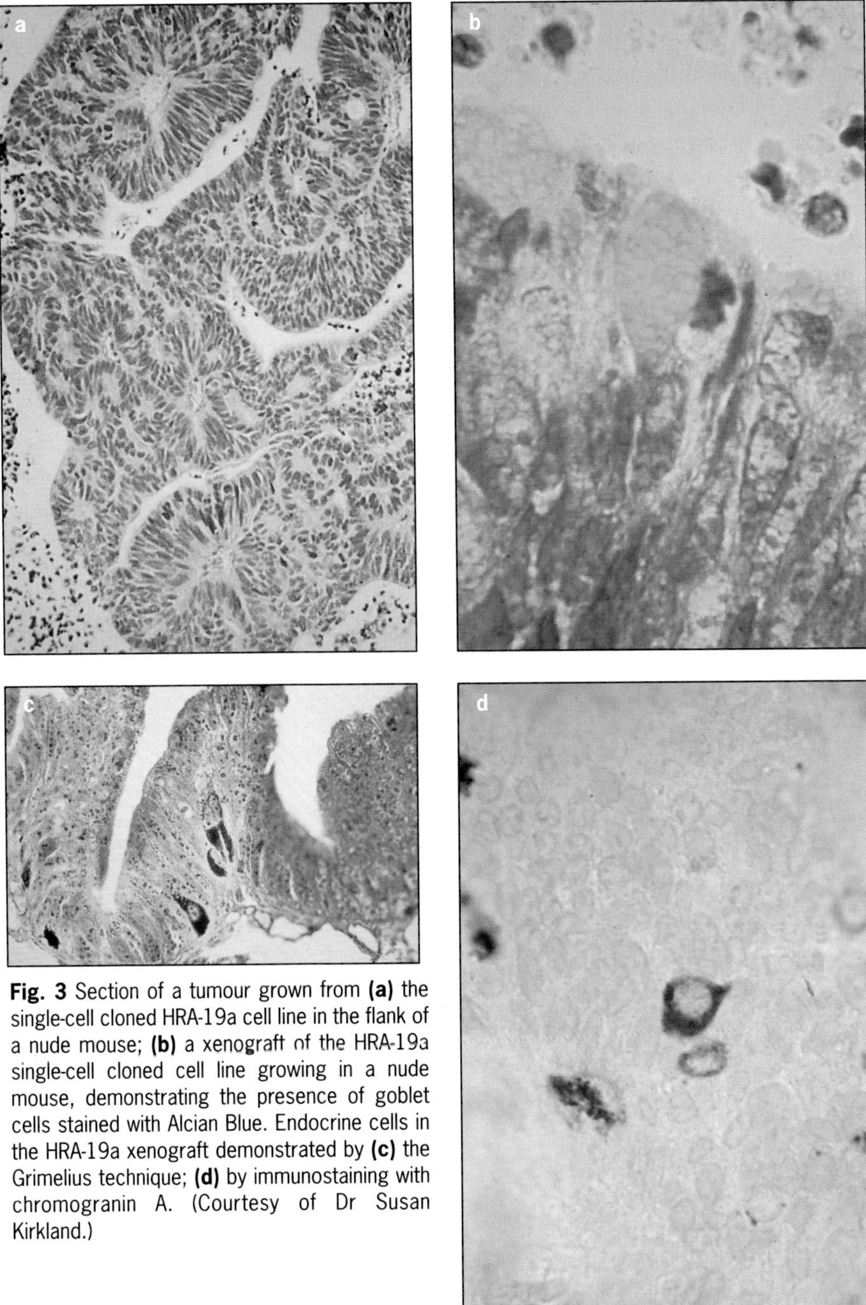

Fig. 3 Section of a tumour grown from **(a)** the single-cell cloned HRA-19a cell line in the flank of a nude mouse; **(b)** a xenograft of the HRA-19a single-cell cloned cell line growing in a nude mouse, demonstrating the presence of goblet cells stained with Alcian Blue. Endocrine cells in the HRA-19a xenograft demonstrated by **(c)** the Grimelius technique; **(d)** by immunostaining with chromogranin A. (Courtesy of Dr Susan Kirkland.)

blood-group antigens on the cell surfaces), while other strains (eg RIII/Lac-*ro* and DDK) do not.

Staining the small intestine and colon of these chimaeric mice with DBA shows a remarkable picture, with each crypt being either positive or negative; no mixed crypts were detected in adult mice after observing tens of thousands of crypts [3] (Fig. 4). Each crypt must constitute a clonal population, being ultimately derived from a single cell; goblet cells and Paneth cells must also share in this clonality (Fig. 4). In neonatal animals (up to two weeks of age) mixed crypts are found, but these quickly disappear. It thus appears that crypts are pleoclonal or polyclonal during development: multiple stem cells contribute to individual crypts which then reorganise themselves to become monoclonal. The mechanisms of 'cleansing' of the crypts are unknown, but may include overgrowth and extrusion of one stem cell lineage by another, or – since there is extremely active replication of crypts by fission at this time – segregation of the lineages could occur at this point.

The concept of the monoclonal crypt implies that a single multipotential stem gives rise to all cell lineages contained in the crypt. Theoretically, however, cells from each partner in the chimaera could segregate independently during development, so that apparently monoclonal crypts might be merely monophenotypic. This view is contradicted by female mice heterozygous for a defective glucose-6-phosphate (G6PD), a gene carried on the X chromosome and therefore subject to random

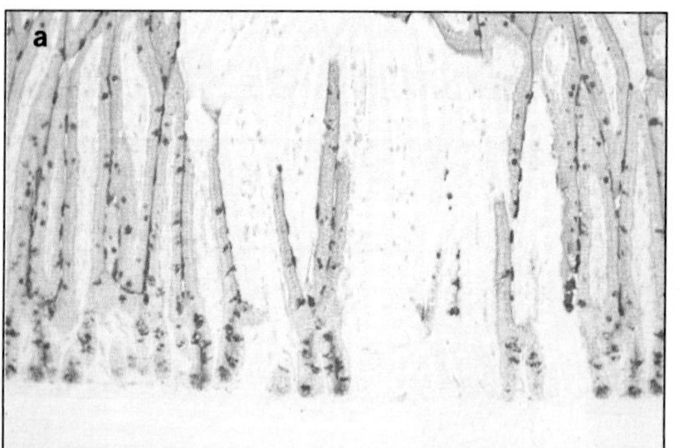

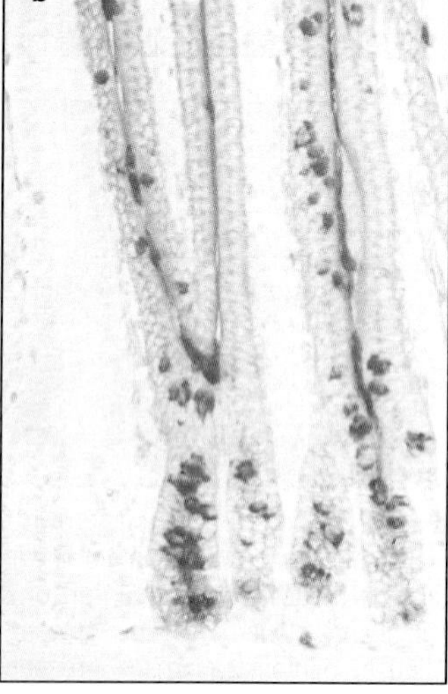

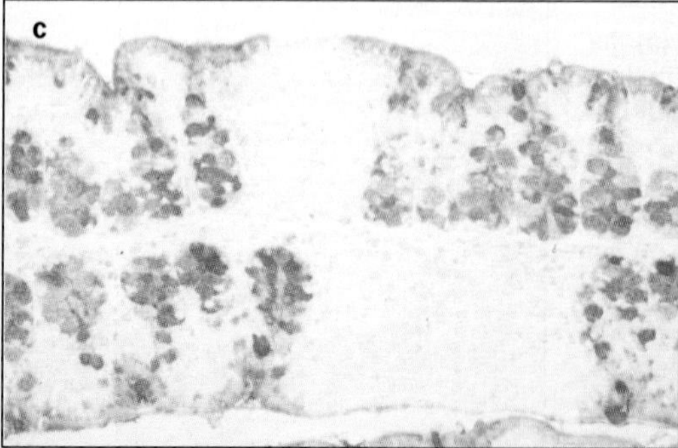

Fig. 4 Section **(a)** from the jejunal mucosa; **(b)** a higher-power view; **(c)** from colon of a tetraparental allophenic mouse stained with the lectin *Dolichos biflorus* agglutinin (DBA) which differentiates between the two types of cells present in the chimaera. In both tissues, each crypt is either totally positive or totally negative, indicating that it was originally the progeny of a single cell or group of cells of the same type. This supports the concept of a clonal origin of crypts. The polymorphism is also shown in the endothelial cells. (Photographed from a preparation made available through the courtesy of Professor B Ponder.)

inactivation of one copy ('lyonisation'). These animals show a crypt-restricted pattern of G6PD histochemical staining; the crypts are also monophenotypic, with no examples of mixed crypts. This confirms the conclusion that crypts are derived from a single stem cell, in this case either showing normal G6PD expression or lacking it.

The same technique was used to address this issue in the stomach. Thompson *et al* [4] employed *XY/XO* mouse chimaeras, and identified the male component of the chimaera using *in situ* hybridisation with a digoxigenin-labelled probe pY 353 that labelled the highly repetitive sequences of the mouse Y chromosome. Figure 5 shows clearly that gastric glands in the mouse, as with intestinal crypts, are clonally derived.

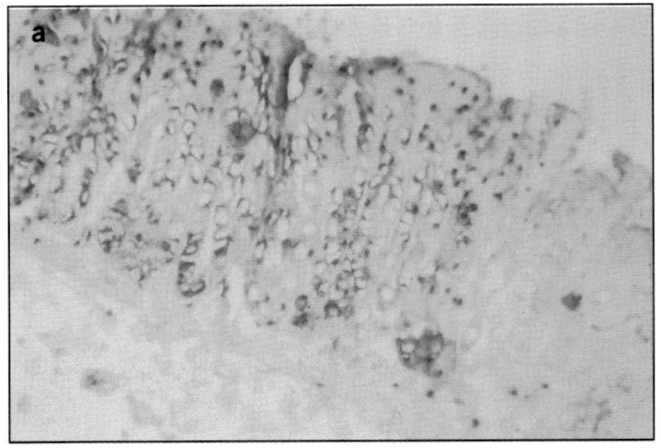

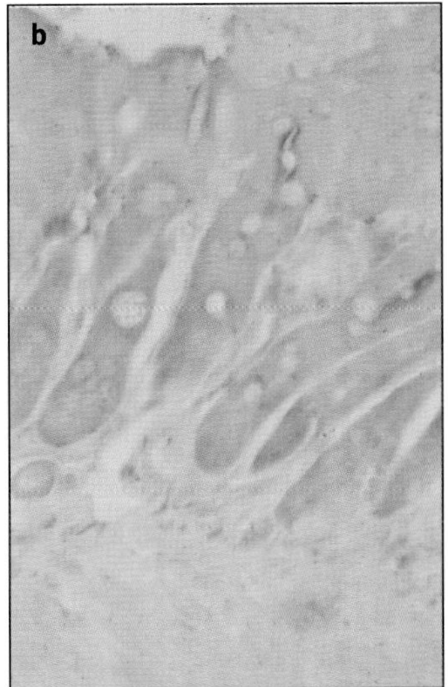

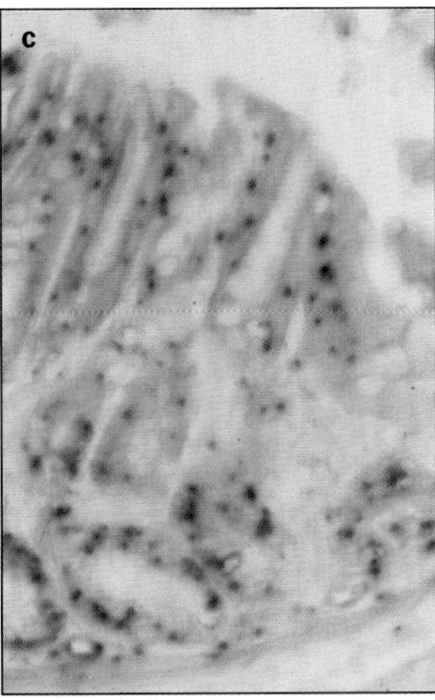

Fig. 5 (a) Low-power view of a section of the stomach of an *XX/XY* chimaeric mouse, with *in situ* hybridisation to demonstrate the highly repetitive sequences in the mouse *Y* chromosome using a digoxigenin-labelled probe (blue spots). Contiguous 'male' and 'female' areas are readily seen. The same technique was combined with immunostaining for gastrin (red) in **(b)** a female area showing endocrine cells which do not bear a blue spot (indicating their female nature); **(c)** a male area containing definitive male endocrine cells. (Courtesy of Dr Mary Thompson.)

Induced stem cell mutations: implications for stem-cell repertoire

The effects of mutagens have also been exploited to study stem-cell behaviour [5]. When mice showing uniform staining for DBA or G6PD are given a single dose of mutagen, over several weeks crypts appear which are apparently composed of cells with a different, mutated phenotype. These experiments initially show a rapid but transient increase in crypts with a partial, or segmented, mutated phenotype (Fig. 6a). Later, there is an increase in the frequency of crypts showing a completely or wholly mutated phenotype, an increase which plateaus contemporaneously with the disappearance of partially or segmented crypts (Fig. 6b). Interestingly, the small intestine and colon show a major difference in the timing of these events: the plateau is reached at 5–7 weeks in the colon but not until 12 weeks in the small intestine. The emergence of the partially mutated crypts, and their replacement by wholly mutated crypts, can be explained by a mutation at the *DlB-1* or G6PD locus in the single stem from which all lineages are derived. The partially mutated crypts may thus be in the process of being colonised by progeny from the mutated stem cell, and will ultimately develop into a wholly mutated crypt. Alternatively, some of these

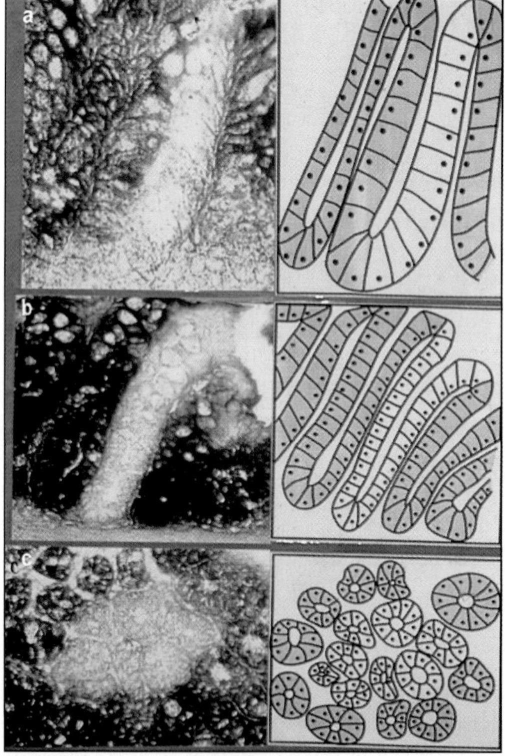

Fig. 6 Sections from the colon of a mouse treated with a single injection of the mutagen ethylnitrosourea (ENU), and histochemically stained for glucose-6-phosphatase activity; **(a)** a crypt in which only a portion stains positive; **(b)** a wholly negative crypt without any positive cells; **(c)** a patch of negative-staining cells. The patterns of distribution are also shown schematically. (Courtesy of Dr Hyun Sook Park.)

partially mutated crypts could derive from mutations in non-stem proliferative cells, which would later disappear as the mutated clone was lost through migration out of the crypt.

These experiments again indicate that a single stem cell can give rise to all crypt lineages, in both colon and small intestine.

Origin of gut endocrine cells

The origin of gut endocrine cells has been disputed for over forty years. As discussed above, endocrine cells in neoplastic tissues can derive from a single epithelial cell (ie an endodermally derived stem cell). This view is supported by classical embryological observations and detailed observations of carcinoid tumours. A unifying concept was proposed by Pearse [6], as part of the 'APUD' cell hypothesis that identified certain cytochemical similarities of apparently unrelated cells, such as fluorogenic Amine content, amine Precursor Uptake and amino-acid Decarboxylase; specific enzymes, notably α-glycerophosphate dehydrogenase, non-specific esterase and/or cholinesterase; side-chain carboxyl groups; the presence of endocrine secretory granules; and specific immunocytochemical reactions, including chromogranin A positivity. Cells with these properties included not only gastrointestinal and pancreatic endocrine cells, but also others of proven neural-crest origin such as phaeochromocytes from the adrenal medulla, cells from sympathetic ganglia and cutaneous melanocytes, and thyroid C cells. This hypothesis proposes that the common properties of these cells indicate a common embryological origin, and that neuroendocrine stem cells from the neural crest colonise the developing gut and maintain the endocrine cell lineage separate from the other crypt cell lineages.

In the above model used by Thompson *et al* [4], gastrin-producing endocrine cells (G cells) in the antral stomach were identified by specific immunostaining. The male and female areas of the chimaeric stomach were easily recognisable by staining for the Y-chromosome. From Fig. 5, it is clear that male gastric glands contained G cells which were exclusively Y-spot positive (Fig. 5a), while female areas contained G cells which were Y-spot negative (Fig. 5c). Gut endocrine cells must therefore share the same clonal origin as the other cell types.

Cell lineage in the human gastrointestinal mucosa

The human gut had not been forthcoming on these issues until a recent report by Novelli *et al* [7] describing a rare, if not unique, individual with both the mosaic genotype *XO/XY* and familial adenomatous polyposis (FAP). This was an extremely serendipitous discovery, as the frequency of this combination of genetic defects is less than 1 in 10^{-8}. This phenotypic male had short stature but no other stigmata of Turner's syndrome. He had undergone a prophylactic total colectomy at 32 years of age, from which archival paraffin-embedded material was available. The clinical diagnosis of FAP was confirmed by mutation analysis of his *APC* gene, which demonstrated a frameshift mutation in codon 1309 in the germline. A combination of karyotyping and fluorescent *in situ* hybridisation (FISH) on the patient's peripheral blood lymphocytes confirmed that he was a mosaic, with approximately 20% of peripheral blood lymphocytes being XO, and also showed the *Y* chromosome to be dicentric. The detailed karyotype was 45,X/46,Xdic (*Y*) (*Y*pter→cen→*Y*q11.23::*Y*p11.3).

In situ hybridisation with *Y* chromosome-specific probes on histological sections of small and large intestine showed that intestinal crypts were composed exclusively of either *XY* or *XO* cells (Fig. 7a). The patches of *XO* crypts were irregular in shape and their size varied widely (mean patch width 1.85 crypts, range 1–14 crypts). Crypts examined at patch borders showed no mixed *XO/XY* cellularity and indigenous epithelial cell lineages could be directly visualised as *XO* or *XY*, including columnar cells, goblet cells (Fig. 7b) and endocrine cells (Fig. 7c). Of the many thousands of crypts examined, four mixed crypts were seen in otherwise pure *XY* patches (Fig. 7d). This recalls the partial loss of O-acetylated sialomucins described in human colonic crypts and in mice given mutagens (see Fig. 6). This rare occurrence of mixed crypts is probably due to non-disjunction and loss of the *Y* chromosome, in a crypt stem cell. Thus, normal human intestinal crypts are clonal populations, each derived from a single, multipotential stem cell.

Histogenesis of reparative cell lineages

Chronic ulcers in the human intestine apparently induce tubular structures containing mucin-producing cells that are different from the indigenous cell lineages. These complex structures are confined to the lamina propria, arise close to the ulcer margins, and produce neutral mucin that stains positively with the diastase periodic acid Schiff (D/PAS) method, in contrast to the acid alcianophilic mucin produced by intestinal goblet cells. These cells have been identified on morphological grounds as 'pyloric' or 'pseudopyloric' metaplasia (or even as 'Brunner's gland' metaplasia), and the production of these cells was suggested in some way to protect the mucosa.

Recent morphological, immunohistochemical and *in situ* hybridisation studies have shown that these cells indeed have novel properties and are not merely metaplastic. They have a distinct life history, during which they sequentially express differentiation antigens that define a specific phenotype; they also synthesise and secrete large amounts of regulatory peptides of considerable interest (see below). The presence of these cells in the ulcerated mucosa appears to induce peptide gene expression in the local intestinal cells, and they also develop their own proliferative organisation [8]. For these reasons, it has been proposed that these cells – although differentiation progeny of the intestinal stem cells – constitute a specific 'ulcer-associated cell lineage' (UACL) in their own right.

On morphological grounds, the UACL clearly arises from intestinal stem cells located in the crypt base. It appears first as small, intensely D/PAS-positive buds at the base of the intestinal crypts adjacent to an ulcer (Fig. 8a). These buds push outwards into the surrounding stroma of the lamina propria as small tubules, which quickly join with tubules from other crypts to form a more or less complex acinar arrangement (Fig. 8b). During induction of this lineage, monoclonal crypts contribute their progeny to form a polyclonal glandular network. It is interesting to

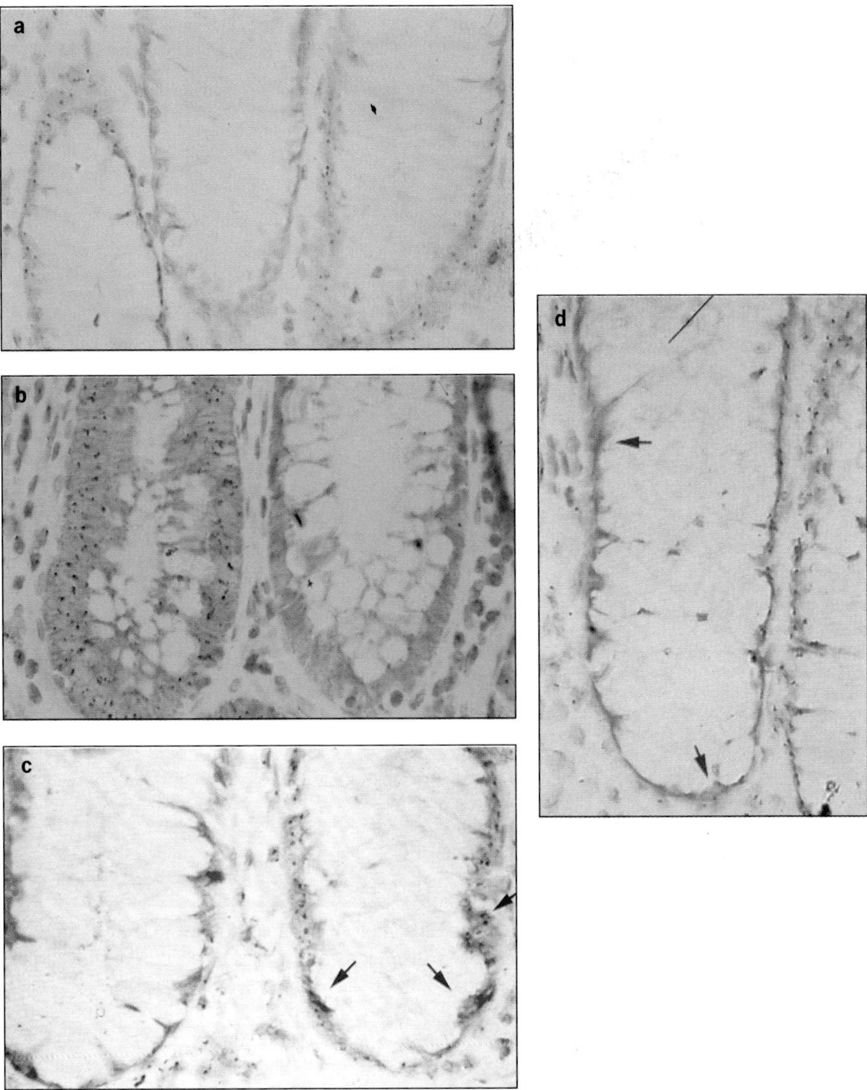

Fig. 7 Sections from a patient with the mosaic *XO/XY* phenotype [7], with the *XY* cell demonstrated by *in situ* hybridisation: **(a)** all cells positive or negative for the *Y* chromosome; **(b)** goblet cell clonality; **(c)** sections stained with chromogranin A for endocrine cells (red), showing clonal derivation; **(d)** a hemi-crypt which has lost nuclear staining for the *Y* chromosome. (Courtesy of Dr Marco Novelli.)

note the buds and acini at this stage are devoid of mitotic figures or proliferative activity, as assessed by specific staining with Ki67 and PCNA. In larger gland formations, ducts are formed by the joining of two or more smaller ductules, and they grow upwards through the core of an adjacent villus towards the epithelial surface (Fig. 8c), where they emerge through distinct pores. The UACL also moves

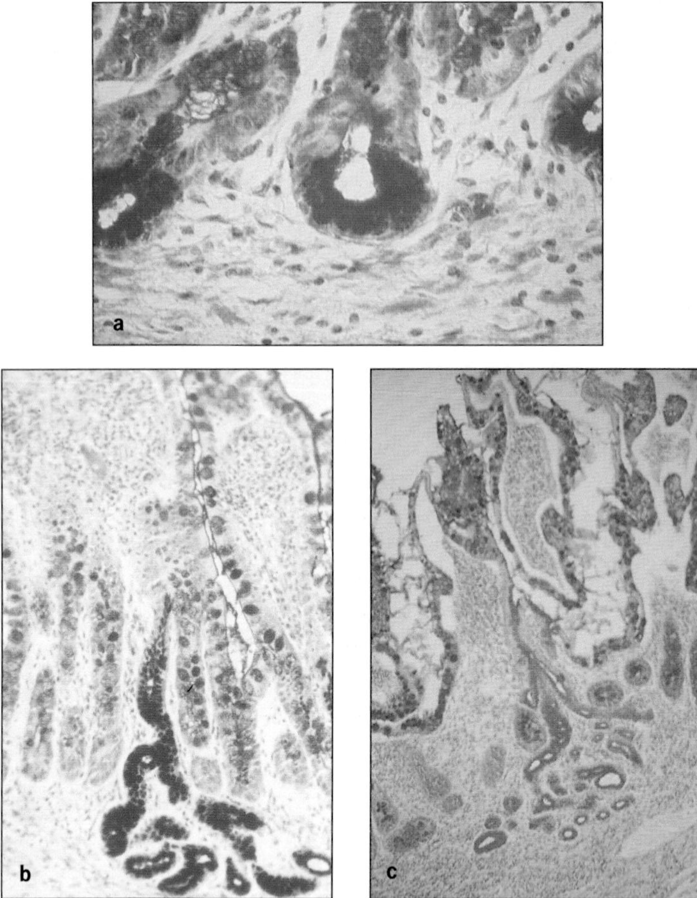

Fig. 8 (a) Early buds of the ulcer-associated cell lineage (UACL) (stained red with D/PAS) growing out of parent crypts close to an ulcerated area of the mucosa in Crohn's disease. Note the abrupt origin of the UACL cells from the stem cell zone and the absence of mitotic activity in the UACL cells; **(b)** a more developed acinar complex, growing as a newly formed gland in the lamina propria; **(c)** a mature UACL complex, showing the acinar area and the duct, with the UACL cells clothing the surface of a villus and displacing the indigenous cell lineages. Note the single goblet cell in the duct area. (Reproduced from Ref 9, with permission.)

out of the tubule and on to the villus surface, where it replaces the indigenous surface cell lineages (Fig. 8c). Ultimately, the entire villous surface can become covered with the UACL cells.

The UACL also express different secretory proteins, again dependent upon the position within the mucosa. The acinar portion contains abundant immunoreactive epidermal growth factor (EGF) [9], which is also found in its secretions and in Brunner's glands in the duodenum; EGF has powerful mitogenic actions on gut epithelial cells in animals and man. In addition, the UACL expresses all three 'trefoil' peptides (TFF1–3) found in the mammalian gut – peptides which have been shown to induce cell migration and may protect the mucosa [10]. The mRNAs for TFF2 (also known as hSP or spasmolytic peptide) and TFF1 (pS2) can be readily demonstrated by *in situ* hybridisation; TFF2/hSP mRNA is seen in the upper acini and lower duct cells, while TFF1/pS2 mRNA and protein are seen in large amounts in the upper duct and all surface cells. TFF3/intestinal trefoil factor (ITF) mRNA is abundant throughout the UACL. A further important protein produced and secreted by the UACL is lysozyme, which has considerable antibacterial action. Both lysozyme mRNA and protein are plentiful in the UACL.

Thus, intestinal stem cells are able to give rise to lineages which produce a range of peptides that help to heal mucosal damage.

□ STEM CELLS GIVE RISE TO NEW CRYPTS

It has been clear for some time that crypt fission is an important mechanism determining the number of crypts in the small intestine and colon. Initial studies indicated its pivotal position in two processes; the massive increase in crypt number which occurs in the post-natal period, and the recovery of the intestine from irradiation or cytotoxic chemotherapy. The morphology of the process can be followed in histological sections, but it is perhaps best seen in bulk-stained, microdissected material (Fig. 9). In many instances, crypt fission begins as an indentation at the extreme base of the crypt, and advances via a vertical split in the crypt which continues until two new crypts are produced. In some instances, the

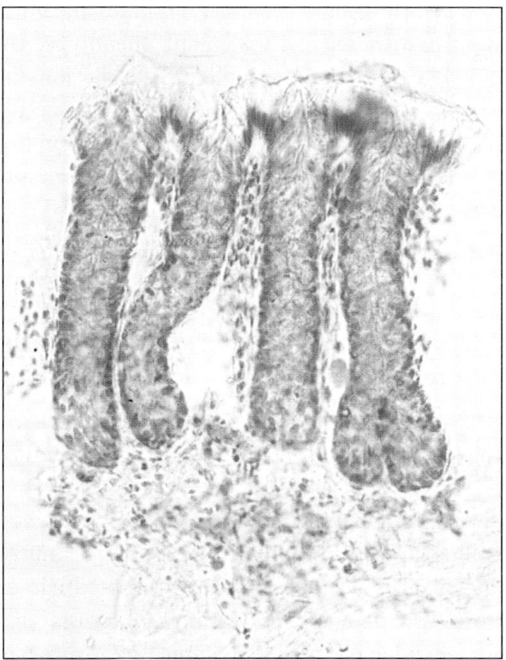

Fig. 9 A microdissected crypt, stained with Feulgen's reagent, showing the mode of crypt fission.

process begins asymmetrically with respect to the crypt axis; this 'budding' can be seen in apparently normal human colonic mucosa, but is more common in precancerous states such as FAP and rat colonic mucosa after systemic treatment with carcinogens such as 1,2-dimethylhydrazine (DMH). In some situations, notably after irradiation, multiple buds can originate from a single crypt.

The dynamics of crypt fission, described in a series of seminal papers by Totafurno and colleagues [11], has led to the concept of the 'crypt cycle'. The crypt, born by fission, gradually increases in size; after about 108 days in the mouse it undergoes fission, a process which takes about 12 hours. Measurements of crypt volume or size show that larger crypts initiate fission, suggesting that they have to reach a certain size before fission commences. This introduces the concept of a threshold size for the number of stem cells, above which crypt fission is initiated. In the human colon, the proportion of crypts in fission (the crypt fission index, *fi*) is small (~0.003%), and the crypt cycle time is apparently about 17 years. While not as clear as in the mouse, there is a tendency for the larger crypts to undergo fission.

We have followed above the changes which occur in the intestinal crypts of mice treated with mutagens such as ethylnitrosourea (ENU) or DMH, showing the gradual emergence of crypts which are partially and wholly negative for G6PD (Fig. 6a and b). It is significant that there is an increase with time in the number of negative patches, defined as a group of two or more negative crypts (Fig. 6c). There is also an increase in the size of the patches, particularly in the colon. It is therefore clear that the mechanism for expansion of these mutated clones is crypt fission.

In ulcerative colitis, dysplasia commonly precedes the carcinoma which is known to complicate the disease. In colonic dysplasia, crypt architecture is preserved, but these crypts are populated by cells of malignant phenotype. Using fluorescence-activated cell sorting (FACS) to analyse single-cell suspensions from these cases, it has been shown that considerable areas of colonic mucosa, exceeding 9 cm in length, contain crypts which have been colonised by the same aneuploid stem. Figure 6c shows that a single mutated clone (ie a crypt which contains a mutation at the G6PD locus) has enlarged by crypt fission to a group of eight mutated crypts. Extrapolation from here to the situation in ulcerative colitis will again lead to the conclusion that mutated clones in the human colon also spread by crypt fission. It is now also clear that the main mode of growth of colonic adenomas in FAP is by crypt fission, this time of the adenomatous crypts [12], providing a further example of a mutated clone spreading by the fission process.

Origins of intestinal carcinomas

Most cells in the gastrointestinal epithelium are short-lived, being destined for loss on the colonic or villus surface. Although the number of mutations necessary to provoke neoplastic change is debatable, the right-shifted age-distribution of the incidence of gastrointestinal neoplasms strongly suggests that this process is protracted. The only cells which remain in the mucosa for such a prolonged time are the self-renewing stem cells, whose progeny will carry the genetic material, including any non-lethal mutations, into successive rounds of cell divisions. Mainly for this reason, stem cells have been considered as carcinogen target cells.

Mutational theories of tumour development suggest that tumours arise from a series of mutations occurring in one cell and its progeny. Other theories argue that tumours are not clonal in origin but require the interaction of multiple cells, and that outgrowth of a dominant clone during subsequent development accounts for their apparent monoclonality. The colon of the XO/XY patient described above [7] contained thousands of tubular adenomas, ranging in size from lesions composed of a single dysplastic crypt (a monocryptal adenoma) to microadenomas 2.5 mm in diameter. Not surprisingly, given the clonal nature of normal crypts, the monocryptal adenomas were entirely *XO* or *XY* in type with no mixed pattern. However, 13 (5%) microadenomas contained a mixture of *XO* and *XY* dysplastic crypts (see Fig. 10), while 13 (76%) of the 17 adenomas containing *XO* dysplastic crypts were of mixed *XO/XY* type and four (24%) were purely *XO* genotype; these results suggested that at least 76% of all the adenomas (above monocryptal size) in this patient were polyclonal in origin. Analysis showed that the random collision of tumours could not account on their own for such high levels of polyclonality.

These results show that colonic tumours can be polyclonal, contrary to popular models of tumorigenesis. Studies of human colorectal tumours using X-linked markers in females and the principle of X-chromosome inactivation have produced conflicting results: isoenzyme studies of G6PD in microdissected tissue from heterozygous black females suggested that a single sporadic colonic carcinoma and seven colonic adenomas from three patients with Gardner's syndrome were polyclonal, while X-linked restriction fragment length polymorphisms suggested 50

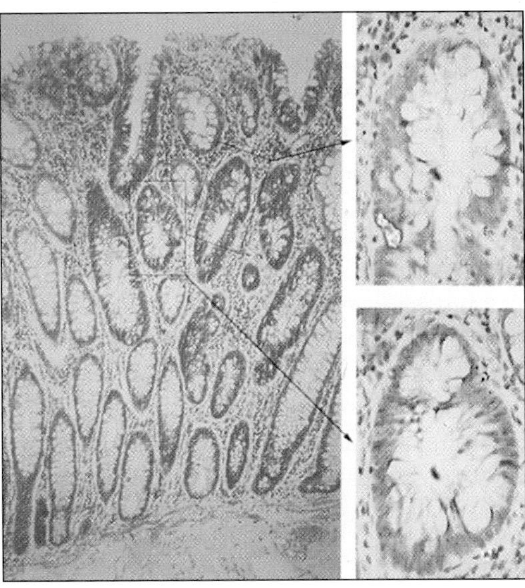

Fig. 10 A microadenoma from the mosaic *XO/XY* patient [7], showing adenomatous crypts in the same lesion which are either positive or negative for the *Y* chromosome. (Courtesy of Dr Marco Novelli.)

human colorectal tumours of both familial and sporadic types were all monoclonal. However, such X-linked markers, with biochemical or molecular analysis of extracted tissues, are probably inappropriate for determining clonality in dissected tissues from primary epithelial tumours: even microadenomas can contain stromal elements and entrapped normal crypts which complicates the interpretation of results. More importantly, patch size can vary widely, and unless those tumours arising at the junction between crypts displaying different genotypes can be directly observed, it becomes difficult, if not impossible, to make meaningful observations on tumour clonality. It follows that only analyses where tissues can be examined *in situ*, as in the patient described above, can conclusively determine tumour clonality. This may explain why results in this individual, with small patch size for the marker used, contrast so starkly with previous results; if the patch size for X-inactivation markers is large, most tumours will appear monoclonal, since they will arise from within the large patches. The chances of finding an adenoma arising at the junction of a patch will be small.

If these results can be generalised, they could have profound implications for our understanding of tumour clonality and the origin of human tumours. They have recently been confirmed [13] in a chimaera made from a *Min* mouse, which has an *APC* mutation, and a *Min*/ROSA mouse; on testing the clonality of the resulting intestinal adenomas, 79% were polyclonal. Novelli *et al* [7] and Merritt *et al* [13] have speculated on possible mechanisms of polyclonality in these lesions. 'Field' effects may cause adenomas to cluster ('non-random collision'), or there may be a passive process involving fusion of two or more *APC*-negative clones early in tumour development; the high frequency of mixed adenomas found in both studies is inconsistent with a random appearance of *APC*-negative clones in the mucosa, and suggests instead that some regions of the intestine have an increased potential for initiation [12]. On the other hand, multiple adenomatous clones may be required for (or strongly favour) early adenoma growth; or, perhaps more likely, early adenomas may induce adenomatous growth in surrounding crypts (this may apply especially in FAP since all cells already have a single *APC* mutation and perhaps some derangement of *APC* function). These latter scenarios imply active cooperation between clones.

The importance of these results, which may have basic implications for more generalised models of tumorigenesis, have been discussed by Merritt *et al* [13]. If an excess of one crypt must be involved to lead to adenoma formation, this would predict that not one but two pro-neoplastic 'hits' would be required in FAP, and four in sporadic adenomas. Adenomas in FAP do not make their appearance until several years after birth, even in an environment where dietary carcinogens are common, and a two- or three-hit model does not fit the age incidence for colorectal cancers. This hypothesis would suggest that at least four hits are required.

□ CONCLUSIONS

The key points of this chapter may be summarised as follows. Gastrointestinal stem cells are pluripotential and give rise to all cell lineages in the epithelium. After damage, gut stem cells produce reparative cell lineages which secrete a wide range of peptides which promote cell proliferation, migration and mucosal healing. An increase in stem cell number is considered to induce crypt fission and the proliferation of crypts; it is also the mode of spread of mutated clones in the colorectal mucosa. Carcinogenesis in the colon occurs through sequential mutations, possibly occurring in a single cell. A case has been made for this being the stem cell, although recent studies indicate that several stem cells may need to be so involved, since early lesions appear to be polyclonal in derivation.

In recent years, much progress has been made in defining the intestinal stem cell's repertoire. There has been much speculation, often on scant and inconclusive data, that 'stem cells' can generate multiple cell lineages in epithelial and other tissues, but it is difficult to show this. The challenge of the next few years will be to define and isolate this elusive stem cell, identify its properties, and define those mechanisms which induce it to produce individual cell lineages at particular times.

REFERENCES

1 Cox WF, Pierce GB. The endodermal origin of the endocrine cells of an adenocarcinoma of the colon of the rat. *Cancer* 1982; **50**: 1530–8.

2 Kirkland SC. Clonal origin of columnar, mucous and endocrine cell lineages in human colorectal epithelium. *Cancer* 1988; **61**: 1359–63.

3 Ponder BAJ, Schmidt GH, Wilkinson MM, *et al.* Derivation of mouse intestinal crypts from a single progenitor cell. *Nature* 1985; **313**: 689–91.

4 Thompson M, Fleming K, Evans DJ, Wright NA. Gastric endocrine cells share a clonal origin with other gastric cell lineages. *Development* 1990; **110**: 477–81.

5 Park HS, Goodlad RG, Wright NA. Crypt fission in the small intestine and colon: a mechanism of the emergence of transformed crypts after treatment with mutagens. *Am J Pathol* 1995: **147**: 1416–27.

6 Pearse AGE. The cytochemistry and ultrastructure of polypeptide-producing cells of the APUD cells series and the embryologic, physiologic and pathologic implications of the concept. *J Histochem Cytochem* 1969; **17**: 303–13.

7 Novelli MR, Williamson JA, Tomlinson IPM, *et al.* Polyclonal origin of colonic adenomas in an *XO/XY* patient with FAP. *Science* 1996; **272**: 1187–90.

8 Patel K, Hanby AM, Ahnen DJ, Playford RJ, Wright NA. The kinetic organisation of the ulcer associated cell lineage (UACL): delineation of a novel putative stem cell region. *J Epithelial Cell Biol* 1994; **3**: 156–60.

9 Wright NA, Pike C, Elia G. Induction of a novel epidermal growth factor-secreting cell lineage by mucosal ulceration in gastrointestinal stem cells. *Nature* 1990; **343**: 82–5.

10 Wright NA, Poulsom R, Stamp G, *et al.* Trefoil peptide gene expression in gastrointestinal epithelial cells in inflammatory bowel disease. *Gastroenterology* 1993; **104**: 12–20.

11 Totafurno J, Bjerknes M, Cheng H. The crypt cycle: evidence for crypt and villus production in the adult mouse small intestine. *Biophys J* 1987; **52**: 279–94.

12 Wasan H, Park H-S, Liu KC, *et al.* APC in the regulation of crypt fission. *J Pathol* 1998; **185**; 246–56.

13 Merritt AJ, Gould KA, Dove WF. Polyclonal structure of intestinal adenomas in APC^{Min}/+ mice with concomitant loss of APC+ from all tumor lineages. ***Proc Natl Acad Sci USA*** 1997; **94**: 13927–31.

Myeloma and other plasma cell dyscrasias: new ideas about pathogenesis and treatment

Charles R J Singer

☐ INTRODUCTION

The plasma cell dyscrasias are a heterogeneous group of disorders characterised by deranged proliferation of a single clone of plasma cells or B-lymphocytes (Table 1) and are usually associated with detectable monoclonal immunoglobulin (M-protein) in the serum or urine. The clinical features of each condition are determined both by the rate of clonal proliferation and by the biological properties of the clone and the M-protein produced.

This review will focus on new concepts about the origins of these diseases, and the treatment of multiple myeloma, the commonest and most important of these disorders.

☐ MULTIPLE MYELOMA

Multiple myeloma is a relatively common haematological neoplasm with an annual incidence of approximately 4 per 100,000. Incidence and mortality rates increased between 1950 and 1980; it is not clear whether this was due to better diagnosis or to

Table 1 Conditions associated with M-protein production.

Stable production

- Monoclonal gammopathy of undetermined significance
- Smouldering myeloma

Progressive production

- Multiple myeloma
  - complete immunoglobulins: IgG, IgA, IgD, IgE
  - free light chains
  - non-secretory
- Plasma cell leukaemia
- Solitary plasmacytoma of bone
- Extramedullary plasmacytoma
- Waldenström's macroglobulinaemia
- Chronic lymphocytic leukaemia
- Malignant lymphoma
- Primary amyloidosis
- Heavy chain disease

a true increase, perhaps related to environmental toxins. The rise is not simply due to an ageing population, as age-specific mortality has also increased. There are racial differences in incidence (African Americans > Caucasians > Orientals). The male to female ratio is 1.5 and the median age at diagnosis is around 65 years. Myeloma is rare below 40 years of age but incidence increases sharply with age to over 30 per 100,000 above 80 years.

Aetiology and pathogenesis

The aetiology of myeloma remains uncertain. Radiation, asbestos, benzene, industrial and agricultural toxins have all been implicated. A small number of familial clusters have been reported, suggesting genetic predisposition. No consistent chromosomal abnormality has been found in multiple myeloma.

Studies of immunoglobulin (Ig) gene rearrangement suggest that the myeloma 'precursor cell' is a B-lymphocyte which has left the germinal centre and has already undergone antigen selection and Ig affinity maturation in lymph node or spleen [1]. Myeloma progenitor cells may migrate via the peripheral circulation before clonal expansion, to the bone marrow where the marrow stromal cells appear to play an important role in creating a microenvironment that favours proliferation of the clone (Fig. 1). Adhesion molecules on myeloma cells induce close cell-cell contact

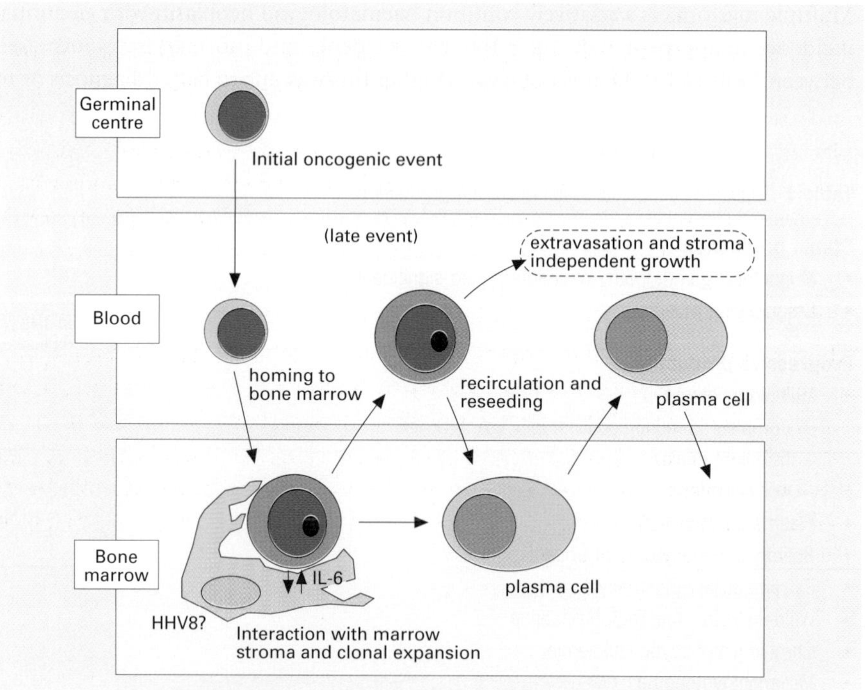

Fig. 1 Schematic representation of the putative phases in the development of multiple myeloma. HHV8, human herpesvirus-8. (Modified from Ref 2.)

with the stromal cells which produce the cytokine interleukin-6 (IL-6); this both promotes proliferation and inhibits apoptosis in myeloma cells. In turn, myeloma cells stimulate an increase in the number of stromal cells and also increase production of IL-6 [3]. They also stimulate production of IL-1β which, together with IL-6 and possibly also tumour necrosis factor β (TNF-β), is a major factor in the activation of osteoclasts and bone lysis, and thus in the development of myeloma bone disease. This permissive bone marrow environment may explain the often widespread bone marrow distribution of multiple myeloma at presentation.

Possible role of Kaposi's sarcoma associated herpesvirus

A herpesvirus first detected in Kaposi's sarcoma (Kaposi's sarcoma associated herpesvirus, KSHV; also known as human herpesvirus 8, HHV8) produces a viral homologue to IL-6 and may be responsible for the production of IL-6 by stromal cells in the bone marrow of patients with myeloma. This virus is related to Epstein-Barr virus and has also been identified in certain HIV-associated tumours, namely pleural effusion lymphoma and multicentric Castleman's disease; like Kaposi's sarcoma and myeloma, these neoplasms are also IL-6 dependent. Using the polymerase chain reaction to amplify a sequence from the KS330 Bam region of the virus, Rettig *et al* [4] identified KSHV in bone marrow dendritic cells from all 15 patients with multiple myeloma studied and from two of eight patients with monoclonal gammopathy of undetermined significance (MGUS; see below). KSHV was not detected in marrow from normal subjects or patients with other haematological disorders, nor was it found in the bone marrow mononuclear cell fraction from myeloma patients which contains the malignant plasma cell population. It is intriguing to speculate that KSHV may play a role in transforming the disordered plasma cell population in MGUS into the fully malignant myeloma phenotype – a notion in keeping with the multi-hit hypothesis of neoplasia. Further studies are in progress to define fully the role of KSHV in the pathogenesis of multiple myeloma*.

Differential diagnosis

Multiple myeloma should be suspected in any person with the clinical features listed in Table 2, especially if elderly, or in whom rouleaux or an elevated erythrocyte sedimentation rate (ESR) or plasma viscosity is detected. Several investigations are required to exclude alternative diagnoses, notably MGUS, smouldering multiple myeloma, primary systemic amyloidosis, lymphoma and metastatic carcinoma (Table 3). Minimal diagnostic criteria have been established (Table 3) as the diagnosis is not always simple [5].

---

* Since the time of writing, subsequent studies at several other centres have failed to confirm this data and cast doubt on the role of KSHV in the pathogenesis of multiple myeloma. Further studies are under way.

Table 2 Clinical features of multiple myeloma (see also Figs 2–7).

Frequent

- Bone pain and pathological fractures: osteoporosis and osteolytic lesions
- Lethargy, anaemia and bone marrow failure
- Recurrent infection due to immuneparesis and neutropenia
- Renal impairment and proteinuria

Less frequent

- Acute hypercalcaemia
- Symptomatic hyperviscosity
- Neuropathy
- Amyloidosis
- Coagulopathy

Table 3 Investigations required and minimal diagnostic criteria for multiple myeloma.

Investigations

Haematological

- Full blood count and film
- ESR or plasma viscosity
- Bone marrow aspirate and biopsy

Biochemical

- Urea and creatinine, uric acid
- Calcium, phosphate, alkaline phosphatase
- Serum protein electrophoresis
- Quantitation of serum immunoglobulins
- Routine urinalysis
- Urine electrophoresis for Bence-Jones protein

Radiological

- Skeletal survey

Minimal diagnostic criteria

- >10% plasma cells in bone marrow, or plasmacytoma on histology
- Clinical features of myeloma
- Plus at least one of:
  – serum M-protein (IgG >30 g/l; IgA >20 g/l)
  – urine M-protein (Bence-Jones proteinuria)
  – osteolytic lesions on skeletal survey

ESR, elevated erythrocyte sedimentation rate.

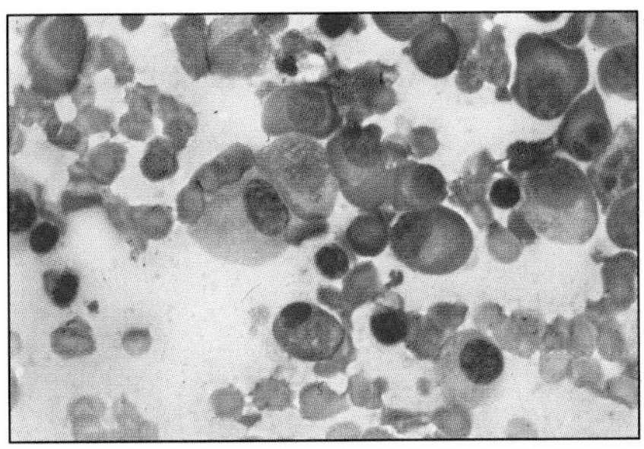

Fig. 2 Medium power bone marrow aspirate showing plasma cell infiltration (Romanowsky stain).

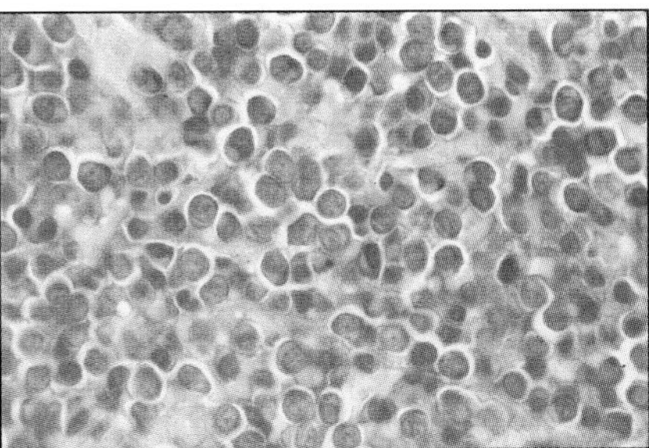

Fig. 3 Medium power trephine biopsy showing extensive plasma cell infiltration (MGP stain).

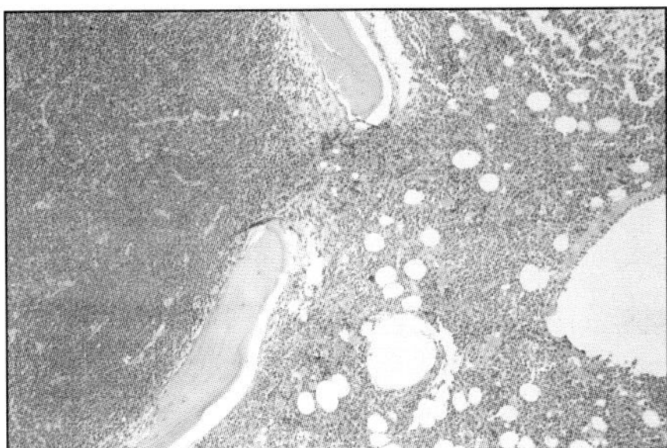

Fig. 4 Low power trephine biopsy showing infiltration of bone marrow (H&E).

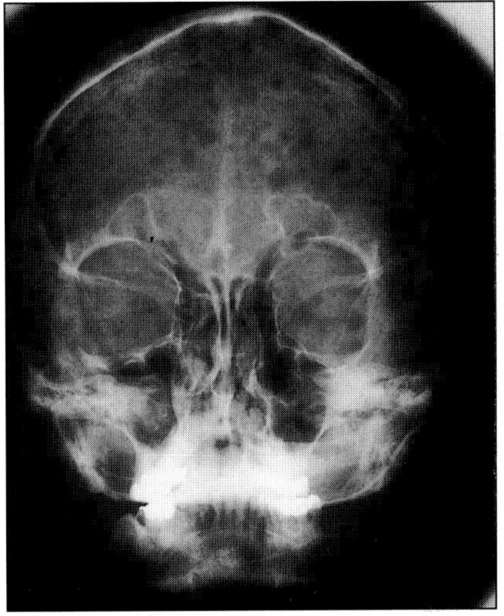

Fig. 5 Skull x-ray showing lytic lesions.

Monoclonal gammopathy of undetermined significance

This term implies the presence of stable M-protein production in an individual who does not have multiple myeloma, Waldenström's macroglobulinaemia, amyloidosis, lymphoma or other related disease (Table 4). The prevalence of MGUS is many-fold higher than that of multiple myeloma, and its incidence increases with age (1% over 50 years of age; 3% over 70 years).

The differentiation of MGUS from multiple myeloma may be difficult. No single test reliably distinguishes the two conditions, although a serum IgG over 30 g/l or IgA over 20 g/l suggests a diagnosis of myeloma rather than MGUS. Various specialised investigations may be helpful (Table 4), but serial measurement of the M-protein in the serum and urine and periodic review of clinical and laboratory parameters over several weeks is often necessary to establish the diagnosis.

No specific treatment is indicated for MGUS, but indefinite follow-up is required as the condition may evolve; multiple myeloma, Waldenström's macroglobulinaemia,

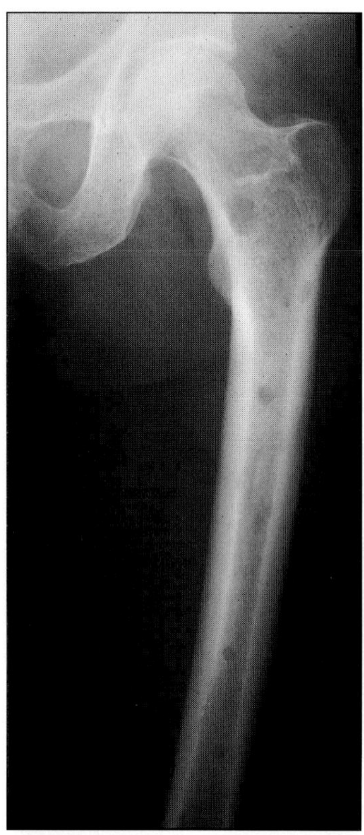

Fig. 6 Left femur x-ray showing lytic lesions.

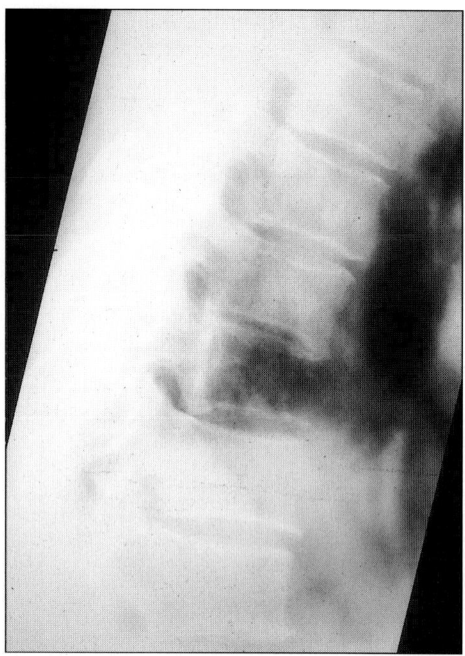

Fig. 7 Lumbar spine x-ray showing wedge compression fracture.

amyloidosis or lymphoma eventually develop in many cases, with an actuarial rate of 16% at 10 years [5]. Once the diagnosis is clearly established, the patient should be reviewed and the M-protein levels re-quantified after six months and annually thereafter, if stable. Patients with MGUS should be instructed to seek early medical review if symptoms develop.

Smouldering multiple myeloma

This term identifies asymptomatic patients with a serum M-protein over 30 g/l and more than 10% plasma cells in the bone marrow but in whom the natural history is that of MGUS rather than multiple myeloma (Table 5). These patients do not have anaemia, renal failure or lytic bone lesions, though there may be modest Bence-Jones proteinuria and immuneparesis, with reduced levels of normal serum immunoglobulins. On follow-up, the M-protein and the proportion of plasma cells in the marrow remain stable. Patients with smouldering multiple myeloma should only be treated if laboratory parameters progress or symptoms of myeloma develop.

Table 4 Basic and additional criteria for the diagnosis of MGUS.

Basic criteria

- No unexplained symptoms suggestive of myeloma
- Serum M-protein <30 g/l
- Less than 10% plasma cells in bone marrow
- Little or no urine M-protein
- No bone lesions
- No anaemia, hypercalcaemia or renal impairment
- Stable M-protein and other parameters on prolonged observation

Additional criteria

- Bone marrow plasma cell labelling index (LI)* <1.0%
- Plasmablasts absent
- No aggregates on trephine biopsy
- No elevation of serum β_2-microglobulin
- No circulating isotype-specific plasma cells
- No light chain isotype suppression

*The plasma cell labelling index is obtained following incubation of fresh bone marrow with bromodeoxy-uridine which is incorporated into the DNA of actively cycling cells in 's-phase' and subsequently detected by a monoclonal antibody. Simultaneous two-colour analysis with an anti-plasma cell antibody (CD38) permits calculation of the proportion of plasma cells in the proliferative phase of the cell cycle.

Table 5 Criteria for the diagnosis of smouldering myeloma.

- No unexplained symptoms suggestive of myeloma
- Serum M-protein >30 g/l
- ≥10% plasma cells in bone marrow
- Little or no urine M-protein (<500 mg/24 h)
- No bone lesions
- No anaemia, hypercalcaemia or renal impairment
- Stable M-protein and other parameters on prolonged observation

Prognostic factors in multiple myeloma

Without treatment, a patient with multiple myeloma is likely to experience progressive bone damage, anaemia, recurrent infection and renal failure, and will have a median survival of only six months. Standard chemotherapy improves the median survival to around three years. However, multiple myeloma is a heterogeneous disease and the survival ranges from a few weeks to over 10 years.

A number of parameters may be used reliably to assess prognosis at diagnosis, including a combination of independent variables reflecting both tumour bulk and proliferation rate (Table 6) [6]. A simpler, widely applicable prognostic index [7] can

Table 6 Features indicating poor prognosis at diagnosis of multiple myeloma.

- Low haemoglobin (<8.5 g/dl)
- Hypercalcaemia
- Advanced lytic bone lesions
- High M-protein production rates
  – IgG >70 g/l; IgA >50 g/l; Bence-Jones proteinuria >12 g/24 h
- Impaired renal function
- High proportion of bone marrow plasma cells
- Unfavourable plasmablast morphology
- Circulating plasma cells in peripheral blood
- High β_2-microglobulin (≥6 mg/L)
- High plasma cell labelling index
- Low serum albumin (<30 g/l)
- High C-reactive protein (≥6 mg/L)
- High serum IL-6

identify three risk groups using generally available serum assays for β_2-microglobulin (reflecting tumour bulk) and C-reactive protein (a surrogate marker for IL-6, reflecting tumour aggression) (Fig. 8). Alternative combinations which provide a similar prognostic stratification are the serum β_2-microglobulin level and plasma cell labelling index or the percentage of circulating plasma cells and the plasma cell labelling index. Assessment of prognosis is increasingly important in selecting the appropriate treatment for an individual patient.

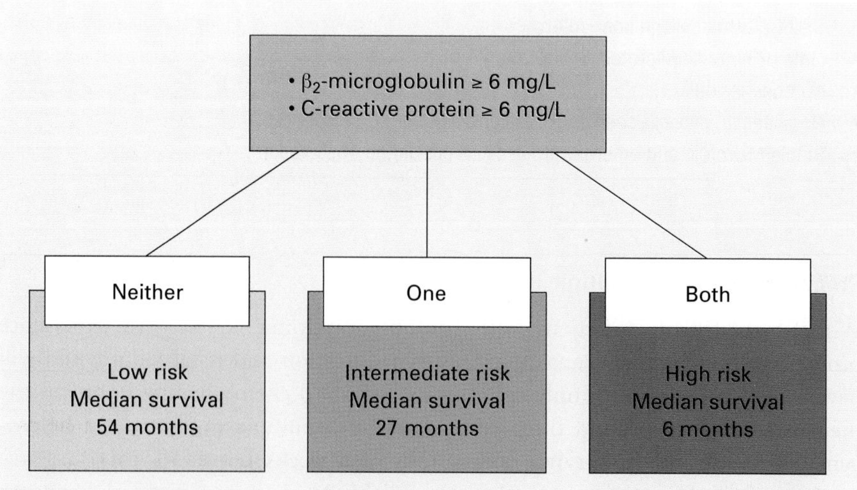

Fig. 8 Prognostic index in multiple myeloma, based on plasma levels of β_2-microglobulin and C-reactive protein. (Adapted from Ref 7.)

□ MANAGEMENT OF MULTIPLE MYELOMA

This review will concentrate on new approaches to the chemotherapy of the myeloma itself, and on the treatment of hypercalcaemia.

Many patients require urgent treatment for the complications of multiple myeloma (Table 7) prior to definitive therapy of the tumour itself.

Chemotherapy of multiple myeloma

Melphalan

Melphalan produces an objective response in approximately 50% of patients when administered at a dose of 6–8 mg/m^2/day with prednisolone (40–60 mg/day) for 4–7 days at 4–6 week intervals (the 'M&P' regimen). Response may be slow and maximum benefit may require treatment for over 12 months; treatment should therefore continue until there is no further improvement, when a plateau phase may have been achieved. Complete response with disappearance of the M-protein and a normal bone marrow is extremely uncommon. The plateau phase may persist without treatment for several months (median approximately 12 months). Patients should be monitored closely during the plateau phase to identify progression early. Many patients who achieve a lasting plateau phase will achieve a further plateau with the same chemotherapy, although resistance to melphalan is the inevitable eventual outcome of this approach in patients who do not succumb to intercurrent complications. Nevertheless, this regimen remains an appropriate option for older patients as it is relatively non-toxic and well tolerated.

Combination chemotherapy

Various combination regimens have been examined in patients with multiple myeloma; the most widely used are shown in Table 8. Although many studies have failed to demonstrate an advantage for combination therapy over M&P, three large multicentre collaborative studies reported improved objective responses, and two also reported improved survival (Table 9). In many studies, the combination regimen appears to be associated with more toxicity in elderly patients but may offer superior results in younger patients and in those with a poor prognosis. Complete

Table 7 Therapeutic considerations in multiple myeloma.

- Analgesia
- Hydration
- Correction of hypercalcaemia
- Treatment of renal impairment
- Treatment of infection
- Local radiotherapy
- Chemotherapy
- Prevention of further bone damage

Table 8 Common combination chemotherapy regimens for myeloma.

VMCP/VBAP	Alternating cycles every three weeks • Vincristine iv, Melphalan po × 5d, Cyclophosphamide po × 5d, Prednisolone po × 5d • Vincristine iv, BCNU iv, Adriamycin iv, Prednisolone po × 5d
VBMCP (M-2)	Every five weeks • Vincristine iv, BCNU iv, Melphalan po × 4d, Cyclophosphamide iv, Prednisolone po × 14d
ABCM	Alternating cycles every three weeks • Adriamycin iv, BCNU iv • Cyclophosphamide po × 4d, Melphalan po × 4d
VAD	Every three weeks • Adriamycin & Vincristine iv infusion × 4d, Dexamethasone po × 4d (Methylprednisolone po × 5d in VAMP)

Table 9 Major randomised trials of combination chemotherapy versus melphalan ± prednisolone.

			Survival	
Study group	**Number of patients**	**Objective responses**	**Median (months)**	**5-year (%)**
SWOG	233			
Salmon *et al.* (1983)				
VMCP/VBAP		53%*	36*	30*
Melphalan & prednisolone		32%	24	19
ECOG	438			
Oken *et al.* (1984)				
VBMCP		72%*	30	26
Melphalan & prednisolone		51%	28	19
MRC	630			
MacLennan *et al.* (1992)				
ABCM		61%*	32*	24*
Melphalan		49%	24	17

Above trials further reviewed in Ref 8.
*p <0.05 vs melphalan ± prednisolone.

response is more common with combination regimens than with M&P but still only occurs in a minority of patients.

High-dose melphalan therapy

A single infusion of high-dose melphalan (100–200 mg/m^2) can achieve a complete response in a high proportion of patients when administered after initial therapy has induced 'minimal residual disease' (Table 10). Doses above 140 mg/m^2 require

Table 10 Results of selected trials of high-dose melphalan therapy in myeloma.

Author	n	Conditioning	Graft	Treatment related deaths (%)	Complete responses (%)	Event-free survival (months)	Overall survival (months)
Cunningham (1994)	53	HDM	BM	2	75	24	80
Anderson (1994)	52	HDM + TBI	BM	2	40	31	50
Harousseau (1995)	133	HDM + TBI	BM/PBSC	4	37	24	46
Attal (1996/1997)	100	HDM + TBI	BM	3	22	27	57
Fermand (1993)	63	HDM + TBI	PBSC	11	20	43	59
Marit (1996)	73	HDM ± TBI	PBSC	3	43	23	60
Jagannath (1997)	231	HDM × 2	PBSC	2	37	43	62

Above trials further reviewed in Ref 9. BM, bone marrow; HDM, high-dose melphalan; PBSC, peripheral blood stem cells; TBI, total-body irradiation.

autologous haemopoietic stem cell (peripheral blood stem cell; PBSC) or bone marrow (ABM) re-infusion to reduce morbidity and mortality. PBSC are best collected once a significant reduction of bone marrow infiltration has been achieved (Fig. 9). The VAD or VAMP regimens are widely used for initial therapy as schedules containing alkylating agents may reduce stem cell yield and quality. Studies of stem cell collections demonstrate frequent tumour cell contamination even after 'purging' or selection procedures [10].

High-dose melphalan or melphalan with total-body irradiation give similar results (Table 10), with a high overall and complete response rate and relatively low toxicity. However, high-dose therapy is not curative in the autologous context; complete responses last a median of approximately two years and are associated with good quality of life. The duration of response and overall survival may be prolonged by maintenance treatment with interferon-α [11]. An important randomised comparison of high-dose and conventional dose chemotherapy showed a significant advantage for high-dose therapy as a component of the initial treatment regimen [12]. This study demonstrated significant improvements in response rate (81% vs 57%), event-free survival at five years (28% vs 10%) and overall survival at five years (52% vs 12%) in patients who received high-dose therapy. Several further randomised studies of high-dose therapy are under way.

Bone marrow transplantation

Allogeneic and syngeneic bone marrow transplantation (BMT) have been undertaken on a relatively small number of patients with myeloma, owing to the patients' advanced age and limited donor availability. Transplant related toxicity is high (up to 50%) and late recurrence occurs, though prolonged disease-free survival has been achieved and some patients may possibly have been cured. BMT should be considered in younger patients (<55 years) with a poor prognosis and a matched sibling donor. A retrospective case-matched analysis of allografts and autografts in

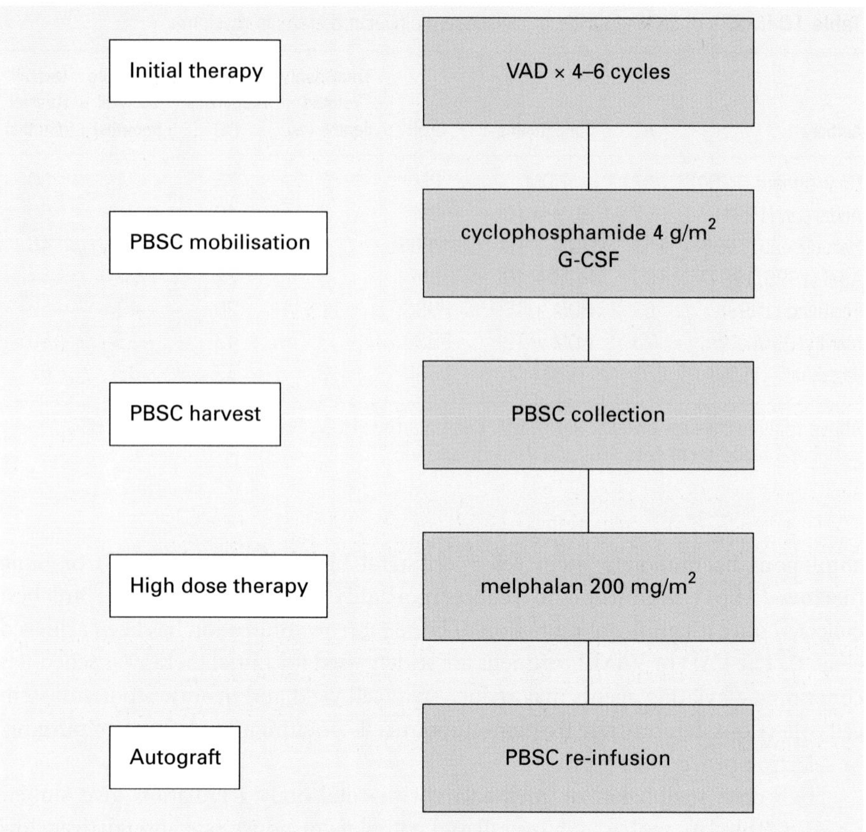

Fig. 9 Outline treatment plan for the use of high-dose therapy as part of the initial management of a patient with high-risk multiple myeloma. PBSC, peripheral blood stem cells.

myeloma carried out by the European Group for Blood and Marrow Transplantation demonstrated a superior overall survival in autografted patients owing to the high early transplant-related mortality in allografted patients which was most marked in males, and was not compensated by the lower relapse rate seen in allografted patients [13]. Reports from single centres confirm a high early mortality associated with allogeneic transplantation for myeloma.

Interferon-α

The addition of interferon-α (IFN-α) to initial chemotherapy may improve the response rate, but adds toxicity [14]. Several studies of maintenance IFN-α have demonstrated prolongation of the plateau phase but only one shows improved survival after conventional therapy (Table 11). None of these studies has been large enough to ensure that a small difference would be detected, and a meta-analysis is awaited. The Royal Marsden group report a significant effect of maintenance IFN-α on response and survival in patients who achieve a complete response with

Table 11 Major randomised studies of interferon-α maintenance therapy.

		Effect of interferon-α	
Author	***n***	**Longer plateau**	**Improved survival**
Mandelli *et al.* (1990)	101	12 mo, $p = 0.0002$	no benefit
Peest *et al.* (1990)	117	no benefit	no benefit
Salmon *et al.* (1994)	193	no benefit	no benefit
Westin *et al.* (1995)	125	8 mo, $p < 0.0001$	no benefit
Browman *et al.* (1995)	176	5 mo, $p = 0.002$	no benefit
Ludwig *et al.* (1995)	100	10 mo, $p < 0.01$	17 mo, $p < 0.05$
Hjorth *et al.* (1996)*	583	6 mo, $p < 0.05$	no benefit
Drayson *et al.* (1997)	284	no benefit	no benefit
Cunningham *et al.* (1998)†	84	19 mo, $p < 0.025$	$p = 0.006$ @ 54 mo

Above trials further reviewed in Ref 14.
*Interferon-α therapy with initial chemotherapy as well as in plateau phase.
†Interferon-α therapy as maintenance of complete response after high-dose therapy.

high-dose melphalan [13]. It is possible that IFN-α may have a greater effect after high-dose therapy when there is minimal residual disease. There is much current interest in the use of immune modulation in an attempt to improve the long-term outcome after high-dose therapy has induced minimal disease.

Bisphosphonates

Several randomised studies suggest that bisphosphonate therapy is beneficial to patients with myeloma (Table 12). Two recent reports suggest that regular use of clodronate or pamidronate not only reduces the incidence of further bone disease but may also improve overall survival of some patients [15,16]. Both studies demonstrated a lower incidence of skeletal fractures, less bone pain and better performance status or quality of life in patients receiving bisphosphonate therapy. Berenson *et al* [16] report improved survival in the group of patients who received bisphosphonate therapy as part of second-line treatment or later. On the other hand, McCloskey *et al* [15], who treated newly diagnosed patients, found the most marked benefit was in those without bone pain or vertebral fractures at diagnosis; these patients, when treated with clodronate, had longer survival, albeit of borderline statistical significance ($p = 0.05$). The possibility that bisphosphonates may have some direct effect on the myeloma clone in addition to their recognised inhibitory effects on osteoclasts has been raised by *in vitro* studies and makes these recently reported results most interesting.

□ CONCLUSIONS

Recent years have brought a clearer understanding of the cellular events in the development of multiple myeloma and an increased number of treatment options

Table 12 Major randomised studies of bisphosphonate therapy.

	Belch *et al.* (1991)	**Lahtinen *et al.* (1992)**	**Heim *et al.* (1995)**	**Berenson *et al.* (1996/1998)**	**McCloskey *et al.* (1998)**
Number of patients	166	336	157	377	536
Drug	Etidronate	Clodronate	Clodronate	Pamidronate	Clodronate
Dose	5 mg/kg/d	2,400 mg/d	1,600 mg/d	90 mg/4 wks	1,600 mg/d
Duration	Until death	24 months	12 months	9/21 months	Indefinite
Skeletal events	0	0	0	+	+
Fractures	0	0	0	+	+
DXT	ne	ne	ne	+	0
Lesions	ne	+	0	0	ne
Pain	0	0	+	+	+
QoL	ne	0	0	+	+
Survival	w	0	0	?*	?*

+, statistically significant benefit; w, worse in bisphosphonate group; 0, no significant benefit; ne, not evaluated.
*Improved survival demonstrated in a subgroup of patients in each study but not in the whole group.

for patients with the disease. There is increasing consensus on general treatment principles (Table 13). Further studies will determine specific points of current controversy, including whether KSHV plays a key role in the aetiology of myeloma, whether maintenance IFN-α is indeed beneficial, whether immunotherapy can improve the results of high-dose therapy and whether allogeneic BMT can cure a significant proportion of patients.

Table 13 Therapeutic guidelines for patients with multiple myeloma.

MGUS or smouldering multiple myeloma
- Watch and wait

Multiple myeloma, age >65 years
- M&P

Multiple myeloma, age <65 years
- Enrol in clinical study
- VAD/VAMP, PBSC collection
- ± Early/late high-dose melphalan

High-risk multiple myeloma, age <55 years, with a compatible sibling
- Consider allogeneic BMT

MGUS, monoclonal gammopathy of undetermined significance; PBSC, peripheral blood stem cells; M&P, melphalan + prednisolone; BMT, bone marrow transplantation; VAD/VAMP, see Table 8.

REFERENCES

1 Bakkus MHC, Vanriet I, Vancamp B,Thielemans K. Evidence that the clonogenic cell in multiple myeloma originates from a pre-switched but somatically mutated B cell. *Br J Haematol* 1994; **87**: 68–74.

2 Van Camp B, Bakkus M, Vanderkerken K, *et al.* Characterisation of the myeloma clone. *Proceedings of the VIth International Workshop on Multiple Myeloma.* Boston: Harvard Medical Press, 1997.

3 Bataille R, Harousseau JL. Multiple myeloma. *N Engl J Med* 1997; **336**: 1657–64.

4 Rettig MB, Ma HJ, Vescio RA, *et al.* Kaposi's sarcoma-associated herpesvirus infection of bone marrow dendritic cells from multiple myeloma patients. *Science* 1997; **276**: 1851–4.

5 Kyle RA. Monoclonal gammopathy of undetermined significance and solitary plasmacytoma. *Hematol Oncol Clin North Am* 1997; **11**: 71–87.

6 Boccadoro M, Pileri A. Diagnosis, prognosis and standard treatment of multiple myeloma. *Hematol Oncol Clin North Am* 1997; **11**: 111–31.

7 Bataille R, Boccadoro M, Klein B, *et al.* C-reactive protein and serum β_2 microglobulin produce a simple and powerful myeloma staging system. *Blood* 1992; **80**: 733–7.

8 Bergsagel DE. Chemotherapy of myeloma. In: Malpas JS, Bergsagel DE, Kyle R, *et al. Myeloma Biology.* Oxford: Oxford University Press, 1995.

9 Jagganath S, Tricot G, Barlogie B. Autotransplants in multiple myeloma: pushing the envelope. *Hematol Oncol Clin North Am* 1997; **11**: 363–81.

10 Samson D. High dose therapy in multiple myeloma. *Curr Opin Hematol* 1996; **3**: 446–52.

11 Cunningham D, Powles R, Malpas J, *et al.* A randomised trial of maintenance interferon following high dose chemotherapy in multiple myeloma: results $5^1/_2$ years after accrual of the last patient. *Br J Haematol* 1998; **102**: 495–502.

12 Attal M, Harousseau JL, Stoppa AM, *et al.* A prospective randomised trial of autologous bone marrow transplantation and chemotherapy in multiple myeloma. *N Engl J Med* 1996; **335**: 91–7.

13 Björkstrand B, Ljungman P, Svensson H, *et al.* Allogeneic bone marrow transplantation versus autologous stem cell transplantation in multiple myeloma: a retrospective case-matched study from the European Group for Blood and Marrow Transplantation. *Blood* 1996; **88**: 4711–8.

14 Peest D, Bladé J, Harousseau JL. Cytokine therapy in multiple myeloma. *Br J Haematol* 1996; **94**: 425–32.

15 McCloskey EV, MacLennan ICM, Drayson MT, *et al.* A randomised trial of the effect of clodronate on skeletal morbidity in multiple myeloma. *Br J Haematol* 1998; **100**: 317–25.

16 Berenson JR, Lichtenstein A, Porter L, *et al.* Long-term pamidronate treatment of advanced multiple myeloma patients reduces skeletal events. *J Clin Oncol* 1998; **16**: 593–602.

□ MULTIPLE CHOICE QUESTIONS

1 Multiple myeloma:
(a) Is increasing in incidence as a result of the ageing population
(b) Is associated with cytomegalovirus infection
(c) Is caused by KSHV infection of the plasma cells
(d) Is associated with exposure to agricultural toxins
(e) Is consistently associated with abnormalities of chromosome 14

2 Myeloma plasma cells:
(a) Only circulate in the peripheral blood in plasma cell leukaemia
(b) Proliferate in the bone marrow as a result of IL-5 secretion
(c) Stimulate osteoblast activity to induce bone disease

(d) Stimulate secretion of IL-6 by stromal cells
(e) Are stimulated to proliferate by IL-6

3 Multiple myeloma:
(a) May be diagnosed in the absence of a serum or urine M-protein
(b) Is rarely associated with bone damage
(c) May cause a coagulopathy
(d) May be diagnosed in the absence of plasmacytosis >10% in the bone marrow or tissue biopsy evidence of plasmacytoma
(e) Is always associated with bone damage

4 Monoclonal gammopathy of undetermined significance (MGUS):
(a) May be diagnosed with bone marrow plasma cells <10%
(b) May be diagnosed if there is immuneparesis of normal immunoglobulins
(c) May not be diagnosed if there is Bence-Jones proteinuria
(d) May transform into myeloma, Waldenström's macroglobulinaemia or amyloidosis
(e) Should only be treated with melphalan and prednisolone

5 A patient aged 65 with high-risk multiple myeloma:
(a) Should receive an allogeneic bone marrow transplant from a compatible sibling
(b) Should receive treatment with a bisphosphonate
(c) Is likely to have a high serum C-reactive protein
(d) Is a candidate for high-dose therapy
(e) Should receive interferon-α as part of initial therapy

ANSWERS

1a False	2a False	3a True	4a True	5a False
b False	b False	b False	b True	b True
c False	c False	c True	c False	c True
d True	d True	d False	d True	d True
e False	e True	e False	e False	e False

Modern drug design: from combinatorial chemistry to high-throughput screening

Colin Dollery

□ INTRODUCTION

Modern therapeutic drugs have come from several different sources. There is a case for arguing that modern therapeutics began with the use of quinine to treat malaria. The Countess of Cinchon, wife of the Viceroy of Spain in Lima, Peru, who was treated with an extract of the bark of the cinchona tree in 1629, may have been the first European to be cured of a deadly disease by a drug [1]. The efforts of chemists to synthesise quinine gave rise to the modern dye-stuffs industry and led, indirectly, to the discovery of phenacetin and aspirin. Many other drugs came from natural sources and were the result of cumulative observation by earlier populations of medicinal activity in plants; examples are digitalis and ephedrine.

The rise of experimental physiology and pharmacology in the first half of the 20th century led to the discovery of hormones such as thyroxine and insulin, and transmitter substances such histamine and adrenaline. These advances in turn stimulated medicinal chemists to try to produce antagonists, resulting in the discovery of antihistamines and α-adrenergic blocking drugs. In the second half of the 20th century, therapeutics has been dominated by partnerships between medicinal chemists and quantitative pharmacologists, such as led to the discovery of propranolol and cimetidine by Sir James Black.

Numerous new leads were founded on astute clinical observation of unexpected effects when drugs were given for another purpose, for example the development of the phenothiazine antipsychotics from the antihistamines. There has also been a significant role for semi-random screening of biological materials for antibacterial and antifungal activity ever since Fleming's chance discovery of penicillin.

None of these methods is redundant as we approach the new millennium but the pressure to innovate faster, combined with the development of novel technologies, is driving drug development in new directions. The traditional and the new strategies for drug discovery are contrasted in Fig. 1.

□ MEDICAL NEED AND COMMERCIAL EXPECTATION: THE 'INNOVATION DEFICIT'

Only an incurable optimist could regard most current medical treatment as the best possible. In the Harveian Oration of 1993 [1], I divided current therapy into five categories of effectiveness that ranged from restoration of normality at the top, to trivial or minor improvement in the lowest rank. The top category included replacement therapy of physiological deficiency and chemotherapy of most bacterial infections; this classification was probably justified for thyroid hormone in

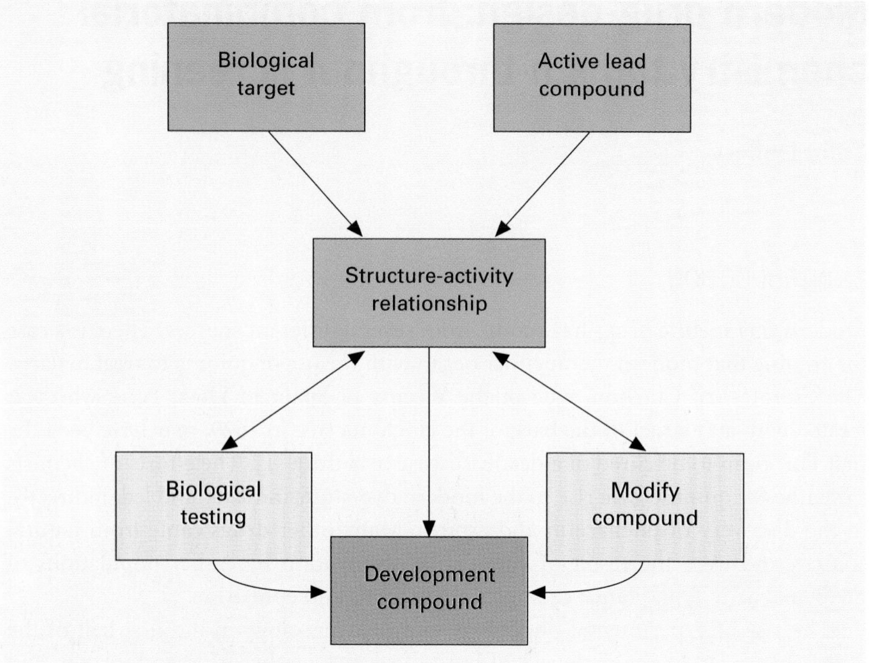

Fig. 1 The 'old' process of drug discovery.

myxoedema or vitamin B12 in pernicious anaemia, but certainly not for insulin treatment in type 1 diabetes. In the bottom category were placed most dementias, most solid tumours, stroke and osteoarthritis. Even in conditions where current treatment is generally regarded as so satisfactory that pharmaceutical companies are scaling back their research and development (R&D) investment (eg hypertension), an objective assessor can see many deficiencies. There remains a great medical need for better treatments across a wide range of human disease.

Pharmaceutical companies have been amongst the most successful new industries of the 20th century. Shareholders have become accustomed to a year-by-year increase in profits of 10–15%, and stock-market analysts project this growth in earnings continuing for years ahead. As the patent life of a new medicine is limited, and the loss in revenue when a patent expires is profound, the pressure on the industry to develop new compounds is very strong. Each of the world's top 20 pharmaceutical companies markets, on average, about one new chemical entity (NCE) per year. Industry calculations suggest that to maintain market position and grow at the rate demanded by shareholders, this needs to be raised to an average of three NCEs per year by about 2005 [2,3]. The industry's response has been to increase efficiency, particularly by shortening overall development time. This gives an important one-off gain by compressing the time-scale of development from 11–12 years to about six years, but leaves unresolved the long-term problem of increasing the rate of innovation. To achieve this gain by traditional ways would mean increasing current R&D expenditure (already 15–18% of turnover) by two- to threefold – which is clearly impractical. Fortunately new technologies have come to the rescue [4].

☐ HUNDREDS AND THOUSANDS: THE GENOMIC FEAST

There is a saying in the pharmaceutical industry that only two things matter in drug discovery: the choice of the target and the choice of the lead compound. Until recently, the number of known targets was the limiting factor, and a reason why different companies tended to produce very similar ('me-too')compounds targeted at the same receptors or enzymes. The situation has been changed radically by genomics – information yielded by the systematic sequencing of the genome of man and other species – and the industry can now contemplate an enormous range of potential targets. It can already be inferred that there are several hundred distinct receptor molecules and over a thousand proteases in the human genome, any one of which could be a prime drug target. The problem is not what to do, but where to start.

An interesting gene, even for a potential drug target such as a 7-transmembrane spanning receptor, is not itself sufficient justification to initiate a drug discovery program. The need is to validate the target both to establish a reasonably secure hypothesis connecting it with the pathophysiology of a disease, and also to minimise the risk of developing an interesting pharmacological or biochemical reagent which is no use as a drug.

There are several possible ways of doing this. One method, particularly applicable to cell surface receptors, is to use the receptor itself as an affinity ligand to try to isolate and characterise the natural ligand. Once this is available, standard methods of physiology and pharmacology can be used. Another method is to knock-out the gene and evaluate the functional disturbance which results [5]. Other methods include evaluating changes in gene expression in animal models of disease or in diseased human tissues. Perhaps the most relevant is to investigate human allelic polymorphisms which predispose to, or protect against, a given disease. For example, the recognition that certain non-functional polymorphisms of the human chemokine receptors provide a high degree of protection against HIV infection opens up the possibility of a preventive strategy based on devising antagonists for those receptors [6,7].

Finding new targets provides a tremendous incentive to the drug hunters, but it is the application of robotics to high-throughput screening that has revolutionised the early stages of industrial pharmacology.

☐ HIGH-THROUGHPUT SCREENING

A pharmacologist using an organ bath containing a piece of tissue such as a guinea-pig ileum can perform only a few tens of assays in a week. By contrast, high-throughput screening can carry out 100,000 assays in a week, with no pharmacologist in attendance.

The principle of high-throughput screening is simple. The assays are based upon expressed human proteins, thus avoiding problems about interspecies differences in the target. Assays are devised to be carried out in the very small volume of the hole in a 96- or 384-well plate, and to have a simple read-out such as a colour, fluorescence or the binding of a radioactive ligand. A simple example might be an enzymatic reaction which yields a coloured product after a short period of incubation; test compounds can then be added to wells to see if they inhibit the formation of the coloured product (Fig. 2).

Test compounds are not added singly but in groups of 10–15 per well and at relatively high concentrations, often 100–1,000 times higher than the activity desired in the eventual drug. The rationale for testing several compounds at once is that the likelihood of a 'hit' is quite low, so the throughput of the assay can be greatly increased by screening mixtures. There is, however, still some controversy about the use of mixtures because of the possible loss of information from interactions in the assay [8]. If a hit occurs, the mixture can be deconvoluted and the responsible compound identified. Alternatively, the target receptor or enzyme can be used as an affinity ligand to pull out the responsible molecule which can then be identified by mass spectrometry [9]. Medicinal chemists then begin the exercise of making analogues to increase the activity and selectivity of the lead molecule.

A more complex example might involve a cell surface receptor and a fluorescent ligand. Cell membranes or whole cells are added with the ligand and a mixture of compounds. After incubation, the cells are filtered and washed, and the fluorescence

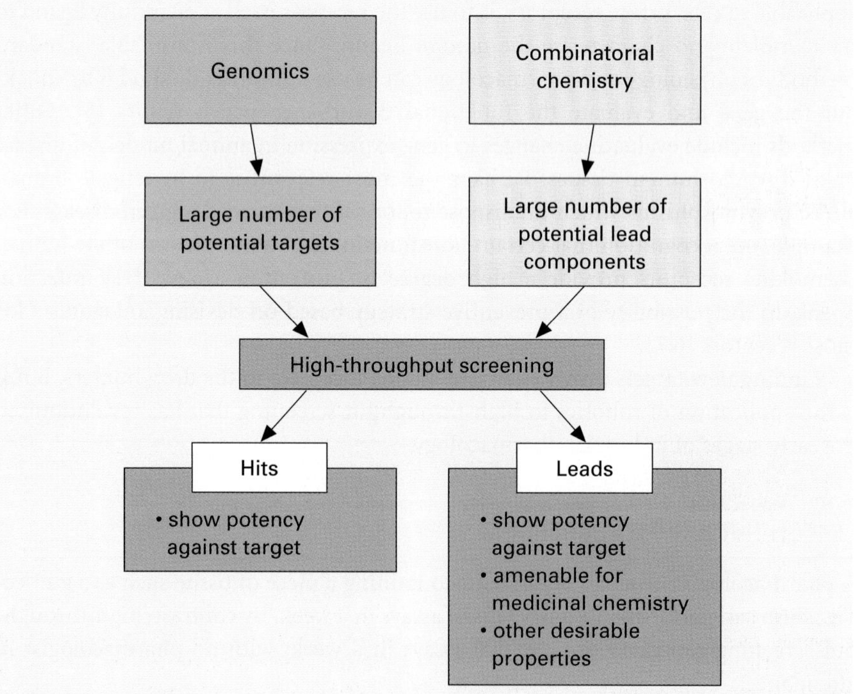

Fig. 2 New technologies in drug discovery: genomics, combinatorial chemistry and high-throughput screening.

is measured using a laser probe. The plates are filled, shaken, incubated, filtered and assayed by computer-controlled automatic devices that move the plates precisely, using a robotic arm running on a track; the system resembles a miniaturised robotic car assembly line (Fig. 3).

These screening systems have several advantages. They have a very high throughput, work 24 hours each day and have very high reproducibility, which can be tracked by routine use of standards. The quantities of reagents required for testing are very small (nanograms), which is particularly important if the source of test compounds is combinatorial chemistry (see below). There is the potential to miniaturise the system even further, with even higher productivity and smaller amounts of reagents needed. The ingenuity of assay designers has raised the possibility of using more complex assays based on reporter genes or measurement of calcium transients in cells.

One obvious consequence of making it possible to screen thousands of compounds each week is that very extensive compound libraries are needed to feed the assays. This need has stimulated the development of combinatorial chemistry (Fig. 1).

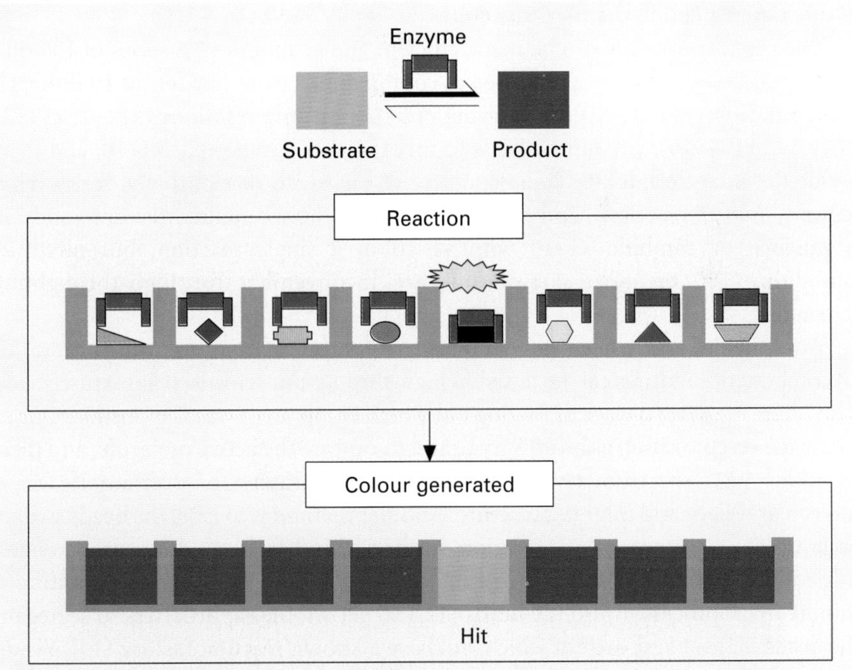

Fig. 3 An example of high-throughput screening (HTS) using a colorimetric reaction, based on an enzymatic reaction which converts substrate (green) into its product (red), to detect inhibitors of the enzyme. The reaction proceeds, generating the red colour, unless an inhibitor of the enzyme is present in the reaction mixture; in this case, the substrate's green colour remains and can be detected automatically by scanning the microtitre plate wells in which enzyme, substrate and test molecules are placed.

☐ COMBINATORIAL CHEMISTRY

When high-throughput screens were first introduced, test compounds came from the archives of major pharmaceutical and chemical companies. A large pharmaceutical company might have 250,000 file compounds that had been synthesised over a period of 25–40 years. This seemingly enormous number can easily be screened by these voracious assays which can quite easily screen a library of that size in only10–12 weeks. Furthermore, the archive may not be quite as useful as it sounds. Some of the compounds will have deteriorated over long periods of storage, and the diversity of chemical structures may be much smaller than the numbers imply; for example, a company with a major interest in antibiotics might have hundreds of beta-lactams in its archives. Other sources of chemical diversity must therefore be found. 'Swap clubs' between companies are one possibility, but only combinatorial chemistry can provide a sufficiently wide range of structures.

The origins of combinatorial chemistry can be traced to the step-by-step, solid-phase synthesis of peptides. The principle is to anchor an amino acid to a solid substrate, usually a resin bead, by a linker molecule and then react another amino acid with the opposite terminus [10,11]. These steps can be repeated, although there is a practical limit to the size of peptide chains that can be produced, as the yield declines with each step. The same process can be used in the step-by-step synthesis of other, non-peptide chemical structures.

The reaction strategy can be made efficient and economical. A series of 100 different molecules could be synthesised as combinations from two sets of 10 different compounds (x1–10, y1–10) by carrying out 100 separate reactions (x1+y1; x1+y2; x1+y3; ... x10+y10). An alternative is to mix together compounds x1–10, and then divide the mixture into 10 aliquots and react each with one of the 'y' series. This requires only 10 reactions, and each reaction vessel now contains 10 compounds; it is possible to combine x1–10 with y1–10 in a single reaction, but mixtures containing 100 or more compounds are inconvenient for high-throughput screening.

After the linker has been cleaved to separate the compound from the beads, the 10 component mixtures can be tested in high-throughput screens. If a mixture yields a hit, there are several ways of finding out which component was responsible. One is to use the receptor itself as an affinity ligand to capture the active molecule, and then to apply mass spectrometry and mass fragmentography to ascertain its exact molecular weight and infer its structure. Another method is to label the beads so that each carries a record of its reaction history; this has been done using oligonucleotides, peptides or other small molecular tags, and even by incorporating a minute microprocessor into the beads [12,13]. Yet another approach is to segregate the beads in 'tea bags', each of which will have a known reaction history [14]. Yields are in low nanogram amounts, but adequate for the tiny samples of chemical required in a high-throughput screen. Robotic devices are available for automating combinatorial chemistry [15] (Fig. 4).

At its simplest level, this may seem a mindless process deserving of the jibes about 'molecular roulette' that were previously applied to 'me-too' compounds in past years. More pragmatically, combinatorial chemistry is a means of speeding up,

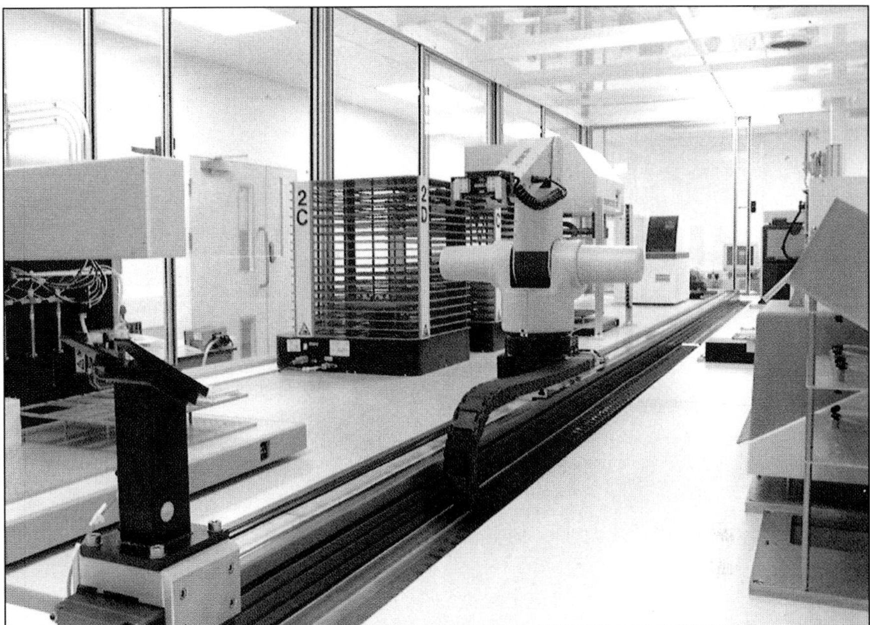

Fig. 4 Robot used in high-throughput screening. Photograph courtesy of SmithKline Beecham, Essex.

a million-fold or more, the natural selection that allowed human beings to identify medicinal herbs over the past 100,000 years. Furthermore, the process can be streamlined by incorporating as building blocks structural motifs with known activity. An example is a chemical structure possessing activity as an inhibitor of serine proteases, exploited in the development of drugs to treat HIV infection.

□ HITS AND LEADS

The threshold set for recognition of a 'hit' in a high-throughput screen is a matter of judgement and statistical analysis of the performance of the individual assay. However, a hit is not necessarily a lead; to become this, it must have additional characteristics. It must be 'drug-like' and have sufficient functional groups with scope for a medicinal chemist to produce many analogues in the laborious process of lead optimisation that may aim to increase the biological activity by 100–1,000-fold. The molecule should not be too large, which might make it too insoluble or impermeable to have good bioavailability. High-throughput screeners and combinatorial chemists may dream of producing a drug directly from a screening hit, but the chances of doing so are very low.

□ THE ROLE OF MEDICINE

Both the greatest bottle-neck and the highest cost in drug development are in the clinical phase. In the large-scale therapeutic Phase III trials, large numbers of

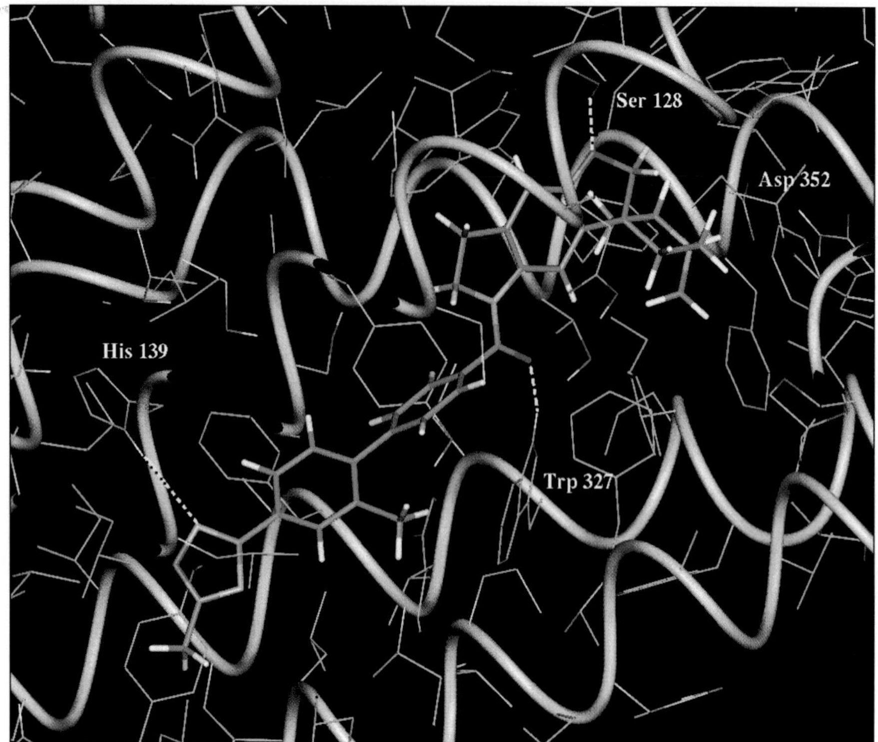

Fig. 5 Molecular modelling, showing a three-dimensional image of a selective 5HT1b receptor inverse agonist, docked into its putative binding site on the 1b receptor. Figure courtesy of SmithKline Beecham.

patients are essential to provide the robust evidence of efficacy and safety required to satisfy the regulatory authorities responsible for licensing drugs, approving therapeutic claims and evaluating safety. However, there is much to be done in the earliest phases of studying new drugs in man.

It is often possible to obtain reasonable evidence about pharmacological action in normal man by techniques such as pharmacological challenge and drug displacement from receptors using positron emission tomography. The greatest problem is to gain an early insight into the likelihood of therapeutic activity when dealing with highly novel targets. Inevitably, many such drugs will fail, and it is in everyone's interest to terminate its career with the minimum of patient exposure and expenditure of time and money.

Clinical pharmacology has been relatively successful, using healthy human volunteers in well designed and safe studies, in delineating pharmacological action in man. Can the same be achieved ethically, safely and expeditiously by asking patients with mild to moderate disease to help with the early characterisation of therapeutic activity? Such studies would not involve large numbers of patients, but would require sophisticated design to extract the maximum possible information from each patient who agreed to participate. This is the antithesis of what often happens with new drugs, which are frequently administered to the most refractory patients who have been unresponsive to other treatments, or to individuals who have become regular participants in multiple trials.

There is a great opportunity for enhanced collaboration between clinical medicine, clinical investigators and the pharmaceutical industry to achieve this aim. Some of the methods, particularly imaging techniques, already exist, while others will need to be developed and validated. In the UK, we are fortunate to have a high standard of medicine, many highly trained clinical investigators ,and strong research-based pharmaceutical companies. Bringing those skills together is essential if we are both to carry forward enough effective new medicines and to retain a strong research-based industry. We must find the will and the way to do this.

ACKNOWLEDGEMENTS

I would like to thank Dr Ken Murray and Dr Peter Machin of SmithKline Beecham for their help with this manuscript. They are the real experts on high-throughput screening and combinatorial chemistry.

REFERENCES

1 Dollery CT. *Medicine and the Pharmacological Revolution.* The Harveian Oration for 1993. London: The Royal College of Physicians, 1993.

2 Drews J. Into the 21st century. Biotechnology and the pharmaceutical industry in the next ten years. *Biotechnology N Y* 1993; **11**: S16–20.

3 Fears R, Ferguson MW, Stewart W, Poste G. Life-sciences R&D, national prosperity, and industrial competitiveness. *Science* 1997; **276**: 759–60.

4 Drews J. Intent and coincidence in pharmaceutical discovery. The impact of biotechnology. *Arzneimittelforschung* 1995; **45**: 934–9.

5 Moreadith RW, Radford NB. Gene targeting in embryonic stem cells: the new physiology and metabolism. *J Mol Med* 1997; **75**: 208–16.

6 Lu Z, Berson JF, Chen Y, *et al.* Evolution of HIV-1 coreceptor usage through interactions with distinct CCR5 and CXCR4 domains. *Proc Natl Acad Sci USA* 1997; **94**: 6426–31.

7 Wu L, Paxton WA, Kassam N, *et al.* CCR5 levels and expression pattern correlate with infectability by macrophage-tropic HIV-1, in vitro. *J Exp Med* 1997; **185**: 1681–91.

8 Murray KJ, Blackburn H, Connolly B, *et al.* In: Dixon GK, Major JS, Rice MJ (eds). *Challenges and Issues in High Throughput Screening.* Oxford: Bios Scientific Publishers, 1998.

9 Kaur S, McGuire L, Tang D, *et al.* Affinity selection and mass spectrometry-based strategies to identify lead compounds in combinatorial libraries. *J Protein Chem* 1998; **16**: 505–11.

10 Tegge W, Frank R. Peptide synthesis on Sepharose beads. *J Pept Res* 1997; **49**: 355–62.

11 Kowalczyk C, O'Shea M. Solid-phase synthesis of neuropeptides by Fmoc strategies. *Methods Mol Biol* 1997; **73**: 41–8.

12 Moran EJ, Sarshar S, Cargill JF, *et al.* Radio frequency tag encoded combinatorial library method for the discovery of tripeptide-substituted cinnamic acid inhibitors of protein tyrosine phosphatase PTP1B. *J Am Chem Soc* 1995; **117**: 10787–8.

13 Nicolaou KC, Xiao X, Parandoosh Z, *et al.* Radiofrequency encoded combinatorial chemistry. *Angew Chem Int* ed 1995; **34**: 2289–91.

14 Pinilla C, Appel JR, Houghten RA. Tea bag synthesis of positional scanning synthetic combinatorial libraries and their use for mapping antigenic determinants. *Methods Mol Biol* 1996; **66**: 171–9.

15 Hardin JH, Smietana FR. Automating combinatorial chemistry: a primer on benchtop robotic systems. *Mol Diversity* 1995; **1**: 270–4.

Chronic fatigue syndrome: a true illness or a social and political issue?

Simon Wessely and Elaine Showalter *(Introduction by Richard Edwards)*

Introduction: the need to widen the debate

Richard Edwards

Attempts to expand our understanding of chronic fatigue syndrome (CFS) have provided many opportunities for the meeting of minds from many disciplines. These have included the meeting in Oxford, where an operational definition was agreed for the purposes of research [1], and the working party responsible for drafting the Royal Colleges of Physicians, Psychiatrists and General Practitioners report [2] which sought to bring clarity to a confused scene. The many challenges of CFS have not yet been resolved to the satisfaction of patients, doctors or health care managers, even though progress is evidently being made.

At the heart of the debate is the issue of whether it is a 'true illness' or a 'social and political issue'. These different, but not necessarily mutually exclusive, viewpoints will be argued respectively by Simon Wessely, a psychiatrist who has made major contributions to the evidence base of knowledge about CFS, and Elaine Showalter, a distinguished writer who has recently been identified as 'hysteria's historian' [3]. My own view is that history may well show that this debate is illusory and perhaps misplaced since both opinions are likely to be at least in part true, and neither alone is a sufficient way ahead to resolve the issues raised by the personal tragedy and health care implications of CFS.

Both Wessely and Showalter emphasise the need for effective management of the person with CFS. Claims for better health care services are understandable and timely in the face of the need for prioritisation in health care. CFS has at least some official recognition in that the Chief Medical Officer in England has announced that CFS is a 'real' disease and that the Department of Health has set up a working party on the condition [4]. I hope an issue to be addressed is the shortage of time for doctors to listen adequately to the patient's complaints and to provide explanations that will help him take part in a treatment plan. Nowadays, such a plan should involve several components: the sympathetic recognition of the patient's illness that is emphasised by Wessely [5], as well as the practical encouragement of measures aimed at restoring normal physiological functioning. Such a treatment process also needs 'to avoid dysfunctional illness behaviour and inadvertent legitimisation and reinforcement of disability' [6]. Failure to do this – whether because of time pressures, narrow professionalism or lack of realisation that CFS inflicts damage – could well be a warning that reductionist twentieth century medical science is not as successful as we would wish in addressing the innermost human fears and burdens which ultimately determine the outcomes of ill health [7]. Doctors and other health care professionals should heed Elaine Showalter's concluding challenge:

> Unless the medical profession is willing to take a convincing stand on the status and dangers of psychosomatic illnesses, CFS and its fellow travellers will continue to escalate [8].

which echoes that of Shorter in his history of psychosomatic illness [9].

Ockham's razor (or the principle of parsimony so beloved of doctors in making a diagnosis) may be too sharp to be applied to separate 'organic' from 'functional' components in CFS. The mind-body dichotomy is illogical and inhumane in people with CFS, as evidenced by the need to provide psychological care for medical patients [10] and vice versa in people with CFS, as has been further explained by Wessely [5]. Disorders of physiology (eg of circadian rhythm [11]) are increasingly reported in CFS, but are not necessarily the appropriate treatment target: the superficially logical response to identifying a relative deficiency of cortisol, that is hydrocortisone replacement [12], may carry a significant risk of harm for only limited benefit. Given that endocrine and metabolic changes can follow alterations in physiological functioning and lifestyle, a scientific holism would suggest the need to demonstrate that recovery of normal physiological functioning in CFS patients is associated with return to normal of the previously abnormal hormonal responses – and this has yet to be done. In the meantime, the need, as Wessely elaborates [5], is for sympathetic but consistent communication about a category of illness which has enormous personal and social costs.

These two challenging contributions will help to broaden the scope of discussion about CFS – an essential step towards better understanding and management of this difficult condition.

REFERENCES

1. Sharpe MC, Archard LC, Banatvala JE, *et al.* Chronic fatigue syndrome: guidelines for research. *J R Soc Med* 1991; **84**: 118–21.
2. *Chronic Fatigue Syndrome.* Report of a Committee of the Royal Colleges of Physicians, Psychiatrists and General Practitioners. London: Royal College of Physicians, 1996.
3. Larkin M. Elaine Showalter: hysteria's historian. *Lancet* 1998; **351**: 1638.
4. Beecham L. *Better services are needed for 'ME'* (feature on Report on NHS services for people with chronic fatigue syndrome/myalgic encephalitis. Bristol: Westcare, 155 Whiteladies Road, Clifton, Bristol BS8 2 RF) *Br Med J* 1998; **317**: 966.
5. Wessely S. Chronic fatigue syndrome: a true illness. In: Williams G (ed). *Horizons in Medicine, No. 10.* London: RCP, 1998: 501–16.
6. Mechanic D. Chronic fatigue syndrome and the treatment process. In: Bock GR, Whelan J (eds). *Chronic Fatigue Syndrome.* Chichester: Wiley, 1993: 318–41.
7. Porter R. *The Greatest Benefit to Mankind: a medical history of humanity from antiquity to the present.* London: Harper Collins, 1997: 717–8 .
8. Showalter E. Chronic fatigue syndrome: a social and political issue. In: Williams G (ed). *Horizons in Medicine, No. 10.* London: RCP, 1998: 501–16.
9. Shorter E. *From Paralysis to Fatigue: a history of psychosomatic illness in the modern era.* New York: The Free Press, 1992: 295–323.
10. *The Psychological Care of Medical Patients: recognition of need and service provision.* Report. London: Royal College of Physicians, Royal College of Psychiatrists, 1995.
11. Williams G, Pirmohamed J, Minors D, *et al.* Dissociation of body temperature and melatonin secretion circadian rhythms in patients with chronic fatigue syndrome. *Clin Physiol* 1996; **16**: 327–37.
12. McKenzie R, O'Fallon A, Dale J, *et al.* Low-dose hydrocortisone for treatment of chronic fatigue syndrome: a randomized controlled trial. *J Am Med Assoc* 1998; **280**: 106–16.

CFS: a true illness

Simon Wessely

☐ SETTING THE SCENE

Chronic fatigue syndrome (CFS), whatever it may be [1,2], is nothing new, and neither is its ability to provoke disputes between patient and doctor and between doctors themselves. In this paper, Elaine Showalter (p. 511–516) and I will address some of these disputes. We agree on many points, notably the importance of social and cultural pressures in determining health and illness, and the assumption that people presenting under the label of CFS are ill and deserve respect and sympathy; we also hope to illuminate some honest differences that emerge from our personal perspectives as a practising clinician and a social historian.

I shall argue that CFS is both a valid nosological entity and a useful concept for doctor and patient alike. Moreover, I submit that the advantages of accepting this diagnostic category outweigh the disadvantages, which are elegantly described in Showalter's paper. Some of the specific points that she and others have raised deserve consideration at this juncture.

There is no diagnostic test for CFS

This remains true; indeed, the literature is scattered with discredited claims for such tests. However, this deficiency is not enough to undermine CFS as a distinct illness, as medicine embraces many entities that lack a truly diagnostic test or that can be diagnosed on clinical grounds when all investigations prove negative; well known examples include irritable bowel syndrome, migraine and some cases of epilepsy.

CFS is not a disease

Critics point to the absence of any demonstrable pathological process underlying CFS, and hence argue that it cannot be considered a valid disease. Again, this situation is far from unique in clinical medicine, and it is more useful to regard CFS as an *illness* (ie causing distress and symptoms, and preventing normal functioning) rather than a *disease* (in which there is a known pathological abnormality). In many settings, notably primary care, I would contend that doctors treat illnesses, not diseases.

It is part of normal experience to feel very tired

This might seem an unfair criticism to anyone with direct experience of CFS sufferers, who report distress and disability that fall well outside normal human experience. Everyone experiences fatigue, but few of us suffer such intense symptoms after minimal activity that most normal life activities become impossible. 'Fatigue', like most variables, is normally distributed in the community [3], and there is no clearcut threshold that defines the fatigue described in CFS; sufferers clearly lie beyond the normal range, but lesser degrees of distress and disability that are common in primary care [4] merge into normal experience. Indeed, all the other symptoms that characterise CFS are dimensional rather than categorical entities, and therefore lack a simple cut-off point to distinguish between CFS, longstanding tiredness and normality.

This argument does not invalidate the concept of CFS as an illness. A good analogy is with hypertension, as there is no particular threshold above which blood pressure suddenly becomes abnormal; instead, there is a continuous distribution of risk, with the threat of complications and the need for treatment increasing progressively as blood pressure rises.

CFS is a damaging diagnosis

Psychiatrists, perhaps more than practitioners in any other branch of medicine, are sensitive to the dangers of diagnostic labelling; in particular, a patient given a label such as schizophrenia may start to conform to the expectations and stereotypes associated with that role. This can undoubtedly happen with CFS, where patients may become convinced that they are in the grip of an invisible virus which is malevolently destroying their immune system, and that the only treatment is bed rest; for them, the chances of recovery are slight. These misconceptions about CFS have been common in the media and popular literature [5], though the situation has fortunately improved in recent years.

The clearest evidence that the diagnosis of CFS can itself damage health derives from the paediatric literature [6,7]. Ever more children are now appearing with the label of CFS. The implication that the child suffers from some mysterious, progressive viral or immunological disorder may cause other potential sources of distress – and attempts at rehabilitation in the family and school – to be ignored. Unsubstantiated statements such as 'ME in children lasts an average of four and a half years' can become a self-fulfilling prophecy, and misinformation and entrenched attitudes can conspire against recovery. The dangers have recently been highlighted of labelling children with a disease that 'has profound implications for their level of functioning in society, especially when the disease is not well defined in childhood and when there are no irrefutable laboratory markers for it' [6], and which is widely regarded as persistent or incurable. Indeed, Plioplys – a committed champion of CFS in adults – has recently suggested that the diagnosis should never be made in children [7], and argues that all the patients he has seen had an alternative and more appropriate diagnosis.

All these points are, quite rightly, grist to Showalter's mill. However, the fault lies not with the basic concept of CFS, but with the connotations it conveys in certain circles [8]. Similar assaults were made previously on the concept of schizophrenia, but did not cause the diagnosis to be abandoned; instead, they made it clear that a diagnosis must not imply certain outcomes or behaviours that cannot be justified. The label of CFS has the advantage of being aetiologically neutral, whereas its close companions 'myalgic encephalomyelitis' (ME) and 'chronic fatigue and immune deficiency syndrome' are inappropriate, because they endorse the existence of pathological processes that simply are not present [1].

The 'CFS' label is undoubtedly used inappropriately in many cases, and can lead to therapeutic nihilism and despair, but I shall argue below that this label can be a constructive and helpful part of the medical consultation.

All those with CFS have known psychiatric disorders

Another criticism of CFS is that it is already adequately covered by existing disease classifications, and that all those who fulfil criteria for CFS can more parsimoniously be given discrete and well known psychiatric diagnoses, namely depression, anxiety and somatisation.

This view invariably infuriates supporters of the CFS concept, yet it may be partly true. Many studies have confirmed an association between CFS and psychiatric disorder, regardless of definition, setting or methodology; these conclusions apply also to community-based surveys and are not attributable to selection bias. The association is too close to be explained as a reaction to physical disability, while prospective studies suggest that pre-existing psychiatric disorder is a risk factor for the subsequent development of CFS.

However, no study has ever shown complete congruence between CFS and psychiatric disorders; consistently, a substantial proportion of subjects fulfil criteria for CFS and no other condition. Furthermore, there are neurobiological differences between the major psychiatric disorders such as depression and CFS, principally in the function of the hypothalamic-pituitary adrenal axis, which may relate to the activity of the serotoninergic input to that system. Classic depression is associated with high plasma cortisol concentrations and underactivity of the serotoninergic system, while non-depressed subjects with CFS show the reverse [9,10]. The significance of such observations remains unclear, and they may simply represent an epiphenomenon due to differences in the sleep/wake cycle [11]; nonetheless, the assertion that CFS is no more than masked or somatised depression cannot be sustained in all cases.

An appropriate analogy may be with post-traumatic stress disorder (PTSD), which has a similar relationship with the formal categories of psychiatric disorder. Most cases of PTSD also fulfil criteria for depression and/or anxiety, while many of the risk factors for PTSD are also those for psychiatric disorder. However, many subjects who develop PTSD do not fufil criteria for depression or anxiety, and attempts to label all cases solely as depressed or anxious will obscure vital aetiological, phenomenological and clinical information.

It is clear that we need improved classification systems for both depression and CFS, and that all CFS cannot simply be subsumed within the category of depression.

□ WHY DIAGNOSE CFS?

A research view

What is the scientific evidence that CFS is a valid concept? Perhaps the most important comes from recent epidemiological surveys, which confirm the existence of a syndrome characterised by easy fatiguability, and that is closely associated with both depression and anxiety, yet is distinct from both [12–15]. Indeed, subjects fulfilling the criteria for CFS are not uncommon in the general population [12,13].

Interestingly, most cases with CFS alone also fulfil criteria for 'neurasthenia' [16–18]. Nowadays, neurasthenia is generally seen as a variant of neurosis, and thus another psychiatric disorder. However, this is a gross oversimplification [13,17]. Historically, neurasthenia was first conceived as a physical, neuromuscular disorder that often arose from a combination of overwork, stress and infection; it was thought to exhaust the body's supplies of energy, and its only solution was rest. It was only in the first half of this century that neurasthenia became accepted as a psychiatric diagnosis, a change that ultimately led to its eclipse. Another finding known to Victorian medicine has also been confirmed, namely that neurasthenia/CFS is a major source of morbidity, albeit not mortality, and that many sufferers are markedly incapacitated in many aspects of their lives [19–21].

Our classifications of illness can therefore accommodate a fatigue syndrome, whether we call it CFS or neurasthenia.

An empirical view

Showalter's view is that there is no such entity as CFS, that the concept must be abandoned, and that the doctor's duty is to refute the label and to focus on the psychiatric disorder that is the real source of the patient's symptoms. This view is shared by many medical specialists; indeed, one clinical consultant reportedly told a medical conference that ME does not exist [22].

This view has potentially serious consequences in dealing with patients who believe that they suffer from CFS. Denying the condition's existence is unlikely to persuade patients to abandon their symptoms and return to work, and neither is the statement that this is 'all in the mind'. People do not generally consider depression to be a legitimate diagnosis without moral overtones [5]; for example, members of an ME support group did not distinguish between malingering and psychiatric illness, tending to assume that 'anyone with depression *wanted* to be ill and taken care of by others' [23]. The use of any psychiatric label is tantamount to calling a person hysterical or work-shy.

Hadler [24] has outlined the dilemma: to get well in these circumstances is to abandon veracity. Patients will be more inclined to get better when they are given explanations for their problems that they themselves find acceptable [25,26]; unsatisfactory explanations may not be merely discarded, as the patient may try actively to prove them false. As patients rarely return to doctors who belittle their illness experience (whether intentionally or not), essential opportunities to treat the patient will be lost.

Disillusioned patients may turn to the alternative therapists, who guarantee explanations in keeping with the patient's own views of illness, but always at a price and with little hope of effective treatment. The patient will conclude that conventional doctors do not understand, reinforcing the ever present polarisation between doctor and patient and the patient's view that they have a disease solely of the body and not the mind; the doctor's suspicion of the key role of the latter may also be confirmed. Mant has pointed out this 'Catch 22' situation: the more the patient denies psychosocial causation, the more the doctor believes it to be present [27].

Patients must have a diagnosis

Several studies of sufferers' views confirm that the act of diagnosis is central to the experience of CFS [28,29]. Without it, the patient feels stigmatised, overlooked and ignored, while the diagnosis brings relief, credibility and acceptance. Some examples graphically capture this paradox: the patient who rejoiced when she learned she had 'an incurable disease' [30], another who felt 'fantastic' on being told that she had ME which would (in her own words) take away her independence and regress her to a baby with little hope of progress [31], and another whose 'mental relief was phenomenal' even though the prognosis was uncertain [32].

A management strategy aiming to help patients must take account of this need for a firm diagnosis – without which they will be unable to organise their dealings with family, friends and work, let alone consider how to get better. There is evidence that patients given a firm diagnosis for non-specific symptoms have a better outcome than those whose consultations expressed uncertainty [33]. If specialists do not provide a diagnosis, someone else will; nonetheless, it is important to avoid the 'contest of diagnosis' [24] from which neither side will emerge the winner.

Patients who say they have CFS may be right

A diagnosis must be acceptable to both doctor and patient; one that satisfies the former but not the latter is unlikely to be helpful. The only situation in which patients convinced that they have ME or CFS should be told that they are wrong is when there is a clearcut alternative diagnosis that requires treatment. Many medical conditions can masquerade as CFS (see Table 1), but most alternative diagnoses can be excluded relatively easily in practice [34].

In all other circumstances, the doctor-patient relationship will be ruined by telling patients that they are wrong and by giving them an alternative, psychological label that is totally unacceptable to them. In my view, the only sensible option is to agree with the patient. CFS is an operational diagnosis; if someone fulfils the appropriate criteria then that is what they have. After all, the alternatives are probably no more valid. Psychiatric diagnoses have a similar status to CFS, in that both are operational criteria that lack external validation. As Komaroff has expressed it: 'One problem is that CFS is defined by a group of symptoms, without any objective abnormalities on physical examination or laboratory testing that readily establish the diagnosis. Another problem is that the same is true of depression and

Table 1 Medical differential diagnoses of chronic fatigue syndrome.

General conditions
Occult malignancy
Autoimmune disease
Endocrine disease (eg Addison's disease, hypothyroidism)
Organ failure: cardiac, respiratory or renal

Neurological
Disseminated sclerosis
Myasthenia gravis
Parkinson's disease
Myositis

Infectious
Chronic active hepatitis (B or C)
Lyme disease
Human immunodeficiency virus

Respiratory
Nocturnal asthma

Chronic toxicity
Alcohol
Solvents
Heavy metals
Irradiation

Sleep disorders
Narcolepsy
Obstructive sleep apnoea

somatisation disorder' [35]. Attempts to replace a solely physical model with an equally monolithic psychogenic explanation are not only doomed to failure but are also misguided and unnecessary.

It is indefensible to give a patient a label that implies a chronic incurable condition or a non-existent pathological process ('encephalomyelitis') whose cure must await a medical 'breakthrough'. A positive diagnosis of CFS has a useful place in clinical practice, provided that it is used constructively; as with fibromyalgia or irritable bowel syndrome, the diagnosis can act as a structure for the patient's understanding and, ultimately, treatment [36]. Indeed, the diagnosis must be viewed as the beginning, not the end, of the process. It is often helpful to begin the consultation by agreeing that the patient has CFS, and then focusing on what can be done about it.

Practical management should begin by broadening the assessment to take account of all the physical, cognitive, emotional, behavioural and other factors that combine to present as CFS. This multidimensional approach has been outlined elsewhere [34,37] and has empirical support as a basis for treatment [38,39]. To improve, patients do not need to (and indeed do not) alter their views that they have ME/CFS or that it began as a physical illness. Instead, improvement requires only a shift in the patient's view on the relative merits of rest and exercise [40]. Most CFS patients believe that rest is the best way of controlling the condition, which they are otherwise powerless to influence [41]. In particular, disability in CFS patients is related to the presence of catastrophic beliefs about the disastrous effect of activity [42]. Effective management involves challenging these damaging assumptions, but not the physical origin of CFS or its status as a genuine disease [38,39].

□ CONCLUSIONS

I therefore conclude that CFS is a valid diagnostic entity, and a useful addition to clinical practice. The drawbacks of using the label in real life come from misinformation and misunderstanding about the meaning and implications of the label, rather than the concept itself. This subject is still replete with ambiguity and uncertainty, but regardless of our personal views, we are obliged to use the concept for as long as patients themselves believe in it. For myself, I believe we can go further, and can now use this diagnostic label – without committing scientific fraud or perjury – in our clinical dealings with these patients, who are often very disabled.

REFERENCES

1 Report of a Committee of the Royal Colleges of Physicians, Psychiatrists and General Practitioners. *Chronic Fatigue Syndrome.* London: Royal College of Physicians, 1996.

2 Wessely S, Hotopf M, Sharpe M. *Chronic Fatigue and Its Syndromes.* Oxford: Oxford University Press, 1998.

3 Pawlikowska T, Chalder T, Hirsch S, *et al.* A population based study of fatigue and psychological distress. *Br Med J* 1994; **308:** 743–6.

4 Wessely S, Chalder T, Hirsch S, *et al.* Psychological symptoms, somatic symptoms and psychiatric disorder in chronic fatigue and chronic fatigue syndrome: a prospective study in primary care. *Am J Psychiatry* 1996; **153:** 1050–9.

5 Wessely S. Neurasthenia and chronic fatigue: theory and practice in Britain and America. *Trans Cult Psych Rev* 1994; **31:** 173–209.

6 Carter B, Edwards J, Marshall G. Chronic fatigue in children: illness or disease? *Pediatrics* 1993; **90:** 163.

7 Plioplys A. Chronic fatigue syndrome should not be diagnosed in children. *Pediatrics* 1997; **100:** 270–1.

8 Finestone AJ. A doctor's dilemma: is a diagnosis disabling or enabling? *Arch Intern Med* 1997; **157:** 491–2.

9 Cleare A, Bearn J, Allain T, *et al.* Contrasting neuroendocrine responses in depression and chronic fatigue syndrome. *J Affect Disord* 1995; **35:** 283–9.

10 Demitrack M. Neuroendocrine correlates of chronic fatigue syndrome: a brief review. *J Psychiatr Res* 1997; **31:** 69–82.

11 Leese G, Chattington P, Fraser W, *et al.* Short-term night-shift working mimics the pituitary-adrenocortical dysfunction of chronic fatigue syndrome. *J Clin Endocrinol Metab.* 1996; **81:** 1867–70.

12 Wessely S. The epidemiology of chronic fatigue syndrome. *Epidemiol Rev* 1995; **17:** 139–51.

13 Hickie I, Hadzi-Pavlovic D, Ricci C. Reviving the diagnosis of neurasthenia. *Psychol Med* 1997; **27:** 989–94.

14 Merikangas K, Angst J. Neurasthenia in a longitudinal cohort study of young adults. *Psychol Med* 1994; **24:** 1013–24.

15 Hickie I, Koojer A, Hadzi-Pavlovic D, *et al.* Fatigue in selected primary care settings: sociodemographic and psychiatric correlates. *Med J Aust* 1996; **164:** 585–8.

16 Farmer A, Jones I, Hillier J, *et al.* Neuraesthenia revisited: ICD-10 and DSM-III-R psychiatric syndromes in chronic fatigue patients and comparison subjects. *Br J Psychiat* 1995; **167:** 503–6.

17 Wessely S. Old wine in new bottles: neurasthenia and 'ME'. *Psychol Med* 1990; **20:** 35–53.

18 David A, Wessely S. Chronic fatigue, ME and ICD-10. *Lancet* 1993; **342:** 1247–8.

19 Buchwald D, Pearlman T, Umali J, Schmaling K, Katon W. Functional status in patients with chronic fatigue syndrome, other fatiguing illnesses, and healthy controls. *Am J Med* 1996; **171:** 364–70.

20 Komaroff A, Fagioli L, Doolittle T, *et al.* Health status in patients with chronic fatigue syndrome and in general population and disease comparison groups. *Am J Med* 1996; **101:** 281–90.

21 Wessely S, Chalder T, Hirsch S, *et al.* The prevalence and morbidity of chronic fatigue and chronic fatigue syndrome: a prospective primary care study. *Am J Public Health* 1997; **87:** 1449–55.

22 Steincamp J. *Overload: Beating ME.* London: Fontana, 1989.

23 Ax S, Gregg V, Jones D. Chronic fatigue syndrome: sufferers' evaluation of medical support. *J R Soc Med* 1997; **90:** 250–4.

24 Hadler NM. If you have to prove you are ill, you can't get well: the object lesson of fibromyalgia. *Spine* 1996; **21:** 2397–400.

25 Brody H. 'My story is broken: can you help me fix it?': medical ethics and the joint construction of narrative. *Lit Med* 1994; **13:** 79–92.

26 Kirmayer L. Healing and the invention of metaphor: the effectiveness of symbols revisited. *Cult Med Psychiatry* 1993; **17:** 161–95.

27 Mant D. Chronic fatigue syndrome. *Lancet* 1994; **344:** 834–5.

28 Woodward R, Broom D, Legge D. Diagnosis in chronic illness: disabling or enabling: the case of chronic fatigue syndrome. *J R Soc Med* 1995; **88:** 325–9.

29 Cooper L. Myalgic encephalomyelitis and the medical encounter. *Sociol Health Illness* 1997; **19:** 17–37.

30 Ames M. Learning to live with incurable virus. *Chicago Tribune* 1985; June 9th (Section 5): 3.

31 Forna A. A real pain. *Girl About Town* 1987; 21st May.

32 Brodie E. Understanding ME. *Nursing Times* 1988; **84:** 48–9.

33 Thomas K. The consultation and the therapeutic illusion. *Br Med J* 1978; **i:** 1327–8.

34 Sharpe M, Chalder T, Palmer I, Wessely S. Chronic fatigue syndrome: a practical guide to assessment and management. *Gen Hosp Psych* 1997; **19:** 195–9.

35 Komaroff A. Clinical presentation of chronic fatigue syndrome. In: Straus S, Kleinman A (Eds). *Chronic Fatigue Syndrome.* Chichester: John Wiley, 1993: 43–61.

36 Goldenberg D. Fibromyalgia: why such controversy? *Ann Rheum Dis* 1995; **54:** 3–5.

37 Sharpe M, Wessely S. Non-specific ill health: a mind-body approach to functional somatic symptoms. In: Watkins A (Ed). *Mind-Body Medicine: A Clinician's Guide to Psychoneuroimmunology.* Edinburgh: Churchill Livingstone, 1997: 169–86.

38 Sharpe M, Hawton K, Simkin S, *et al.* Cognitive behaviour therapy for chronic fatigue syndrome; a randomized controlled trial. *Br Med J* 1996; **312:** 22–6.

39 Deale A, Chalder T, Marks I, Wessely S. A randomised controlled trial of cognitive behaviour versus relaxation therapy for chronic fatigue syndrome. *Am J Psych* 1997; **154:** 408–14.

40 Deale A, Chalder T, Wessely S. Illness beliefs and outcome in chronic fatigue syndrome: is change in causal attribution necessary for clinical improvement? *J Psychosom Res* 1998; **45:** 77–83.

41 Clements A, Sharpe M, Simkin S, *et al.* Chronic fatigue syndrome: a qualitiative invesitgation of patients' beliefs about the illness. *J Psychosom Res* 1997; **42:** 615–24.

42 Petrie K, Moss-Morris R, Weinman J. The impact of catastrophic beliefs on functioning in chronic fatigue syndrome. *J Psychosom Res* 1995; **39:** 31–7.

CFS: a social and political issue

Elaine Showalter

□ INTRODUCTION

In this paper, I shall argue that chronic fatigue syndrome (CFS) is a psychosomatic illness with hysterical symptoms, the contemporary version of the 19th century neurasthenia. In many respects, this view shares common ground with that of Simon Wessely (p. 503–10). However, I shall concentrate on the social and political issues that – unlike the case of neurasthenia – have encouraged CFS to escalate into an epidemic in the USA and many European countries.

It is hard to say how many people actually suffer from CFS. Advocates for CFS claim that it is a worldwide infectious pandemic affecting four million people. However, these apparently authoritative 'statistics' are only estimates, extrapolated from self-reported symptoms, and may have been exaggerated in order to raise the profile of CFS and strengthen the case for research funding. As Wessely points out, people with chronic tiredness who fulfil minimum diagnostic criteria for CFS are common in the community, at least in the UK, although far fewer claim to be disabled by their symptoms. More stringent diagnostic criteria yield a very different picture: in a recent study in the USA, only one case out of 13,000 diagnosed on clinical grounds satisfied the research-orientated definition proposed by the Centers for Disease Control (CDC) [1]. In the USA, we know that CFS is a disorder of white people and of women. In summer 1997, according to the CDC, 84% of American patients were female, and 94% were white.

□ CAUSES OF THE CFS EPIDEMIC

Whatever its precise numbers, there can be no doubt that CFS has been an increasing illness category since its reappearance in the early 1980s. Its predecessor, neurasthenia, was a relatively limited illness culture in the 1890s, but CFS is enjoying epidemic status during the 1990s because of four significant social factors:

- □ the influence of the mass media;
- □ the example of AIDS;
- □ the exploitation of disability insurance;
- □ the Internet.

To these major influences can be added millennial paranoia, New Age alternative medicine, religious fundamentalism and the growing culture of patient self-help organisations.

The mass media

In contrast to the 1890s, the mass media – newspapers, magazines and television –

have played a major role in propagating the mythology of CFS. They have circulated stories about the syndrome and have reinforced anti-medical and anti-psychiatric thinking, particularly about its possible causes. Although they readily admit to the presence of stress factors in their lives, CFS patients react with outrage to suggestions from doctors that their symptoms are psychological rather than organic. Encouraged by the media, patients blame organophosphates, chickenpox and other viruses, mobile phones, electromagnetic fields – indeed, anything but their feelings and conflicts. In my view, the media have helped to strengthen the CFS sufferer's programmatic resistance to psychological explanations, diagnoses or treatments, which I feel is one of the most characteristic traits of these patients.

Building on the example of AIDS

The American Chronic Fatigue Immune Dysfunction Syndrome (CFIDS) Association groups have deliberately adopted the strategies of AIDS groups to get attention, funding and respect for their illness, adopting the now familiar framework of an auto-immune disorder, and even arguing that CFS is caused by a variant of HIV. CFIDS literature is full of emotive comparisons with AIDS, including the statement of an American infectious diseases specialist that 'a CFIDS patient feels exactly the same every day as an AIDS patient feels two months before death' [2].

CFS groups imitate the organisation of the AIDS activists, calling themselves PWCs (people with chronic fatigue), wearing blue ribbons, and demonstrating through the action group of the CFIDS Association of America, C-ACT. Government attitudes to CFS have been unfavourably compared to those during the early stages of the AIDS epidemic [3]. With scare headlines, innuendo, inflammatory rhetoric, and a detailed history of medical investigations and dead-ends, this analysis has brought chronic fatigue into the spectrum of contemporary epidemic-conspiracies.

The exploitation of disability insurance

Disability insurance has also been a significant factor in the rise of CFS and other self-reported somatic illnesses. Between 1989 and 1993, claims to American insurance companies for CFS quadrupled. In 1996, UNUM, the largest provider of group disability insurance, attempted to limit benefits for self-reported illness to a maximum of two years, a move that has led to increased CFIDS lobbying. North American courts and judges have been validating CFS as a 'real' disease rather than a 'psychoneurotic disorder' in some cases involving massive disability payments, including US$1.3 million payable (by his employer) to a broker with CFS, and long-term disability compensation awarded to an employee of an insurance company. These rulings delighted activist groups. In France, sickness has been described as the new form of labour protest [4]. Indeed, for many, in the modern post-industrial welfare state, absenteeism and chronic illness have become a way of life, a kind of activity and identity – even a career.

Help from the Internet

Unlike AIDS groups or trade unions, CFS groups are virtual communities. Davidson and Pennebaker [5] have noted a quiet revolution taking place within the support group movement since 1992, with individuals turning to the computer world of the Internet in addition to traditional group meetings. CFS patients used the Internet well out of proportion to their numbers or to the severity of their symptoms, making more posts (entries) during the two-week sampling period than the combined total of five other chronic-illness groups, namely heart disease, breast cancer, prostate cancer, arthritis and diabetes. Moreover, CFS patients registered among the longest average posts [5]. Davidson and Pennebaker concluded that, of all the chronic illness groups, CFS sufferers held the most rigid views about illness prototypes – which seems ironic, as CFS remains a diagnosis of exclusion. Contributors' posts indicate that they are familiar with the latest research and discussions about chronic fatigue; authors who allude to suspected psychological factors or psychosocial treatment strategies are anathema, and 'practically subhuman in their callous and ignorant statements' [5].

Because patients communicate through the Internet, the group has little control over its members, whose antagonism towards dissenters can be extreme. The campaign organised against my book, *Hystories* [6], by the CFIDS Association (whose stated wish is for decorum and civility) led to hate mail, death threats and efforts to deface or destroy the book itself. In general, CFS patients appear to be easily won over to conspiracy theories that explain all disagreement with their beliefs as a plot.

☐ A DISEASE IN SEARCH OF A NAME

Following the history of AIDS and HIV infection, the major project of the American CFIDS Association for most of 1997 was to have the term 'chronic fatigue' changed, since they felt it deprived them of dignity and legitimacy. 'The name of this disease is an atrocity' wrote one nurse in the *CFIDS Chronicle*, while another activity has noted that 'anger about the name is as high as it's ever been'.

Some new names proposed in a member survey are listed in Table 1. These choices illustrate some fundamental misconceptions about the condition. 'Myalgic encephalomyclitis' (ME) and 'myalgic encephalopathy' are misnomers, because there is no evidence for inflammatory or other disease of the central nervous system. Neither is there a proven immune disorder to justify 'CFIDS'. Melvin Ramsay was the British doctor who described the Royal Free epidemic in the 1950s, while Peterson and Cheney were American doctors who treated an outbreak in Nevada in 1984. Sir William Osler was the turn-of-the-century doctor who advocated that physicians should listen to their patients. Nightingale and Darwin are two famous historic figures who had undiagnosed debilitating illnesses.

CFS patients have been urged by the CFIDS Association to write to the US Secretary of Health, 'making a strong case about how the name of this illness affects your life and that of others and how it holds back medical research', and this has been a strong theme for lobbying the US Congress on CFIDS/CFS/ME Awareness Day. At present – owing both to the inability of patients to agree on a new name and to an internal battle among American doctors who wanted it named for them – the

Table 1 Some alternative names proposed for chronic fatigue syndrome (CFS).

- Myalgic encephalomyelitis (ME)
- Myalgic encephalopathy
- Chronic fatigue immune dysfunction syndrome (CFIDS)
- Ramsay's disease
- Peterson-Cheney (or Cheney-Peterson) disease
- Osler's syndrome
- Nightingale's disorder
- Darwin's disorder

Change-the-Name project has been set aside 'until future scientific research may merit a name change for the illness'.

☐ CFS AND CULT STATUS

In the late 1990s, CFS has become a quasi-cult, complete with gurus, prophecies, group pressures, and powerful anti-medical and anti-psychiatric taboos. This cult is most active in North America but has strong links in Britain, Australia, South Africa and the Netherlands. The mystical element is illustrated, for example, by a CFS sufferer reported in a feminist self-help book [7] who describes reading an article in the *Observer* as her epiphany: 'I had a flash of recognition akin to a religious conversion'.

CFS patients enthusiastically embrace quack remedies and faith healing, including those endorsed by the self-named 'Duvet Women' (who are notably scornful of medicine and science) [7]. Some are listed in Table 2. In 1997, a woman in England with CFS even claimed to be cured after bumping heads with a dolphin named Funghie. Many sufferers are also convinced that they have allergies to dietary components such as wheat, sugar, salt, dairy products, chocolate, coffee, red meat, fizzy drinks and white bread.

Role of doctors in the CFS cult

As with other cults, CFS groups maintain their state of intensity through regular predictions of medical breakthroughs. In the USA in particular, many doctors have jumped on the CFS bandwagon and attract desperate private patients for expensive, idiosyncratic and unproven treatments. These include: the weekly 'Meyers Cocktail' of magnesium, vitamin B_{12}, and calcium, topped off with oestrogen; biaxin 100 mg/day to clear infection with *Mycoplasma fermentans incognitus*; and ampligen, a very expensive (£6,000 per year) immunomodulatory drug which is produced in Belgium and is not approved in the USA or the UK.

Patients are also being enthusiastically investigated (at further cost) for supposed medical disorders, including impaired blood flow to the brain, disorders of melatonin, steroids and other hormones, candida and bacteriological infestations of the gut, and vitamin and micronutrient deficiencies.

Table 2 Some treatments currently recommended by CFS self-help groups. Adapted from [7].

Homoeopathy	Chinese herbs	Hugging
Reflexology	Kombucha fungus	Chanting
Acupuncture	Organically grown vegetables	Stroking a cat
Shiatsu massage	Anti-candida diets	Cetacean contact
Astrology		
Aromatherapy		
Jin Shin Jyutsu		

Survival of the CFS cult

Cultural anthropologists explain that discredited prophecy is a characteristic of cult organisation: 'prophetic failure will be followed by increased conviction and vigorous proselytising, especially when there is undeniable evidence that prediction was wrong, and when members have social support from fellow believers' [8]. If a cult predicts the world will end next Tuesday, and it doesn't, believers congratulate themselves on the faith that has spared mankind, and eagerly reschedule the date.

Similarly, when CFS prophecies of discovery or cure are discredited, patients' conviction increases. In autumn 1997, government researchers from the CDC announced that a study of a supposed biological marker for CFS [9] could not be replicated, and that many CFS patients tested negative for the test while false positives were also common. Nonetheless, CFS groups continued to insist on the Internet that 'the research was still very impressive despite the new clarifications' [10].

□ THE WAY FORWARD?

CFS patients and their families are obviously suffering, but their pain does not originate from a mysterious virus, a genetic predisposition or a neurological flaw. The endless quest for an organic cure postpones or prevents the likelihood that patients and their families will seek effective psychiatric therapy (behavioural, cognitive and physical rather than psychoanalytical) as well as antidepressants and other forms of appropriate medication.

Dealing with hysterical epidemics will demand not only courage from doctors but also a set of profound changes from society. A century after Freud, psychogenic illnesses are still stigmatised and penalised, and there remains great reluctance to accept, name and seek help for hysterical disorders; for example, we have yet to see the day when an American political candidate can admit publicly to having been treated for depression without sacrificing his or her career.

The expert recommendations of Simon Wessely and his colleagues seem ideal for the effective and sympathetic medical management of patients with CFS [11]. However, there is an inevitable conflict between the desire to avoid confrontation with individual patients about their disease beliefs and failing to state an overall position on the pathological causation of the disorder. Unless the medical profession is willing to take a convincing stand on the status and dangers of psychosomatic illnesses, CFS and its fellow travellers will continue to escalate. Moreover, there is good historical evidence that when doctors finally do firmly discredit a hysterical illness, it declines.

I have no doubt that the first step towards the future is for doctors to speak up. Without strong and clear statements from the medical profession as a whole, the CFS epidemic will continue to gain momentum and to attract both converts and fanatics.

REFERENCES

1 Price RK, North CS. Reported in *USA Today* February 1993.
2 Loveless M. Literature distributed by the CFIDS Association.
3 Johnson H. *Osler's Web: Inside the Labyrinth of Chronic Fatigue Syndrome.* New York: Crown, 1996.
4 Ferro, M. *Les Sociétés Malades du Progrès.* Paris: Plon, 1998.
5 Davidson KP, Pennebaker JW. Virtual narratives: illness representations in online support groups. In: Petrie K, Weinman J (Eds). *Perceptions of Health and Illness: Current Research and Applications.* London: Harwood Academic Press, 1997: 463–86.
6 Showalter E. *Hystories: Hysterical Epidemics and Modern Culture.* London: Picador, 1997.
7 March C (Ed). *Knowing ME: Women Speak about Myalgic Encephalomyelitis and Chronic Fatigue Syndromes.* London: Women's Press, 1998.
8 Black RW, Dimitrovich J, Mahnke BL, Morrison V. Fifteen years of failed prophecy. In: Robbins T, Palmer SJ (Eds). *Millennium, Messiahs, and Mayhem: Contemporary Apocalyptic Movements.* New York and London: Routledge, 1997: 73–92.
9 Schmidt P. Protein marker for CFIDS closer to reality. *CFIDS Chronicle* Summer 1997: 17.
10 Klimas V. *Suhadolnik Research Related at Government Meeting* (CFIDS Internet post). 12 January 1998.
11 Wessely S, Hotopf M, Sharpe M. *Chronic Fatigue and Its Syndromes.* Oxford: Oxford University Press, 1998.

Gene therapy: the beginning of the end or the end of the beginning?

David J Weatherall

□ INTRODUCTION

Ever since the seminal studies of Avery, McLeod and McCarty on DNA-mediated genetic transformation, geneticists have realised that it might be possible to transfer genes into cells for the treatment of inherited disease. In the late 1970s, following the advent of recombinant DNA technology, it became possible to isolate human genes and to learn at least something about their regulation, and thoughts then naturally turned to the exploitation of this remarkable new facility for the development of gene therapy. Articles describing promising approaches started to appear in the literature, usually accompanied by editorials proclaiming 'gene therapy just round the corner', or something similar. However, 15 years have passed and the promise has yet to be fulfilled.

Where does gene therapy stand today? Was it a myth created by overenthusiastic molecular biologists in the heady days of the 1980s following the first characterisation of monogenic disease at the molecular level or, given time and some luck, will it make a genuine impact on medical practice?

□ ROOTS OF CURRENT SCEPTICISM ABOUT THE FUTURE OF GENE THERAPY

Like many new approaches to the treatment of human disease, gene therapy got off to a bad start. In the late 1970s, an American scientist decided to attempt to treat β thalassaemia by inserting a normal β-globin gene into marrow cells using a viral vector. When he was unable to obtain permission from his own institutional ethics committee, he carried out the experiment in another country; it did not work, but caused no harm to the recipient. This experiment raised considerable concern in the biomedical field, which fortunately led to serious and extended debate on the ethics of gene therapy on both sides of the Atlantic. The conclusion was that somatic cell gene therapy does not raise any major new ethical issues beyond those relating to the evaluation of the safety and risk/benefit of any novel form of treatment.

Once research workers were given the go-ahead to proceed with research into human gene therapy, the field rapidly expanded and achieved an enormous momentum of its own. The vast amount of animal and human experimentation was reflected by the publication of two new journals devoted entirely to the field; it became the subject of large international meetings, and even managed to generate at least two accounts of its history before there had been one genuine clinical success. Yet serious problems were encountered at every step. Although it was possible to isolate human genes and their major regulatory regions, it proved extremely difficult to construct vectors with which to transfer them into the appropriate cell populations at anything like the level of efficiency required. Even when cells were successfully transfected, the genes often did not function for very long in their new home. Moreover, it proved difficult to isolate the target cells in sufficient quantities or purity to offer any hope of correcting a genetic disease.

Over the past 20 years, the initial dreams of gene therapy have been transformed into the reality of more than 175 clinical trials and over 2000 patients treated, but there is not yet conclusive evidence for efficacy. To reconcile the hyperbole with the continued lack of success, the Director of the National Institutes of Health (NIH), Harold Varmus, set up a committee under the chairmanship of Dr Stuart Orkin to review the whole enterprise. Its report, published in 1997, concluded that in essence researchers in the field had tried to run before they could walk and that a great deal more basic science would be required before success was likely. It stressed the importance of further research and suggested that fewer patient protocols should be developed until more was understood about the biology of the problems involved.

Few would doubt that the message from the NIH working group is correct or that workers in the field of gene therapy have been victims of naivety. However, this remains an approach of enormous promise for the future, not only for the management of at least some monogenic diseases, but also for the development of new strategies to tackle some of the more intractable chronic diseases of Western society.

□ PRESENT STATUS OF GENE THERAPY RESEARCH

In briefly reviewing the current status of gene therapy research it is important to take a broad view of the technology, which encompasses any form of genetic manipulation designed to control or cure a disease.

It is vital to distinguish between germ cell and somatic cell gene therapy. Germ cell therapy involves the insertion of genes into fertilised eggs for the correction of a genetic disease. Because these genes are dispersed throughout the tissues of the egg, they end up in the germ cells as well as the somatic cells of the fetus, and hence are passed on to future generations. This approach has been banned in most countries, for complex reasons, involving both ethical and safety issues. Furthermore, there does not seem to be any pressing reason for pursuing research into this form of therapy for the immediate future. The remainder of this discussion will therefore be confined to somatic cell gene therapy, ie the manipulation of the genetic machinery of cells other than germ cells.

Strategies

The general approaches to somatic cell gene therapy are outlined in Table 1 and have been the subject of several recent reviews [1–3]. Ideally, gene therapy should emulate transplantation surgery, by removing a mutant gene and replacing it with a normal one. Since this is not technically possible, another way of achieving the same end – gene correction – would entail the specific alteration of a mutant gene sequence using nature's way of exchanging material, that is by site-directed recombination. In

Table 1 Methods for gene therapy.

Viral transfer
• Retroviral vectors
• Other viral vectors
Physical methods
• Direct injection of DNA
• Calcium phosphate transfection
• Electroporation
• Liposome-mediated DNA transfer
Receptor-mediated gene transfer
Targeted gene transfer
Artificial chromosomes
Activation of genes of related function

many respects this is the best approach to correcting a genetic defect or otherwise altering the function of a gene, and it has been achieved in cultured cells; however, current approaches have such a low level of efficiency that it may be a long time before this approach can be used in practice.

Because of these technical difficulties, much current research is directed towards gene augmentation, that is introducing a gene into cells in a way that will allow it to produce enough of its product to compensate for the lack of expression of its defective counterpart. At the same time, and particularly in the settings of cancer and infectious diseases, attempts are being made to interfere with the expression of genes in order either to modify the behaviour of cells or to kill them.

Finally, because certain genetic diseases are due to mutations in genes that have counterparts that are active at earlier stages of development, there is growing interest in the reactivation of these 'fetal' genes to take over the role of their defective adult homologues.

Vehicles for gene transfer

The major approaches to transferring genes or other agents designed to interfere with gene function into cells are summarised in Table 1; they fall into two broad classes, viral and non-viral [3,4].

Several classes of viral vector have been subjected to clinical trial. Because retroviruses integrate DNA into the genome, much early research focused on vectors derived from retroviruses from which many of the viral genes had been removed or altered so that no viral proteins could be made in the cells that they infected. Viral replication functions are provided by packaging cells containing helper viruses that produce all the viral proteins required, but which themselves have been altered so that they are unable to produce infectious viruses. A great deal of experimental work has been based on the Mouse Moloney Leukaemia virus. Vectors constructed from this virus transduce cells in culture but, as most cells *in vivo* are quiescent and because this virus only invades dividing cells, it has limited uses for gene therapy. More recently, a chimeric Moloney-human lentiviral vector has been constructed that can transduce at least some quiescent cells, including neurones.

Because of these problems, human adenoviruses have also been exploited as vectors for gene therapy, particularly for the treatment of cystic fibrosis and cancer. By eliminating a particular region of the viruses, it is possible to insert human genes and to render the viruses incapable of replication and spreading after gene transfer. The main problem with this family of vectors is that they produce antigens that elicit an immune response which tends to eliminate the transduced cells and hence the inserted human gene. However, a considerable amount of work is continuing in an attempt to prevent the production of these immunogenic proteins.

Another family of viruses that is showing considerable promise for gene transfer is the adeno-associated viruses (AAV), which appear to be able to transduce brain, skeletal muscle and other cells. Their major disadvantage is the relatively small amount of foreign DNA that can be inserted. A variety of other viral vectors are being explored, including those based on Epstein-Barr virus, herpes, simian virus 40 and papilloma virus. To date, however, the ideal retroviral or viral vector for gene therapy has still not been developed.

Most work with the non-viral vectors listed in Table 1 has been directed at cationic lipid-based delivery systems called liposomes, in which the genes to be transferred are enclosed within a lipid envelope that can fuse with the cell membrane. Liposomes have the advantage that they are relatively easy to prepare, do not evoke an immunogenic response and do not carry the dangers (particularly the oncogenic potential) of retroviruses. On the other hand, they are a relatively inefficient way of transferring genes into the nucleus, and it is not possible to target them at specific tissue. Under experimental conditions, DNA can also be introduced directly into cells by microinjection; by complexing it with calcium phosphate to form aggregates that are taken up intracellularly; or by permeabilisation of cell membranes using electric currents (electroporation).

Receptor-mediated gene transfer

Most experimental work involving the use of gene-transfer vehicles outlined in the preceding section has been carried out by transfecting cells *ex vivo*; the growing realisation that this will always be inefficient and inapplicable in the case of many organs has fuelled much interest in the concept of receptor-mediated gene transfer. In theory, this would entail designing a vector that could be injected into the blood stream and would home in on an appropriate tissue.

Because the liver is of such central importance in metabolism, and is therefore an obvious target for gene therapy, much work has focused on hepatic-specific receptors, in particular the asialoglycoprotein receptor (ASGPr). Transferrin-polylysine-DNA conjugates, which bind transferrin receptors, have been constructed for this purpose. DNA is packaged in an electrostatic complex using asialo-orosmucoid-polylysine in place of lipid. This conjugate efficiently binds to ASGPrs on the surface of the liver and can be administered intravenously. The problem encountered with this approach is that, after they enter the hepatocytes, the conjugates fuse with vesicles to form endosomes, within which the DNA is largely degraded. Hence a variety of ingenious approaches are being explored to avoid the endosome shuttling stage.

A related method involves the use of the haemagglutinating virus of Japan (HVJ; a form of Sendai virus). This attaches to the plasma membrane at the cell surface, after which fusion occurs and releases the viral contents directly into the cell cytoplasm. Although transient expression is still a major disadvantage of the HVJ-liposome systems developed so far, a variety of other ways to improve its utility are being explored.

Targeted gene therapy

As mentioned earlier, the use of homologous recombination to make alterations in gene structure offers the most specific approach to gene therapy. Although this has been achieved in human cell lines and non-transformed primary human cells, the efficiency is still very low. Methods that are being explored to solve this problem have been reviewed recently [5].

Interfering with gene function [6–8]

Because of the different objectives involved in controlling cancer or infectious disease, a number of approaches are being explored which aim to alter the function of particular genes that are involved in neoplasia or in the virulence of infectious agents.

Several techniques are being investigated that aim to manipulate the genes of cancer cells in an attempt to restore a normal phenotype. Some forms of neoplasia reflect defective function of tumour suppressor genes, including *TP-53* (the protein product of which is p53), *MTS-1*-p16, *RB-1* and *APC*. *TP-53* and *MTS-1*-p16 are defective in various tumours, while *RB-1* mutations have been implicated in retinoblastoma, prostate carcinoma and osteosarcoma. *APC* mutations predispose towards adenomatous polyposis and a proportion of sporadic colorectal tumours. A variety of attempts are being made to replace these defective tumour suppressor genes with the normal 'wild-type' genes, and some successes have been achieved, at least in cultured cells.

Another approach to modulating the expression of oncogenes is through the use of 'antisense agents', short complementary single-stranded oligonucleotides that interfere with gene function by binding specifically to their target cellular mRNA partners; the complex may then be broken down by ribonuclease H. A related technique involves the specific binding of oligonucleotides to gene targets, so forming a triple helix that blocks transcription of the gene. Other attempts are also being made to attack the transcription machinery of cells, including the use of ribozymes, agents that are able to cleave pre-mRNA at specific sites. All these approaches have been used to interfere with oncogene function in malignant cell lines, while antisense and ribozymal technologies are also being applied to the treatment of viral infections, notably HIV.

Cell destruction by genetic manipulation [6–8]

In the field of cancer and infectious disease it is becoming clear that the most effective treatments will involve destruction of the target cells rather than short-term manipulation of their genes. A variety of ingenious ideas are being explored.

One of the most promising approaches to cancer therapy is to utilise transcriptional differences between normal and cancer cells to drive the selective expression of a metabolic 'suicide gene' to confer sensitivity to a pro-drug. For example, the herpes simplex virus thymidine kinase (HSV-TK) converts ganciclovir into its active form. The idea is to target a viral vector carrying this particular gene to express itself in malignant tissue. There are two methods: transduction targeting, which relies on preferential gene delivery to actively dividing cells using a viral vector; and transcriptional targeting, which depends on unique tissue-specific or tumour-specific transcriptional elements to drive the expression of a toxic protein only in cells that contain factors capable of activating the promoter elements. These techniques have been combined and have shown considerable promise for the management of brain tumours in experimental animals. A number of human trials have been established. One of the unexpected benefits of this type of therapy is the 'bystander effect', in which non-transduced cells are killed as well as those that have been transduced; a variety of ways are being explored to take advantage of this unexplained phenomenon.

The other general approach to killing cancer cells is to attempt to increase their immunogenicity or to introduce cytokines and thus stimulate the immune system to reject the tumour without systemic toxicity. A number of experimental systems have demonstrated that the growth of tumours can be inhibited by the insertion of genes encoding different agents of this type [8].

Artificial chromosomes [9]

The transfer of a large genetic unit containing a particular gene and its control regions in the form of a self-replicating molecule – an artificial chromosome – would have obvious advantages over other forms of gene therapy. It would overcome limitations on the length of DNA that can be inserted and, theoretically at least, not be associated with the dangers of inserting material into nuclear DNA. Considerable progress has been made in this field, particularly with respect to the creation of appropriate telomeric sequences; the centromere remains a problem, though this is likely to be overcome. The major difficulty will undoubtedly lie in devising methods to try to transfer such large constructs into cells at the high frequency required for effective gene therapy.

Reactivation of fetal genes

Interest in this form of gene therapy has been mainly confined to the field of haemoglobinopathy, although a similar approach has recently been explored for the management of Duchenne muscular dystrophy.

Most of the important inherited disorders of haemoglobin are due to mutations at the β-globin gene locus. In fetal life, this only functions at a low level and the γ-globin genes of fetal haemoglobin are active. The switch from fetal to adult haemoglobin production is a reflection of the neonatal decline in γ-chain synthesis and the full activation of β-chain production. It has been known for many years that individuals with sickle cell anaemia or β-thalassaemia who show persistent γ-chain synthesis are partly or even completely protected from the effects of their disease. Thus attempts are being made to try to reactivate or increase the activity of γ-chain production in adult life.

Several agents are capable of stimulating fetal haemoglobin production in adults [10], including the demethylating agent 5-azacytidine, hydroxyurea and several butyrate analogues. A recent clinical trial reported that the administration of hydroxyurea reduced the frequency of painful crises in patients with sickle cell anaemia, while at the same time almost doubling their steady-state fetal haemoglobin levels [11]. This remarkable result cannot be attributed entirely to the elevation of fetal haemoglobin, but it shows that the approach is viable. Similar studies in β-thalassaemia have been less successful, though a few cases with particular underlying mutations have responded spectacularly well to a combination of hydroxyurea and butyrate analogues [12].

It has recently been found that dystrophin, the protein that is defective in Duchenne muscular dystrophy, has a fetal counterpart called utrophin. Recent work suggests that the latter can 'make up' for a deficiency of dystrophin in mice with muscular dystrophy [13].

□ POSTSCRIPT

It seems very likely that at least some forms of gene therapy will start to make a genuine impact on clinical practice in the not too distant future. At first this will probably involve short-term genetic manipulation for the management of different forms of cancer, and possibly for other acquired disorders such as vascular disease; it may also be possible to apply the same approach for the management of certain infections. Next we are likely to see the successful management of a few monogenic diseases due to disorders of housekeeping genes, that is genes that do not require tight regulation and are expressed in most cells. In the longer term, and only when we can really understand the ways in which genes are regulated, and have produced completely new varieties of vectors or have learned how to scale up the efficiency of site-directed recombination, we may see the management of monogenic diseases due to mutations at genes that require extremely tight, tissue-specific related regulation. I suspect that, along the way, methods for reactivating fetal haemoglobin genes in the disorders of β-globin production will improve and assume more wide clinical use. It will be a slow road, but we shall undoubtedly see successes in the future.

REFERENCES

1 Weatherall DJ. Scope and limitations of gene therapy. *Br Med Bull* 1995; **51**: 1–11.
2 Lemoine NR, Cooper DN (Eds). *Gene Therapy.* Oxford: BIOS Scientific Publishers, 1996.

3 Kay MA, Liu D, Hoogerbrugge PM. Gene therapy. *Proc Natl Acad Sci USA* 1997; **94**: 12744–6.

4 Schofield JP, Caskey CT. Non-viral approaches to gene therapy. *Br Med Bull* 1995; **51**: 56–71.

5 Yáñez RJ, Porter ACG. Therapeutic gene targeting. *Gene Ther* 1998; **5**: 149–59.

6 Culver KW, Vickers TM, Lamsam JL, Walling HW, Seregina T. Gene therapy for solid tumours. *Br Med Bull* 1995; **51**: 192–204.

7 Martin L-A, Lemoine NR. Cancer gene therapy. I. Genetic intervention strategies. In: ref [2]: 255–75.

8 Galea-lauri J, Gäken J. Cancer gene therapy. II. Immunomodulation strategies. In: ref [2]: 277–99.

9 Huxley C. Mammalian artificial chromosomes: a new tool for gene therapy. *Gene Ther* 1994; **1**: 7–12.

10 Olivieri NF. Reactivation of fetal hemoglobin in patients with β-thalassemia. *Semin Hematol* 1996; **33**: 24–42.

11 Charache S, Terrin ML, Moore RD, *et al.* Effect of hydroxyurea on the frequency of painful crises in sickle cell anemia. *N Engl J Med* 1995; **332**: 1317–22.

12 Olivieri NF, Rees DC, Ginder GD, *et al.* Treatment of thalassaemia major with phenylbutyrate and hydroxyurea. *Lancet* 1997; **350**: 491–2.

13 Tinsley JM, Potter AC, Phelps SR, *et al.* Amelioration of the dystrophic phenotype of mdx mice using a truncated utrophin transgene. *Nature* 1996; **384**: 349–53.